From the editors of *Nursing* magazine

NURSE'S BOOK of
ADVICE

An encyclopedia of answers to hundreds of difficult
questions–ethical, legal, moral, technical, and professional

Springhouse Corporation
Springhouse, Pennsylvania

From the editors of *Nursing* magazine

NURSE'S BOOK of
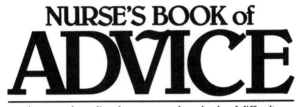

An encyclopedia of answers to hundreds of difficult
questions–ethical, legal, moral, technical, and professional

Springhouse Corporation
Springhouse, Pennsylvania

Staff

Executive Director, Editorial
Stanley Loeb

Executive Director, Video and Related Publications
Jean Robinson

Clinical Director
Patricia Nornhold, RN, MSN

Art Director
John Hubbard

Editor
Susan L. Jackson

Consulting Editors
Joan Cassin, Susan Doan-Johnson

Copy Editor
Mary Hohenhaus Hardy

Designers
Stephanie Peters (associate art director), Mary Stangl

Art Production
Robert Perry (manager), Anna Brindisi, Donald Knauss, Tom Robbins, Robert Wieder

Typography
David Kosten (director), Diane Paluba (manager), Liz Bergman, Joyce Rossi Biletz, Phyllis Marron, Robin Rantz, Valerie Rosenberger

Manufacturing
Deborah Meiris (manager), T.A. Landis, Jennifer Suter

Production Coordination
Aline S. Miller (manager), Colleen M. Hayman

This book is dedicated to Jeanmarie Coogan, who served as Editorial Director of *Nursing75* and the magazine's succeeding issues until *Nursing89*. Her intelligence, cleverness, and caring attitude helped generate a wealth of good advice for a host of problems. She not only launched an interesting editorial feature; she also touched the lives of many readers with valuable advice over the years.

Advisory board

About this book

Nurse's Book of Advice is the first of its kind! It deals with over 800 real-life problems, conflicts, dilemmas, and concerns, giving you common-sense, insightful, and usable solutions.

Sure, there have been *other* reference books, but never before has one addressed so much of the *human* side of nursing. Everyone knows by your title "nurse" that you're someone who cares deeply for others, cares about life, and has the unique blend of personal characteristics to fulfill your professional role. You help a lot of people and you probably save a lot of lives.

Sometimes it's easy for others to take your expertise for granted. But we at *Nursing* magazine recognize that you, as a person first and a nurse second, may need someone to talk to, to listen to you, and to help you. That's why we offer you this book—an expression of our respect for you as a *person*.

Actually, we have to extend our gratitude to hundreds of nurses across the country for helping us create this book. It consists of hundreds of questions they wrote to us over the years that we published in our *Advice, p.r.n.* column. Answers have been carefully prepared by seasoned nurses and experts from many fields. The answers consist of practical advice you can actually use. And it's advice that'll stay solid for years!

Here's how to use *Nurse's Book of Advice*. Look up a subject, like "Socializing" for example, and you'll find questions such as *What are the risks of romantic involvement with a staff doctor? ... What's the risk of attending a wine-and-cheese party while on duty? ... Is it okay for a nurse to have a sandwich with her patient's husband? ... Is having an off-duty drink with a patient unprofessional? ... Could a nurse be fired if she refused to agree to never socialize with patients?*

You'll find sound, practical advice for these intriguing and difficult situations!

You'll find what you want fast because of the book's alphabetical arrangement, tabs, table of contents, and index, complete with cross-references. You may find yourself reading about something you *weren't* even looking for because the questions and answers are so interesting and captivating. We'll bet you won't want to put the book down!

Indeed, we think *Nurse's Book of Advice* will be a constant counselor.

The Editors

Contents

1	Abortion	19	Apgar scores
1	Accreditation	19	Apnea monitoring
2	ACLS test	20	Arterial puncture
3	Admissions	20	Aseptic technique
3	Affection	20	Assessment
4	Agency administration	21	Assisting friends
4	Agency nursing	21	Autologous blood transfusions
5	AIDS	22	Baccalaureate exam
8	Alcoholic doctor	22	Barium preparations
10	Alcoholic nurse	23	Bathing
11	Alcoholic patient	23	Bed linens
12	Alcoholic visitor	23	Benadryl
13	Allergies	23	Bladder drainage
13	Allergy bracelets	24	Blind nurse
13	Allergy shots	24	Blind patient
14	Allergy testing	24	Blood pressure
14	Aloe plants	25	Blood transfusion
15	Alternative therapy	27	Boards
15	Alzheimer's disease	27	Body donation
15	Ambulance	27	Body odor
16	Ampules	28	Bomb threats
16	Amputee nurse	28	Borrowing medication
17	ANA code	28	Breaks
17	ANA exam	29	Burnout
17	Anesthetics	30	Call lights
18	Anger	31	Cancer
18	Angioplasty	31	Cancer treatment
18	Antibiotics	32	Cardiac care
19	Antiembolism stockings	32	Career choices

33	Casts	60	Cremation
33	Catheterization	60	Crowding
33	CCU	61	CT scanning
34	Central line	61	Cytomegalovirus
34	Chart access	61	D&C
35	Charts	62	Deaf nurse
35	Chemotherapy	62	Death
38	Chicken pox	64	Defibrillation
38	Child abuse	65	Degrees
39	Childbirth	65	Departmental hierarchy
40	Cleaning	66	Deposition
40	Clinical experience	66	Depressed nurse
41	Code	67	Depression
41	Code yellow	68	Dermatitis
42	College applicants	68	Diabetes educator
42	College infirmary	68	Diabetics
43	Communication	69	Diarrhea
44	Compliance	69	Dictation
45	Computerization	70	Difficult co-worker
45	Confidentiality	72	Difficult doctor
49	Consent	74	Difficult nurse-manager
56	Consultation	75	Difficult orderly
56	Contact lenses	75	Difficult patient
56	Contamination	75	Difficult unit
56	Continuing education	76	Discharge
57	Copyright	78	Discharge orders
57	CPR	78	Discharge planning
58	Crab lice	79	Discouraged nurse
59	Crash cart	82	Discretion

82	Discrimination		122	Enemas
84	Dismissal		122	Enteral feedings
85	Dispensing		122	Epidural catheters
86	Divorce		123	Epileptic nurse
86	Doctor-patient relations		124	Equipment bag
86	Doctor's behavior		124	Euthanasia
87	Doctor's orders		124	Exhibitionism
94	Documentation		125	Expiration dates
105	Draft		125	Externs
105	Drainage tubes		126	Eye patch
105	Dress code		126	Eye trouble
106	Dressings		126	False accusation
107	Drug abuse		127	Falsifying records
108	Drug-addicted nurse		127	Family members
108	Drug addiction		128	Family questions
109	Drug administration		128	FDA
110	Drug incompatibilities		128	Feeding tubes
110	Drug samples		129	Felony
111	Drug screening		130	Fetal monitoring
111	DTP vaccines		130	Fibrosis
112	Dying patient		130	Fingernail polish
113	Education		130	Fingernails
114	Elder abuse		131	Fire drills
114	Electrocardiograms		131	Flexion deformity
115	Emergency department		131	Flirting
117	Emotional involvement		131	Floating
118	Emotional support		132	Florence Nightingale
119	Employee problems		133	Fluid intake
119	Employment		133	Flunking
120	Endoscopy		134	Foot care
120	Endotracheal intubation		134	Forced absence

134 Forced labor

135 Forcing treatment

135 Formula feedings

135 Gastrostomy tubes

136 Generic substitutes

136 Geriatric nursing

136 Gift giving

137 Gloves

137 Glucose levels

137 Good Samaritan

138 Gossip

139 Graduate nurses

139 Grief

140 Guardianship

140 Guest-patient

141 Handiwork

141 Harsh treatment

141 Heel sticks

142 Hematoma

142 Heparin injections

143 Heparin locks

143 Hepatitis B

145 HIV antibody test

146 Home health care

148 Homicide

149 Homosexuality

149 Hospital manual

149 Hypnosis

150 Hypochondria

150 Hypothermia blankets

150 ICCU

151 ICU

153 ID badges

154 ID bracelet

154 I.M. injections

154 Incident report

155 Incompetent colleague

156 Incompetent patient

156 Incontinence pad

156 Indwelling urinary catheter

158 Inexperience

158 Infection control

161 Informality

162 Injections

162 Injured nurse

163 Innovation

163 Inquisitiveness

164 Insecurity

164 Instructor's liability

165 Insulin

167 Insurance

167 Insurance physicals

168 Interviews

169 Intuition

169 Isolation

169 I.V. bag

170 I.V. infusion pumps

170 I.V. lidocaine therapy

170 I.V. therapy

173 Jehovah's Witness

173 Job application

174 Job benefits

174 Job change

174 Job description

175 Job dissatisfaction

175 Job evaluation

177 Job hunting

179 Job rejection

179 Job responsibility

185 Job selection

185 Job title

186 Jurisdiction

186 Kerosene heaters

186 Kidnapping

187 Laboratory values

187 Language barrier

187 Lateness

188 Law practice

188 Lawsuits

189 Laxatives

190 Leadership

190 Liability

192 License

193 License reinstatement

193 License revocation

195 Lie-detector test

195 Life support

196 Lonely patient

197 LPN image

197 Male student

197 Management

198 Manipulative patient

198 Marijuana

199 Married couples

199 Medical assistants

200 Medical student's orders

200 Medicare

200 Medication

201 Medication change

201 Medication confusion

201 Medication errors

203 Medication orders

207 Medications

209 Mercury

210 Mood swings

210 Morale

211 Multidose vial

211 Mycostatin oral

211 Names

212 Narcotics counts

212 Narcotics record

212 Nasogastric feeding

213 Nasogastric tubes

213 Nasopharyngeal airway

214 Negligence

215 Negligent doctors

216 Neonatal ICU

216 Nipple pinching

217 "No code" orders

223 Noises

223 Nuclear accident

224 Nurse-doctor conflict

224 Nurse practitioners

225 Nursery

225	Nurses' pledge
225	Nurses' titles
225	Nursing
226	Nursing home
227	Nursing responsibility
227	Observation
228	Obstetric nursing
230	Occupational health nursing
231	Off-duty nursing
231	On-call policy
231	OR
232	Organ donation
233	OR nurse
233	Ostomy
233	Otoscopes
234	Overbearing nurse
234	Overdose
235	Over-the-counter products
236	Overtime
237	Oxytocin drips
237	Pacemaker
238	Pain medication
238	Paramedics
238	Parenting
239	Parking
239	Patient abuse
240	Patient advocacy
241	Patient-centered nursing
242	Patient injury
242	Patient privacy
244	Patient's rights
244	Patient teaching
245	Patient transfer
245	Pay
246	Payroll deduction
246	Pediatric oncology unit
246	Peer evaluations
247	Personal disability
247	Personal journal
247	Photographs
248	Picketing
248	Piggybacking
248	Pilfering
249	Placebos
249	Postop hemorrhage
250	Postpolio syndrome
250	Preemployment exam
250	Pregnant nurses
251	Pressure sore
251	Prison nursing
251	Private-duty nursing
253	Prolixin
253	Promotion
254	Pronouncing death
254	Psychiatric nursing
254	Psychiatric patient
255	Psychiatric problems
255	Pulmonary artery catheter
256	Pulse dosing
256	Pupil size
257	Quadriplegia
257	Quota system pay

258 Radiation monitoring

258 Radium implants

258 Recreation program

259 References

260 Refusing nutrition

260 Relatives

261 Religion

261 Relocation

262 Report

262 Reporting

262 Reputation

263 Resentful doctor

263 Responsibility

264 Restraints

265 Retirement village

265 Return to nursing

266 Right of refusal

267 RNLP

267 Robots

267 Safety straps

267 School nursing

268 School's medication policy

268 School transcripts

268 Scrub gowns

269 Search

270 Secrets

270 Sedation

271 Self-confidence

271 Self-discharge

271 Self-esteem

272 Self-medication

272 Shoplifting

272 Sick leave

274 Signature

274 Silver nitrate

274 Sleep

276 Smoking

276 Socializing

279 Social workers

280 Spelling

280 Sphygmomanometer

280 Sponge count

281 Sports medicine

281 Staff development

281 Staff relations

282 Standards of care

282 Staph infection

282 Stat doses

283 Status epilepticus

283 Sterilization

284 Stethoscopes

284 Stomatitis

284 Stress

285 Student health problems

286 Students

286 Substance abuse

286 Substitutions

287 Suctioning

287 Suicidal nurse

288 Suicidal patients

288 Suicide

289 Sump tubes

289 Supervision
289 Supervisor
290 Surgical lifts
290 Suturing
291 Talwin
291 Tape recording
292 Telemetry system
292 Telephone advice
293 Telephone orders
294 Telephoning
294 Terminal illness
295 Termination
295 Test anxiety
295 Tetanus injections
296 Theft
296 Time
297 Time clocks
297 Time off
298 Tipping
298 Tongue blades
299 TPN
300 Tracheostomy
300 Tranquilizers
301 Treatment delay
301 Treatment error
301 Treatment refusal
303 Troubled husband
304 Truthfulness
304 Tube feeding
304 Tuberculosis
305 Tuition assistance
305 Twins

306 Understaffing
309 Unemployment compensation
310 Uniforms
311 Unit manager
312 Unlicensed nurse
312 Vacation
313 Vaccination
313 Vaginitis
313 Ventilator patients
314 Verbal abuse
314 Verbal orders
316 Vibrators
316 Visitation rights
316 Visiting hours
317 Visitors
319 Vital signs
320 Vocal cord paralysis
320 Volunteering
321 Waiting
321 Walking report
321 Wandering patient
322 Water pitchers
322 Weapons
323 Weight loss
323 Withholding information
324 Withholding treatment
325 Witnessing
325 Work load
327 X-rays
328 Youthful appearance
328 Z-track injections

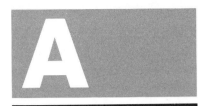

Abortion

Can a nursing student be excused from observing one during her rotation?

Q I'm a nursing student, and I'm afraid I'll have to observe an abortion during my surgical nursing rotation. I have a moral objection to abortion. Could I ask to be excused?

A Yes, you could, but observing an abortion probably isn't required in any nursing school. If yours is an exception, talk with your nursing instructor. In a polite, nonjudgmental way, ask to be excused and request a different assignment to complete your surgical rotation.

Remember, patients who undergo abortions have rights, too. No matter how you feel about abortion, you're morally obligated to care for a patient after the procedure and to provide the same emotional support you would for any patient.

What are a nurse's legal responsibilities when a live fetus is delivered after a saline-induced abortion?

Q Recently, a 20- to 24-week-old fetus that was being aborted was delivered with a strong heartbeat. He wasn't resuscitated despite his efforts to breathe, and he died 45 minutes later. The doctor had left after starting the procedure, so the charge nurse actually delivered the fetus. She never informed him of the live birth when he came back to sign the stillborn certificate. Some of the nurses are concerned about our legal responsibility in a situation like this. What should we have done?

A This is a very difficult situation with tremendous moral and legal facets to it.

Simply put, a fetus that is live-born following or during an attempted abortion must be accorded all appropriate resuscitation measures. Period. Various states have specific statutes that deal with this issue. Among them are California, Pennsylvania, and Missouri.

> *"The nurse who delivered the fetus that was being aborted never informed the doctor of the live birth."*

This issue will become more and more difficult as medical technology moves the limits of fetal viability closer and closer to the point of conception. State abortion laws will probably be revised to reflect fetal viability limits.

The nurse's duty here was to inform the physician that the infant had been born alive. In addition, the nurse had the obligation to call a physician for assistance in resuscitating the infant. (The term "infant" is appropriate because the fetus was live-born.)

Finally, physicians have been charged with manslaughter or infanticide when, following a live birth during the course of a hysterotomy, saline, or prostaglandin abortion, they smothered the infant with the placenta or poured water into the waste bucket into which the infant had been placed. The issue here wasn't that these were second trimester abortions—which were permitted by statute—rather, the issue was failing to resuscitate the live-born infant.

Proper nursing practice dictates that a nurse remain with a patient who is undergoing a second trimester abortion by saline or prostaglandin induction. The nurse acts to minimize trauma to the patient, assist with delivery, and resuscitate the infant when necessary.

What can a nurse do if she's morally opposed to abortions?

Q When I first started working on a women's surgical unit, my unit manager told me I wouldn't have to assist with urea abortions if doing so were against my convictions. At the time, I had no particular opinion about the procedure, so I agreed to participate. But after 6 months, I found the practice abhorrent. I discussed this problem with my unit manager, but she said that I'd have to continue and that I'd "get over it."

I asked to be transferred to another unit, but I'm still waiting. How do I deal with my assignments? Do I have the right to ask for other patients, as I was originally promised?

A You have the right to express your objections, no matter how you felt 6 months earlier. First, contact your personnel department to find out if the hospital has a written policy regarding assignment changes. Then, put your objections in writing and give them to your manager, director of nursing, and personnel department. Because you're locked in a painful and complicated conflict between your rights and your employer's demands, you may have to rely on the personnel department to provide objective counseling. If you have a staff ethicist, enlist her aid, too.

If you still aren't satisfied, check with your nurses' association. Your state may have legislation that permits you to withdraw from procedures that are morally unacceptable to you.

Accreditation

Could a nurse be in legal trouble if she lied to the JCAHO?

Q The day before the Joint Commission on Accreditation of

A

Healthcare Organizations (JCAHO) came to inspect the hospital where I work, our manager asked me if I was certified in cardiopulmonary resuscitation. I told her that I had been, but my certification had lapsed. She said I should tell the JCAHO inspector that I'd left my card at home.

Luckily, he didn't ask. But if he had, I wouldn't have lied.

This situation has made me wonder: Could I—or the hospital—have been in legal trouble if I'd deceived the JCAHO?

A Theoretically, yes. When you lie, you face three legal risks: a civil lawsuit, if the party to whom you lied was injured; criminal prosecution, if the lie constitutes criminal behavior; or administrative (license-related) censure, if the lie was unethical.

As a practical matter, though, it's unlikely anyone would go to the trouble of suing you or your hospital, prosecuting you, or revoking your license for a lie like the one you describe.

A spokesperson said the JCAHO expects hospital personnel to be honest, and most are. But if inspectors discover that they're being deceived, they can withhold a hospital's accreditation until the situation is corrected. In an extreme case, the hospital might lose its accreditation altogether.

Why does the JCAHO announce the date of a visit to a hospital beforehand?

Q Can you tell me why the Joint Commission on Accreditation of Healthcare Organizations (JCAHO) announces the date of a visit to a hospital beforehand?

Time and time again, I've seen hospitals shape up just before the visit, then fall back afterward into old habits.

I think a hospital would be more likely to keep up higher standards if the JCAHO visits were unan-

nounced. Why doesn't the JCAHO use surprise visits?

A It's more cost effective to notify a hospital beforehand; the proper personnel and records will be available when the JCAHO surveyors arrive. Here are some more reasons why the JCAHO announces its visits:

• Any hospital could easily figure out about when the next survey might be scheduled, since the surveys are currently done every 3 years.

• The month's advance notice the JCAHO gives the hospital is probably not time enough to "doctor" 3 years' worth of records—especially since the JCAHO inspection of the hospital is painstakingly thorough.

• JCAHO is neither a punitive agency nor a regulatory agency of the federal government. Any power JCAHO might have to change hospital conditions comes solely from its right to withhold accreditation. Even the accreditation is a voluntary process: No hospital will be visited unless the survey is requested.

Before the surveyors arrive, a hospital is asked to post a notice announcing that a public information interview will be held in conjunction with the survey. At the meeting, an interested person—any present or former patient or health care professional—can ask questions, make comments, or offer opinions.

The JCAHO also leaves another option open. Let's say you have something important on your mind but don't wish to speak up in public: You can write to the JCAHO survey program directly, providing all possible documentation on the issue you've raised.

Although a JCAHO representative may call you to verify the documentation, the commission assures you your anonymity will be maintained. If you feel strongly that conditions in your hospital need improving, the JCAHO seems willing to listen.

ACLS test

What should an ED nurse do if she fails the test?

Q I've just turned 50 and have passed the 10-year mark working in the emergency department (ED) of a university medical center. My personnel file is full of complimentary reports on my patience and my willingness to teach and help others. I've been able to think of myself as an asset to the department. But now my confidence is shaken, and I'm embarrassed in front of my co-workers. The reason: I just failed the written exam for Advanced Cardiac Life Support (ACLS). However, I did pass the practical part of the exam.

I could take the test again next month, but I'm not sure I want to put myself through the stress and distress involved.

I'd value your objective viewpoint: If I don't take the test, or if I should fail again, should I leave the ED? Not that I'm looking forward to starting all over again, but I'm concerned. Should an ED nurse be ACLS certified?

A Certainly, failing an exam can rock your confidence. But many good nurses have failed written exams.

If you decide to take another crack at the exam—for your own pride and sense of self-worth—ask your instructor about better ways to study. You may just be out of the habit of studying after so many years.

Certainly it's more desirable to have the ACLS certification, but perhaps your hospital doesn't require it.

Try to look upon your first try at the written exam for ACLS as a temporary setback. In the meantime, shore up your morale by thinking of the many patients you've helped in your 10 years in the ED.

Whatever your decision, good luck.

Admissions

Who's liable if a patient's condition deteriorates in the waiting room?

Q Before a patient is admitted to our emergency department (ED), an admissions secretary interviews him for about 10 minutes, recording the patient's chief medical complaint and personal and billing information. Then the patient sits in the waiting room until a nurse can see him. Can I be held liable if the patient's condition deteriorates while he's waiting?

A No, because you haven't started treating the patient. But your ED's protocol could cause legal problems for the hospital.

An admissions secretary, who's often the first person emergency patients see, should record the patient's name and billing information only. Then a triage nurse or doctor—not the admissions secretary—should question him about his medical problem.

That's not the case at the hospital where you work. If a patient is injured, the hospital will most likely be liable for misdelegating authority or for failing to provide an adequate admitting protocol for the ED.

Affection

Isn't it okay to encourage visitors to touch and hold loved ones in the hospital?

Q I'd like your opinion on an incident that happened last week in our surgical department.

A woman in her late 20s was admitted and scheduled for a biopsy of the axillary nodes to detect any remaining cancer cells following a recent lumpectomy. She was scared and showed it. We were all relieved when her husband arrived to keep her company.

The patient asked her husband to lie beside her on her bed, above the covers. They held hands and watched television. Noticing the couple on the bed, our supervisor strode into the room and snapped, "This behavior is totally unacceptable." She ordered the husband off the bed "immediately." He not only got off the bed, he also left the hospital before visiting hours were over.

We staff nurses couldn't believe our ears. You'd think the supervisor found them doing something outrageous. As far as we were concerned, she acted like this because of her own hang-ups—not for the patient's best interests. We feel that if anything, nurses should encourage people to touch and hold their loved ones in the hospital to ease their natural anxiety. Do you agree?

A Like 100%. The behavior you describe is nothing to be uptight about.

Before wagging a finger at the supervisor though, suppose the couple chose more ardent lovemaking. Or they weren't married. Or they were adolescents. Or they were the same sex. Or they were severely handicapped. And so on. How would you and other staff nurses react then? A bit differently, possibly, because you all carry around highly individualized feelings about sexuality, propriety, and privacy. And you have to come to terms with your feelings before you can deal with other people's feelings.

But come to terms you must because nurses—not doctors— form the first line of compassion, objectivity, and defense when it comes to dealing with patients' sexuality.

Your whole department could probably benefit from an open discussion on this topic. You know, it's not so long ago that even the holistic approach to nursing virtually ignored patients' sexuality as a legitimate nursing matter.

So why don't you try to get the discussion going? And be sure to invite your supervisor.

Will embracing make a nurse-patient relationship look improper?

Q I'm a male nurse working in a busy psychiatric emergency department, and although we have several nurses on staff, the patients—both male and female—seem to single me out when they have problems. And many of them ask me for a kiss or a hug just before they're discharged. In my family, hugging and kissing relatives and friends of either sex comes naturally, and I'd never want any patient to feel rejected. But I don't want my nurse-patient relationship to look improper, either. What should I do?

A Surely a sincerely meant hug or kiss good-bye for a scared or depressed patient seems natural now and then. But if this is happening regularly and you feel vague, nagging doubts about it, pay attention to them. Ask yourself whether you're just a nice person or you're actually encouraging more dependence and familiarity than called for. Better still, ask a co-worker whose judgment you trust for his opinion on how you're coming across to the patients.

Because you're obviously someone who inspires trust, you can help any patient who's looking for emotional reassurance by steering him to a support group in the community. In these groups, close relationships often develop among members. Gradual reciprocal affection and support can develop over time and spring from self-confidence rather than dependence. These will do more for your patient over the long term than any fond farewell.

Would kissing a patient be "professionally inappropriate"?

Q In my 10 years as an emergency department (ED) super-

A

visor, I've never heard any complaints about my professionalism. Until last week, that is. An 8-year-old child, suffering from renal failure, was brought in by her parents. At first the child was unresponsive, but gradually her condition stabilized. The pediatrician decided to send the child to a dialysis facility.

After preparing the child for transfer, I said good-bye and kissed her lightly on the forehead. Both the assistant director of nursing and the ED administrator said my gesture was "professionally inappropriate." They added that I shouldn't handle the direct care of children until I could be "more objective." I don't see anything unprofessional about giving a child some reassurance. Do you?

A You'd find two sharply divergent points of view on this seemingly minor issue.

One nursing administrator, who understood what was upsetting your ED administrator, might say "A kiss usually connotes affection—not just reassurance." She would suggest more appropriate, more subtle ways of expressing your concern: a touch on the patient's arm, a squeeze of the hand, or a verbal reassurance. She'd admit that your concern for the child was heartfelt but that "a nurse should keep her care—and her caring—professional."

> *"They said I shouldn't handle the direct care of children until I could be more objective."*

Another experienced nurse would say something like this: "This is a hard one to call. I can't believe an occasional kiss is something to be criticized. I think the child warmed you at that moment—and your kiss was a natural response. If I'd been a parent watching, I'd have said, 'Get me that nurse for my child.' "

Agency administration

Do you know of any master's degree programs that might fit the bill?

Q Several doctors at our community hospital are planning to open a home health agency as a private business venture. They've approached me with an offer too good to refuse. The agency administrator job is mine—if I return to school for my master's degree. The doctors will pay half my tuition.

I'm single; I have a little nest egg saved; and I'm at that stage of my nursing career where I'm torn between being cautious and taking a gamble on something I'd enjoy. From what I've been reading, diagnosis-related group (DRG) regulations assure a bright future for home health care.

Do you know of any master's degree programs that might fill the bill for me?

A The University of Michigan School of Nursing started the first organized master's degree level program designed specifically for home health agency nurse administrators. This program leads to a master's in community health nursing with a concentration in home health care. Besides a strong emphasis on management theory, the curriculum includes principles of marketing, quality assurance, staffing, and personnel management.

You're on target about the growth of home health care, and DRGs are only one factor contributing to this momentum. Advances in medical technology enable nurses to administer at-home treatments previously performed only in hospitals; many items are now portable and usable outside the hospital setting, including dialysis and respiratory equipment. And by the year 2000, 32 million Americans will be over

65 years old—the age group most in need of nursing care.

So you won't exactly be throwing caution to the winds by getting your master's degree at this time. In fact, you could be making a sound investment for your own future—one with accruing and lasting interest.

For more information about the master's program, contact: University of Michigan School of Nursing, Ann Arbor, MI 48109-2007.

Agency nursing

Can they sue a nurse for breach of contract if she accepts a permanent job?

Q For a year or so after my son's birth, I worked for an agency doing occasional shifts in area hospitals. About 3 months ago, one of the hospitals offered me a permanent job with flexible scheduling and a great salary, so I took it.

Now the agency is suing me for $5,000—for breach of contract. An exclusivity clause in their contract prohibits any employee from accepting a nursing job in the area for 1 year after the contract is terminated. My new employer is anxious to keep me working and offered to pay the agency $1,000 to release me from my contract.

I knew about the agency's policy when I signed on, but I didn't take it seriously. I never expected them to raise such a fuss over one employee accepting a permanent job that she needed. Now, I'm not sure what to do, and I don't have the money they want. Do other agencies act like this?

A Most agencies hiring nurses as employees rather than private contractors write a 6-month exclusivity clause into their contracts. One year seems unduly long, but they have your signature on the dotted line. And with the current highly competitive job market, the stakes are high, so there's no telling how far they'll pursue this.

Set up a meeting right away with the hospital's attorney and administrator to find out just how actively they'll negotiate with the agency in your behalf. If they want you badly enough, they may increase their offer. The agency would be better off getting a good settlement from the hospital quickly than going through a lawsuit with a disgruntled employee. But don't count on anything; get your own lawyer. If the agency won't negotiate with the hospital, you could end up with a lien on your personal property. Take this seriously.

How can someone start an agency business?

Q After doing some informal market research, I found a significant need for a nursing service agency in my community.

I have the necessary funds to start up the agency, but my one problem is my lack of business experience. What do you suggest?

A First off, bravo. You've taken your first entrepreneurial step—finding a service community members need and a way to provide them with it.

Now get down to (your) business. Hiring a lawyer and a tax accountant is always a good idea, because once you start your agency, you'll be an employer—and subject to all the requirements of that role. For example, you'll need to set up a tax account with the federal government and follow all the rules concerning employee withholding and Social Security taxes.

You'll also need to establish operational space for your business (anything from a spare room to a commercial office is fine), recruit nurses, buy liability insurance, and determine your fee structure. Then you'll be ready to go out and get accounts.

For additional information, send for copies of the Joint Commission on Accreditation of Healthcare Organizations (JCAHO) and American Nurses' Association (ANA) standards on supplemental nursing services. You can write to JCAHO at its Nursing Service Section, Dept. N90, 875 N. Michigan Ave., Chicago, IL 60611, and to the ANA at Dept. N85, 2420 Pershing Rd., Kansas City, MO 64108.

Should a nurse point out a discrepancy in technique?

Q As an agency nurse, I've worked at several area hospitals. On the unit where I'm currently assigned, I've noticed discrepancies in technique among the staff nurses. I'd like to call this to someone's attention, but the nurse-manager seems to accept what's going on. Should I get involved in this situation?

A That depends. Do these differences endanger patients? If so, document the problems in a memo to nursing administration and give a copy to your supervisor at the agency.

If such prompt action isn't necessary, ask yourself whether the care you perceive as inconsistent is really just different from what you're used to. In other words, would uniformity in technique improve patient care? If you believe it would, make a list of your recommendations, the reasons behind them, and the benefits for the unit and patients (cost effectiveness, time savings, and so on).

Before sharing your list with the unit's nurse-manager, review hospital policy on agency nurses' responsibilities. Then, ask for feedback on the list from your agency supervisor. If she feels you have some good suggestions, request a meeting with the unit's nurse-manager to share your ideas. Keep the tone positive and constructive. Remember, the information you present should focus on facts, numbers, and specific techniques, not on names, personalities, and value judgments.

What do you think about staffing solely with agency nurses?

Q What do you think about units staffed solely with agency nurses? I'm an agency nurse who works the third shift. Recently, I've been assigned to various units with only agency nurses. Is this legal?

A Legal, yes, but not always conducive to quality care.

If the hospital gives the agency responsibility for staffing certain units on a prearranged basis, the chances for careful planning and for orientation of the agency nurses are greater. But if the staffing pattern is happenstance, patient care could suffer.

The nurse shortage undoubtedly accounts for staffing with agency nurses. And the pattern's bound to become even more common as the shortage becomes more critical.

However, the reason for the problem doesn't help you. You're still responsible for giving quality care, which will take some "preventive nursing." When you arrive on a new unit, check to see where the emergency equipment is located. Take the time you need to become familiar with the working of the unit. Make sure that your co-workers do the same. This will mean some time away from patients, but it will pay dividends in your self-confidence and nursing preparedness.

AIDS

Can a nurse really tell her patients who need blood transfusions that there's no risk at all?

Q I read recently that screening tests have virtually eliminated the possibility that blood positive for the human immunodeficiency virus (HIV) will be accepted for donation to blood banks.

A

Can I really tell my patients who need transfusions that there's no risk at all?

A If a patient asks, tell him that it's extremely rare, but not absolutely impossible, for HIV positive blood to pass undetected through the screening tests. These tests detect antibodies to HIV, but because newly infected people don't develop antibodies for many months, blood from a newly infected person could pass the screening process.

For patients who have the time and opportunity, though, you might suggest an autologous transfusion—a practice that's becoming more routine as the AIDS crisis expands.

Can self-healing work?

Q My son, who just learned that he has acquired immunodeficiency syndrome (AIDS), has heard about a woman in California who promotes self-help and healing techniques for AIDS patients. Now he wants to go out there and consult with her. What do you think about this?

A Your son is probably referring to Louise Hay, who is doing some incredibly inspiring work. She draws hundreds of people like your son to her weekly meetings called the Hayrides. At the meetings and in her books, she teaches them about the link between the body and the mind.

Louise reminds patients that they deserve to find happiness. People with a feeling of self-worth can heal themselves, she says. Not enough of us take that kind of responsibility for our own sickness and wellness.

What's convincing is that Louise's motives are pure—she refuses to become a guru. She doesn't claim to heal these people. She'll place a mirror in front of a young man's face and say, "I'm not the great healer.

Let me show you who is." And, of course, the mirror reflects the man himself.

Louise teaches 10 basic points to help patients learn how to love and forgive themselves. She tells them to:
• stop criticizing themselves and others.
• accept themselves lovingly.
• comfort—not scare—themselves.
• create an image they love, then grab hold of that image whenever they allow a negative thought to scare them.
• be gentle, kind, and patient with themselves.
• accept their minds.
• praise themselves.
• support themselves.
• take care of their body by eating the right foods and exercising.
• do mirror work; that is, look in the mirror at least twice a day and say, "I accept you. I love you. What can I do for you today?"

Does the law allow a nurse to inform her co-workers about a patient's history?

Q Because I work for several nursing pools, I sometimes care for the same patients in different hospitals. Recently, I recognized a former patient of mine who was admitted for substance abuse to the unit where I'm working now. I know he tested positive for the human immunodeficiency virus in another hospital, but he denies it and refuses to be tested again.

This patient has bowel incontinence and a speech problem that makes him spit when he talks, so I'm worried that he'll infect someone else. To protect the hospital staff and other patients, does the law allow me to inform my co-workers of this patient's history?

A No. In at least one state—Texas—you could face civil and criminal liability for a breach of confidentiality related to testing for the

acquired immunodeficiency syndrome (AIDS) virus. You owe this patient the same confidentiality you gave him when you first learned of his test results, even though you now work at a different hospital.

The Centers for Disease Control (CDC) hasn't documented a single case of AIDS transmission from contact with feces or saliva. Still, health care professionals must minimize any risk by taking blood and body fluid precautions with *all* patients, as the CDC recommends.

How can a nurse help a friend find the will to live?

Q One of my dearest friends was recently diagnosed with acquired immunodeficiency syndrome (AIDS). Since then, he's lost the will to live. Although his general condition is good, he sits home alone waiting to die. He lets me visit, but he won't see any other friends. And he's forbidden me to tell anyone about his diagnosis. How can I make him see that he still has a lot of living to do?

A You can't make your friend do or feel anything other than what he chooses. It's understandable that you're frustrated, but the bottom line is this: You aren't responsible for your friend's happiness—or for saving his life. He's probably not even asking that of you.

He's grieving for a life-style that will never be the same and for a life that will be severely shortened. And that's natural, because AIDS is such a nasty, deadly disease.

Remind him that even though he's ill, he's at home—that's certainly an encouraging sign. Many AIDS patients require intensive care for complex medical problems. And some die within months of diagnosis because they don't respond to treatments.

Right now, he is grieving. You can't compare him with anyone else. He's unique and that gives him the right to deal with his grief in his own way.

Patients can live or die despite medical intervention. Researchers have reported on patients with full-blown AIDS who are alive and well after 5 years.

Why have these patients lived while thousands who received the same treatments have died? The power of the spirit enters the picture. These patients believed, unequivocally, that they could turn their disease around, that they could move mountains. And they did. That's the only difference between the ones who lived and the ones who died.

You can't make your friend believe. He has to find that himself—within himself. Keep visiting and caring about him. He needs your love, regardless of the outcome he chooses.

How can nurses get volunteers to help care for AIDS patients?

Q The hospice where I work depends on volunteers for many patient-related services. With more and more acquired immunodeficiency syndrome (AIDS) patients to care for, we've run into a problem because most volunteers refuse to have anything to do with them. They say they're afraid they'll catch the disease or pass it on to their families.

No matter how much we explain that AIDS isn't transmitted through casual contact, they don't seem to believe us. How can we convince our volunteers to care for patients with AIDS?

A You shouldn't try to "convince" volunteers to give care to any patients they're not comfortable with—for the patients' sake

as well as their own. Instead, give the volunteers the opportunity to observe the professional caregivers; in time, some of them may resolve their fears or prejudices about helping with AIDS patients; others won't. Respect them for their gift of time and energy, and make them feel valued for the work they're already doing. Assign them to other patients, and look for alternative caregivers for the AIDS patients.

Here are some suggestions: Ask the patients' relatives and friends to donate their time. Check with area churches, clubs, and schools for people who'll volunteer to care for AIDS patients. Contact local gay organizations to see if they provide volunteers for AIDS patients. If they don't, offer to help them form a group that your hospice can contact on a p.r.n. basis. Don't lose heart: One New York City hospital has prepared enough volunteers to work with more than 200 AIDS patients. Perhaps your hospice can do something like this on a much smaller scale.

Is it okay to give a combination of diazepam and morphine?

Q One of my acquired immunodeficiency syndrome (AIDS) patients was receiving morphine every 4 hours. He was dying, and his respirations were slow and labored. When he began having seizures, his mother and friends asked me to do something. I got an order for diazepam (Valium) I.V. push. Both the doctor and I knew the patient could die from the combination of diazepam and morphine. When I explained that to his mother and friends, they told me to go ahead and give it to him. So I did. He died later during my shift.

Although I was unsure at first, I think I did the right thing in this situation. Could you comment?

A If relieving a patient's suffering was what you intended, then yes, you did the right thing. But choices of this kind are never easy when you're the one holding the syringe.

In such cases, you might consider the ethical principle of double effect. According to this principle, an action (giving the diazepam) that achieves a good effect (relief of suffering) only at the risk of causing unintended but unavoidable harm (death) is morally acceptable.

Honestly explaining the treatment and possible consequences to the patient's mother and friends was important because it gave them a chance to participate in decision making. This can prevent or ease the guilt that families of dying patients sometimes feel.

Should a nurse continue to help on an AIDS support committee if her opinions are ignored?

Q For the past 2 years, this hospital has sponsored an "I Can Cope" education program for people with acquired immunodeficiency syndrome (AIDS) and their families. Every year, the same RN supervisor and her assistant run the committee. The program is good PR for the hospital, so it gets a lot of attention throughout the community.

At the urging of my manager on the medical/surgical unit, I joined the committee this year. Before long, I realized the coordinators didn't want any help, suggestions, or interference from me. In fact, one of them stopped me in the hall after our first meeting and accused me of talking too much and trying to "take over."

Now I feel like a fool. This committee position is part of my bid for promotion, and my manager won't like it if I quit. But why should I stay if nobody's going to listen to me?

A You've already given your reasons for staying—and they're strictly business. So don't hurt yourself by taking this criticism personally and exaggerating its sting.

You do have to find out what your role on the committee's going to be. Ask the team leader for a specific responsibility so that you can work on it and report back. Take notes at the meetings, jot down your ideas, and listen. But don't jump in with your opinions until you learn the ropes.

You can also learn a lot about group dynamics and what makes a meeting productive. Involving everyone and giving credit can be just as important as identifying problems, establishing goals, writing agendas, and setting deadlines.

Try to hang in there. Your manager's confident that you have something valuable to offer the committee. But what you hear, observe, and bring back in experience will help you on the unit—and when you're promoted.

Should a nurse share her concern over an unapproved drug for AIDS?

Q I'm caring for an acquired immunodeficiency syndrome (AIDS) patient who I believe is treating himself with ribavirin on the sly. He has hemolytic anemia—a common adverse reaction to this drug—which can't be explained by his prescribed therapy. And yesterday, I overheard him talking to his friends about their recent trip to Mexico, where I know ribavirin is available over the counter.

I'm concerned that this drug will compromise his treatment, so I'd like to talk with him about it. How do you suggest I approach him?

A Before talking with your patient, share your concerns with his doctor. Then, gather appropriate pamphlets and teaching materials on AIDS therapy and drugs and the effects of hemolytic anemia on the body. You might also call a community AIDS hot line and ask what advice would be offered to an AIDS patient who was thinking about using ribavirin.

Identify the people your patient trusts. These may include his spouse or lover, family members, a minister, or a therapist. They're potential allies, so tell them what you suspect and give them the facts about the dangers of self-treatment. Then, ask them to back you up after you talk with the patient.

When you speak to him, keep your tone matter-of-fact and non-threatening. Nurses routinely ask patients about their medications, so you might include ribavirin in your assessment. If he admits to taking the drug, ask him other routine questions, such as: How long have you been taking ribavirin? How has it helped you? Have you noticed any side effects? Did you know that ribavirin can cause anemia? Your questions may encourage him to talk about his reasons for using the drug, his fears about AIDS and his current treatment, and his psychological needs. You should also urge him to talk with his doctor.

Suppose he denies using ribavirin? Leave the door open to future discussions by acknowledging that some AIDS patients take ribavirin and offering to answer questions. Have your pamphlets and other information ready. Even if he's not ready to confide in you, he may be willing to read about AIDS therapy, call a hot line, or talk with a friend. Then he may turn to you for advice.

Should a nurse who didn't wear gloves be concerned about contracting AIDS?

Q For the past 5 years, I've worked on a postpartum unit in a county hospital and have been exposed to a lot of blood and body fluids. Until recently, I didn't always wear gloves. And although I don't have any symptoms or any specific reason for worrying, I can't stop thinking that I might have contracted acquired immunodeficiency syndrome (AIDS) from one of my patients.

Am I worrying over nothing?

A The chance that you've contracted AIDS is extremely small. But who can say positively one way or the other unless you have an AIDS-screening test?

Worrying won't help. Why not arrange for a screening test and find out, as the saying goes, if there's more fear than the facts warrant?

Alcoholic doctor

How can he be helped?

Q For the past 18 months, I've been office nurse for a highly skilled doctor. I respect, admire, and love the man. He has no personal life anymore. His wife is an alcoholic. He drinks much too heavily, too, but he was always able to maintain his practice until about 6 months ago.

Then, he began missing appointments and staying home without good reason. He became irritable, indecisive, and paranoid. About 4 months ago, I noticed the narcotics count was off. Things are getting worse. We've lost almost half of our patients in the past 3 months. I can't tell him my suspicions because I know how he'll react—mad!

I wouldn't want to report him to the medical society. But I want to help him, not hurt him. Any other suggestions?

A Flat out, the first thing you must know is that if you do not report a suspected narcotics law violator, you could be held criminally liable. You could also be subjecting yourself to disciplinary action by your licensing board.

As a fact of human nature, however, official statutes tend to influence you less than your own private code of law—your conscience. So look at it from that point of view.

Here's a man you admire who's bent on destroying himself and his career. In so doing he could be jeopardizing *your* career. (With the expanding role of nurses, courts have indicated increasingly that a nurse may be liable for malpractice she might have prevented).

Most important, he could be jeopardizing his patients' lives—those lives you've sworn to protect. Can you in conscience let this continue?

You *must* report the doctor's aberrant behavior. Under the doctrine of qualified privilege, your anonymity will be protected.

> *"The doctor's missing appointments, staying home without good reason and becoming irritable, indecisive, and paranoid."*

Further, and perhaps just as difficult for you, you probably should resign. There are simply too many perils involved for you to continue in this situation. Before you leave, however, talk to the doctor.

You don't have to confront him about your suspicions of his drug taking. Instead, perhaps as part of your notice of resignation, you could discuss the changes you've noticed in his personality. Show him your records of his missed appointments and failing practice. Tell him you feel he has problems that have become too serious for him to handle alone. Urge him to seek psychiatric help.

But what an exquisite relief it will be for him when he finally sees the downward spiral of his life stop. And he can start looking up to the time when he will again be the man and doctor a co-worker or patient *should* respect, admire, and love.

You know the expression you often give patients, "This will hurt a little in the beginning—but it'll do so much good." Time to apply this thinking to your feelings about the doctor.

What can be done about an alcoholic doctor?

Q A recent incident in our intensive care unit has me angry—and frustrated—and I don't know what to do about it.

A 57-year-old man had been admitted in respiratory distress secondary to congestive heart failure and pulmonary edema. He was placed on a ventilator, then on a T tube and, tolerating that well, was then extubated. Shortly after extubation, though, he began to get restless, tachypneic, and confused.

By the time I came on duty (4 hours after the patient was extubated), he was cyanotic, clammy, tachypneic, bradycardic, and nonresponsive to verbal stimulation. I started to manually ventilate him while the charge nurse went to call the doctor.

She said the doctor, who sounded foggy, refused to reintubate. At the time, I didn't know where to turn to have this doctor's order questioned or overruled.

Within 20 minutes, the patient had a cardiac arrest. He's now on a ventilator, has lost renal function, and lacks cerebral response.

There's one more thing: This doctor is a known alcoholic, whose orders are often vague or suspect.

What could I have done in this situation? And what action should I take now?

A First things first. After the charge nurse received the doctor's negative reply, you could have asked her to continue manually ventilating the patient while you called the doctor back to question his decision, assuming this patient was a candidate for resuscitation.) If the doctor still refused to give an order to reintubate, you could then have contacted the nursing supervisor, explained the situation, and

said something like "The doctor on this case seemed a little 'foggy' and I'm not sure he understood what I said." His reputation would have done the rest for you.

The nursing supervisor could have then contacted the unit's medical director. Remember, one doctor is never the final authority—especially if he has the reputation you say he has.

If you plan to take action about this incident, you must act promptly...but wisely. Get all the facts before you make any formal complaint, and elicit peer review from the nursing and medical staffs.

Why? For one thing, you received a patient who was in acute distress. For another, because that patient is now on a ventilator, some doctor had to have made a late decision to reintubate.

When preparing your documentation, include only facts and observations (no opinions or conclusions) and consider the following questions:
• What actions had been taken by the previous shift?
• When your charge nurse called the doctor, what did he say other than "don't reintubate"?
• Did the charge nurse question the doctor on his decision?
• Did she think the doctor sounded intoxicated?

Then send your complete report up through proper channels.

You're in a very touchy situation, and it's not likely to get better until this doctor gets better. He needs help. Your report should prompt hospital administration to take action that will protect the doctor's other patients.

P.S. You have great spirit!

What can be done about an anesthesiologist's drinking problem?

Q While scrubbing for emergency surgery early one morning, I started talking with the anesthesiologist. His speech was slurred, and he

A

had alcohol on his breath. I informed the surgeon, who got another anesthesiologist. Later, I talked with the surgeon about the situation. He told me the anesthesiologist was trying to overcome his drinking problem and said we shouldn't make it harder for him. But I think someone should be told about what happened. What should I do?

A You were right to act as you did. Obviously, the surgeon (and probably other colleagues) are aware of the anesthesiologist's problem. Now you need more information before going further.

Is the anesthesiologist in a program for impaired professionals? Has the medical staff taken steps to protect surgical patients? Or was this patient just lucky that you noticed the signs of intoxication and spoke to a surgeon who was willing to act? What if other nurses aren't as observant or as bold?

These are questions you should ask the surgeon. Then, offer to work with him and your manager to set up a system for protecting patients.

But if he's not willing to take action that will guarantee patient safety, tell him and the anesthesiologist that you're going to notify your manager and the director of anesthesiology about what happened. Assure them of your concern for the anesthesiologist as well as your patients.

Alcoholic nurse

How can it be proven?

Q We feel sure that our night supervisor is abusing alcohol, but we can't prove it. She often comments how the antibiotic she takes smells like alcohol, as if to explain away any alcohol on her breath. A co-worker and I mentioned our concern to the nursing home's administrator, and he asked her to take a

blood alcohol test. She refused and went home for 3 days on sick leave. Now she's back on the job, but the administrator said he can't do anything without more to go on than our suspicions. Unfortunately, he's not around when she's working.

What do you say?

A Your administrator's right. Vague suspicions and rumors about alcohol on her breath won't get the supervisor off the job and to the recovery program she needs. Those of you who actually observe her behavior will have to give the administrator something more to go on, in writing. For instance, look for and report specific behavior: increased tardiness, Monday absences, disappearing in the middle of a shift, sleeping or dozing on duty, inability to meet schedules, withdrawal from others, inappropriate responses, errors of judgment, irritability with patients and staff, deteriorating personal appearance, slurred speech, or unsteady gait. Even if your evidence is only circumstantial, you're justified in reporting it.

Recruit at least one co-worker to verify your observations and join you in signing. (Some administrators won't consider a complaint valid unless those making it are identified.) And if nothing changes, get back to the administrator again. Remember, you're not trying to punish the supervisor; you're trying to get her the help she needs to avoid more serious consequences.

Is it okay for a recovering nurse to counsel alcoholic patients?

Q I just got a job as an LPN after being out of work for several months because of alcoholism. Thanks to Alcoholics Anonymous (AA), I'm back on my feet.

We often have alcoholic patients on our unit. I have to bite my tongue

to keep from telling them my own story and how AA changed my life.

My employer doesn't know my history. Would I lose my job or my license if I tried to counsel these patients?

A The danger is not that you'll lose your job or license because you're a recovering alcoholic. But, on the job, even well-meant proselytizing is out of line. You may offend a patient who's denying he's an alcoholic. Worse yet, your advice may conflict with his doctor's treatment plan.

Without realizing it and without using words, you're probably already communicating special caring and encouragement to your patients. And when you've been a recovering alcoholic a while longer, then speak up—to your unit manager and the doctors on staff. Ask them how you can use your own experience with this disease to help their alcoholic patients achieve similar success in their battle against it.

Is there anything a nurse can do if her supervisor ignores the situation?

Q My question is whether to tell or not to tell. I'm worried about the one (and only) nurse who works the night shift on our hospital's special care unit. (I work the evening shift on the same unit.)

I suspect the night nurse is an alcoholic. She often comes to work moody, smelling of liquor, and saying she "doesn't feel like working."

Despite this, her supervisor lets her work—maybe trusting that the night nursing assistant can cover for anything that might go wrong. And believe me, a lot could go wrong. Our patients are often critically ill, and any mistake in judgment could cost them unnecessary suffering or even death.

Please don't think I'm unsympathetic to this nurse's problems. She's a divorcée trying to support two children. Still, I don't feel her patients should be jeopardized.

Is there anything I can do if her own supervisor ignores the situation? Though most of the other nurses know, I don't think our director of nursing does. Should I go to her, even if I have only suspicions—not concrete proof—to back up any accusation?

A Tell! The night nurse you describe has no business coming into the unit if she cannot deliver care. And you should get your priorities straight. Your first obligation is to the patients; *then* you can sympathize with the troubled nurse.

A director of nursing cannot act in this situation unless she has evidence. As a nurse, you have a duty to give your supervisor documented accounts of a co-worker's questionable behavior—if that behavior endangers patients. With proof in hand, your supervisor's obliged to act.

But until you can *document* your suspicions, proceed cautiously and say nothing. Once you do have evidence, follow the hospital's chain of command. Begin with your supervisor. If she does nothing, talk to the night supervisor. Next, approach the director of nursing; and then, if necessary, her immediate superior.

When you've protected the patients, you can then turn to the nurse's problems. This divorcée needs help badly. Have you ever talked with her yourself? Perhaps you could persuade her to go to the director of nursing and discuss her problem—before you have to. Perhaps you can offer her encouragement, tell her there is help.

None of this will be easy. In fact, if you pursue the matter, you may find you've antagonized not only the night nurse herself (alcoholics are notoriously hard to help), but some

of your co-workers, who'll look upon you as a company spy.

What should a nurse do if she fears her alcoholism will be revealed to the unit manager?

Q About a year ago, I realized my social drinking was becoming more than just that—although in my own defense, I never, never came to work under the influence. I quit drinking and joined Alcoholics Anonymous (AA) before the addiction got too strong a hold on me. No one I work with knows I ever had a problem—until last week, that is.

Like a fool, I made the mistake of confiding to a co-worker (who is herself a recovering alcoholic) that I go to AA meetings twice a week. I thought this bond between us might help us both. Imagine how I felt when she said that she intends to inform the unit manager and the coordinator about me. Because, as she explained, they should know right away that I'm an impaired nurse before rumors get back to them.

Instead of the feeling of pride I felt for doing something positive about facing my drinking problem, I'm now nervous and disillusioned. What's your opinion?

A There's no explaining why someone you'd expect empathy from would act so uncool. Confession may be good for the soul, but keeping mum about personal problems is the best (make that safest) policy at work.

Don't let this unexpected setback throw you out of focus. You're the same person now as you were last week, with the same courage, smart thinking, and stick-to-itiveness to win a hard battle.

Act positively. If you've the gut feeling that your co-worker will indeed report you, beat her to the

punch. Make an appointment with the unit manager and coordinator. Tell them your situation, and invite them to take a close look at your nursing care. Request that they review past performance evaluations as proof of your continuing excellent nursing performance.

And give yourself a pat on the back for handling your problem like a true professional. Good luck.

Alcoholic patient

Could a private-duty nurse be blamed if a drunk patient falls down and fractures her hip?

Q I'm an RN doing private duty for a patient who's a heavy drinker. She's usually intoxicated when I arrive, and she continues to drink while I'm there. I've called her doctor, who said she could have two drinks a day, but he refused to put anything in writing. When I relayed his message to the patient, she just laughed it off. She said she's in her own home and can do whatever she wants.

I actually feel sorry for her; my own father died an alcoholic. But I'm worried that she'll fall down and fracture her hip while she's drunk and I'll be blamed. What do you suggest?

A You've talked with the patient and her doctor. Now you must watch out for yourself by taking the following steps and documenting that you have done so:
• Discuss the implications of her drinking with the patient, and stress the potential hazards, such as falls.
• Report the problem to the appropriate people—the patient's family, her doctor, and your agency.
• Do your best to protect your patient during your shift—clear her paths, remove scatter rugs, and warn her to be careful.
• Ask someone in her family to come stay with your patient if you have to leave when she's drunk.

A

• Teach her family safety tips and—one more time—don't forget to document that you have done so.
• Send copies of your documentation to the doctor and to your employer, but keep the original.

Bravo for sticking with this difficult patient.

How can he be helped?

Q One of the patients on our busy medical/surgical unit is an alcoholic. When he's intoxicated (which is much of the time), he becomes agitated and abusive. One day he grabbed an empty irrigation bottle and threatened to hit a staff member with it. He refuses all meals, medications, and treatments. In fact, some of the nurses no longer think it's worth offering anything to him.

We seem to be standing by, watching this man drink himself to death. As concerned health professionals, we wonder: What can we do? We don't want to abandon him just because he's an alcoholic. We want him to have the therapeutic environment and help he needs.

We also have to face the potential danger in this situation: The longer he's on our unit, the greater the likelihood that he'll injure himself or one of the staff.

Do you have any suggestions?

A You have every right to be concerned: You have a tough situation on your hands. Understandably, with the pressures of a busy medical/surgical unit, you have no way of giving this patient the time and thought he requires. Nor do you have the proper environment or professional preparation for treating this highly specialized patient problem.

Here are some steps that could help:
• Ask to have this patient transferred to a less busy unit—preferably one better equipped to deal with an alcoholic patient's difficult behavior.
• Until he is transferred, you need help: Ask a psychiatric nurse consultant or other qualified counselor to give your staff some insights into the handling of an alcoholic patient. Also review the techniques for protecting yourself against an abusive patient.
• Try to locate and control the source of the patient's liquor. But bear in mind that cutting off the patient's supply of alcohol could bring on a whole new set of problems, including the onset of alcohol withdrawal syndrome. Here again, request the services of a skilled professional—one who should be on call in the event of a crisis.

In the potentially explosive situation you've described, protect yourself against possible legal recriminations. Put the details of the situation and your concerns in writing; send copies of your memo to the patient's doctor, to your own nursing supervisors, and to the hospital administrators. Keep a copy for yourself.

This patient's lucky to have a staff like yours—nurses who obviously care.

What should be done about an alcoholic patient who's ruining morale?

Q I have a morale problem. My usually super staff nurses are very unhappy—starting to call in sick, talk of transfer to other units. And it's all over one patient. This woman has a chronic problem (nothing serious) and is hospitalized periodically. The minute she signs in: Trouble. Her husband brings in liquor daily and they both drink all the time he is there. She becomes abusive, demanding, and treats the staff as if they were her personal maids. I have told her doctor about this and asked that he prohibit the liquor, but he's an old friend of the husband's and minimizes the problem. Any suggestions?

A Since you say, "my staff," you're probably a unit manager or supervisor. Dear lady, where have you been? Nurses are *not* personal maids of the doctor and his friends, and it's a sorry lot who let themselves be put in that position. Think of what it says for their leadership!

When you got nowhere with the doctor, you should immediately have taken this problem to your unit-managers meeting. If that didn't get results, then to the director of nursing...right up to the chief of medical staff. The doctor would be reprimanded and the patient, discharged pronto. Patients—like the proverbial poor—we have always with us. Not so a super staff. Act now.

Alcoholic visitor

How can a nurse protect a patient from her alcoholic husband?

Q I'm a private-duty LPN. For the past 5 months, I've been caring for a woman with right hemiparesis and aphasia caused by a cerebrovascular accident. She's showing much improvement, but she has a problem I can't deal with.

The problem's her husband. He's an alcoholic. Every day he drinks himself into a stupor. He falls, talks to himself continuously, uses foul language, and even urinates on the floor.

He interferes with his wife's care and orders her to "talk right." If I try to reason with him, he seems to drink even more.

When he drinks, he neglects his wife. For instance, he allows her to smoke in bed, and she has, on occasion, burned herself.

I was trying to cope with the situation by myself, until a recent incident made me realize I couldn't handle this alone. I walked in and found something burning on the stove and two smoke alarms blaring. My patient was in her bed, crying. She'd pulled the cover over her head. The husband had passed out on the floor.

I immediately turned off the stove and got my patient outside until the smoke cleared.

But this woman needs help...more than I can give her. She has no one she can turn to. Who can help me get her out of this intolerable situation?

A You're right: She needs protection. Her life could be in danger. Get in touch with your county's office for older adults—they may be able to apply legal pressure to change the situation. The local chapter of Alcoholics Anonymous and Al-Anon might have some useful advice. Or you could ask your department of public health for their suggestions.

One more thing: Try to enlist the help of your patient's doctor. He'll have to back up your account of the patient's predicament when you apply to the various agencies for help.

The agencies may take some time before acting, so you'll have to work with the situation in the interim. Position the patient so she has the phone close to her—on her unaffected side. Also, try to arrange for neighbors to make checks until something more basic can be done.

You certainly did take more than you bargained for. But congratulations for your good effort—and your good heart.

Allergies

Does a nurse have to give up nursing if she's allergic to penicillin?

Q What a problem for a nurse: I've developed a severe allergy to penicillin. In the intensive coronary care unit where I work, I've been reasonably well protected thus

far. My co-workers have been very cooperative, and I've been extremely careful not to be the one who prepares the penicillin.

The trouble comes when I float to other units. Since our hospital is small, floating's fairly frequent. I'm all right if I'm sent to the emergency department, but I'm not all right when I'm sent to medical/surgical units, where penicillin is commonly administered.

I've had a couple of severe allergic reactions already, but luckily they didn't go beyond hives and some chest pain. Both responded well to antihistamines.

I've seen an allergist at the hospital's request and at my expense. He recommends staying away from penicillin, which is easier said than done, and undergoing desensitization, which frightens me.

Any suggestions before I'm forced to give up nursing?

A Reconsider the advice about desensitization. As a nurse in a critical care setting, you should be able to handle and administer penicillin.

If you're allergic to penicillin, you could also be allergic to a long list of penicillin derivatives; among these are nafcillin, cloxacillin, oxacillin, cyclacillin, amoxicillin, ticarcillin, carbenicillin, and many others. You could also be allergic to cephalosporins, such as cephalothin (Keflin) and cefazolin (Ancef).

Unfortunately, there's probably no hiding place out there. If you really want to stay in nursing, think again about desensitization—it might be the only sensible choice.

Allergy bracelets

Should registration clerks ask outpatients if they're allergic to anything?

Q As a nurse at an acute care facility, I question a policy that

has the registration clerk asking outpatients if they're allergic to anything and then giving them bracelets identifying their stated allergies. I think a nurse should do this.

A You're right. As a nurse, you could make an insightful assessment that a clerk couldn't. The clerk could prepare the bracelet identifying the patient's allergy, but you should double-check it.

Allergy shots

Could a nurse legally charge a small fee to give them?

Q Before moving to this farm district, I worked for an allergist in another part of the state. I had a special interest in my work because my whole family and I are allergic and, with my doctor's permission, I'd always given us our shots.

> *"Now that I can give allergy shots myself, the whole neighborhood wants to come to me"*

In our new home, we are 15 miles from the nearest doctor—who is so overworked he refuses to take on any new patients. As a consequence, we had to drive a 100-mile round trip to the nearest city for our weekly allergy injections. I now have permission from my new allergist to give our family injections.

Neighbors who know of this and who want to avoid the long trip are now asking me to give them their injections. Would it be legal for me to give them their injections? Would it be legal for me to do this in my own home? Could I legally charge a small fee? Could I advertise this service?

A

A Professionally and legally a registered or graduate nurse may give allergy injections to her *immediate family* if the administration is based on an order by a physician licensed to practice in that state.

A nurse may legally give injections to the *public*, however, only if she is licensed in that state—and, of course, if the injections have been ordered by a physician who is also licensed to practice in that state.

So, providing you get written approval from the attending physician of each patient, you can give allergy injections to your neighbors. You may also charge them for it.

You may *not*, however, advertise your service because that is considered unethical and could subject you to disciplinary action by your state licensing board.

Should the syringe be aspirated?

Q I am one of four nurses working in an allergist's office. We figure that together over the years we've given thousands of subcutaneous injections.

When I give an injection, I don't aspirate the syringe, but the other nurses do. They maintain that aspiration is necessary to check whether they hit a blood vessel. What's the right method?

A No single absolutely right method exists. Like your co-workers, some nurses aspirate the syringe, and others don't. Many reference books recommend this practice except for injecting certain drugs such as heparin or insulin.

Those who subscribe to your method and omit aspiration for subcutaneous injections say the negative pressure that aspiration creates can cause unnecessary trauma to healthy tissue cells. Hitting a major blood vessel is unlikely, they also say, because you're injecting the

needle into the subcutaneous tissue beneath the skin.

Look at it this way: If you and your co-workers have already given thousands of problem-free injections, you must all be using the technique that's right for you.

Allergy testing

Is it okay to do when the doctor's out of the office?

Q I'm an RN working part-time for an allergist. My duties include complete allergy workups—taking patient histories, giving injections of various allergens, and so on.

Although I know the allergy-testing technique is quite safe—and I'm very careful—I'm worried because the allergist isn't always at the office during the testing. Other doctors have offices in the building, but I'm still nervous about the injections: What if I come across a very sensitive patient or give someone a dose from the wrong vial? (We have vials for over 300 patients.)

The other staff members, an LPN and medical technician, say I'm looking for trouble—they've been doing the testing for the past 6 years without a doctor on call. Am I overanxious?

A You may not be "looking for trouble," but your chances of finding it are fairly good. Administering allergy tests without a doctor close at hand is risky. As you well know, severe allergic reactions can lead to swelling and possible closure of the airway; an emergency tracheotomy may be necessary. How quickly could the other doctors in the building respond to your emergency call?

Voice your concern about patient risks to the allergist; perhaps some rescheduling can help. Setting up blocks of hours specifically for al-

lergy testing, for example, could make the testing more convenient for the allergist—and safer for the patients. Knowing the allergist is there to help in an emergency should help you breathe easier, too.

Aloe plants

What are the ethics of suggesting a patient use aloe products?

Q Products derived from the aloe plant work successfully on abrasions, sores, cuts, and burns at home. But can I use the same products safely in the hospital or suggest their use to patients?

I work largely with isolation cases, where I often see allergic responses from antibiotics. Sometimes only minor results are achieved with the expensive preparations prescribed.

> *"I'd like to suggest aloe products to my patients but I'm afraid of being charged with practicing medicine."*

I'd like to suggest aloe products, which I believe could be beneficial, but I've not yet seen any of the aloe derivatives listed in the *Physicians' Desk Reference.*

Can you tell me: What are the ethics of my suggesting a patient use an aloe product?

A In a nutshell: "Don't." Do not suggest or recommend aloe products, not while you're on duty—and not while your professional responsibilities are on the line. Natural products can be as potent and dangerous as any classified drug; in fact, many potent drugs were originally derived from plants.

The same regulations prevail with aloe products as with any other drug—which means a doctor's order is necessary.

Your intention was generous. But even more admirable was your professionalism—which made you check before you acted.

Alternative therapy

How can a nurse be sure she's steering her patient in the right direction?

Q The parents of a young cancer patient I'm caring for have lost faith in medical treatment. The child is making some progress, but we've told them she has only a 50/50 chance of recovering. They want to discontinue chemotherapy and start her on a diet that's supposed to work wonders for cancer patients. They've also asked for my advice. I'm a great believer in alternative therapies, but I don't want to steer them wrong. What should I do?

A You need to keep the lines of communication open and encourage these parents to share their hopes and fears with you and the doctor. You could say: "Your concern about the diet and your daughter's therapy tells me you want to make wise choices. We can talk about the pros and cons of the diet, and I'll try to answer your questions."

This doesn't have to be an either-or situation. Find out what your patient's parents already know about the diet. If elements of it can be incorporated into your care plan, offer to discuss it with the doctor and the dietitian. But if you believe the diet is potentially harmful, offer to help them find objective research that presents both sides of the issue. Document your conversations, and make sure you keep the doctor informed of this family's wishes.

Sometimes, family members worry about biting the hand that feeds them when they inquire about alternative therapies: They're afraid their questions will turn the pa-

tient's caregivers away from him. So reassure your patient's parents, and encourage them to ask as many questions as they want.

Finally, listen to your patient. If she's old enough to understand the basics of her treatment, how does she feel about the choices? What are *her* hopes and fears? If she can't articulate her feelings, watch her play and let her body language speak for her. Document your findings and relay the information to her doctor.

Alzheimer's disease

Any suggestions on how to handle patients with the disease?

Q I recently began working in a skilled nursing facility and am finding it extremely frustrating to care for patients with Alzheimer's disease.

Communication problems are the worst. Sometimes I spend 5 minutes or more explaining a simple procedure to a patient, only to discover he hasn't understood a word I've said.

I've been yelled at, kicked, scratched, and bitten. I realize the patients aren't responsible for their actions, but I can't help feeling discouraged and angry, and I hate feeling this way day after day.

I really love nursing and wouldn't give it up for anything. But I need advice on how to handle these difficult patients and the stress I'm under when caring for them.

A Your feelings aren't unusual. But showing your anger and frustration in front of a patient will only threaten him and increase his agitation. Instead, when you become irritated, leave the patient's room and express your anger to another nurse. (Let your peers come to you for support, too.) Once you've regained your perspective,

you'll be able to return to the patient and calmly give him the understanding care he needs.

For more help, read as much as you can about how others cope with the frustrations of caring for—and communicating with—Alzheimer's patients. An excellent source to help you through days that sometimes seem endless is *Understanding Alzheimer's Disease* (Miriam K. Aronson, ed. New York: Charles Scribner's Sons, 1988). The authors suggest ways to manage the stresses of caring for patients with Alzheimer's disease. Though written for families of these patients, the book is valuable for anyone who wants to understand the troublesome behaviors that makes this disease so mysterious and threatening.

Ambulance

How can a nurse listen to her patient's apical heart rate and blood pressure with the noise and vibrations during the ride?

Q I work with a local ambulance service escorting critically ill children or adults to the appropriate medical facility. A routine trip from our small town to the nearest big medical center may take 40 minutes or more.

But we have a nursing problem along the way: The noise and vibrations during the ride make it almost impossible for me to listen to my patient's apical heart rate and blood pressure. Palpation is difficult, too. Is there a solution to this problem?

A Several instruments could resolve your problem. When transporting adult patients, one possible solution would be for the ambulance service to buy a portable cardioscope, which permits visual monitoring, and a portable blood pressure unit, which provides a digital readout. The blood pressure unit doesn't require a stethoscope and would be unaffected by the noises and vibrations you mention.

When transporting an infant or child, you could use a portable unit now available that is designed to monitor the heart rate, respiratory rate, and blood pressure of young patients in transit.

These pieces of portable equipment have proven successful not only for ground transportation, but also for air transport. (They work equally well for fixed-wing or helicopter flights.)

Perhaps other ambulance nurses have found their own ways and means of solving problems involved in transporting their patients, so why not exchange ideas with the ambulance nurses in your general area?

One more suggestion for further advice: Get in touch with the director of professional activities at the Emergency Nurses Association (ENA), 230 E. Ohio, Suite 600, Chicago, IL 60611.

Ampules

If paint falls into the solution, could this in any way alter the drug's action?

Q Where I work, we use injectable drugs packaged in glass ampules. Some ampules are scored with a band of paint at the breaking point. Quite often, when snapping one open, minuscule particles of paint or glass fall into the drug. I worry that some might be drawn up into a syringe, even if a very small-gauge needle is used.

Although I'd like to discard the ampule and start over, this isn't always possible. If paint falls into the solution, could this in any way alter the drug's action? And how harmful are glass particles if they are accidentally injected, especially I.V.?

A Particulate matter is unnecessary, unwanted, and possibly detrimental to the patient. But, after years of study (which, incidentally, was initiated by two Australian doctors), the subject remains controversial. Some experts believe particulate matter injected I.V. is harmful, some don't.

Small paint particles from the band probably won't alter the drug's action. And of all materials injected I.V., glass particulate is probably the least harmful.

> *"Sometimes minuscule particles of paint or glass fall into the drug and I'm worried this could be harmful."*

Whenever you snap an ampule open, some glass particles might fall into the solution. Try to avoid aspirating these particles into your needle and syringe by tilting the ampule at about 20 degrees above horizontal and inserting the needle tip at the shoulder of the ampule just above the deepest point of fluid. That way, you'll avoid drawing up the largest glass particles, which should fall to the deepest point when you tilt the ampule. Don't try to withdraw every drop of drug from the ampule—there's always a slight overfill anyway. As an alternative, you can use a filter needle to withdraw the drug, then replace it with a regular needle for the injection.

Amputee nurse

Can a nurse with an amputated leg carry out her duties satisfactorily?

Q A young woman who lost a leg in an automobile accident is now applying for admission to our nursing program. She doesn't wear a prosthesis but gets around quite well on her crutches. She seems highly motivated, and we think she possesses many characteristics desirable in a student nurse.

We have an associate degree program in a community college with an open-door policy. If the applicant meets our physical and academic requirements, we'll have to accept her. But how can we determine whether she can carry out her nursing duties satisfactorily?

We need your advice on how to handle this sticky situation.

A Your situation—and the applicant's—is a difficult one, but not hopeless.

Sit down with the applicant and explore the possibility of a prosthesis. Assuming she's a candidate for one, a prosthesis could be the solution to both your problems.

If she isn't a candidate for a prosthesis, or if she rejects the idea, explain the energy and mobility requirements for nursing. Nursing means hard work, often amid such routine obstacles as crowded rooms, hectic schedules, and unforeseen emergencies. Also, many procedures require two hands, stability, and strength.

Suggest she get some practical experience before entering the program. Would an area hospital hire her as a nursing assistant?

How about arranging to have her meet the program's faculty and a nursing representative of a hospital where you have student practicums?

The faculty should think about how they would teach and evaluate her in situations where she'd be at a disadvantage. Also, how will the faculty and other students deal with the extra time and attention this applicant may need to handle a difficult curriculum? And what about patient reactions?

You should also consult your school's guidelines for disabled-student applicants and talk with the school's lawyer.

In the long run, this situation could provide a unique learning experience for everyone involved.

ANA code

Can a nurse lose her license if she violates the ANA code?

Q Does the American Nurses' Association's (ANA) Code for Nurses carry any legal weight? Can a nurse lose her license to practice nursing if she violates that code?

A No, you won't lose your license if you don't comply with the code. Membership in the American Nurses' Association is voluntary, and therefore, not all nurses can be bound by the ANA's code.

However, the 10-point code clearly sets out standards of conduct and practice in professional nursing. If you conform to these standards, you'll be unimpeachably professional. Copies of the code are available from the ANA at 2420 Pershing Road, Kansas City, MO 64108. A single copy is free.

ANA exam

Is it recommended that a nurse be certified as a maternal-child heath nurse?

Q I'm certified by the American College of Obstetrics and Gynecology as an inpatient obstetric nurse. I'm also certified by the American Nurses' Association (ANA) as a community health nurse. And in October this year, I could take the ANA exam to be certified as a maternal-child health nurse. Should I?

How much certification does one nurse need? All of these exams pertain to my professional practice, but what are the chances that a prospective employer may think I'm overdoing it with three certifications?

A Certification is a wide-open matter at this time. Very few people get either extra pay or extra

benefits because of certification. One of the arguments is that a certificate is not a degree. With certain groups—the Emergency Nurses Association and the American Association of Critical-Care Nurses, for example—certification carries peer prestige.

The theory is that there are levels of practice. Your certification attests that you've reached a higher level of competence and knowledge. Bearing this in mind, and even taking account of your other certifications, why not go for the third certification? That is, if you have the time, the money, and the energy. You're bound to add to your information and skills. Who could fault that? Certainly not a prospective employer.

If you want to look ahead, add a degree to the certification; the combination will certainly lead to career advancement.

Anesthetics

Is injecting the drug into the catheter considered practicing medicine?

Q I'm a staff nurse in a 137-bed general hospital. Since a new anesthesiologist began practicing here a few months ago, we've had some cancer patients (especially the debilitated ones) come back from surgery with epidural catheters providing continuous anesthesia. The doctor stipulates the amount in his orders.

Since this procedure's new to us, the anesthesiologist has given us detailed instructions and a demonstration on how to inject the anesthetic into the catheter.

But we have no confirmed hospital policy to guide us—even though our staff development director did write up the procedure.

We're concerned: If we inject the drug into the catheter, are we prac-

ticing anesthesiology, or is this a legitimate nursing procedure?

We've checked with other area hospitals and with the public health officials who investigate hospitals. What should we do?

A You're checking with the wrong sources. To find out whether injecting an anesthetic into the catheter *is* a bona fide nursing procedure in your state, check with your state board of nursing. If the board has approved this practice for nurses, take three precautions before you start doing the procedure:
1. Be sure you've received sufficient training in injecting the anesthetic into the catheter under the direction of clinical instructors of anesthesia.
2. Be sure written hospital policy lists this as a nursing procedure.
3. Be sure you have both hospital and personal liability insurance to cover this procedure.

Is it legal for nurse anesthetists to administer anesthetics?

Q In my hospital we don't have an anesthesiologist on staff. A nurse anesthetist administers all anesthetics. Is this legal? I thought the nurse had to work under the direction of an anesthesiologist.

A In most states, a nurse anesthetist must work under medical supervision—but not necessarily under an anesthesiologist's supervision.

In the situation you describe, the nurse anesthetist is probably working under the supervision of the doctor doing the surgery. This doctor is responsible for writing and signing the anesthesia orders. As long as the doctor accepts this responsibility, as well as responsibility for monitoring the nurse anesthetist's performance, your hospital's practice is perfectly legal.

A

Anger

How can a nurse help a nursing assistant with personal problems?

Q My children are all in school, so I'm back working full time as an RN at a 300-bed nursing center for the aged. Each RN has three nursing assistants working for her. My problem is an 18-year-old nursing assistant I'll call Mary. Mary, who comes from a problem family, resolved her difficulties by quitting college and leaving home. She's lost all contact with her family and, until 2 months ago when he split, she was living with a kind of hippie young man.

Mary is attractive, gets long well with co-workers, but loses her temper with patients. This has happened four times that I know of. Afterwards, she's always remorseful and full of apologies. And, she's never physically abused anyone. I haven't mentioned any of this to the director lest she fire Mary, and I don't know if this young woman could handle another problem in her life. Am I doing the right thing?

A You may be back at work, but you sure haven't left your mothering instincts at home. And you're to be commended for taking such a kindly interest in your young nursing assistant. Certainly, from your description, she needs all the understanding she can get.

Your other consideration, of course, is your responsibility to your charges. Anyone who "loses her temper" with patients—especially when they're old and helpless—is not fitted for that work.

Encourage this girl to seek counseling. She may not realize she needs it—and she may not know how to go about getting it. You might be able to ease her way by doing a little preliminary legwork. Call your community health agency.

Explain the kind of help you're looking for; find out what resources are available; then support Mary in a decision to seek help.

Remind her that, although you didn't report her misconduct in the past, you can no longer continue to ignore your responsibility. And if another episode of temper does occur, report her immediately to the director. Your first obligation is to your patients.

Angioplasty

Is it legal for a nurse to assist with certain parts of the procedure?

Q I'm a scrub nurse in a cardiac catheterization laboratory where doctors perform percutaneous transluminal coronary angioplasty. One of the doctors asks me to advance a guide wire down the artery and across the lesion while he advances the balloon catheter. I'm concerned that this procedure goes beyond my professional responsibility. But the medical director assures me he's ultimately responsible for anything that goes wrong.

Am I just a worrywart, or are my concerns well-founded?

A Pull out your license and take a good look at it: There's only one name on that license, and it's not the doctor's. No matter what he tells you, a doctor's presence in the room doesn't insulate you from liability.

Manipulating a guide wire, with all its inherent dangers (vessel perforation, plaque dislodgment, and so on), is clearly beyond the scope of nursing practice. Just think of what's required: sophisticated knowledge of anatomy, familiarity with reading the viewing screen, and coping with any complications that arise. Only doctors with spe-

cialized training are qualified to deal with this.

Again and again, nurses need to be reminded not to take on procedures when they can't take full responsibility for their actions. Follow your instincts and refuse to continue this practice.

Antibiotics

What if cephalexin seems to be overused?

Q At the nursing home where I work, the director of nursing firmly believes we should start residents on cephalexin (Keflex) at the first sign of a cold—even when no complaints exist. I'd prefer to follow the home's standing orders for aspirin or acetaminophen. Prescribing cephalexin seems poor medical practice as well as an unnecessary expense for the resident.

The doctor on call for the nursing home (the only doctor in this small town) doesn't give me much support on this issue. He usually orders cephalexin as often as the director of nursing requests it. Besides, he's in the habit of giving 95% of his medication orders over the phone (generally to me) without examining the residents.

Last week my concerns over the routine use of this drug came to a head. One of the residents had chest congestion, nonproductive cough, and low-grade fever. She was put on the usual cephalexin regimen. When her fever shot up to 101° F (38.3° C) one night, the director of nursing called the doctor, who ordered another antibiotic.

The next morning, before giving the new antibiotic, I questioned whether the cephalexin was to be continued. Although the director of nursing said, "Of course," I still wanted a doctor's say-so. When I finally reached him, he rather testily told me to continue the cephalexin *and* to give the new drug as ordered.

The whole situation has me very frustrated. Was I right to be worried about the combined use of the two antibiotics?

A Antibiotics are used together effectively in some situations, but it's understandable you're frustrated with the nursing home's current medication policies. Both the director of nursing and the doctor seem to have a "dependency" on cephalexin.

Prescribing shouldn't be a reflex action. But what is worrisome is that the doctor is prescribing without examining the patients. As you know, a doctor is responsible for assessing a patient's new, changed, or persistent symptoms before prescribing medication.

How can you improve the medication practices at the home? Try a direct, assertive approach. For instance, you might say to the doctor when he calls: "I feel uncomfortable with the prescription you've ordered for Mrs. Smith. I'd like you to see her before I give her any medication."

If the doctor persists in his phone prescribing habits, make an appointment with the director of nursing and the doctor to air your concerns. This won't be easy—especially in a one-doctor town. But you have a nursing responsibility. That responsibility means doing your best to have the doctor do his best.

Antiembolism stockings

Do they serve a real purpose?

Q On the medical/surgical unit where I work, we automatically put antiembolism stockings on every patient who's confined to bed rest. And many of them complain about the discomfort. Do these stockings serve a real purpose? Or is their use just a ritual from the past that we've never abandoned?

A Probably just about every order for antiembolism stockings is based, at least in part, on the old chicken-soup principle. That is, they won't harm the patient (if they're fitted correctly) and they could help. Studies show that stockings with a pressure gradient diminishing from 18 mm Hg at the ankle to 8 mm Hg at the thigh can help clear venous blood more rapidly from the lower legs. That, in turn, reduces venous stasis and decreases the incidence of deep vein thrombosis, a potentially serious condition.

Of course, as with any therapy, you must tailor the routine for your particular patient and his degree of risk. For a patient confined to bed rest, the usual practice calls for applying antiembolism stockings, elevating his legs, teaching him how to perform passive exercises, and, when the time's right, getting him out of bed to walk.

So stick with the stockings for your patients—and maybe the chicken soup, too.

Apgar scores

Should the test be repeated until the score reaches 10?

Q At the hospital where I work, we always take Apgar scores at 1 and 5 minutes after birth. As long as the score is at least 7, we don't repeat the test.

A new staff member has suggested that we test infants at 1 and 5 minutes—and then every 10 minutes until the score reaches 10. We don't think that's necessary. Do you?

A No. Although a score of 10 at 1 minute after birth indicates the best possible condition, an infant scoring 8 or 9 is in fine shape. As a matter of fact, an infant scoring 7 isn't necessarily in trouble.

The rating scale runs like this: 0 to 3 indicates severe distress; 4

to 6, moderate difficulty adjusting to extrauterine life; 7 or above, the absence of difficulty adjusting to extrauterine life.

Of course, you should repeat the test more frequently if the score falls within the low range of the scale. But repeat it until every infant scores 10? No, that's not necessary.

Apnea monitoring

If a nurse does it for a neighbor's baby, could she be liable?

Q I'm an experienced nurse on a leave of absence to spend some time at home with my family.

One of my neighbors, who's also a nurse, just had a baby—her second. Her first child died of sudden infant death syndrome, so this baby came home from the hospital with an apnea monitor. My neighbor's maternity leave will be up soon, and all the usual baby-sitters in the area are afraid of this machine and its implications. In desperation, she turned to me, and I impulsively agreed to care for the baby 12 hours a week.

Now I'm having second thoughts. My neighbor asked me to do this basically because I'm a nurse, although I won't be paid a third of what I'd make nursing in a hospital. If I establish that I'm employed as a baby-sitter, not a nurse, could I be liable as a nurse anyway?

> *"What bothers me is having to worry about liability at all when I know I could be helping out someone who needs me."*

What bothers me is having to worry about liability at all when I know I could be helping out someone who needs me. What do you say?

A

A Let your good instincts prevail. Take the job—but use caution.

First of all, you're responsible as a nurse whether you're receiving whole pay, half pay, or no pay. And although it's unlikely one nurse would sue another for malpractice under these circumstances, strange things happen when children or insurance are involved. So you should definitely have your own malpractice insurance, and check with your carrier to make sure this type of activity is covered.

Then, back to basics. Review both the operating manual for the monitoring equipment and basic life support techniques for infants before the first day on the job. Check the equipment to be certain it's functioning properly each time you mind the baby. Ask your neighbor for any records she's been keeping on the baby's progress, and keep records of your own. And make sure she leaves you the phone numbers for the doctor, the supplier of new electrodes, and the monitor repairman.

Then breathe easy and be the good neighbor you are.

Arterial puncture

Who should complete the procedure—the nurse or the lab technician?

Q At the acute care hospital where I work, we've run into a situation that's rapidly becoming a real sore spot between the nursing staff and laboratory personnel.

After withdrawing a blood specimen for arterial blood gas (ABG) analysis, the lab technician expects a nurse to take over and finish the procedure. His excuse is that he must rush back to the lab (although the specimen's put on ice as soon as it's withdrawn). We nurses say that if he draws the specimen, he should apply pressure to the site and make sure no bleeding occurs afterward.

We look upon this as just one more example of somebody else delegating to nursing. To check it out, we surveyed area hospitals and found them evenly divided on who completes the procedure, the nurse or the lab technician. What is your opinion?

A It's surprising that in half the hospitals you surveyed the nurses were willing to take over for the lab technician. Whoever draws the ABG specimen should be responsible for the entire procedure from start to finish.

There's more than just inconvenience involved here. Suppose a lab technician damaged an artery while taking an ABG specimen. It could be your word against his on whether you applied pressure too late, not long enough, or not at all.

To be fair, the lab technician will need some help. A trained nursing assistant can maintain pressure at the ABG site while he puts the specimen on ice—a matter of seconds. The assistant can then take the specimen to the lab while the technician continues to check for bleeding and maintains pressure for 8 to 15 minutes.

Stand firm on this. You already have enough to do without taking on another department's responsibility.

Aseptic technique

How can a nurse make sure the doctor complies?

Q One of our surgeons constantly breaks aseptic technique in the operating room—and he ignores me when I remind him of it. Last week, he wore the same surgical gown for two successive operations, even though plenty of gowns were available. I took him aside and pointed this out, but he just brushed me off. I'm concerned about patient safety. What can I do?

A You've already taken the first step—speaking directly to the doctor when the problem occurred. Now you have to pursue the matter through channels.

First, check the policies and procedures manual for hospital guidelines on maintaining aseptic technique in the operating room. Then, document your concerns about this surgeon—including what happened and when, what you said to him, and how he responded to you—and take them to your manager.

Together, you should go to the unit's medical director. He's responsible for enforcing the policy, not you. But you're all responsible for patient safety, so you're right to insist that this surgeon mend his ways.

Assessment

Can a nurse legally perform an initial psychiatric assessment?

Q The head of administration at this 95-bed psychiatric facility is asking the evening and night supervisors to evaluate "walk-in" patients seeking admission. (We're getting this additional duty because the medical staff doesn't want to sleep at the hospital in order to take calls. Instead, the medical staff will be brought in only to handle emergencies or to see someone who we feel needs admission.)

Although administration claims the evaluations are "nursing" assessments, we're not sure we have the skills to make these judgments.

Some of us are experienced in psychiatric nursing—some of us aren't. Some of the patients are already known to us—some are not. What if we should decide that a patient doesn't need admission or immediate treatment, but after leaving the facility, he were to kill himself or someone else?

Can we refuse to do the psychiatric evaluations? Or should we consider the evaluations within the bounds of nursing assessment?

A Yes, you can say no to taking on this extra duty—but not all your co-workers will want to take this stand. Here are some factors your nursing staff should consider in making their individual decisions:

Most states permit RNs to do nursing assessments in the five areas of nursing expertise: medical, surgical, obstetric/gynecologic, pediatric, and psychiatric nursing. But you must be able to answer yes to these two questions: (1) Are the assessments really nursing, not medical, assessments? (2) Do you have the education and experience to perform these psychiatric assessments competently?

Bear in mind that the regulations on this score vary from state to state. In some states, only psychiatric nurse clinicians with MSN degrees may perform psychiatric evaluations. In other states, nurses may make nursing assessments only in conjunction with mental health personnel who have the proper credentials—and with a doctor on call. Therefore, each nurse must be familiar with the regulations that apply in her state.

If you do say yes to this added responsibility, consider buying personal malpractice insurance. If you say no—because you feel illprepared for the task—don't feel that your co-workers who have said yes are more professional than you.

Being a professional means making choices—choices based on your education, your background, and your patients' best interests.

That's an answer to your immediate problem—but in the long run, you and your co-workers must face a bigger question: Must the doctors' scheduling problem become your problem? This is the fundamental issue: If you do tackle it, try working through your nursing director first. Eventually you should aim for a joint committee of doctors and nurses who will put the responsibility where it belongs.

Should a newly admitted patient be assessed right away or during any shift within 24 hours of admission?

Q On the medical/surgical unit where I work, we can't agree on when a newly admitted patient must be assessed by a nurse. Should it be right away—during the shift the patient's admitted—or during any shift within 24 hours of admission?

Those who say right away maintain that a patient's condition can change too radically between his admission and his assessment one or two shifts later. Others say that as long as we do an admitting assessment within 24 hours, we're covered legally.

What do you think?

A A new admission should receive a basic nursing assessment within 1 hour. A more detailed assessment and completion of the long assessment form should be performed within 24 hours.

Under diagnosis-related groups, every patient's hospital stay is now considerably shorter, so your care plan must be more exacting on a day-to-day basis. A full day is a lot to lose.

Assisting friends

How far does a nurse's responsibility go for her friendly advice?

Q Last week, my neighbor's husband was discharged from the hospital with a tracheostomy. Because she's squeamish about suctioning him and changing his dressing, she frequently calls me over to help her

Her husband also has diabetes and, since arriving home, has started on insulin. So now I'm also involved with educating them both about diabetes—self-injection, diet, exercise, and so forth.

The patient's doctor says I have his "blessing," but that seems to be all.

Several times after reporting to him about the patient's condition (pain or elevated blood glucose readings), he's taken no action. So far, no apparent harm's resulted, but I feel uneasy. How far does my responsibility (if any) go for my friendly advice? What do you think?

A You've obviously entered into a nurse-patient-family relationship. And we mean a professional relationship, with all the responsibility that word implies and without any of the protection usually accompanying such an arrangement.

Halfway positions are weak and confusing. So for your own good (and the patient's, too, in the long run), either drop back to a loving support role only or work out a more formal arrangement for care giving, education, and record keeping that's agreed to by the patient's doctor and the patient. If you want to work gratis, that's up to your good nature. Just as long as you make sure your malpractice coverage is current, you're using established nursing procedures, and you have a listening ear at the doctor's end of the telephone.

Autologous blood transfusions

Are nurses expected to take vital signs?

Q We recently transfused a patient with blood he had donated himself before surgery. This was a first for our unit. And because of the acquired immunodeficiency syndrome crisis, we expect more

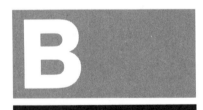

patients will request such autologous transfusions.

We're not sure if it's necessary to take vital signs during these transfusions because the patient's receiving his own blood. Can you tell us the protocol?

A According to guidelines from the American Association of Blood Banks, you should take the same precautions for autologous as for homologous transfusions. This means taking vital signs before the transfusion starts, every 15 minutes for the first 30 minutes of the transfusion, and every 30 minutes thereafter until the transfusion is over.

Although autologous transfusion virtually eliminates the risk of infection or immunologic complications, others can occur. For instance, the blood could have been contaminated during either collection or transfusion. Also, fluid overload or just plain anxiety could lead to still other complications. And there's always the possibility of error: You could make a mistake and administer the wrong unit of blood.

You can't consider any transfusion trouble-free until it's over. So take care—and take vital signs.

Baccalaureate exam

Isn't there something radically wrong with any program that has only a 10% passing record?

Q I enrolled in the Regents College Degrees program offered by the University of the State of New York, hoping to obtain a baccalau-

reate in nursing through their external degree program.

All went well until I reported for on-site clinical exams. After completing a series of not particularly difficult (although for me, stressful) clinical situations, the examiner told me that I had failed—but that I could appeal. I decided not to appeal after a fellow student told me that 90% of the candidates fail the clinical aspect at least once. It seems to me that something's radically wrong with any program that has only a 10% passing record.

Any comments?

A The statistics you heard are way off the mark. According to the program's consultant, 93% of the RNs taking the baccalaureate clinical exams (and 80% of LPNs taking the associate degree clinical exams) pass the first time around— no mean feat when you consider that a perfect score is required as the passing grade.

> *"After I completed a series of stressful clinical situations, the examiner told me I had failed the exam."*

When you get over your initial disappointment, remember that you have 30 days from the exam date to send a typed explanation of why you think your grades should be reconsidered by a review panel. Don't be foolish and let the appeal opportunity go by unless you yourself are convinced that, for whatever reason, you just bombed the test. The review panel reports back within 90 days, and they also tell you what clinical areas need remedial reviewing for next time around.

Yes—next time around. You've already put too much into it to let this one blockbuster disappointment keep you from seeing the program through to success.

Others interested in the external degree program should contact: Re-

gents College Degrees, The University of the State of New York, Dept. N86, Cultural Education Center, Albany, NY 12230.

Barium preparations

Should nurses be expected to give them?

Q Until recently, the radiology technicians at the hospital where I work always administered barium preparations before abdominal computed tomography scans. Now they want us to do it, so we're administering an oral mixture three times within 2 hours during our morning rounds.

Frankly, I'm peeved—the X-ray technicians are saddling us with their responsibility—because we're pushed as it is to keep up with a hectic schedule. What do you think of this practice?

A Sounds great for the patient. He'd certainly be more comfortable receiving the contrast media in his room instead of waiting around in the radiology department.

But transferring the responsibility for the barium preparations to the nursing department won't help you—especially when these preparations must be administered during your busiest hours. Also, with an arrangement like this, you're being drawn into fulfilling part of another department's procedure. Does this mean you'll share the responsibility as well if the radiology staff makes an error or change—say, in scheduling—without notifying you? Better sit down now and talk this over with representatives of both departments.

As an alternative, why can't the X-ray technicians come to the patient to administer the preparations? This way, the patient can remain comfortable and in your care until it's time for the scan, and the technicians will be overseeing their department's procedure from start to finish. Best of all, in the enlightened spirit of diagnosis-related groups, both departments will be working together to give the patient the best possible care during his shortened hospital stay.

Bathing

Should a foreign nurse be expected to conform to draping policies?

Q Recently, I was preceptor for a foreign-educated nurse. She's a superb nurse, so I gave her a favorable report. But I have a nagging doubt about her bathing technique. After she removed a patient's gown and sheet, she began the bath without draping him first. Thinking she'd just forgotten, I handed her one to cover him. She put it aside and went on with the bath. I was surprised, but decided not to say anything in front of the patient. Later, she explained that she never drapes male patients and that none has ever objected or seemed uncomfortable. Should I have done more than inform her that our customs are different from hers?

A For three reasons, she should go by the book and keep her patients covered during their baths. First, privacy is more than a matter of custom or how a nurse was educated. It's a fundamental right for every patient, so physical examinations, treatments, and baths should be done discreetly. Second, covering the patient during a bath prevents chills. And finally, using a drape protects the nurse against allegations of sexual impropriety.

Review hospital guidelines on bathing patients, then share your rationale for covering patients with the nurse you oriented.

Should hexachlorophene preparations be used?

Q We use a hexachlorophene preparation for bathing our infants in the small hospital where I work. If my memory serves me correctly, I heard some caution against this practice a few years back. Should we be using hexachlorophene preparations? If not, what should we use?

A Don't use hexachlorophene preparations for routine bathing of infants, especially premature or low birth weight babies. They're particularly susceptible to hexachlorophene absorption, and studies show a positive correlation between hexachlorophene baths and brain lesions.

Plain warm water should do the job nicely. An infant's slightly acidic skin surface has bacteriostatic effects, and water won't alter the skin's pH (which is about 5 soon after birth). If you feel you must use soap, choose one that's pH-adjusted (neutral or slightly acidic pH).

Bed linens

How often should they be changed?

Q Do you think we need to change hospital beds linens every morning, even for patients up and about most of the day?

I realize my question's not earth shaking, but we're trying to save nursing time and money—and every little bit helps.

A Changing bed linens every day is a nursing ritual from a past era—before escalating costs, diagnosis-related groups, and nursing shortages forced us to take a closer look at what's really necessary for quality patient care.

You must change a patient's bed linens every day, or even more often, when they're wet or visibly soiled. Otherwise, it's largely a matter of aesthetics. You can limit the changes to twice a week, which should save nursing time (and dollars) for more important tasks.

When you think about it, we go to great effort to make hospital care as much like home care as possible. And how many people change linens at home every day?

Benadryl

Couldn't it mask a transfusion reaction?

Q One staff doctor orders 25 mg diphenhydramine (Benadryl) I.V. injected into the I.V. tubing before infusing blood. Some of us nurses feel the Benadryl could mask a transfusion reaction and harm the patient. Is this a common practice?

A This practice is both common and recommended. Although some doctors prefer that the Benadryl be administered orally, the rationale's the same and sound: to prevent (not mask) an allergic reaction to the transfusion.

Bladder drainage

Does draining a distended bladder risk causing hemorrhage and edema?

Q At the hospital where I work, we've been taught that in catheterizing a patient whose bladder is distended, we should not drain the bladder completely.

We've been told that complete drainage might cause bladder hemorrhage and edema as a result of rapid decompression. In fact, our hospital policy specifically prohibits complete drainage in this situation.

But now I'm in a quandary.

Our staff urologists claim that, contrary to what I was taught, draining a distended bladder com-

B

pletely does not entail the risk of hemorrhage and edema. We frequently see our staff urologists doing a complete drainage.

Which do you consider the correct procedure—complete or partial drainage?

A The urologists' information seems to be more current than your hospital policy and the method you were taught. Urologists used to believe that draining a distended bladder completely could result in hemorrhage and edema. But recent studies have shown just the opposite. The more accepted practice today is drainage to avoid problems brought on by prolonged urine retention. These include infection, sepsis, and possible reflux to the kidneys.

However, as a precaution, some hospitals still limit drainage to 700 to 1,000 ml at one time. Your hospital may be one of these. This could leave you in a quandary. So ask your procedures committee to give you a clear directive—and some peace of mind.

Blind nurse

Where can a blind nurse get cassettes or tapes of nursing magazines and textbooks?

Q One of our home care patients, a graduate nurse, was recently blinded in an accident. Because she hopes her sight will return, she's trying to keep up with the latest in nursing. To help out, some of us on the nursing staff take turns reading the journals and textbooks to her. However, the independence she'd get with a tape recorder, replaying what she wants, when she wants it, would probably do wonders for her sense of self-sufficiency. Where can she get cassettes or tapes of nursing magazines and textbooks?

A Several "talking books" programs might help your determined patient find the cassettes or tapes she needs. One, Recording for the Blind, provides talking textbooks for blind students and professionals. Your nurse patient may find some nursing literature among the organization's 50,000 textbooks. Write to the agency at 20 Roszel Rd., Princeton, NJ 08540. Or call (609) 452-0606.

Another organization, Associated Services for the Blind, will gladly lend your patient any nursing textbook on hand. If they don't have a specific book on tape, they contact other organizations. If the organizations don't have the tape, Associated Services will tape the book on request. (This service is free if your patient returns the tape within 1 year. If she decides to keep the tape, the fee is $2.) For more information contact Associated Services for the Blind at 919 Walnut St., Philadelphia, PA 19107. The number is (215) 627-0600.

And according to the American Foundation for the Blind, nearly every state has a Library for the Blind. In your state, the Library for the Blind and Physically Handicapped (919 Walnut St., Philadelphia, PA 19107) will also record a specific book on request, if the book isn't in their, or another group's, archives.

Many hospital supply companies have tapes and will make them available for a limited time—without charge.

Blind patient

Should a sign be placed at a patient's door or bedside indicating that he's blind?

Q The nurses on the ophthalmology unit of our hospital wonder: Should we or shouldn't we place a sign at a patient's door or bedside indicating that he's blind? (We're including those patients who

are, for all practical purposes, almost blind—even though this could be a temporary situation.)

Our staff nurses and the families of our patients with vision problems are divided: Some think the signs would help, others find the idea distasteful and humiliating for the patient. The nurses who favor the idea argue that the signs would cue everyone entering the room to follow our established "treat as blind" procedures.

We've even checked with a hospital where they've tried out such signs; nurses there tell us the signs did help in coordinating care, but (and this is a big but) where the signs were posted, thefts of the "blind" patients' belongings increased dramatically. You can see we need a bit of guidance.

A Even if arguments for the signs sound convincing, never label patients as blind. Men and women who are blind or have poor sight want to be considered as normal as possible, and they struggle against being labeled blind. Aim at assisting each patient as much as you can, yet allow him to retain as much of his independence and self-respect as possible.

Blood pressure

Should it be taken in the patient's left or right arm?

Q Sometimes we care for patients who previously had mastectomies, either simple or radical. I was taught that I should never take a blood pressure or start an I.V. line in the arm on the affected side, but my co-workers don't agree. Am I right?

A If your patient had axillary nodes removed during a previous radical or modified-radical mastectomy, don't use the arm on her affected side for either measuring blood pressure or starting an I.V. line. Because of her surgery, her immune responses are compromised and lymph drainage is impaired for the rest of her life.

However, for most other patients, you should measure the blood pressure in both arms as part of your initial assessment so you can determine if one arm has a higher pressure. Then always use that arm. Document this in the patient's chart so that everyone else who takes the patient's blood pressure during his hospital stay will use the same arm.

What's the proper position for the cuff?

Q When using a wall unit for taking blood pressure, is it all right to turn the cuff upside down with the tubing up over the patient's shoulder? This would certainly be more convenient for patients in bed.

A Here's a more convenient—and excellent—technique. Just make sure that the center of the cuff bladder is placed over the artery being measured.

Blood transfusion

Can blood be administered without first running a starter I.V. solution?

Q I recently started working on the night shift in a small hospital. Last night we received an order for one unit of packed red blood cells for a patient who had no I.V. running and no order for one. Both the procedure and the policy manuals say the doctor must order an I.V. if it's to be used with the blood.

I felt uncomfortable about this because where I worked before, we always ran an I.V. of normal saline with blood administration. So I

called the supervisor and she advised me to "just run the blood slowly." (The night nurses aren't allowed to phone the doctors.)

The patient was fine—I watched him like a hawk. So I'm wondering if I'm wrong to be concerned? If no I.V. line is already established when blood is ordered, can the blood be administered without first running a starter solution?

A Although rarely done, blood can be administered without another I.V. running. Most hospitals, however, have standing orders to run an I.V. of normal saline with blood administration—for a number of reasons. If an adverse reaction occurs, for example, and you must stop the blood, you can quickly switch to the saline I.V. and keep the vein open for administering the drugs needed to counteract the reaction. (An adverse reaction, if one is going to occur, usually happens within the first 10 to 20 minutes of blood administration.) Keeping the vein open after completing blood administration can save the patient another stick if his hemoglobin and hematocrit haven't increased enough and if more blood must be infused. Last but not least, many manufacturers of these blood filters recommend a saline flush before and after blood administrations; otherwise blood may remain in the filter and the patient won't receive all of it.

Procedure manuals aren't carved in stone. When you identify a procedure that needs updating, speak up to avoid the same dilemma next time around.

Is administering blood to a febrile patient considered acceptable practice?

Q I recently started working in the medical/surgical unit of a small community hospital.

Last week, one of the doctors ordered three units of blood for a post-

operative patient whose hemoglobin was down from 10 g/dl to 9 g/dl and whose temperature was elevated to 102° F (38.9° C). Is administering blood to a febrile patient considered acceptable practice?

A If the temperature elevation is secondary to infection and the patient's hemoglobin is down, the patient needs the blood to increase oxygen and carbon dioxide carrying power. You should use such measures as antipyretic drugs, soaks to the axilla and groin, and forced fluids to bring the temperature down before and during the blood administration. Of course, the doctor should know about the patient's condition and what you're doing about it.

If the patient's temperature continues to rise while you're administering the blood, stop the transfusion and assess the patient carefully. Check for other signs and symptoms of a transfusion reaction: itchiness, chills, rash. If a transfusion reaction isn't causing the temperature elevation, the patient's underlying problem could be worsening.

Either way, be sure to notify the doctor at once.

Is infusing blood from an unlabeled bag all right in a life-and-death situation?

Q I work in the emergency department of a small hospital. Last week, a doctor ordered a stat transfusion of O-negative blood before the patient's blood could be typed and crossmatched. The unit of blood we received for the transfusion had no label.

Is infusing blood from an unlabeled bag all right in a life-and-death situation?

A Never. You don't know for sure what's in that bag. But you can infuse O-negative blood as long as it's properly labeled. The label

B

should clearly state what type blood the bag contains and the patient's assigned identification number plus his name, if possible.

When the lab sends a unit of typed and crossmatched blood, you can begin to administer that.

Is it acceptable to infuse blood through small-gauge needles?

Q Nurses at the hospital where I now work routinely administer blood through any size needle the blood will drip through. I was taught that you should use only an 18G catheter or a 19G butterfly needle to infuse blood—and that the blood should never hang for more than 2 hours. Then, as I understand it, if the nurse cannot successfully insert the needle, she should call a doctor to do a cutdown.

When I started my 3-to-11 shift one day, I found packed cells being infused through a 22G needle. The blood had been hung at 1:30 in the afternoon, and the infusion wasn't completed until 5:30 that evening.

The patient's doctor had ordered another unit of packed cells, so I used an 18G needle for this infusion. After I hung the second unit, I put in a call to the doctor and left word about what I'd done.

The next day my charge nurse was angry, and the doctor told me he didn't understand why I called. I explained that I was taught blood will hemolyze if pushed through too small a needle and that this could be fatal to the patient. Both the charge nurse and doctor brushed off my explanation.

A few days later, a similar incident took place. A doctor ordered 2 units of packed cells for one of my patients. Because this woman was obese and had very bad veins, I called the I.V. team to insert an 18G needle. The I.V. nurse said I should use the 22G needle already inserted. I refused and asked her to try an 18G.

She argued. But when I insisted, she inserted an 18G needle, and I then started the infusion.

Am I outdated in my thinking—is it now acceptable to infuse blood through small-gauge needles? And is it correct to let blood hang for over 2 hours? I don't like refusing to use small-gauge needles without solid evidence to back me up.

A Most of medical and nursing literature confirms your belief. The 18G catheter and 19G butterfly needle *are* most often recommended for transfusions. If a smaller needle is used, the red cells could be damaged. (And of course, a smaller needle slows the flow of blood.)

Most authorities recommend running blood at a slow rate (20 to 40 drops/minute) *only for the first 15 minutes.* (Transfusion reactions, if any, usually occur during this time.) If the patient shows no reaction or if his condition doesn't warrant a slow infusion, you can then infuse the blood at 80 to 100 drops/minute.

Generally speaking, an infusion should never last longer than 2 hours; the longer the blood hangs, the warmer it gets, increasing the threat of bacterial growth.

Yes, in short, you *do* have the right to refuse to do any procedure you're justifiably uncomfortable with. And you used good judgment to not compromise your standards of good nursing care.

But you're not finished; now you should try to convince the hospital to revise its policy on blood transfusions.

Will the hospital allow a nurse to refuse to give a blood transfusion?

Q I'm a nursing student who can't take an active part in administering blood transfusions for religious reasons. So far, this

restriction hasn't created any problem because I haven't worked with the critically ill.

As I move closer to graduation and the job market, I'm wondering if hospitals will have a "conscience clause" that will protect my job if I refuse to help administer a blood transfusion.

A Before you're hired, check with the hospital's personnel office to see if there is a policy that fits your situation. You probably won't find a specific policy on refusing to give transfusions, but look for a general policy on the employee's right of "conscientious objection" to refuse to participate in any practice that is against personal, moral, or religious beliefs.

Examine the policy carefully and ask how it has been applied and interpreted. In some hospitals, a nurse cannot be required to participate in the procedure of abortion (she has the right to refuse without fear of losing her job), but she cannot refuse to care for women admitted for abortions. A nurse's religion or personal beliefs may prohibit the practice of homosexuality or I.V. drug abuse, yet the nurse can still be required to care for acquired immunodeficiency syndrome patients. Make clear in your own mind the difference between doing a procedure or treatment that you believe is wrong and caring for the patient receiving that procedure or treatment, especially a patient who does not believe that procedure or treatment is wrong.

Then check with knowledgeable church leaders for an accurate position statement on blood transfusions. Some Jehovah's Witnesses, for example, now accept autologous blood "transfusions" through a closed-system chest tube drainage and reinfusion process. Be sure you can clarify where you stand on specific technologies, artificial blood products, and so on.

Boards

How can a nurse face taking them again after flunking the first time?

Q When I finished my nursing program, I thought everything would be great. Instead, I failed the boards, and everything fell apart. My co-workers started avoiding me. They must have thought I was stupid to have failed the boards.

I'm still on the same unit, but I've been demoted to nursing assistant. And now that I have to face taking the boards again, I don't know what I'll do if I flunk. Any advice?

A Try to get a new fix on what happened. Failing boards was (notice the past tense) a short-term episode in your life. And you're not alone. Last summer, nearly 17% of those taking the 2-day test for the first time failed, and probably each one of them can relate to your feelings. But being overly embarrassed or anxious doesn't help anything, so calm down and concentrate on passing next time around.

Some suggestions: Go back to your nursing school and ask the faculty for some study guidelines. If one area—for example, pediatric nursing—is causing you problems, ask that instructor to recommend review material. Get out notes you took, then test yourself on the content you've gone over by answering practice questions in a state board review book, such as the *American Nursing Review for NCLEX-RN* by Carol J. Bininger, et al. (Springhouse, Pa.: Springhouse Corp., 1989). If you feel you lack test-taking skills, consider a state board review course that helps with these techniques—one that guarantees that you'll pass or you'll get your money back.

At work, attend staff development sessions on various nursing pro-cedures. Watch an experienced co-worker so when you're asked about certain procedures on the state boards, you'll remember the steps she followed. Ask her to help you.

Most important: Don't lose heart. You can pass the boards.

Body donation

What's the name of an organization that helps do this?

Q On occasion, patients ask me for the name of the national organization to which they can will their bodies after death. Through such a bequest, they hope to aid research and to save their families the expense of burial. Do you know the name of such an organization?

A Most such programs are state-chartered and empowered to pay the costs of shipping and preparation of a body only within the boundaries of that state.

There is, however, one nonprofit, charitable organization that acts as a sort of registry for all 50 states so that no matter where you live—or die—they will contact the proper authorities to see that your request is carried out.

For further information, contact: The Living Bank, P.O. Box 6725, Houston, TX 77265.

Body odor

How should a nurse be dealt with who gives excellent patient care but has poor personal hygiene?

Q A nurse on our unit who gives excellent patient care has poor personal hygiene. Her hair looks unwashed, her uniforms are unkempt, and she has a strong, unpleasant body odor. Everybody's talking about the problem, but nobody's doing anything about it. Even the unit manager is at a loss.

We know the woman has a tough life, with seven children and a philandering husband. But we have to consider our patients and professionalism.

How can we deal with this without being hurtful?

A In the long run, you're not being kind by permitting this nurse to continue her poor hygiene. Eventually, she could be hurt by overhearing a disparaging remark.

If no one on the unit feels comfortable discussing the problem with her, ask your supervisor to handle the situation. If the supervisor's at all sensitive, she'll explore possible causes for the nurse's poor hygiene: depression, exhaustion, hostility—or even a medical condition.

After exploring all possible "good" reasons for the poor hygiene, the supervisor should state that this will be their only discussion of the matter, and the nurse will be expected to change. The supervisor should also state that her door will be open for discussion of the nurse's personal problems.

The situation is a supersensitive one. Good luck reaching an effective and sensitive solution.

What can a nurse do if she gets queasy when a patient has BO?

Q I'm in an embarrassing predicament: I'm an LPN with a queasy stomach. I get sick—I mean sick enough to throw up—if I'm attending a patient with a bad body odor resulting from poor personal habits. I stay in the room with the patient as long as I possibly can—then I have to dash for the hall bathroom.

Does this make me less of a nurse, or perhaps no nurse at all?

A Yes, your predicament's a bit unusual, but nurses are human, too. Anyone can be so sensitive to odors that she becomes physically ill.

Certainly don't leave nursing on that account. If the problem becomes troublesome enough, ask not to be assigned to the patient who's the cause of the problem. Or try to trade off this patient to another staff member who doesn't react so strongly to odors; take one of her patients that she has a problem with and you don't. This kind of exchange is frequently done. Or why not have another staff member stop in the room with a deodorizer before you go in to give patient care?

Your getting sick in front of the patient or leaving the room abruptly in the midst of giving care because you're sick to your stomach won't help anyone—certainly not the patient. So avoid the whole problem. Stay away, if you possibly can. As long as you're conscientious and concerned on other scores, this one vulnerability can be more than canceled out.

What can be done about a staff doctor who has terrible body odor?

Q One of our staff doctors, a well-loved and respected man, has gotten very careless about his appearance and has developed terrible body odor. Patients and staff alike have mentioned this. What can be done?

A On television, this problem keeps popping up in those "even-your-best-friend-won't-tell-you" commercials. And maybe there's a clue here. Perhaps you've been unable to deal with this because you're viewing it personally.

Try assessing the situation *professionally.* Here's a man who has suddenly become indifferent to his appearance and intimate hygiene. Such behavior often heralds the on-

set of an emotional or physical illness—and *he* could be needing a doctor. Further, consider the damage being done to his personal and professional image by this aberration. When a patient is acutely ill, even unconscious, we are still careful about his hygiene so that his ego integrity will not suffer once he becomes conscious of his former condition. Surely this doctor deserves as much consideration.

Go to your director of nursing and ask her to discuss the odor problem with the doctor's partner, or, if he hasn't one, with the medical director. Don't expect them to thank you for "thinking of them" in this assignment. The last person to be called "lion hearted" died in the 12th century. And it *is* a touchy situation. But if they, too, can look at it professionally rather than personally, it should help.

Further, until the looked-for changes come about, be very circumspect in your discussion even among yourselves. And never encourage patients' conversation about this.

Bomb threats

Are nurses supposed to search for the bomb?

Q I was taken aback last week when I came across a memo in the procedure manual of the small community hospital where I work. The memo states that in the event of a bomb threat, the staff nurses are supposed to search for the bomb.

Who said there's nothing new under the sun? This is certainly an unusual nursing assignment. But I'd like to know: Can I be fired for refusing to comply?

A Your hospital would be ill-advised to fire any employee for refusing to participate in a dangerous action for which that em-

ployee has not been trained. If the employee were hurt in that action, the hospital could be held liable.

Your hospital would be wiser to draw up an evacuation plan for just such an emergency. In fact, if the hospital doesn't have a plan already, it could be in violation of the local fire code.

You'd better take this issue up through proper hospital channels right away. Nursing's hard enough without assigning us to the bomb squad.

Borrowing medication

Is it acceptable to borrow some ointment from another patient?

Q In the nursing home where I work, an elderly woman was diagnosed as having conjunctivitis. Her doctor ordered erythromycin ophthalmic ointment applied twice a day for 5 days.

The pharmacy couldn't send up a new tube until later in the day. So a co-worker decided to borrow some ointment from another patient for the time being. I told her this was wrong. Am I right?

A Right you are. Where ophthalmic ointments are concerned, "neither a borrower nor a lender be." A patient should never share ophthalmic ointment with someone else—or even use her own leftover medication for a new eye infection.

Breaks

Doesn't the law require breaks in an 8-hour shift?

Q When a nurse asked about half-hour meal breaks on her shift, you said the law doesn't require any breaks in an 8-hour shift. Is that true in all states?

A First, no *federal* law requires meal breaks. That part of our answer stands.

However, a few states do require *some* employers to give *some* employees a meal break and a rest break in an 8-hour shift. In some states (Ohio, for example), the law requiring breaks for women is antiquated, probably discriminatory by today's standards, and—more pertinent—excludes nurses from its rulings. The Ohio Nurses' Association negotiates meal breaks in all collective bargaining agreements.

In a few other states, such as California, some industries must provide meal and rest breaks during 8-hour shifts. However, the California law applies only to nurses who work in private hospitals. County, state, and federal hospitals decide on their own meal-break policies.

In Canada, the law varies from province to province.

In short, depending on your state or province and employer: You may not get a break; you may get an unpaid break; you may get a paid break. In states that don't require meal breaks, you may have to rely on "power breaks," with the power coming from your state or provincial nurses' association.

To find out whether you're getting a decent break, check your hospital's administrative manual or contact your state nurses' association.

Before leaving the subject, consider one other aspect of meal breaks: a federal law on compensating for meal breaks. By federal law, you *must* be paid during your meal break if you aren't relieved of all duties during the break and you aren't free to leave your post of duty.

So, *if* your state law or contract requires meal breaks, and *if* you have to brown bag your meals at the nurses' station, your employer has to pay you for that time.

What can a nurse do for meal breaks?

Q What should a nurse do when the hospital practice is not to relieve her for coffee and meal breaks? Our supervisor says it's okay to leave the patients alone with just a nursing assistant on the floor because a nurse on the next unit will come in to check.

> *"How can I possibly take a break when I know if I do my patients won't be taken care of properly?"*

She knows as well as I that half of the time they don't even make an appearance. The rest of the time, they don't make patient rounds but just put a casual "How's everything?" to the nursing assistant.

A Staffing patterns for most hospitals are based on the needs of patients in certain units. Since you expect your reliever to make patient rounds, you're probably not on a subacute unit working with seriously ill patients. Here are some thoughts to guide your actions.

The law, in general, requires the hospital organization to provide adequate and competent personnel in accordance with the needs of the patients at any given time. The Joint Commission on Accreditation of Healthcare Organizations and some state hospital codes also have this requirement. If the hospital fails to provide a sufficient number of competent personnel and a patient sustains an injury as a result of the inadequacy of the staff, the hospital will be found liable in negligence.

If a nurse, knowing that the condition of her patient requires her attention, abandons that patient who sustains an injury as a result, then the nurse also will be considered liable in negligence.

How about that for a comforting appraisal of the situation to help you relax on your breaks? Your present arrangement won't do. Nursing is demanding enough without having worry and tension accompany you on your relief periods.

Get together with other nurses who feel the same as you about your present working conditions. Write it all out and present it to your supervisor.

If you don't get a satisfactory response within a reasonable time, ask for a meeting with the administration and the insurance carrier for the hospital. Understaffing, with its resultant increased exposure to liability, would be of great interest to the carriers, who would surely bring pressure to correct the situation.

Burnout

Any suggestions for coping?

Q As a staff nurse on a critical care unit for 5 years, I always performed competently and received excellent yearly evaluations. For the past 6 months, though, I've been tired, irritable, and depressed. I didn't know what was wrong, but finally I realized I was burned-out.

My supervisor suggested that I take a leave of absence until I get hold of myself. Now I feel like a failure. And I'm afraid my career is in jeopardy.

I'm trying to "think positive," but I don't feel up to it. I guess I just don't know what to do.

A Here's one thing not to do: Don't give up! Removing yourself temporarily from a stressful situation is smart and the first step toward replacing the energy and enthusiasm you've lost. But rather than take a leave of absence, couldn't you transfer to a less hectic unit for a while? Discuss this option with your supervisor—she should understand that you're still able to give nursing care.

Perhaps your expectations of yourself were too high; high achievers are frequent burnout victims. Or maybe you became so committed to work that you neglected other aspects of your life—recreation or exercise—that help relieve anxiety and stress.

Other nurses have found that coping techniques such as using positive imagery, rescheduling their time and tasks, taking mini-vacations, or setting new career goals can help them gain control again.

You could also consider starting an informal support group: Post a note on the hospital bulletin board inviting nurses to participate in a discussion on burnout. You'll probably find that many of your colleagues have felt some of what you're feeling and can offer solutions that worked for them.

How long can a hospice nurse last?

Q I've worked on a medical center hospice unit for several years. In the beginning, I loved my job. But lately, I've been feeling tired and irritable, snapping at my patients and co-workers alike. Many mornings, I wake up in the early hours and have trouble getting back to sleep.

I recognize the symptoms—I'm starting to burn out. I don't know how much longer I can last.

A It sounds as if you need a break. Caring exclusively for dying patients is emotionally and physically exhausting. In fact, some experts suggest working with the dying for only 6 months out of a year.

If possible, work in another area where you help patients recover and walk out of the hospital.

Watching a patient recover from gallbladder surgery *is* rewarding. You see improvement daily, so you feel your care is doing some good.

Death and dying are different. You may never be sure that your skills and caring helped. Co-workers and families can be difficult, and they may care more about prolonging life than about providing relief.

The job is a tough one, and it takes a special person to do it. You have to be assertive. Defend your patients' rights and yours, too. You're entitled to a break from death-bed duty. But it's your responsibility to ask for that break.

Your patients deserve to have competent, loving care provided by a stable, healthy nurse. Exhausted, suffering martyrs aren't helpful to them.

That's another reason why you should play as hard as you work. Take walks, work out, read, laugh, go to the movies—anything that allows mental escape from thoughts of death and dying. If you focus your attention on a ballet or a mystery, or if you just try to remain upright on a pair of roller skates, your mind simply won't have the room for the worries of your job. So, get out there and have some *fun*.

Should a nurse fight for better conditions?

Q I've become so disillusioned with nursing that I've changed jobs five times in the last 2 years. Each hospital offers me challenging clinical work, but I've been disappointed by short-staffing, disorganization, and unreasonable demands from administration. When the situation becomes unbearable, I leave. But I still wonder: Should I stay and fight for better conditions?

A Most nurses enter the profession with high ideals. Sadly, hospital politics, shrinking budgets, and administrative red tape often squelch enthusiasm. That can cause stress and burnout. Like many others, you're doubting yourself, the value of what you're doing, and the possibilities for change.

Before you decide whether to leave or to stay, ask another nurse—one whose style of nursing and professional savvy you admire—to help you explore your hopes and doubts about nursing. A psychiatric clinical nurse specialist or a counselor could also help you develop insights into the reasons you became a nurse, your hopes for the future, and your vision of success. By talking about these values, you may see your choices more clearly.

Values motivate all behavior, including change. A technique called values clarification can bring your unconscious values into focus for examination and possible change.

For more on this, you might want to consult a book called *Values Clarification in Nursing,* by Shirley Steele and Vera Harmon (Norwalk, Conn.: Appleton & Lange, 1979). It can help you discover more about your own nursing values, giving you a clearer idea of what you'd be willing to risk if you decided to stay and fight for better conditions—and what you'd hope to gain for yourself and your patients.

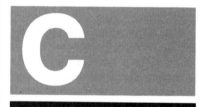

Call lights

What should be done if they're not watched?

Q On our medical/surgical unit we have an unwritten agreement that one staff nurse will voluntarily stay overtime to watch the call lights if shift report runs late. Sometimes, however, I've come out of the change-of-shift meeting only to find all my co-workers gone. I'm worried that an emergency might occur when the call lights are left uncovered. How do you suggest I avoid such a problem?

A You're wise to worry about this problem. Covering call lights is no light matter. Put the unwritten agreement aside and draw up a nursing policy that calls for posting the responsibility on the assignment sheet—with a specific nurse's name next to the assignment each day. This'll avoid those all-too-common excuses: "Oh, I thought Sally was supposed to cover today, or "I didn't know it was my turn."

But more important, when the assignment's put down in black and white, you can feel secure: It should mean a nurse will always be available in case of emergency.

Cancer

How can a nurse encourage a pediatric patient to talk about his illness?

Q Many of my pediatric patients who have cancer undergo frightening procedures, only to die. I'm worried that those children never have a chance to express their feelings about death. How can I get them to talk?

A Working with dying children is just plain tough. Too many nurses and doctors believe children won't grasp what's going to happen. But that's simply not true.

All patients—young and old alike—need to be given the opportunity to share their feelings if they want to.

Playtime presents a good arena for expression. Many children turn to dolls, stuffed animals, or puppets just for fun. But after a while, they're sharing their own thoughts and feelings through those little friends. With practice, you can encourage and participate in that dialogue.

Just being in the hospital is scary. To sense something bad might happen—something so bad people won't even talk about it—is even worse. So, please be warm and real with your patients. Use bears, bunnies, and dolls.

But most of all, use your heart.

Cancer treatment

How can an "abused patient" be persuaded to seek proper treatment?

Q My brother was recently a patient in a large cancer-treatment center. I was surprised by how poorly run it was. First, his records were mixed up with those of another patient with the same last name. Then, he had to undergo a painful procedure twice because his test results had been lost. He ended up signing himself out without receiving any treatment. How can I convince him that he should return?

A You can't. Although you mean well, you aren't responsible for judging what's best for another person.

Unfortunately, your brother has experienced what sometimes is called "bureaucratic pain"—that is, pain and frustration caused by bureaucratic bungling, delayed diagnoses, slow insurance payments, and doctors swamped by the health care system. Nurses can contribute to this pain by misplacing narcotic keys, returning late from lunch or meetings, or answering call lights slowly.

The bottom line is that because of bureaucratic pain, your brother is missing out on important and urgent medical care. Your best bet is to be his advocate. Talk to his doctor about what happened and ask him if he'd be willing to discuss the problems with people in charge at the cancer center.

Also, find out if that center is notorious for these types of errors. If so, change to another hospital. Remember, many institutions can treat cancer appropriately, and most doctors have admitting privileges at more than one hospital.

But if these were isolated incidents, your brother has to make a choice. Encourage him to discuss his feelings about his cancer. Without downplaying the fears and frustrations associated with bureaucratic bungling, your brother may have used the problems as an excuse to avoid treatment. Unconsciously, he may have been trying to leave the cancer behind.

Wherever he decides to go for treatment, visit him often. Be his troubleshooter by asking a lot of questions. And don't stop asking until you have satisfactory answers.

That's one of the best ways you can help your brother help himself.

Wouldn't the patient be better off without the treatments?

Q One of my home care patients is dying of cancer, but she's still getting chemotherapy. After her regular Monday treatments, she's sick for several days. By the weekend she feels better, but the next Monday the whole process starts again.

She knows the chemotherapy isn't working. Wouldn't she be better off if she stopped the treatments?

A She might be. But right now, she may be doing exactly what she wants to do. Legitimate or not, that's her choice.

Perhaps your patient feels pressure from her loved ones. Or maybe she wants chemotherapy so she'll feel she's doing *something*. Or she might not want to miss out if a cure for cancer is around the corner.

Some patients take chemotherapy to please their doctors. They feel obligated, they say, because their doctors have put so much time and energy into their cases. They don't want to seem unappreciative.

How sad that is. But what's even sadder is that not all doctors allow their patients to make a choice.

C

Of course, many people are alive today because of chemotherapy. But how many of them sat down with their doctors to discuss all the details, all the facts, all the benefits, all the options—and then decided if it was worth the risk?

So, talk to your patient. Find out *why* she's continuing her treatments. Make sure she has all the information she wants about her cancer. And tell her you'll support her no matter what she decides.

Cardiac care

Should a nurse tell patients they'd be better off in a medical center?

Q Until recently, the small community hospital where I work sent all cardiac patients to a larger medical center about 20 miles away. Now, administration has hired a young cardiologist who wants to keep the patients here. The patients love the idea of staying near their homes, of course. But we don't have enough cardiac monitors or backup equipment, and we can't give them the same high-quality care they'd receive at the medical center.

We know the new cardiologist is doing his best, but we feel dishonest about not telling patients that they'd be better off in the medical center. What should we do?

A You have valid concerns that your manager should share with the director of nursing. Together, they should request a meeting with hospital administrators and the cardiologist to determine what the nursing staff's responsibility is for cardiac patients.

Do hospital administrators plan to duplicate the equipment and services already offered at the larger medical center? If so, that hardly makes sense in today's economy.

Instead, they should concentrate on upgrading the equipment they already have and providing backup. That way, patients with less complex problems could stay close to home while more seriously ill patients go to the medical center for specialized care.

To that end, hospital and nursing administrators should provide you with a policy for triaging patients according to severity of problems, need for nursing care, and availability of facilities, equipment, and staff.

Once the hospital formulates a policy, you can use it to help patients and their families make choices. Many will opt for the familiarity and convenience of the community hospital, even if that means accepting some risks.

But before your patients can make an *informed* decision, they need to know which resources they're likely to need—and which institution can best provide them.

Career choices

What should a nurse's aim be when she is middle-aged?

Q Shortly after getting my BSN 23 years ago, I married and had two children. Through the years, however, I always kept my hand in nursing (part-time, private duty, volunteer work). And I'm lucky I did because nursing was the only thing that kept me going when, in a period of 18 months, my children left home to get married...and my husband left home to get a divorce.

A second lucky thing happened to me when I went back to full-time nursing. I discovered I love obstetrics and perinatology. Now, since I no longer have family obligations to keep me here and I have enough money to go back to school, I feel I'm ready to make the decision of my middle years: what to do with the rest of my life.

I guess my overall aim is to be well-qualified in a field of nursing that's not overcrowded and where my age won't be held against me.

Keeping that aim in mind, do you think I should stay in obstetrics and perinatology? Should I take courses to become a nurse clinician in that field—or go on for a master's degree? I'll appreciate any thoughts you have on this.

A Despite your personal problems (everybody has *them*), you're quite right to consider yourself lucky. Anyone who has found a field she loves, and has the means to pursue it, is one lucky lady.

Obstetrics and perinatology (O & P) is a beautiful specialty. You should be prepared, however, (if the birth rate continues to fall) for the possibility of an oversupply of nurses in O & P. But that musn't be your first concern. Be prepared—not *daunted*.

If O & P is what you want to specialize in, then do it! A person's success in any endeavor is almost directly proportionate to his love for that work. So you'd do well no matter how crowded the field might become.

As to whether you should become a nurse clinician or go for a graduate degree, only you can answer that. Ask yourself all the pertinent questions—how long do you want to study; do you want to work directly with patients or would you prefer to teach, and so on. Write to nursing schools at the university level and see what's being offered in specialty courses and graduate programs. Then, make your decision.

As to your age, here's a quote from the directors of a nurse practitioner program at a midwestern university: "We give preference to the mature candidate. The nurse who brings both life and work experience with her is significantly better able to identify and meet patient needs. In addition, she usually has a stronger concept of herself as a nurse and as a woman, both of which can be threatened in the evolution of a new role."

Get ready for your new role...and good luck.

Casts

Are nurses legally qualified to remove them?

Q I'm an RN working in a small-town emergency department. Recently, my supervisor said that from now on, when ordered by a doctor, we RNs will be expected to remove casts. In fact, even our emergency department LPN and nursing assistant may be asked to do this.

Are we legally qualified to remove casts?

A As an RN, you're *legally* free to remove casts when ordered to by a patient's doctor—provided you have the training and skill to do the job. But as a protection, try making sure your job description calls for you to remove casts. If it doesn't, ask your supervisor to revise the description accordingly.

> *"I can't believe that RNs, LPNs, and nursing assistants are expected to remove casts."*

But in the case of your LPN and your nursing assistant, they—or your supervisor—should check with the state board of nursing. Since state regulations vary, there's always a chance that in your state the LPN or the nursing assistant is prohibited from removing casts. The supervisor should review *their* job descriptions as well as yours—at the same time, making sure the LPNs and the nursing assistants know how to remove casts safely.

Now that *your* question is answered, here's a question for you:

Why can't the doctor do his own job of removing casts so the nurses can do their job of nursing?

Catheterization

Is using clean, not sterile, technique okay?

Q I've worked as a school nurse for the past 8 years. This semester, several disabled children who must be catheterized have been mainstreamed into our general school population. According to our administrator, I'm to use clean, not sterile, technique for this procedure.

I was taught that catheterization is always done using sterile technique. I'm not sure how to proceed.

What's the thinking nowadays on this?

A What you learned still goes. Although self-catheterization may be done with clean or sterile technique, catheterization of another person demands sterile technique. So much for a practical answer to a practical question.

Now, here's some information on the changing philosophy of school nursing—especially for the 8 million disabled children in the United States today.

Experts in nursing and education now see the school nurse's role as educating the disabled, not just caring for them. Eloise Jones, RN, EdD, an authority in special education, says, "Special education is instruction. It is not therapy. Most of all, it is not custodial care. Retarded or distorted development and physical disabilities are not conditions simply to be managed; rather, they represent problems to be reversed, drastically reduced, or compensated for, with the goal of successive steps toward normalization."

With that in mind, perhaps some of the children you mentioned, who

weren't ready for such instruction before, can be taught self-catheterization. This would reduce the chance of urinary tract infections and help them achieve a degree of physical independence in the day-to-day school experience and for the future. When you stop to think about it, the school nurse, better than anyone, can effectively teach many self-help skills properly and without embarrassing the children.

What a wonderful opportunity you have to contribute in a special way to these special children's lives. Even a small measure of progress in self-care can be enormously rewarding for them.

Which is the best type of catheter to use for long-term catheterization?

Q At the home health agency where I work, we're reviewing our policy on long-term catheterization. And we're trying to find out which type of catheter is better for long-term catheterization—fluorocarbon resin- or silicone-coated. What's your expert's opinion?

A When a patient will be catheterized for months or years, try using the lower-cost fluorocarbon resin-coated model first. If crystal precipitation and encrustation becomes a problem, switch to the silicone-coated catheter. The silicone coating will reduce urethral irritation and encrustation, and the catheter will last longer.

CCU

How frank should a nurse be with a cardiac patient?

Q My brother-in-law, who was recovering from a coronary, met one of his coronary care unit (CCU) nurses in the hospital corridor.

As part of an otherwise cheerful conversation, she said: "Boy, we had a tough time pulling you through. You almost didn't make it."

Is this an appropriate comment to make to a cardiac patient who's still convalescing?

A The nurse should have bit her tongue after that uncalled-for statement. And she should have been warm and supportive in nonverbal ways, which *might* help a little with the problems she stirred up.

Allowing the patient to "replay" his experience in the CCU can have great value. A nurse who was with a patient in intensive care can help him afterward to clear up episodes he remembers indistinctly or incorrectly.

If the patient himself *wants* to talk about how close to death he was, let him talk. Explore the experience with him. He needs to relive it—to come to terms with it. But telling a patient he "almost died" can only feed and fuel the anxieties he's already coping with.

Central line

Should the jugular or the subclavian vein be used for insertion?

Q One of our anesthesiologists always uses a patient's jugular vein to insert a central line. This is very uncomfortable for the patient, and we have a terrible time withdrawing blood. Unfortunately, we haven't much clout with this doctor because his department is an independent service. But, in our opinion, he should be using the subclavian vein when he inserts a central line.

Do you agree with us?

A Yes, 100%. Many experts say the subclavian vein is the better choice for inserting central lines for both the reasons you give. Also,

when a central line is inserted in the jugular vein, any movement by the patient can increase the risk of infection and may dislodge the line. Doctors know this, which is why most of them will use the subclavian vein for central lines.

Alert the medical chief of surgery. He has clout.

What's the procedure for checking blood return?

Q Is it necessary to routinely check for blood return in a central line? Some of my co-workers say yes, others say no. We'd like to hear an expert opinion.

A It's necessary to check for good blood return only when the central line is inserted and when blood is drawn. Routine checks aren't necessary; in fact, avoiding extra manipulation will cut down the chances of line-related infections.

Arrange for an X-ray when the line is inserted to confirm correct placement. And, of course, always observe the patient's chest or neck near the insertion site for swelling, discomfort, and redness.

Chart access

How can a nurse keep an administrator from reading his fiancée's chart?

Q One of our hospital administrators is engaged to a patient on our medical/surgical unit. He visits her every day, brings flowers, and has stopped by our desk on his way out to say jokingly, "Take good care of the mother of my future children."

Yesterday, he came onto the unit when we were all away from the nurses' station. From the corridor, my co-worker and I saw him slip

behind our desk and read his fiancée's chart—without anyone's permission. We couldn't believe his boldness, but we didn't stop him. Instead, we asked the patient if she'd given anyone permission to read her chart. She said no, so we told our charge nurse, and she called the supervisor, who told her not to rock the boat.

What would you do?

A Make waves. Reading the patient's chart without permission is an invasion of her privacy. And, while hospitalized, only she can legally give permission for someone not directly involved in her care to read her chart. This includes her fiancé—whether he's an administrator or chairman of the board. (Of course, if she were unconscious or incompetent and he were her legal guardian, he could see the chart.)

Now that you know the administrator's tactics, be ready for him. Before his next sneak attack, ask the patient if she wants him to read her chart. If she says no, then you'll have to play a David versus Goliath. Make sure you're armed with a written policy on who can review a patient's chart. Clearly one is needed.

If a nurse-patient is allowed complete access to her chart, won't other patients request the same privilege?

Q Whenever a nurse from our own staff is admitted as a patient to our medical/surgical unit, we extend her the VIP treatment she deserves. Recently, however, one nurse-patient requested that her chart and Kardex be kept in her room "for confidential reasons." The administrator okayed this move, which meant that everyone assigned to her had to borrow the records when they needed them.

With all respect to confidentiality, this arrangement seems unprofessional, if not illegal, to me. If we allow this patient complete access to her chart, what's to stop other patients from requesting the same privilege?

I'd be interested in your comments. Personally, if I wanted to restrict information about my hospitalization, I'd go to another facility where nobody knows me.

A Join the crowd. One survey showed that many nurses would choose not to be a patient at the hospital where they work. To your hospital's credit, this nurse-patient felt differently. Still, you can't blame her for protecting her privacy. And if the attending doctor and administration okayed the rooming-in privileges for her records, what's the big deal?

Be prepared for more and more patients (consumers) exercising their right—guaranteed by law in some states—to see their charts and be clear about what's written. True, the hospital may own the physical record itself, but the patient (who's paying) owns the information.

Should the chart be made available to the patient or not?

Q When I was in school, we were taught that a patient's chart is available to him upon request after discharge from the hospital. After all, it's his chart. Now, I'm told I'm wrong. Will you please set this straight? Must the chart be made available to the patient or not?

A The hospital owns the hospital medical records, and the doctor owns his office records, according to court decisions. Generally, the courts have decided that a patient sees a doctor for diagnosis and treatment, not to obtain records for his personal use.

The second issue the courts had to resolve involved access. While granting ownership of medical records to doctors and hospitals, the courts have expressed their own right to get the records anytime they need them for case review.

For this reason, any patient in any state can file a lawsuit to subpoena his medical records. But some court decisions and some states' laws have given patients the right to direct access. Nine state laws guarantee a patient's right to his medical information. And in states without such laws, the courts have recognized a patient's right to see this information.

In *Cannel v. Medical and Surgical Clinic S.C.* (1974), the court ruled that a doctor had the duty to disclose medical information to his patient. However, the court said doctors and hospitals needn't turn over the actual files to the patient. Instead, they need only show the complete medical record—or a copy—to the patient.

Charts

Is borrowing a page from a chart over a weekend so bad?

Q With only 1 week left of my assignment as a traveling nurse, I ran into a problem with a co-worker on the next shift. She told me a patient complained that I took her call light away during the night and shouted at her. I admitted I was exasperated and probably abrupt, but that was all—no big deal. Later, I found out she charted just what the patient said anyway.

The entry she wrote started a new sheet. I wanted the supervisor's advice on this, so because it was the weekend, I removed the page from the chart, intending to keep it with me until the supervisor came in on Monday. On Saturday night, the director of nursing knocked on my

door, demanded that I hand over the page, then fired me on the spot without giving me a chance to explain.

Is borrowing a page from a chart over a weekend so bad?

A Bad? Maybe. Dumb, yes. The medical chart, which is hospital property, is a legal document. You destroy its integrity by erasing, backdating, tampering with, removing, or throwing away anything written in it.

Faced with the circumstances, you might have telephoned the supervisor and asked for the proper form to document your version of the incident in the patient's chart. And while we're discussing proper procedure, we're less than impressed with a director of nursing who would fire someone without discussion. But all that is Monday-morning quarterbacking.

By now, you've probably started your next assignment. At least write a documented note of explanation to the director of nursing and ask that it be placed in your personnel file.

Chemotherapy

How often should someone handling chemotherapeutic drugs have physical examinations?

Q As an oncology nurse in a large community hospital, my duties include preparing and administering drugs used in cancer chemotherapy.

Although I'm very careful about using proper technique, I'm worried that daily exposure to these drugs over a number of years will eventually affect me.

How often should someone handling chemotherapeutic drugs have physical examinations? Could physiologic changes caused by exposure to these drugs be detected during a routine medical examination?

A Medical checkups are always a good idea. But don't count on them to detect physiologic changes caused by handling chemotherapeutic drugs—at least not at the present time.

Small wonder that you and other nurses handling chemotherapeutic drugs feel anxious about long-term risks. The Oncology Nursing Society (ONS), provides the following information and guidelines in their publication *Safe Handling of Cytotoxic Drugs:*
• Employers must inform employees about the potential hazards of exposure to cytotoxic agents.
• Employee health departments should keep a current list of employees who are routinely involved in handling cytotoxic drugs or waste.
• Employees who are pregnant, breast-feeding, or trying to conceive should follow previously identified procedures for maximum protection.

You can write to the ONS at 1016 Greentree Road, Pittsburgh, PA 15220-3125 or call them at (412) 921-7373 for a copy of *Safe Handling of Cytotoxic Drugs.*

Should administering it be a nursing responsibility?

Q I recently accepted a position as an oncology nurse. My duties on the new job include preparing and administering drugs used in cancer chemotherapy. To be properly qualified to do this, I attended special classes on chemotherapy.

But now I'm wondering whether administering these drugs should be nursing responsibilities? I'm also worried about the possible dangers involved in working with these drugs. Have I got good reason to worry?

A Taking your first question first: Administering chemotherapeutic drugs is a legitimate nursing responsibility as long as you've been properly prepared. You certainly seem to qualify on that score.

But now for your question about any possible dangers: You have grounds for worrying. Preparing these drugs does have potential risks.

You probably know about the risk of skin irritation from direct contact with one of these drugs—but you can easily avoid this danger by wearing gloves or taking precautions to protect other areas of your body that are exposed. But did you know that some of these drugs are dispersed into a fine mist (atomized) during preparation? This can happen when you transfer a chemotherapeutic drug from the vial to the syringe, or when you expel air from a filled syringe. Invisible droplets of the drug enter the atmosphere and can be inhaled by the preparer.

The greatest danger here is chromosomal damage from long-term inhalation of chemotherapeutic drugs in their atomized form.

The best way to protect yourself, according to the latest studies, is to prepare these drugs in a Class II biologic safety cabinet (also known as a vertical hood). Note that a standard laminar air flow hood (also known as a horizontal hood) offers no protection; it just circulates the drug droplets toward the preparer. A Class II hood, on the other hand, provides a noncircular vertical air flow, which prevents the droplets from reaching the mouth or nose of the preparer. The hood usually comes with a glass barrier, which gives the additional protection of separating the preparer from the drug.

Certainly other nurses out there are asking the same questions you've asked. Thank you for bringing up this important subject.

Should ED nurses be expected to administer chemotherapy?

Q I work in a fairly busy emergency department (ED) averaging about 30 patients every shift. Two oncologists recently joined the hospital staff, and both of them brought several chemotherapy patients to our facility. Administration decided that we ED nurses will handle the chemotherapy for these patients plus take care of our own patients. All without extra staff, of course. Already an ED patient had to wait while we administered chemotherapy. Worse still, we nurses have little experience in handling these drugs and no written policies or procedures.

Granted, ED nurses deal with a wide variety of medical problems—but this is getting ridiculous. Don't you agree?

A Like 100%. Administering chemotherapy is not a recognized role in the core curriculum for ED nurses. Chemotherapy treatments are usually given in an outpatient setting by specially prepared staff.

If you're stuck with this assignment—even temporarily— here's what you need: written protocols on the drugs themselves with easy-to-use drug charts; written protocols on patient management; written policy on ED priorities—the needs of the oncology patient versus the needs of a routine ED patient. And here's the big one: staff-development programs on administering chemotherapy. These drugs are dangerous to both patients and staff.

Additionally, only a specific few ED nurses, possibly volunteers, should be prepared and assigned to administer chemotherapy drugs during certain hours on the day shift (when on-call help is easily available from oncologists, pharmacists, and oncology nurse specialists). Establish wide-open lines of communication with administration, and provide continual feedback on your professional and personal concerns.

Shouldn't knowing the current bone marrow status be routine during chemotherapy?

Q On the oncology unit where I work, we have patients coming in for "day care" (about 8 hours). Frequently, one of the oncologists orders chemotherapy without ordering a hemogram (white blood cell count and platelets). When we ask him about the lab work, he either says that the patient was in the hospital several weeks earlier and the blood picture was okay, or that the blood work was done in his office a day or so before and it's safe to administer the drugs.

We don't feel comfortable infusing the drugs without knowing the current bone marrow status— especially for outpatients who will be discharged in a few hours. We've tried telephoning the doctor's office for the lab results (he doesn't like this at all). But between busy signals or people out to lunch, too much time is taken away from the little we have to accomplish our work.

Why do we have so much trouble getting the information we need?

A Sounds like a classic case of tunnel vision. The doctor sees only his responsibility for his patient; he's obviously lost sight of what you need for your nursing assessment and documentation.

Why hassle over a procedure that should be routine? Ask administration for a written policy spelling out that either lab work for outpatients should be done on the unit before the chemotherapy is administered or the results of previous lab work must accompany the chemotherapy order.

Time's a wastin'—and it's yours.

What should be done when a supervisor orders administration in violation of hospital policy?

Q I'm a new nursing graduate, working the night shift on an oncology unit. Maybe because this is my first nursing job, I've read the hospital's policy manual carefully and I try to follow instructions. But not everybody does the same.

According to our hospital's written policy, only trained (certified) chemotherapy nurses may hang (or give as an intravenous push) any chemotherapeutic drug. This regulation also stipulates that if a chemotherapy nurse isn't available, the attending doctor must administer the drug himself.

The policy couldn't be more clear. But on our floor, when a chemotherapy nurse isn't available, uncertified nurses *do* hang 5-fluorouracil (5-FU).

I checked with my supervisor about this practice, and she took out her policy manual. Sure enough, it said that only chemotherapy nurses may hang or push chemotherapeutic drugs.

My supervisor's stand was: "Look—everyone else hangs 5-FU. It's not a potent chemotherapeutic drug and won't cause damage if it should infiltrate. If we don't have a chemotherapy nurse available, the attending doctor isn't about to come in to hang a bottle of 5-FU at midnight."

She was telling me, without using the words, to hang the drug if I had to—despite what the manual said.

What should I do now? If I follow my supervisor's advice and I run into trouble, will my malpractice insurance protect me?

A You're in a precarious position—and you're right to be concerned. If a written hospital policy says one thing and a nurse does another, she has no excuse. She's legally liable for any trouble that may arise. Nurses have been sued

for administering a drug improperly. What's more, if a nurse is acting contrary to hospital policy, she's not acting as an agent of the hospital. Therefore, the hospital's insurance doesn't have to cover her.

If you're going to correct this situation, you'll have to document and report all the facts. Then take your documentation through channels to the top and to the hospital's policy committee.

To alert other nurses to the problem, urge your supervisors to hold a staff development program on hospital policies; that'll be your opportunity to discuss who originates policy and what happens in cases of noncompliance.

As a new nurse and a new employee questioning an entrenched hospital practice, you'll feel very alone and very uncomfortable. But someone has to question the practice before a patient is injured.

Where can nurses get information on protection from chemotherapy?

Q On our unit, we administer chemotherapy to cancer patients. Because exposure to these drugs can be hazardous to us, we wear gloves to prevent contact with the patients' body secretions and use specially labeled waste bags for their trash.

My concern is that we simply flush the feces, urine, vomitus, and saliva of these patients down either the toilet or sink. And we send their sheets for regular laundering with the other linens. No one around here seems to know whether we're following safe practices. Where can I get information on this?

A Flushing excreta, vomitus, or other body fluids (such as blood or cerebrospinal fluid) down the toilet or sink is currently accepted practice. For your protection, wear latex gloves during this procedure. The committee also recommends that disposable pads or sheets be used for patients who are incontinent or likely to vomit. The nondisposable sheets you're using require special attention. When contaminated, they should be placed in a specially marked impervious bag and laundered according to procedures used for other contaminated linens.

You can get a copy of *Safe Handling of Cytotoxic Drugs* from the Oncology Nursing Society, 1016 Greentree Road, Pittsburgh, PA 15220-3125 or by calling them at (412) 921-7373.

Chicken pox

Is it really necessary to "air" the showers for at least 8 hours?

Q In the college infirmary where I work, we assign students with varicella (chicken pox) to a separate room. But because we have limited facilities, all patients must use the same shower stalls.

A co-worker insists that for infection control the showers must "air" for at least 8 hours after the patients with chicken pox use them (which means they have to wait until everyone else is finished). The calamine lotion we apply for itching can be a terrible irritant, especially bothersome when the patients must wait to shower for relief.

Is it really necessary to "air" the showers that long?

A A spokesperson at the Centers for Disease Control says "airing" doesn't really do anything. Instead, disinfect the showers after the patients with chicken pox use them.

You might also try using something less irritating than calamine lotion, such as a paste of baking soda and water, Burow's solution compresses (two to four times a day

for 15 to 30 minutes), or wet compresses with isotonic saline or tap water. If these measures don't relieve the itching, the doctor may order a 0.5% hydrocortisone cream.

Child abuse

Could a parent sue if the nurse wrongly accused her?

Q Yesterday, a woman brought her 18-month-old son to the emergency department because she couldn't wake him up. She said she'd rubbed whiskey on his gums because he was teething. As I undressed him, I noticed faint bruises on his legs and hips. When I asked his mother about them, all she said was, "He falls a lot."

A toxicology screening showed that the boy had a negligible blood alcohol level. By then, a few hours had passed and he was more alert. So I warned the mother against giving the boy alcohol and sent them home.

> *"I suspect that the mother had deliberately given the boy more than a little alcohol to quiet him."*

I'm still uneasy about the incident. I suspect that the mother had deliberately given the boy more than a little alcohol to quiet him. Maybe she or someone else in the household was beating him, too. But I didn't report my suspicions because the evidence was inconclusive.

If I'd reported this case and had been wrong, would the mother have had grounds to sue me?

A You should always call local authorities when you have reasonable evidence—conclusive or not—of child abuse. In fact, you could be fined for failing to report your suspicions. As a matter of pub-

lic policy, health care professionals are immune from lawsuits brought by parents wrongfully accused of child abuse.

Did you have reasonable evidence in this case? Yes. The mother's explanation for the bruising was unconvincing. Her story about anesthetizing the gums was questionable, too—an 18-month-old child should already have most of his primary teeth. Certainly the boy's sedated condition was consistent with significant alcohol ingestion.

In the future, follow these guidelines:
• Request toxicology studies on the blood and urine of any child you suspect has ingested drugs or alcohol, as you did this time.
• Ask the doctor to order a total body X-ray to check for recent and healed fractures.
• Obtain an order for a blood coagulation study if the child has severe bruises, to rule out a bleeding disorder.

You have a legal and ethical duty to protect the victims of child abuse. Contact local authorities whenever you suspect abuse.

How should a nurse handle a suspected case of it?

Q One night, a 12-year-old girl and her mother came into the emergency department (ED). The girl was sobbing and holding a wet washcloth to a large hematoma on her right lower jaw. The mother explained that the girl had been fighting with her 11-year-old brother, but I thought the injuries looked rather severe for a brother-sister squabble.

Before I could examine the patient thoroughly, the doctor arrived and the mother repeated her story. After palpating the bruised area and giving the girl an injection, the doctor discharged her.

To me, there was something suspicious about the case. I feared the girl was a child-abuse victim. So I called the doctor at home and told him how I felt. *He* didn't think it was child abuse but promised to "look into the matter and notify the authorities if necessary."

Because *my* name was on the record, I felt I should protect myself, so I wrote "Dr. Smith assuming responsibility for notifying proper authorities." Then I signed my initials.

The next day, I was reprimanded by the assistant administrator of our hospital. The doctor had called him and claimed that my written comments left him, the doctor, "wide open for a lawsuit."

A "Yes" to the first question. "No" to the other two. All states have laws requiring doctors and nurses to report suspected child abuse. In fact, you're *breaking* the law in some states if you *don't* report such cases. (In many states there are forms on hand for this purpose.)

Sounds as though your hospital needs a written policy stating who's responsible for reporting suspected child abuse. But until such a policy's written, you'll have to continue protecting yourself by making notations on the chart.

One last thought—next time you care for a child you suspect has been abused, try to examine her more thoroughly. Tell her mother (or whoever's with her) that you'd like the child to be alone for a brief period so she can rest and calm down. Then you can check the child more carefully. Even if you don't find anything suspicious, you'll be able to record the condition more accurately.

Childbirth

How can a nurse protect a patient from being pressured?

Q Recently, one of our obstetricians was in a hurry to leave the hospital, so he urged a woman to take drugs to speed up her de-livery. I was shocked when she finally agreed, because she was prepared for natural childbirth. Later, she was angry that she'd given in. How can I prevent something like this from happening again?

A You can protect a patient when she's being pressured by taking the following steps:
• Carefully document her requests, prior health education and preparation (such as natural childbirth), expectations, and objections to any procedures.
• Relay her objections to the doctor. Explain, for example, that she's prepared for natural childbirth and is opposed to using drugs. Ask him if he has explained why he wants to prescribe drugs, then document your conversation.
• Show your patient a copy of the American Hospital Association's Patient's Bill of Rights, and remind her that she has the right to refuse the drugs (and to be informed of the medical consequences of her decision).
• Inform the doctor of your own objections, and document that conversation.

If you're sure that your patient's treatment had no medical justification, you and your manager may want to take the case to the hospital's ethics committee.

How dangerous is applying fundal pressure?

Q I'm a nursery nurse in a small hospital. Occasionally, when I'm called to the delivery room to care for newborns, I'll be present during deliveries. Several times I've heard one of the obstetricians tell the delivery room nurses to apply fundal pressure when he wasn't satisfied with the patient's pushing.

I was shocked when I saw a nurse climb right up onto the delivery ta-ble and use the full weight of her body to help force the baby out.

I realize fundal pressure may sometimes be called for. But in the case I observed, the fetus wasn't in distress and the labor hadn't been overly long.

> *"I was shocked when I saw a nurse climb right up onto the delivery table and use the full weight of her body to force the baby out."*

Doesn't this practice seem excessive—and potentially dangerous?

I'm especially concerned about all this because I'm expecting my first baby in 6 months—and the obstetrician I'm talking about is my doctor.

A The scene you described sounds like the stuff childbirth nightmares are made of. The patient must have been horrified to have a nurse climb onto the delivery table.

Gentle fundal pressure is certainly used safely in labor and delivery. And even the extreme pressure you described may be called for in an emergency situation. But it shouldn't be used as a routine procedure to hurry along delivery or to compensate for poor coaching or pushing techniques.

To remedy the pushing problem, join with other nurses who share your concern, and prepare a documented memo on what you've all observed. Send the memo up through nursing channels so nursing administration can take up the matter with the medical staff.

And for your own state of mind, talk with your doctor about your anxiety. Don't wait until you're on the delivery table—when you should have confidence in your doctor.

What can be done about medical residents who force patients to deliver naturally?

C

Q The family-practice residents at our hospital are so sold on natural childbirth that they're convinced a mother and child can bond effectively only if the mother has a natural delivery.

For patients who want natural childbirth (and who've taken the necessary childbirth courses), this is fine. But what about the patients who come into the hospital thinking they'll get a saddle block and who are 8 cm dilated when the resident tells them they'll "go natural"?

These patients—many with low incomes and little education—usually haven't taken the preparatory childbirth classes. When they suddenly face enforced natural childbirth, they object—loudly. They become so uncooperative that sometimes they literally have to be held down during the delivery.

I don't want to assist at such deliveries. Do you blame me?

A If you're giving all the facts, you can't be blamed for being angry and upset with the situation you describe. These residents are turning the childbirth experience into a nightmare for the patients, whose rights are being abused—and for you, forced to take part in these deliveries. These residents are badly informed.

A maternal-child health specialist advises: "A saddle block numbs the mother from the waist down—not from the waist up. The mother's fully alert (she just can't feel her toes) when her child is born and able to handle her new infant.

"What a crime," she says "that these patients are being denied the delivery of their choice. Besides, this practice could result in a lawsuit—since patients' rights are being abused and refused." She suggests that the hospital take immediate steps to correct the situa-

tion—before a judge makes the hospital take steps.

As the nurse in the situation, you can't change things singlehandedly. Go to your nurse-manager and then to the director of nursing for administrative support.

But you can also take the following steps:
1. Find out who's telling these residents that a mother can properly bond to her infant only when she's had no anesthesia.
2. Get several copies of the Pregnant Patient's Bill of Rights (available from International Childbirth Education Association, Dept. N81, P.O. Box 1900, New York, NY 10001) and show item number 7 to the residents involved (this paragraph clearly says that the patient has the right to decide whether she wants a procedure).
3. Persuade the residents to look through a copy of *Parent-Infant Bonding,* by Marshall H. Klaus, and John H. Kennell (2nd ed. St. Louis: C.V. Mosby Co., 1982). This book spells out the bonding process and will clarify any misinterpretation residents may have.
4. Check on whether your delivery room's policy and procedure manual is up to date—and whether the residents have ever read it.

When your patients come from a low-income group and are neither well educated nor well informed, they have a great need for your services and your genuine concern. Your role as their advocate can make a difficult experience easier for them. And you'll find a deep satisfaction in protecting these patients and their rights.

Cleaning

How should a mortar and pestle be cleaned?

Q How should a mortar and pestle be cleaned? Where I work, some people wipe both with an alcohol sponge; others rinse them with water.

A There are three types of mortar and pestle available: ceramic, porcelain, and glass. Wiping with an alcohol sponge isn't good enough to clean any of them.

Glass is nonporous, so thoroughly rinsing in water is probably okay. But both ceramic and porcelain may be porous, so these types should always be washed with soap and water first, then thoroughly rinsed. The point, of course, is to prevent contamination by any drug previously mixed in the mortar and pestle.

Clinical experience

How much is enough for an AD program?

Q I just finished my third term in an associate degree nursing program. And although I'm not an A student, I devoted a lot of time to my studies and maintained a respectable average. My main worry is that my clinical practice at school (twice a week) isn't enough. Currently, I work as a part-time sales-clerk to earn spending money. I was thinking of quitting and working as a nursing assistant in a nursing home to get more clinical experience, but only full shifts on weekends are available. And some friends who have jobs like this say they're usually too exhausted to open a book.

My nursing professors say to stop worrying—that I'm getting enough clinical experience and I shouldn't squander my energy and jeopardize my marks.

I'd appreciate your views.

A Listen to your teachers: School is your top priority. What good will extra clinical practice do if you flunk your courses?

Look into job options you can handle. For instance, a job as unit secretary would help you learn the inside ropes at a hospital. The pace is fast, but the physical demands wouldn't be exhausting. Or if you'd rather work as a nursing assistant, apply at hospitals. They're usually better staffed than nursing homes, so flexible, part-time hours might be possible. If you're still concerned about your clinical skills when you graduate, look for a job at a hospital with a strong internship program.

For now, stop worrying about the future and concentrate on your studies. That's good use of your time.

Code

How can a nurse be more confident during a code?

Q Since I passed my boards 4 months ago, I've been working the night shift on the intensive care unit. Two months ago I was made charge nurse, and only now am I beginning to feel comfortable in that role. Last week my nurse-manager told me I'd been "elected" to the code team that responds to cardiac and respiratory arrests within the hospital. I protested all up the line and got nowhere. "Someone has to do it. You'll do fine," my nurse-manager told me. Fine? With a half-hour training session? Every time I sleep, I dream that I'm freezing up in a code situation. What do you think about this, and what can I do?

A Stop worrying that you'll freeze. Nurses are instinctively action-oriented; when the demand arises, we guarantee you'll act. The nightmare here is just how well you'll act. A half-hour's training is demonstrably inadequate—and code time is certainly no time to be learning. Added to that, you'll probably be the code leader until the doctor arrives.

Please spare yourself more bad dreams. Pressure administration in

writing (and keep copies for yourself) for proper training. You should have:

• basic life support and advanced cardiac life support certification
• protocols to use until the doctor arrives
• special preparation sessions.

If you're not experienced at starting I.V.s, go to the operating room, where you can practice under an anesthesiologist's supervision. Review defibrillation skills, and familiarize yourself with the medications on the crash cart. And remember, this kind of orientation is periodic, not a onetime thing.

So back to the pressure—pressure on administration, that is. With the appropriate training and experience, you'll do just fine.

How can nurses protect themselves from AIDS?

Q According to hospital policy where I work, the nurse calling a code gives mouth-to-mouth resuscitation until the crash cart arrives. These days, with identified (and possibly some unidentified) acquired immunodeficiency syndrome (AIDS) patients on our medical/surgical unit, I'm very hesitant about resuscitating a patient without a manual resuscitation bag or some protection. Yet these supplies aren't always available.

At a recent staff meeting, we discussed ordering more bags or resuscitation masks. But our unit is on a profit-sharing plan, and the majority vetoed spending extra money on these devices.

I'm a single parent, so perhaps I'm more worried about keeping myself healthy for my young daughter's sake. What can I do?

A There's nothing wrong with your wanting to stay healthy for your child's sake.

There is something you can do: You can buy a simple oral airway

with a nonreturn valve for less than $20. A local drugstore or your hospital's central supply department should carry this product. Just slip the airway into your pocket so it's available for an emergency. And breathe easier.

Code yellow

Should a male nurse be expected to respond along with security guards and orderlies?

Q Last night, we had a code yellow at the hospital where I work. A code yellow summons help when disoriented patients, unruly visitors, or hostile intruders threaten the safety of other patients or staff. Because our hospital's in a populous (albeit seedy) tourist area, we see more than our share of all three.

As a male, I'm expected to respond to the code with the security guards and orderlies. Last night I didn't and was read the riot act by my supervisor. I asked her who would take care of my 12 patients while I was out doing battle? Our other nurses (females) all had full assignments too. As far as I'm concerned, I'm employed as a nurse and should be valued for my nursing skills, not my muscle mass.

I'd hate to lose my job or, far more than that, my license because of code yellow. What do you say?

A Bravo for you. No matter what administration calls it—code yellow, mauve, or cerise—quelling disturbances is a security enforcement problem and not a nursing responsibility. You're not hired, prepared, insured, or compensated to perform defense or attack activities. (In fact, even for code blue, only designated nurses respond, never anyone whose patients won't be covered in the interim.)

Don't waste more words with your supervisor. Send a note to administration through channels (including the medical head of the department); ask for a stat review of code yellow. Any administrator worth his salt should realize that you're trying to avoid trouble, not start it. In this litigious climate, the hospital could wind up liable for injury to unattended patients, to bystanders, to you, or even to the attacker, when people untrained to handle security problems get involved.

College applicants

Should psychiatric patients be admitted into a community college program?

Q I teach a training course for nursing assistants and orderlies at a community college. Before being admitted, applicants must have an interview with me and take a personality test.

Here's the problem: last week, I interviewed two men who're currently under psychiatric care and are taking "heavy" medications. One applicant had been diagnosed as manic-depressive, and the other's an alcoholic who admits he's still drinking. Both showed "undesirable tendencies" on the personality test. But their psychiatrists felt it'd be "good therapy" for the men to work as orderlies.

But what about the patients? Will it be good therapy for *them*?

College administrators told me we *had* to admit these men, or we'd be risking a lawsuit for discrimination. We're more sympathetic than we may sound, but we're afraid of letting ourselves in for some serious problems.

Do we *have to* admit these students and their problems?

A You do, and then, you don't. You can't refuse admission to these applicants because they have psychiatric problems—that'd be discrimination. They could sue and win.

But you *can* refuse them admission if you truly feel they're not qualified to handle the responsibilities of the job. For instance, the Supreme Court recently upheld a nursing school's decision *not* to admit a deaf student, on the grounds that her disability would prevent her from meeting the job requirements.

If your college had more stringent screening criteria, you might not be in such a jam now. A personality test and an interview are not sufficient criteria for judging applicants. An interest and ability test would be more to the point.

But what's even more basic is the school's need for admission guidelines which clearly state that a person with a *current* problem of alcoholism or a serious emotional disturbance is not an acceptable candidate for the program.

Is there no place in the health care field for those with overwhelming problems of their own? How can they be therapeutic to others when they're in trouble themselves?

Even if you *have to* accept these applicants, don't panic. The problem will probably work itself out—although things may get worse before they get better. It wouldn't be surprising if your "problem" students were to be frequently absent from class, or to have difficulty getting along with co-workers and patients. If these students don't meet the accepted standards of performance during their training, you'll have grounds to dismiss them. (Document any incidents, and try to have a witness for the record.)

Throughout the training period, the door stays open for the students as well as the school. Each student has the right to leave the program at any time during the probationary period without explanation or damage to his personal file. And the school has the parallel privilege of dismissing any student during probation.

If the two students in question *do* get through the training without

dismissal, they'll probably have trouble finding jobs; their past records seem to promise future trouble for an employer.

College infirmary

How can a nurse make it more enjoyable to work there?

Q Last week a student complaining of mild abdominal pain came into our college infirmary. I telephoned the on-call doctor, and he said the patient should go directly to the hospital—30 miles (48 km) away. My supervisor vetoed calling an ambulance because the situation was not an emergency. So I tried (unsuccessfully) to get someone from campus security to drive. In the end, another student took the patient in his car.

As things turned out, they just about made it to the hospital's emergency department when the patient's appendix ruptured. Later, we were told that his father might sue us because no officially designated personnel had accompanied his son to the hospital.

I thought working in a college infirmary would be a piece of cake. Now I'm not so sure. What do you say about this?

A Every nursing job comes with its own set of problems. The small college infirmary harbors many legal hazards: So much rests on your assessment and what you report to the doctor. That's why you need written administrative policies to spell out the circumstances requiring an ambulance.

Consider following these guidelines:
• Call an ambulance if the student is in acute distress.
• Consider the distance to the hospital before ruling out the need for an ambulance, even for lesser complaints.
• Never drive or let patients' friends drive to the hospital. Have security

personnel (who should have basic first aid and cardiopulmonary resuscitation training) drive. When they're not available, call the local police.

• Check back with the doctor when you're not sure what to do, and document what he advises.

Nobody earns high marks without guidance and support—all the more reason why you need the doctor, security, and written policy to back you up.

What can be done about an understaffed service?

Q I'd like your opinion on a priority problem in the college health service where I work. I'm one of three nurses at the service, but at times, one of us could be on duty alone. Yet, we're expected to answer emergency calls on campus, *even if it means leaving patients in the health service unattended.*

The situation troubles me. We've been told that the emergency takes priority—that we *must* answer the emergency call, no matter how sick the students in the infirmary are.

If I'm the only nurse on duty, I might have to leave my sick patients in the care of a nonmedical person, or perhaps even without supervision of any kind while I'm responding to the emergency call. To make matters worse, many of the "emergencies" prove to be unwarranted. Calls will come from nonprofessionals—untrained people who panic all too easily.

If something happens to an unattended student while the only nurse on duty is called out on an emergency, what legal problems could arise? What if an infirmary patient were to fall out of bed or have a seizure? Could I be sued for *not* being there? And how about the students? They're admitted for our care and supervision. Should they be told beforehand that they'll be receiving something less than 24-hour care?

I feel trapped by my situation. What advice can you give me?

A Your dilemma and your concern are understandable. You must certainly use discretion before leaving your patients unattended in the infirmary to go out on emergency calls. Standard nursing practice holds that once a nurse has accepted responsibility for a patient's care, she *can't* leave the facility or the patient until someone else takes over. Although there's no *specific* law covering the situation you cite, standard nursing practice *is* the basis for many court decisions. In your predicament, get a job description and malpractice insurance.

In spite of this somewhat discouraging answer, here are some solutions to your problem:

1. Get campus security to bring in the emergency patient; or, if the case sounds severe enough, call an ambulance right away. Other possibilities: call the community paramedics or the local ambulance service. (The school will probably reimburse the service for picking up and delivering an emergency patient.)

2. Head off the situation in two ways *before* it happens. First, train the dormitory counselors in first aid and cardiopulmonary resuscitation. This training should be mandatory for the job and could eliminate some of the unnecessary hurry-up calls you receive. Second, very ill students shouldn't be in a health-service facility. They should be in a hospital or at home with their families.

3. Although you shouldn't leave your patients, if you *must* answer an emergency call on campus, why not use bed rails or other means to secure the infirmary patient you're anxious about?

4. Present the problem and your suggested solutions to your administration. Let them know what other colleges do in *their* campus emer-

gencies and ask for a revision of your policy—in writing. While you're at it, tell the administration you could use one more nurse.

Communication

Can you recommend an English-Spanish guide that's geared to medical personnel?

Q I work in the emergency department of a large metropolitan hospital. Lately, we're treating an increasing number of Spanish-speaking patients, many of whom understand no English whatsoever. Not being able to communicate with these patients really frustrates me; what I remember of my high school Spanish is very little help.

Can you recommend an English-Spanish guide that's geared to medical personnel?

A Chances are, you're communicating more caring than you realize. But to help you with your Spanish, try the expanded fourth edition of *Que Paso? An English-Spanish Guide for Medical Personnel,* by Martin P. Kantrowitz, et al. (Albuquerque, N.M.: University of New Mexico Press, 1984). You'll find vocabulary and terminology lists plus essential phrases and questions and answers that will help you to assess over 20 of the most common patient complaints. And because the authors want to retain the characteristic politeness of the Spanish language, they make a special point of emphasizing form instead of sticking with a literal translation.

¡Buena suerte!

Should a nurse give bad news over the phone against the doctor's wishes?

Q When one of my patients died of cancer recently, her doctor asked me to call her husband to the hospital so he wouldn't have to hear the news over the phone. As the doctor suggested, I told him that his wife had taken an unexpected turn for the worse and that he'd better hurry to the hospital if he wanted to see her alive. Now I feel bad about lying—especially because I'd grown so close to the patient and her family.

A Your concern is understandable. The patient had already died, so you created a false expectation by lying to her husband. Along with his grief, he may now have an extra burden of stress or guilt. For example, he may feel he let his wife down by not getting to the hospital in time to comfort her or to say good-bye.

In a situation like this, you could ask the doctor to make the call. Let him know that family members will have concerns that he'll need to address. Their safety, peace of mind, and ability to cope with a crisis should guide his decision about how much to tell them over the telephone.

If you contact a family member, start with what he already knows or expects. For example, you could say, "After you left, your wife slept until about 8 p.m. Then she started to have difficulty breathing and her blood pressure dropped. We didn't expect this, so I'm calling to ask if you'd like to come back to the hospital now." Pause and wait for questions. Then answer truthfully, and be prepared to give facts that will comfort him on his drive back to the hospital: "She didn't feel any pain," "I held her hand as she died," or "Her struggle with cancer is over now, as she wished."

Should the doctor have given bad news over the phone?

Q One of my patients, who was scheduled for a lung biopsy, had been worried about her condition. When I went in to administer her evening medication, I found her collapsed on the floor and in hysterics. After I calmed her down and helped her back into bed, I asked her what had happened. She said she'd just called her doctor, who told her that the chance of malignancy was 90% and that he'd probably have to remove her lung.

I don't think he should have given her information like that over the telephone. How should I handle a situation like this?

A Your patient has a right to information about her diagnosis and prognosis, so if the patient insisted, the doctor responded appropriately. The "how to" of sharing this type of information depends on many factors: how much time was available, the doctor's assessment of his patient's coping skills, and their relationship.

> *"I couldn't believe the doctor told his patient over the phone that the chance of malignancy was 90% and that he'd have to remove her lung."*

You responded well, too, by calming her and assessing the situation. Your letter doesn't indicate what steps you took after talking with her. Did you find out why she was on the floor? If she'd fallen, you'd need to fill out an incident report. Also, did you, another nurse, or the hospital chaplain stay with her to determine her risk for attempting suicide? You could have asked her if she wanted you to call in a family member to stay with her.

Finally, you should have notified her doctor of his patient's response to the phone call and of your nursing interventions. Naturally, you'd chart this information, including how you found the patient

and her emotional response to the news from her doctor.

Your patient needed more information than the doctor gave her, though. In the future, make sure patients understand that they have choices about their treatment. Otherwise, they can't give informed consent for surgery.

Compliance

What if a cultural difference affects potential compliance?

Q I've been working on a Navaho Indian reservation for about 2 months and I think I may be in over my head. Just the other day, I went to see a man who has heart disease. Although he understands that he's ill, he won't take his medication—he says it's against his religion. How can I convince him to comply with treatment?

A Without pressuring your patient, ask him to talk to you about his health, his use of medications, and his expectations for treatment. Look for cultural biases that may explain his resistance to medical treatment. In some American Indian cultures, for example, the person who tells the patient he has an illness is believed to be the one who gave it to him. For this reason, your patient may mistrust his doctor and think that taking medication prescribed by the doctor will worsen his disease.

After talking with your patient, consult a respected medicine man about the tribe's religious and cultural traditions and healing techniques. Your willingness to seek his advice will honor him and help you gain your patient's trust.

To head off noncompliance in the future, you might also consider sharing your patient care with the medicine man. Sometimes, a Navaho medicine man will agree to set up his hogan next to a hospital so patients can see both the nurse and the medicine man during their appointments. That helps patients understand the collaborative relationship.

Remember, your patient has the right to refuse treatment. Assure him that no matter what he chooses, you'll be available for him.

Computerization

Would computerized care plans be a good idea?

Q If our hospital computers are smart enough to streamline the work of billing, payroll, and medical records, why couldn't they help nurses write care plans? Getting this time-consuming task done more efficiently would be a real blessing for our busy 35-bed medical/surgical unit.

A The innovative nursing department at Long Island Jewish-Hillside Medical Center is using computers to develop nursing care plans on the unit. Nurses no longer have to write care plans in patient charts by hand, and the consistent entries make evaluating patient progress easier.

Computerized Nursing Care Planning—Utilizing Nursing Diagnosis—A Handbook by Joan M. Crosley, et al. (Washington, D.C.: Oryn Publications, Inc., 1985) details how the center's nursing task force modified IBM's Patient Care System (PCS) software package to develop its own computerized program. Other hospitals can adopt these easy-to-understand techniques using any computer equipment.

Now that diagnosis-related groups are here, your role in writing detailed patient care plans is more important than ever because you'll be documenting your contribution to efficient, cost-effective patient care.

Confidentiality

Can a drug-abusing nurse be helped by a colleague?

Q I've got quite a dilemma: A 28-year-old woman recently came to the emergency department where I work after an accidental overdose. She told me that she, too, is a nurse. Then she confessed that she has a drug-dependency problem. She also said that she works for three nursing pools, so she has easy access to drugs. I think she needs professional help, but I'm reluctant to betray a patient's confidence—or to turn in a fellow nurse. What should I do?

A By abusing drugs, this nurse is risking her health and her life. If she's practicing while impaired, she's also jeopardizing her patients. For those reasons, you're ethically bound to take action. Depending on the circumstances, that may mean breaking a confidence.

Contact the nurse and tell her that you want to help her. Explain that because you're concerned about her dangerous behavior, you can't promise to keep her secret if she refuses to get help. Then refer her to a drug hot line or a peer assistance group.

If she won't get help, inform a peer assistance program about her problem so people with expertise in drug problems can intervene. If they're successful, she may be able to enter a treatment program on her own before she's reported to the state nursing board. If peer assistance volunteers can't convince her to get treatment, they may report her to the state board, which could suspend or revoke her license.

Like a suicidal patient who says he plans to kill himself, this nurse is crying out for help. Don't turn away from her. Your intervention could help her take that important first step toward recovery.

Can a nurse release information about patients to other doctors' nurses?

Q As a nurse at a doctor's office, I'm frequently called by other doctors' nurses for information about patients who've been referred for treatment. I'm concerned about confidentiality. Should I be releasing this kind of information?

A Only if the patient has signed a form authorizing you to do so. Unless this form is in his medical record, he could argue that you and the doctor breached your duty of confidentiality.

The same is true of information requested by insurance companies. Most provide a standard release form. Make sure the patient has signed it before you give an insurance company any information about diagnoses or treatments.

How can a nurse get a doctor to inform his patient's family about his condition?

Q I'm frustrated by a patronizing doctor who won't give family members information about my patient's condition. I'm tempted to talk with them myself. I don't want to violate doctor-patient confidentiality, but I'm concerned about leaving them in the dark. What advice can you give me?

A You should start by assessing three things: what family members already know, what they want to know, and what the patient wants them to know. Remember, family members don't have an automatic right to confidential information about your patient. So you should keep quiet unless he allows you to discuss his condition.

You should also talk with the doctor about the situation. He may have

C

some information that will explain why he doesn't want to inform the patient's family. If a personality conflict is clouding your relationship with this doctor, talk with your manager. She may be able to help you approach the doctor for more fruitful discussions.

What if the patient can't speak for himself? Then you—or the doctor—could ethically discuss the diagnosis and prognosis directly with family members. They'd need this information to make informed decisions about aggressive versus palliative care and withholding or withdrawing treatment. If they seem uncomfortable, you might involve a chaplain or ethicist who could help them deal with whatever feelings are making them reluctant to become surrogate decision makers.

How can it be protected?

Q At the nursing home where I work, we occasionally receive detailed psychological records of patients. These records often contain intimate information.

Recently, a social worker, looking through the charts of a new admission, announced to the nursing assistants (within earshot of some residents) that we were getting a psychiatric patient. Immediately, there were complaints and wisecracks about "the nut case."

This violation of the patients' right to privacy concerns me deeply. Why can't we divide patients' charts into a general summary of pertinent information for everyone to use and a more detailed record that will be available for those who need this information?

What do you think of this idea?

A Your idea is excellent. The more detailed record you envision could be kept in a locked file with access on a "need to know" basis. This would substantially limit the number of people who share

confidential information. That's the easy part—the paperwork.

The harder part is the "people work"—changing the staff's attitude toward the patient's right to privacy. Surely, when a patient has so few comforts left, his rightful expectation of professional confidentiality should not be denied him.

The staff appears to need a staff development program on this, and you appear to be the person to run it. Think about this—it's not as hard as you might think.

One sourcebook is the second edition of *Privacy and Confidentiality of Health Care Information* by JoAnne C. Bruce (Chicago: American Hospital Publishing, Inc., 1988). As the author points out, "The health care institution's position on patient rights should be part of employee confidentiality training and should be included in a staff handbook on privacy protection."

Is filming in the hospital breeching confidentiality?

Q A few months ago, a local television station was doing a story on acquired immunodeficiency syndrome (AIDS). Our public relations director allowed a reporter and camera crew into the clinic to interview some of the nurses, doctors, and patients. They wanted shots of a doctor examining a patient and of a nurse counseling another patient. We convinced two patients to participate by promising them that the camera angle would disguise their identities.

Now one patient is suing us. He says he *is* recognizable, so he claims we breached our duty to keep his treatment confidential. What do you think?

A He's right. Implicit in your nurse-patient relationship is the assumption that you won't disclose confidential information about

his treatment—or even that you're treating him. Some patients simply don't want anyone to know that they *are* patients.

A court in New York supported that right in a similar case brought against a hospital, nurse, and doctor. An AIDS-infected man had been photographed for a newspaper article on AIDS research at the hospital. The nurse and doctor told him he'd be photographed from behind so no one could recognize him. But when the article appeared, he was clearly identifiable.

Ruling in his favor, the court said he hadn't consented to publication of a photograph in which he was recognizable. In fact, he hadn't even consented to having a reporter and photographer in the waiting room at the hospital. Just by being present, they violated his right to privacy.

Should an AIDS patient's diagnosis be told to his church?

Q We care for many acquired immunodeficiency syndrome (AIDS) patients at the outpatient clinic where I work, and we're very careful to keep our records confidential. So I was disappointed and angry to learn that a co-worker who attends the same church as one of our patients had disclosed the man's AIDS diagnosis to their minister and a few members of the congregation. Our patient is understandably hurt and embarrassed. What's more, he no longer seems to trust us.

My co-worker defends her actions by saying she wanted to make sure he'd have the prayers and support of the congregation as his disease progressed. I told her what she did was wrong. What do you think?

A In general, nurses shouldn't disclose a patient's diagnosis (or any other private information about him) to his friends, his employer, or his co-workers without his permission.

The only exception—and it doesn't apply to this situation—is when protecting the patient's privacy might endanger others. Before disclosing any information, though, you would have to consult with your manager, hospital chaplain, an ethicist, or the hospital's lawyer to decide on the best way to proceed.

Why do nurses violate patients' confidences? Some may use privileged information to gain power or to impress others. In this case, though, your co-worker probably had good intentions. She hoped that those who knew the patient's diagnosis would rally around him. Unfortunately, all she did was alienate the patient.

Should a nurse answer a state trooper's questions about a patient?

Q I work in a doctor's office. Recently, a young man with lacerations on his arms came to the office for treatment. He joked about running his truck into a lake after he'd had "one too many" at a party with some friends. Although he smelled of alcohol, I couldn't tell if he was intoxicated.

Later, a state trooper called the office and wanted the man's name, address, phone number, employer, and "other pertinent information." I told him what he wanted to know, but I didn't mention the alcohol smell or what the man had said to me.

Now I have two questions: First, should I have given the officer the information he asked for? Second, am I guilty of withholding evidence?

A You present a fascinating issue: Can you balance your desire to be a good citizen with your role as a health care professional? The answer is surprisingly direct—in a case like this, your professional responsibili-

ties come first. By giving out *any* information about this patient, you violated his right to privacy and confidentiality.

A person seeks medical care with the understanding that he'll be treated in confidence. Even the fact that he's been treated shouldn't be revealed. (Giving information about treatment to a third-party payer is an exception to this rule, but you'd do this only if you'd first obtained the patient's consent.)

You say you received a telephone call from a state trooper. How do you know the person really was a trooper? The call could have been from anyone. Even if the trooper had come to the office, you shouldn't have told him anything about the patient unless he presented a warrant for the information.

Should a nurse break confidentiality if an unborn baby's life is at stake?

Q I get to know the patients pretty well at the small obstetrics clinic where I work, and many of them confide in me. Last week, one pregnant woman told me she'd had an illegitimate baby when she was a teenager. Knowing she's Rh-negative, I asked her whether she'd received $Rh_0(D)$ immune globulin (RhoGAM). She said she didn't think so.

Now I'm worried about her unborn baby's health. But she refuses to let me tell anyone—including the doctor—for fear that her husband will find out about her first pregnancy. What should I do?

A For the sake of this woman and her unborn baby, the doctor must be informed about her history. Remember, you have a professional duty to safeguard *both* of your patients.

Speak to her again and explain why the doctor must know her secret. Reassure her that he'll protect

her privacy and that her medical records will remain confidential. Then invite her to go with you when you speak to the doctor.

Nobody likes breaking a confidence. But in this case, the patient probably wouldn't have confided in you if she didn't want you to help her. You can't do that by keeping quiet.

Should a nurse send a child's file to her father's lawyer?

Q I've just started working in a small clinic. A woman who brought her 3-year-old daughter in for treatment listed the child's father as the "financially responsible party." So we sent the bill to him (he lives in another state). A few days ago, we received a letter from a lawyer stating that the mother had run off with the child. He said he was representing the father, who was trying to locate his daughter. He demanded her address and all pertinent information from our files. The medical director of the clinic decided that we should send him the file. Is that the right way to handle this situation?

A This is a very difficult situation. By providing payer information to your clinic, the mother essentially authorized the release of information to a third party—but only upon the production of a duly signed authorization or release form. The medical director should have required a written request from the father and authorization from the mother prior to the release of information. Without these documents, the child's records shouldn't have been released.

Whenever the financially responsible party is in another state, a local address and phone number should be obtained from the custodial parent. This can help protect your clinic from fraud.

Should a nurse tell her friend about her boyfriend's syphilis?

Q My friend's boyfriend just came to the clinic where I work to be treated for syphilis. He hasn't listed my friend as one of his contacts, but I know she's at risk. Should I talk with her about this?

A You have two obligations here: to protect your friend's health and to maintain a patient's confidentiality. To meet them both, proceed carefully.

Talk to the patient first. If you spoke with your friend instead, you'd betray confidential information.

Discuss your dilemma with the patient and make sure you have the facts straight. Then ask him how he'd like you to handle the situation. Offer him two choices: to add your friend's name to his list of contacts or to have you discuss the situation with her.

If he rejects both options, ask your manager or the medical director of the clinic for guidance.

Should a nurse tell on a co-worker who has had three staphylococcus infections?

Q One of my co-workers confided to me that she's had three staphylococcus infections in the last 6 months. But she hasn't stayed home because she's already on probation for taking too many sick days. She says I'm the only person she's told.

I don't want to betray her confidence, but I'm afraid she's a health hazard. What should I do?

A Your concerns are well-founded, and you should act on them. Anyone who has recurrent staph infections could transmit the disease, even between flare-ups.

This nurse is endangering her immunocompromised and surgical patients.

Try to deal with the problem in private. Take your co-worker aside and encourage her to do two things: visit your employee health department or clinic for treatment, and confide in your manager. If she says she's afraid she'll lose her job, remind her that she's a serious health threat to her patients and co-workers.

What if she refuses to seek treatment or confide in your manager? Then the next move is yours. Tell her that for the patients' protection, you must inform your manager. If that statement doesn't get her moving, then follow through. But when she's faced with the choice of acting or having you act, she may take the initiative herself.

Your manager should understand her dilemma and encourage her to seek treatment without penalty. Until your co-worker is infection-free, your manager could assign her to duties that don't involve direct patient care.

Betraying your co-worker's confidence, if it comes to that, will be painful. But in this case, the patients' health must come first.

Should a nurse who was treated for an alcohol and drug overdose be reported?

Q I'm the supervisor of an emergency department (ED) in a rural hospital—the only hospital in a 45-mile radius. While reviewing charts last Saturday, I noticed that one of our LPNs had come into the ED during the night as an alcohol and drug overdose patient. She'd been given ipecac, lavaged, referred to the mental health clinic, and advised not to work that day. You can imagine my surprise when I saw her working on her unit, as if nothing had happened, only 6 hours after her discharge.

Torn between reporting her to administration (How could she take proper care of her patients?) and respecting her right to medical confidentiality, I chose not to report her—this time. But what if there's a next time?

A Your question's a toughie. Under ordinary circumstances, all patients have the right to medical confidentiality. However, in special circumstances like this, the employer-employee relationship alters the duty of confidentiality. Hospitals must deliver a reasonable standard of care for every patient; part of this duty includes providing competent personnel. Therefore, the employee-patient's right to confidentiality is superseded by the hospital's need to know what may affect safe and adequate care.

But you shouldn't be deciding when or whom to report. Ask administration for a written policy on this. To ensure safe patient care, emergency treatment of any staff member for substance abuse should be reported to administration. And the employee should be offered an appropriate course of treatment and follow-up care without fear of dismissal. This policy should apply equally to all hospital employees, from the housekeeping staff right up to the chief of the medical staff.

Should the nurses have revealed so much about a patient who was recently charged with murder?

Q A former nursing home patient was recently charged with murder, and our local paper published several interviews with nurses who had known him in the home. The articles gave the nurses' names and quoted them directly.

These nurses gave very personal information about their patient, which I considered a breach of professional confidentiality. I was so upset that I called the newspaper editor and asked him about the ethics of publishing the interviews. He said that the nurses interviewed no longer worked at the home, so they were free to say whatever they wished. Is this true? Does confidentiality end with the job? Aren't all health employees bound by confidentiality? What's being taught in nursing schools today?

A Nursing schools are still teaching what you learned: that no nurse is free to reveal information learned in connection with patient care without the patient's permission. Both the nurses and the editor were wrong in thinking that this responsibility ends when the patient is discharged or the nurse changes her job.

Unfortunately, some professionals, including nurses, do reveal confidential information. But they never do so ethically when professional confidences are concerned.

Was it improper to give an insurance representative information?

Q Recently, I received a call from an insurance company representative who said he needed information about one of my patients for billing purposes. He said the patient's doctor had suggested he call our unit for the information. I answered questions about the patient's medications, treatments, and physical therapy, thinking I was following the doctor's wishes.

Can you imagine how I felt when, later that day, the patient summoned me to her room. She was furious—and so, she said, was her doctor. It turns out that he hadn't instructed the insurance representative to call the unit. Using the information I supplied, the representative called to notify her that his company could not justify payment for any further hospitalization.

What do you think about this?

A What a bummer. Sounds like you were finessed by a fast-talking insurance investigator who's expert at getting this type of information. In the future, you'll remember to never, never give out patient information to anyone who's not directly responsible for the patient's care. All requests like this should be routed to the financial office, period.

Discussing confidential information with a third party can also get you into legal trouble: It's a breach of confidence and a violation of the patient's privacy.

While you can't get much consolation from this answer, you're reminding other nurses to watch what they say—and to whom.

Consent

Are nurses allowed to obtain it?

Q I'm a part-time RN in the intensive care unit of a small community hospital. A recent incident put me in disfavor with one of the staff surgeons and resulted in an uncomfortable working relationship between us.

Here's what happened. After giving report at 3 p.m., the charge nurse told me to obtain a consent-to-operate signature from a patient scheduled for a cholecystectomy at 7:30 the following morning.

> *"The surgeon became upset, demanded my name, and insisted I'd better get the consent signed or else."*

I'd always understood that nurses in this hospital couldn't obtain the necessary consent from the patient. The other nurses agreed with me. Both the nursing supervisor and the chief of staff said I was correct. I found the final verification in the hospital's policy manual.

I then called the surgeon and explained why I couldn't obtain the consent. I suggested he get the necessary signature in the morning before the operation. The surgeon told me: "You'd better get that consent signed," and threatened to call the hospital administrator.

A short time later, the surgeon called back to say he'd spoken to the administrator and to ask if I'd gotten that signature yet. I said I hadn't, and that legally I couldn't obtain it even with the administrator's approval.

The surgeon became even more upset, demanded my name, and insisted I'd better get that signature or else.

I told the supervisor, who called the director of nursing, who called the administrator. The upshot was that the patient signed the consent form in the surgeon's presence, after the surgeon had explained the operation to her. Her operation took place as scheduled.

Obviously, this incident caused a lot of unnecessary, unfortunate commotion for all concerned. I think I followed safe, legal practice, but how can I prevent another such incident?

A Congratulations for standing firm in a situation where other nurses might have backed down. You acted properly and professionally, but the experience must have been disturbing and disruptive.

How can you protect yourself and forestall further incidents? Try submitting a written report of the incident to your director of nursing and then request that a copy be placed in your personnel file. (Keep a copy for yourself.)

The director of nursing has to get the word to the doctors that her staff nurses must follow hospital policy—not whatever arbitrary directions a doctor may issue.

You acted professionally in this incident; your co-workers would be wise to follow your example in similar situations. You deserve a pat on the back.

C

C

Can a homosexual lover give consent?

Q Like most nurses in the New York metropolitan area, we see a lot of acquired immunodeficiency syndrome patients. Among other issues, we're concerned about consent for treatment when the patient is incompetent. Recently, a gay patient's lover of 5 years insisted that he had the right to sign the consent form because he was the patient's only family. Most of the nurses agreed—we've seen this happen so many times before. But the doctor and hospital administrator wouldn't allow him to sign. Now we're wondering: Does a patient's live-in lover have the same rights as a family member? Can he give consent for treatment?

A No—not unless the patient signed a durable power of attorney for health care designating him the surrogate decision maker. Otherwise, only a relative (spouse, parent, or sibling, for example) or a court-appointed guardian can give consent for treatment or for withholding treatment. When the patient has no family, not even a friend of many years can legally dictate medical or nursing actions.

When you're caring for a patient who hasn't designated a surrogate decision maker, try to find out who his next of kin is. If he says he doesn't have a family, you could suggest that he consider granting durable power of attorney to someone he trusts—such as his lover.

Can a live-in partner legally authorize emergency treatment?

Q I recently attended a seminar on legal problems in nursing, sponsored by a local medical college. An emergency department (ED) nurse raised an interesting

question: Citing the growing number of men and women living together, she wondered if one of the live-in partners could legally authorize emergency treatment for the other.

The ED nurse presented a hypothetical situation: A young woman requiring an emergency appendectomy is brought to the ED by her live-in partner. The admitting doctor wants her to have surgery immediately.

Can her partner legally authorize this emergency treatment? We all aired our opinions on this question, but no one could come up with a definitive answer.

After the seminar, we were all still talking about the question. We wondered: What do you say?

A This question can't be answered with a simple yes or no.

The law governing consent to treatment involves the *patient's* consent. In other words, no one but the patient himself can legally consent to treatment. The exceptions to this law apply to patients not of sound mind and to children who haven't reached their majority. There's also an exception in the case of a true emergency.

The law defines a true emergency as a situation where the patient may die or suffer permanent bodily harm. In this case, consent is *implied,* and therefore, treatment can be started without waiting for consent from anyone involved.

In the case you described, the doctor could proceed with the appendectomy if he decided this was a true emergency. But if he decided the situation was less than a true emergency, he'd have to obtain the woman's consent to perform the surgery. If he couldn't obtain it from the woman, he would try to get it from her next of kin. Since the woman's live-in partner has no legal relationship with her, he *cannot* give any consent on her behalf. Marriage is a different matter.

Can a nurse refuse to help obtain the patient's consent if he's incompetent?

Q An 80-year-old-man, admitted to our surgical unit a week before surgery, was so confused and disoriented that we nurses decided he was legally incapable of consenting to major abdominal surgery. Unfortunately, no near relative could be found to give the doctor an informed consent.

> *"The doctor wanted us to obtain consent from an 80-year-old patient who was confused and disoriented."*

On the day of surgery, the doctor asked one of us to help him obtain consent from the patient—that is, have the patient sign the release form.

We all refused, except the unit manager. She did as the doctor asked because she believed the patient was lucid. But then she reported us to the supervisor for not doing our job properly.

Were we right in refusing to help obtain the patient's consent? What legal responsibility does our unit manager have in case of a lawsuit?

A You were right not to get involved. Your hospital needs a written policy that spells out *who's* legally allowed to obtain and witness surgical consents. Actually, the doctor should ask a resident before he asks an RN or unit manager.

But prepare yourself before a case like this occurs again. Make sure your hospital policy specifically states whether or not you (or the unit manager) *can* witness consent.

Also, keep in mind that, even as the witness to consent, you could be asked to testify in court that the patient's consent was given voluntarily, and that he was informed and able to give the consent. Therefore, be sure you document how well the patient could comprehend when you help to obtain or witness his consent. If you feel compelled to refuse a doctor's request to obtain or witness the patient's consent, document your refusal and your memory—should you ever be required to testify.

If you get involved in another case like this, follow the hospital policy as written, with *supercaution.*

Can a patient be sedated before he signs a consent form?

Q We've developed an ongoing conflict with the anesthesiologist on our short-stay surgical unit. What happens is that, on occasion, a patient arrives for surgery without his signed consent form. His doctor's afraid the patient will forget the form, so the doctor himself brings the permit to the hospital just before surgery.

This would be okay with us— except that the anesthesiologist wants to sedate the patient before the doctor arrives with the consent form. We nurses contend that we can't sedate the patient before we see the signed permit.

The anesthesiologist argues against our withholding sedation; he says if the patient's not sedated, he's not properly prepared for general anesthesia. We maintain it's not quality care to sedate a patient preoperatively without a signed operative permit.

Does our responsibility end when we inform the anesthesiologist there's no permit? Must we then give the sedation as ordered, or can we refuse to sedate the patient until the signed permit arrives?

A If your hospital policy includes a preoperative checklist that states a signed operative permit must be present before a patient is

sedated (most hospitals stipulate this), then the patient's doctor, the anesthesiologist, and you must abide by this policy.

Therefore, your responsibility includes refusing to sedate the patient until you see the signed permit. Obviously, if a patient signs a permit after he's been sedated, that permit is virtually worthless.

The solution to this problem doesn't seem too complicated: If the doctor is really afraid the patient will lose the permit, why not have the doctor's secretary deliver it early enough to allow the anesthetist to sedate the patient?

Document your concerns in a memo and send a copy to your nursing supervisor. If the hospital policy is indeed being ignored, the administration should know about it.

Can a patient's relative sign consent for his treatment?

Q We have a blanket policy at the hospital where I work: Any person may sign a consent form for treatment, including surgery, for any family member. Is this good policy?

A No. If the patient is competent, nonemergency invasive procedures shouldn't be done without his consent—whether or not a family member has signed. Without his consent, the hospital and the doctor could be held liable if he sues later. (You'd probably have little or no liability.)

If the patient isn't competent, a family member can make treatment decisions if he's the patient's legal guardian or if he has a durable power of attorney. Practically speaking, though, the next of kin will routinely make health care decisions for an incompetent patient who doesn't have a guardian. Appointing a guardian may take up to 21 days, which could be too long to wait.

Can a patient who's been premedicated legally sign?

Q When a patient who was scheduled for surgery questioned something on her consent form, I immediately notified the surgeon and my manager. But because of a mix-up, the patient was taken to the operating room and premedicated. The surgeon answered her questions there, then called the hospital lawyer to find out if the patient's husband could sign the consent form. The lawyer said he could. So after the surgeon again explained the procedure to the patient and her husband, they both signed it. Was this consent valid?

A That depends. Was the patient capable of rationally weighing the pros and cons of surgery? If so, then yes, it was valid.

You don't say what she questioned, though. Did the surgeon merely clarify a point they'd already discussed? Or did he disclose new information—such as a major risk of the surgery—that the patient hadn't known about before? In the latter case, the consent might be invalid. In any event, you should have documented the patient's level of consciousness and her responses to the discussion.

One more thing: You say the patient's surgery was *scheduled,* not an emergency. A patient's spouse can consent for surgery only in an emergency. So if her husband alone had signed the consent form, it wouldn't have been valid.

Does a patient whose surgery was canceled and rescheduled need to sign another consent form?

Q As a staff nurse, I make it a practice to see that a patient signs any necessary consent forms within the 72 hours before a scheduled operation.

C

We now have a patient who'll stay on our unit until his canceled surgery is rescheduled. Should he be counseled again, then sign another statement? Our hospital has no policy on this.

My unit manager says that as long as the surgery or procedure itself remains the same, the signed consent's valid, even if the procedure is performed more than 72 hours after the consent was signed.

A Your question leaves a question: Are you talking about your obtaining a patient's consent signature—or about checking to be sure the consent form has been signed and is in order?

If you're asking for details about how a nurse should obtain a consent, the answer is: Don't. Nurses shouldn't be obtaining consents. Only the surgeon who's scheduled to do the procedure is qualified to obtain the consent for surgery. The doctor can't delegate this responsibility.

However, you could be called upon to make certain a consent form's in order: You must then be sure the form's been properly signed; the date's still effective; and the procedure hasn't been revised since the original signature was obtained. To do a proper check, you should know your hospital's policy.

Since your hospital's policy hasn't been formulated yet, if there's any question about the validity of a consent (like that of the patient now on your unit), the entire health team, the hospital, and certainly the patient will be better off with a freshly signed consent form.

Doesn't a patient have the right to know what his surgery entails?

Q As an operating room nurse, I have the job of explaining preoperative procedures to patients scheduled for surgery the next day.

Recently I stopped in to see a middle-aged man scheduled for a bilateral orchiectomy. I explained the preoperative procedures to him, and then, almost routinely, I asked if he had any questions. Unbelievably, he asked, "Exactly what is a bilateral orchiectomy?"

When I explained that it was removal of both testicles, the patient was clearly shaken. He hadn't fully realized what the surgery involved, he told me, because the doctor had described the procedure so vaguely.

I tried to reassure the patient and advised him not to sign the surgical consent form until after he'd talked to his doctor again.

I reported this episode to my nurse-manager and my supervisor, and they advised me to call the doctor at once and explain the problem to him.

The doctor was wild. He accused me of "practicing medicine" and said he had told the patient "all he needed to know." "If you ever overstep your bounds again," the doctor warned me, "I'll file a complaint against you."

I can't believe I was in the wrong. Suppose the patient had signed the consent form and gone into surgery without realizing what it entailed? Couldn't he then have sued the doctor and the hospital? (By the way, the patient did sign the consent form, but I understand that the doctor had a lot of talking to do first.) What's your viewpoint?

A The doctor should have thanked you, but that's beside the point. The real issue is: Were you overstepping your bounds? The answer is no—a very definite no. The patient could've looked up "orchiectomy" in a medical dictionary, but he didn't. He asked you, and you did the only thing you could. You answered him truthfully.

According to *The Law and the Expanding Nursing Role,* edited by Bonnie Bullough (New York: Appleton-Century-Crofts, 1980), the doc-

tor is responsible for getting the patient's consent. So the doctor took a big risk when he didn't explain the procedure adequately. If the patient had signed the form without knowing what the operation involved, the consent would certainly not have been "informed." The patient might have sued—and won.

If you encounter this problem again (and chances are you will), do just what you did before. Reassure your patient, then tell him not to sign the consent form until he talks to the doctor again. Make sure, as you did, that the nurse-manager on the unit, your supervisor, and the doctor all know about your actions. Next time, take things one step further and document everything in your nurse's notes.

Chances are the doctor won't thank you next time, either. But he might be less inclined to reprimand you if you've put everything in writing—in the right place.

Is it legal for a doctor to write embarrassingly simple explanations of procedures on a consent form?

Q I recently began work in a small community hospital where one of the doctors, an orthopedist, is put on a pedestal by some of the staff and all of the patients. Perhaps this explains his cavalier attitude toward operative permits, or maybe he believes it when he says, "These people couldn't understand the medical jargon anyway." On the permit form, under procedure or operation, he simply writes, "Remove a disk from my back" or "Fix my knee as best you can."

What do you think about these permits, and what's the liability of the nurse witnessing such a permit?

A The whole purpose of the consent form, as you well know, is to document that the patient agrees to a specific procedure with a full understanding of the goals, risks, and possible complications associated with this procedure. In knee surgery, for instance, the patient should know that knee fusion can lead to loss of range of motion of the knee, whereas knee arthroplasty, which may preserve range of motion, carries a higher risk of infection.

As for your role as witness, when a nurse performs the function of a "witness" on an operative consent form, this is only an acknowledgment that the patient signed the form in the presence of a witness. It doesn't in any way attest to the contents of the discussion or accession on the part of the patient. If the patient later expresses doubts or misunderstanding about the procedure, however, the nurse's duty is to notify the doctor and document that she did so.

You said that you began working at this hospital only recently. Once you're there long enough to feel comfortable with the human dynamics of the situation, maybe you'll be able to share your concerns with the doctor and coax him down from his pedestal.

Is it legal to alter an operative permit?

Q I am a staff nurse in a busy operating suite that handles 35 to 40 cases a day. My problem concerns altering an operative permit. Here's what happened.

The operative permit read: "Adrenal exploration—remove tumor or kidney as indicated." It did not, however, specify the right or left side. The X-ray report stated "Mass in left adrenal-kidney area," and the patient, who had already received preop medication, agreed his problem was on the left side.

The charge nurse took it upon herself to add "left" to the permit and signed her initials. She did not include her title, the date, or time,

nor did she make a notation in the nurses' notes. I'm wondering about the legality of altering an operative permit in this fashion. I was taught that a permit could be altered only if the patient was not premedicated, if he concurred with the change, if he signed the permit next to the correction, and if two proper witnesses also signed.

Your opinion, please.

A In the first place, nurses shouldn't be obtaining informed consent for surgical procedures. And in the second place, they shouldn't be adding information to incomplete forms. Those actions are the responsibility of the doctor.

How many times have you heard or read of surgery being performed on the wrong area? The charge nurse in this case would certainly share some measure of liability if the surgery proceeded on the left kidney and this was later proven to be wrong. Additionally, a plaintiff's lawyer could argue that any permit signed by a premedicated patient is generally considered legally invalid; verbal information obtained under these same circumstances would be similarly questioned.

When you find that a change is called for in an operative permit, contact the doctor; he's responsible.

Is it legal to present blank forms to patients for their signature?

Q Several surgeons in our hospital make a practice of presenting blank preoperative consent forms to patients for their signatures. Only after the operation does the doctor fill in these forms. Is this illegal and, if so, what should we do about it?

A You personally should neither solicit or witness a patient's signature on a blank consent form. Neither should you stand by and let

a doctor treat a patient this way. The possible legal liabilities definitely involve you.

Why should you risk a law suit and possible loss of your license because careless practices have been allowed to take hold at your hospital? You've got to reverse this trend immediately and your best bet for success is to make it a group effort. Go to your supervisor and ask her to relay your position to the director of nursing—or to the surgeons themselves. And stand firm.

Isn't it risky to obtain consent from a patient who seems mentally incompetent?

Q I've just started working at a psychiatric hospital. Recently, a psychiatrist wrote in his progress notes that a patient who'd been diagnosed as paranoid schizophrenic was competent—even though 5 days earlier this patient had been hallucinating. He was scheduled for an invasive test, so his doctor explained the procedure to him. Then I obtained his consent. Within the next 2 hours, he asked me three times to explain the test. I'm concerned about obtaining consent from patients who don't seem competent.

A Check the hospital's policies and procedures manual for guidelines. As you know, the purpose of consent is to ensure that the patient is making an informed decision about his health care. To do so, he must be alert and oriented when the procedure is explained and when he signs the consent form. And of course, information about his state of mind must be charted.

In this case, the doctor felt your patient met the criteria, but you didn't. You should have shared your assessment with the doctor and asked him to reevaluate the patient. Remember, consent is invalid if a patient is incompetent when he gives it.

C

Should an intoxicated patient be allowed to sign a consent form?

Q When a patient is admitted with a blood alcohol level that classifies him as legally drunk, can his signed consent for treatment be considered valid and legal?

How about the signed consent of a patient on mind-altering substances?

A That old saying, "the Lord looks after drunks and babies," would seem to get some backing from earthly legal authority, too. When a person is rendered incompetent (because of drugs, medication, intoxicating substances) and obviously cannot render proper consent, the law then turns that protection over to a responsible person—the health care provider.

A nurse need have no fears legally of rendering care to such a patient, then, even though she doesn't have his specific consent.

Shouldn't consent forms be more specific?

Q A patient who was having surgery for carpal tunnel syndrome in her right wrist had signed a consent form. But because the form didn't specify which wrist, I was concerned about its legality. When I spoke with my manager about it, she said I shouldn't worry; the patient's history and physical noted which wrist was to be operated on. Is she right?

A She is, to a point. The form probably meets the minimum requirements of informed consent.

But you're right, too: It lacks an important detail, which could lead to serious problems. Because doctors and nurses often check the consent form to verify patient and procedure, it can serve as a valu-

able safeguard against errors. In this case, that safeguard was missing. Suppose the doctor had filled out the history and physical forms incorrectly (doctors are only human, so this could happen). The patient could have undergone unnecessary surgery and the hospital could have faced a negligence lawsuit.

Given the possibility for error, amending the current forms seems reasonable. First, find out what the hospital's policy and procedure manuals say about the consent form. Then, talk with your manager again about the problems ambiguous information could cause. With her, request a meeting with the director of surgical services. Revising the form to include important information should be a fairly simple matter.

In the meantime, you'd be wise to confirm the surgical site with the patient—especially if a limb is involved.

What are the legal issues in making tape recordings?

Q We're a group of RNs who've returned to school for our BSNs. For our community health course, we're required to tape-record our patient interviews during three home visits. We've been issued a standard consent form used by the university's psychology and sociology departments for similar interviews. The form states that the tape recording is simply being used to evaluate the student's work; will be heard only by the student and her instructor; and will be erased as soon as the instructor finishes her evaluation. Does such a simple form sound adequate?

Our second question has to do with possible liability. As RNs, we know we're fully responsible for our practice. If malpractice difficulties arise, we feel that we can't count

on the school's assuming legal responsibility for us the way they could for students who are not yet RNs. We all carry our own malpractice insurance, incidentally. What do you think of this?

A The patient consent that is implied when a nurse records necessary information in the patient's record does not extend to tape recording. So you are quite right to get the patient's *specific* consent for the tape recordings.

The consent form, as you describe it, would seem to be adequate, and only one consent would be needed for as long as you continue the care.

Your first responsibility, then, is to make certain that the patient honestly understands what he is signing. As a matter of fact, your explanation of the consent form might be a good way to start your interview.

Your second responsibility is to make sure that the recording is not heard by anyone other than the instructor, as promised on the consent form, since that could constitute a breach of confidentiality.

If any question of malpractice did arise, the responsibility would almost certainly rest with the school. In any event, you have the best protection going—a strong sense of personal responsibility, and your own malpractice insurance coverage.

What can a nurse do if she disagrees with a doctor's explanation?

Q One pediatrician at my hospital routinely tells his patients' parents that a lumbar puncture is no more dangerous than a blood test. The parents then consent to the procedure without understanding the risks for their children.

I often assist this doctor with lumbar punctures. If something goes wrong, could I be liable for failing to inform the parents about the risks involved?

A Legally, the responsibility for informing a patient (or in this case, a minor's parents) about medical procedures and their risks belongs to the doctor, not you. But if the parents ask you a question that's within your scope of practice, you're legally obligated to answer them. If you can't answer the question, refer them to the doctor.

This doctor has put you in a difficult position. If a child suffers serious complications, his parents could sue you, along with the doctor and hospital. You may be found liable if you knew that the parents weren't informed of the risks and you didn't try to stop the procedure. Under these circumstances, the courts may say that you breached your duty to the patient.

> *"The pediatrician tells his patients' parents that lumbar puncture is no more risky than a blood test."*

So, talk to the doctor about your concerns immediately. If he refuses to give parents the information they need to make an informed decision, pursue the matter through nursing and medical channels.

Failure to obtain informed consent is one of the leading causes of malpractice lawsuits today. Don't let this doctor put you and your hospital at risk any longer.

What should a nurse do when a doctor refuses to inform the child's family?

Q A woman brought an 8-year-old boy to the emergency department for treatment of a badly lacerated knee. She said that she was his neighbor and that his parents were out of town. She gave me the name and telephone number of his aunt, who she said could give us consent for treatment. But the doctor told me not to call. He sutured the knee and asked me to give the boy a tetanus shot, which I did.

I'm uncomfortable with the way this was handled. What should we have done?

A Ideally, you'd want consent from a parent or guardian before initiating treatment. So under the best circumstances, you would have obtained permission from the boy's parents—not his aunt, unless she had a written document giving her temporary guardianship.

But realistically, sometimes you have to use common sense. This boy's welfare was your most important consideration. He needed treatment to stop the bleeding. Ordinarily, cleaning a wound, suturing it, and even administering a tetanus shot wouldn't be a problem.

If the boy had required surgery or invasive diagnostic tests, you would have had to make every effort to contact his parents or guardian. If that had failed, administrators would have asked for a court order to permit treatment.

What should nurses do when children and their parents don't agree on treatment?

Q I care for many cancer patients on the pediatric intensive care unit where I work. Hospital policy requires parental consent for treatment (and for discontinuing treatment), and the children don't seem to have any say in what happens to them. I don't feel right continuing treatment for a dying child—especially a teenager who knows that chemotherapy is prolonging his dying, not curing his illness.

What should I do when children and their parents disagree?

A In these situations, you need to keep the lines of communication open. Often, parents are unwilling to admit how much their child knows about his illness because they're too frightened to face his impending death. The child, sensing this, thinks talking about his illness and his feelings is taboo. So he also keeps quiet.

What can you do? Get them together and encourage them to discuss those difficult subjects. When a child tells you what he wants and why he wants it, talk to his parents and the doctor so everyone knows. Then make every effort to follow his wishes.

If the hospital doesn't have a support group for parents and seriously ill children, you might consider starting one. When parents meet with others in the same situation, they become more willing to openly share their problems and fears.

What should we do about a school's consent forms that were signed years ago?

Q As a school nurse, I question our school's policy of giving aspirin to students for headaches or minor pain. While we're careful not to give aspirin unless we have a signed permission form from the child's parent or guardian, some of these signed forms are up to 5 years old.

A Save yourself a headache. Just make sure you have signed forms for all the students and that the forms are updated *annually*. Anything can change in 5 years' time—especially a health history.

If you have a freshly dated permission slip the next time you give a student aspirin, you won't get an attack of conscience or a phone call from his parents.

Consultation

How should a nurse handle it when a doctor changes his mind?

Q I was recently trapped in a frustrating situation between an attending doctor and a neurologist. Here's what happened. The attending doctor told a patient whose right arm was numb that he'd request a neurology consultation. When the neurologist hadn't arrived by the end of my shift, I called him. He said the attending doctor had asked for some advice—which he gave over the telephone—but not for a consultation. He said I should tell the patient that her doctor hadn't asked him to examine her.

I relayed this information to the patient, who asked me to find out why her doctor had changed his mind. When I contacted him, he said to tell her that the neurologist didn't think he needed to see her.

By then, the patient was just as confused and angry as I was. How could I have handled this situation better?

A Unfortunately, nurses are frequently caught in the middle when attending and consulting doctors are unclear about their responsibilities to a patient.

To avoid future traps, review—and, if necessary, clarify—hospital policy on consultations. It should require that the doctor write (or dictate and sign) an order in the patient's medical record when he requests a consultation. He should also write an order to cancel the consultation if it's not needed.

If the attending doctor followed this procedure, you could have said something like this: "I see that your doctor wrote an order to cancel the neurology consultation. I'll talk with him and ask him to share his reasons with you." Then you could have gone to the doctor and said: "Your patient has some questions about your decision to cancel the neurology consultation. She'd like to talk with you."

That approach takes you out of the middle. And it focuses on the patient's need to know *why* the consultation was canceled, not on who canceled it.

Contact lenses

What if keeping them in too long causes pain?

Q Last week my son telephoned me from his senior class ski trip asking for advice. One of his friends had worn hard contact lenses all day skiing and all night partying. Now his eyes hurt. What to do?

Rather than make a mistake, I advised the friend to get in touch with his doctor. But for my own information, I'd like to know the answer to this in case it comes up again.

A And well it might. High school and college students are infamous for leaving their contacts in too long for cramming...or partying. Calling the doctor is always a good answer, especially if the pain is severe or if the discomfort lasts longer than 24 hours. For immediate relief, of course, the patient could lie in a darkened room with cold compresses or an ice pack applied to his eyelids. He may require some eyedrops and an analgesic for pain management. This condition is usually self-healing, and the patient can wear the contact lenses for limited periods after several days of being asymptomatic.

Contamination

Are light handles on OR lamps a source of contamination?

Q I have a new job in the operating room (OR) of a famous university hospital and wonder about light handles on the spotlights. The surgeon can adjust the lights to suit his purposes without having to repeatedly ask the circulating nurse to adjust them.

But one of the senior nurses on our team refuses to use light handles because she claims they're a source of contamination. I've tried to persuade her that with proper care they can be kept free from contamination in the same way that basins, trays, and instruments are managed.

But this nurse is adamant. She says no, she won't use them.

Can you throw some light on the subject?

A Light handles on the spotlights are designed to prevent contamination, not to cause it, if you're using proper technique. That means washing and sterilizing the light handles along with other OR equipment, and being certain that whoever screws the handles onto the light fixtures before the surgery is both gowned and gloved. Although the part of the light handle that touches the fixture itself will be contaminated (there's no way around that), the long handle that the doctor reaches for during the surgery will be sterile.

The Association of Operating Room Nurses (AORN) hasn't done a study on this and so hasn't taken a stand. A spokesperson did say "each individual institution should establish its own policy."

Continuing education

Can you come up with some good reasons for home study?

Q In our special unit of the Navy Reserve Nurse Corps, we have a flexible program that allows us to substitute 16 hours of continuing education (CE) in nursing each month for the required weekend duty at the reserve unit. Ideally, this will accomplish two goals—expand our nursing knowledge and attract more nurses to join the corps.

To date, the Navy hasn't permitted us to use home-study CE courses to fill even part of the requirement. I like taking these tests and feel I get more out of them than attending seminars and staff development programs. So with the Navy's permission, I'm writing a justification paper to request approval for using home-study CE courses. As providers, can you help me come up with some good reasons?

A When your whole program is based on flexibility, you shouldn't have too much trouble selling the merits of home-study CE courses, because flexibility is their major appeal. Explain in your letter that finding a seminar on a topic that will help you and one that fits into your nursing schedule is really tough if you're working rotating shifts and weekends and live far from a big city. With home-study CE courses, you can study what you want and when it's best for you, take a test that's independently graded, and—most important of all—end up with written proof that you've learned something, not just attended a course.

Note too that reputable home-study CE courses are accredited by professional nursing organizations. And states that have mandatory CE contact hours for license renewal accept home-study credits for part or all of the required hours.

How will home study CEUs and those earned for attending courses and seminars be applied to dual licenses?

Q Last year, I moved to a New Mexico town near the Colorado border, and I'm licensed in both states. New Mexico requires 30 con-

tact hours of mandatory continuing education units (CEUs) within the 2-year license renewal cycle; Colorado requires 20 contact hours. How will home study CEUs and those I earn for attending courses and seminars be applied to my name in each state? And who keeps track of how many CEUs I earn?

A You do. When you attend courses and seminars or complete any approved CE offering, the provider should give you a certificate granting a specified number of contact hours. Make sure that you get one, and keep it for your own records. In New Mexico, your home state, you must list your CEUs on the state board's license renewal form and attach photocopies of the certificates. Colorado limits the number of home study offerings to 5 hours in each 2-year period. Just list your CEUs on the back of the renewal form. Then, if you're included in the state board's random postrenewal audit, you'll have to send in photocopies of your certificates for approval.

For someone like you who's licensed in two states with mandatory CE requirements, record keeping can be a little tricky—but twice as necessary. You're responsible for knowing the exact requirements of each state and fulfilling them.

Copyright

When and how should a nurse go about getting it?

Q I've developed an activity book that's so popular at the nursing home where I volunteer I'd like to have it published.

Is it better to find a publisher for my book first and then get a copyright, or vice versa? And how do I go about getting a copyright in the first place?

A You automatically own the copyright interests for any work you've created—just by the act of creating it. And you don't need a registered copyright to protect most unpublished works. When you submit your activity book to a publisher, signify your copyright by writing the statement: Unpublished work, the word copyright or the copyright symbol ©, the year, and your name at the bottom of the first page. Simple? Yes, but true.

Of course, if you want to, you can register any unpublished book or manuscript with the Copyright Office. The U.S. Government Printing Office publishes a booklet, *Copyright Basics* (Circular R1), that outlines the procedure. You'll also need application form TX.

To get the forms and circulars, telephone the Copyright Office hot line: (202) 707-9100, or write: Copyright Office, LM 455, Library of Congress, Washington, DC 20559.

CPR

Could a nurse be charged with giving medical advice without a doctor's license?

Q I've had considerable experience with cardiopulmonary resuscitation (CPR) and, over the years, I've seen some gross errors committed by well-intentioned people. (Most recently, I saw a large, muscular man vigorously administer CPR to a person having an epileptic seizure.)

I wrote an article, addressed to the layman, on the hows, whys, and whens of CPR. A newspaper syndicate has accepted the article for publication. Now, I'm having second thoughts.

Could I be charged with giving medical advice without a doctor's license? Are there any other legal considerations for a nurse writing such an article?

A Your article is obviously an expression of your opinions based on your experiences. That part of the First Amendment directed to freedom of speech protects your right to publish such an article.

You are not prescribing therapy for an individual, but merely imparting professional information, which is within the accepted expertise of a nurse—especially one with your training and experience. In no way can you be considered to be practicing medicine.

Write on!

How can an instructor be sure the people she teaches are really qualified?

Q I teach cardiopulmonary resuscitation (CPR) at a psychiatric hospital. Instead of paying overtime so nurses can take the required American Heart Association (AHA) course, administrators allot 30 minutes for instruction—which I must squeeze in between patient care.

All nurses at the hospital have to be certified in CPR, yet only 10% of those I teach are actually proficient. If they pass the written examination, though, I feel compelled to certify them so they don't lose their jobs. What can I do to remedy this situation?

A Voice your objections in a memo sent up through channels. Outline the AHA requirements and why you believe the 30-minute program is insufficient—and dangerous. You might want to ask some graduates of the 30-minute course if they feel qualified to perform CPR and include those comments in your memo. Also, document the outcome of codes to help administrators assess the hospital's needs.

If administrators won't budge, you could substitute a series of continuing education programs that would culminate in a hospital certificate of training. During those sessions, you could teach them the skills they need to become proficient at CPR.

Should a nurse have been reprimanded because she refused to do it on an infant?

Q I'm supervisor of our hospital's coronary care unit, but right now I'm in hot water. Last week, the director of nursing asked me to accompany a critically ill infant in respiratory distress to a hospital 25 miles (40 km) away. She felt I was qualified because I was a cardiopulmonary resuscitation (CPR) instructor. Since I rarely care for infants, and since I knew nothing about the baby's history, I refused to go in the ambulance.

I was reprimanded by the director for having a poor attitude and setting a bad example. I don't think the punishment fit the crime. In fact, as far as I'm concerned, there *wasn't* any crime. I was totally within my rights. What do you think?

A Some would say you were right to tell the director of nursing about your limitations—and that she shouldn't have been so hard on you. In fact, she should have been relieved that you recognized your limitations before you went into the ambulance. On the other hand, the director had some logic on her side when she assumed you could handle an emergency. You *are* a CPR instructor, which means you teach others how to give CPR to adults, children, and infants.

But others would say that if a baby is critically ill and a candidate for respiratory distress, the personnel and equipment going with it should be far more than just a nurse trained in CPR. Treating a patient in respiratory distress in a moving vehicle is a special situation—and takes special training as well as special transportation facilities.

Also they might ask why the baby wasn't prepared beforehand: that is, recognized as a high-risk baby and intubated before making the move to another hospital. They feel a nurse should never have gone in that ambulance with the baby. There are people and facilities to do this job. Use them. Working in a moving vehicle is a whole different ball game from working in a hospital.

Everyone panics when there's a baby in the picture. So the best advice is: Keep your head—then you can use it to analyze the situation and make sound decisions.

Crab lice

Should a nurse have been fired for not telling the director of nursing?

Q The other evening when I got home from work, I felt a sudden severe itching in my pubic area. It turned out to be *Phthirus pubis* (crab lice). I didn't call my doctor because I identified the crab lice by checking my microbiology book.

As a single parent who enjoys disco dancing, I assume I caught it from a heavily used disco bathroom. I ruled out my male friend, since I hadn't had sexual relations with him during the incubation period.

As soon as I discovered the infestation, I rushed out and bought a liquid which I applied to the pubic area, and a special spray which I used on the mattress and furniture. I laundered my bed linen along with the clothing I'd been wearing.

The next day, I went to work. I did *not* mention the condition to my supervisor. However, I observed carefully. None of the patients had been infested, but several employees had.

The director of nursing heard of my problem through the grapevine and asked me point blank if it was true. "I don't have crab lice now," I told her, "but I did have them." She suspended me on the spot. Shortly afterward she fired me on the grounds that my handling of the situation proved my incompetence as a nurse.

Out of work, I face not only a battered ego, but a serious financial predicament. I don't qualify for unemployment benefits, and I'm at risk for losing my car and my house.

Did I mishandle the situation? Or do you think I was right in my effort to spare the staff and the patients undue alarm?

A You should have gone posthaste to your doctor and director of nursing about the contamination. But your employer overreacted to the situation. You can be fired only for just cause but your case doesn't fall into this category. A reprimand should have sufficed—unless, of course you've had repeated hygiene problems and, even then, the director of nursing should have followed the established grievance procedure.

What happened to the other employees with the same problem? Did they report to the nursing administrator? Did they get fired?

Fighting to get your job back could take months or even years. but if you decide that's what you want, start with your nearest American Civil Liberties Union office, or your state's Department of Human Rights to determine possible recourse.

If, on the other hand, you decide to call this job a loss, try to switch to another job without going into detail about this past problem. If you have to discuss it with a prospective employer, be discreetly open; explain your thinking at the time and admit that, in retrospect, you probably should've worked through your doctor and director of nursing.

If misery does indeed love company, you may be interested to learn that the problem is not uncommon. Recently *every* nurse on a unit of a large inner-city hospital caught the "bug" from one of the patients.

Crash cart

Shouldn't a crash cart be readily accessible in acute care hospitals?

Q I'm a manager on a skilled nursing unit that's attached to an acute care hospital. The hospital has four code levels, from "full code" to "no code", that apply to my unit, too. But we don't have a crash cart on the unit, and I'm the only nurse certified in advanced cardiac life support. If a patient codes, we have to call the hospital to request the crash cart; then the house supervisor takes over. I think we're putting ourselves in a very tenuous legal position. What do you think?

A If you're going to call codes on your unit, you need the right equipment, as well as staff prepared to intervene.

As nurses, you and your colleagues have a legal duty to provide a reasonable standard of care. This "reasonable" standard is usually open to interpretation, but not in this case. To fulfill your legal and nursing obligations, you must be ready to implement any of the code levels included in unit policy.

That couldn't possibly happen for the reasons you've given: You're the only nurse on the unit qualified to assist with a code, and a crash cart isn't readily accessible. Besides endangering patients who may need advanced life support, this situation puts the staff and administration in a legally precarious position.

To correct the problem, a crash cart must be made available and staff nurses must be educated to use it during a code. Talk with the unit's medical director and nursing and hospital administrators—they should begin correcting this risky situation at once.

Shouldn't there be one on each surgical unit?

Q At the hospital where I work, one crash cart serves three units: It's used by two separate surgical units and by the gynecologic unit that connects them. I think it's absurd not to keep a crash cart in each surgical unit—but even more absurd to keep the one cart, as we do, on the gynecologic unit, which has very few codes.

Just last week when a code was called on one of the surgical units, at least 4 minutes elapsed before a nurse could push the cart to the scene. I consider this arrangement dangerous. Do you agree? If you do, how would you go about improving the situation?

A Yes, the arrangement is dangerous. But this is one battle you shouldn't have to fight alone. So here's what you can do.

Begin by writing a memo stating your concern and the reasons for your concern; send it through the appropriate channels. Of course you should cite the recent delay in getting a crash cart to the scene when a code was called. If you've had other incidents of the same sort, list them with documented facts.

Ask all the nurses in the three units involved to sign the memo. Also ask the doctors and respiratory therapists involved to sign.

After you've allowed time for your memo to go through channels, ask for a meeting of all those who've signed: Request that the nursing supervisors of the three units, the director of nursing, and other department heads attend the meeting.

Explore solutions to the problem with your colleagues before the meeting. As further preparation for

C

the meeting, find out about the crash cart arrangements in other area hospitals. You'll want to marshal the best possible support for your arguments.

Let's hope that when the powers-that-be see how many people are concerned about the irrational placement of this critical emergency equipment, they'll become the powers-that-do...something about it.

Will it contain everything we need in the right place?

Q According to a new hospital policy, the pharmacy department will soon take over full responsibility for maintaining all crash carts, including ours on the intensive care unit (ICU). Pharmacy technicians will lock our cart with a registered plastic lock that only they can supply, so none of us have access to any of its contents except during a code, when we break the lock. We'll have an "educational cart" on the unit to be used only for staff review.

Now that we're "locked out," how can we be sure that everything we need will be in the right place? We'd rather trust ourselves than the pharmacy technicians—we've got the experience with codes, they don't; besides, we've never had any problems maintaining our own cart. Do other hospitals have this policy? Are we overreacting?

A Perhaps your administrator is the one overreacting. In some hospitals, policies like yours are in effect in hectic departments where there's rampant "borrowing" from crash carts. But any policy that keeps ICU nurses from double-checking the supplies on their crash cart is borrowing trouble.

Here's a better system: After a code, the pharmacy department should be responsible only for replacing any drugs used during a

code and for checking the expiration dates of those on hand. At least once a shift, you or another designated ICU nurse should verify the technician's inspection. Check other equipment that's not usually pharmacy's responsibility (pacemaker, lab tubes, arterial blood gas and respiratory equipment), including their expiration dates, then lock the cabinet. If the cart isn't used during your shift, the next shift's nurse can leave it locked and use a checklist for drug expiration dates and equipment and document that the cart's contents are intact. Routine checking—and the weight of responsibility for getting it right—are far more instructional than a "sample" cart.

Get back to administration. Although the new policy is most likely well-intentioned, it needs rethinking.

Cremation

Shouldn't the patient's wishes be respected?

Q You wouldn't believe the family ruckus my father caused by announcing that he wants his body cremated when he dies. My brothers say they won't allow it, and my mother refuses to take a stand.

I think my father's wishes should be respected. How can I help him?

A Tell him to continue expressing his wishes, especially to your mother. She's the key player here.

At one time, it was thought that cremation inhibited healthy grieving because it didn't allow widows to participate in traditional funeral rituals. But Joy Ufema, RN, a thanatologist, questioned 70 widows; half had cremated their husbands and the other half had buried them.

Results were surprising: Women whose husbands had been cremated *hadn't* had difficulty grieving.

Not only did they agree with their husbands' decision, but they planned to choose cremation for themselves, too.

You could advise your father to sit down with your mother and have a chat about his feelings—and hers. She may agree with his wishes.

But even if she doesn't, he still has two options.

He could continue to plead his case—in time, she might understand his position and change her mind.

Or he could let it go. After all, once his spirit leaves his body and "crosses over," how his old coat is discarded may not be important to him.

Crowding

What can be done if the hospital insists on admitting another patient to an already full room?

Q As nurse-manager on a 44-bed orthopedic unit, I'm sometimes required to admit a fifth patient to an already full four-patient room. Written hospital policy allows this as a temporary arrangement, but I still feel the practice is unsafe.

> *"I feel that admitting a fifth patient in an already crowded four-patient room is dangerous but my department head insists I must."*

My department head told me in no uncertain terms that I cannot refuse to admit the fifth patient. What's my responsibility in this situation?

A Because your hospital has a written policy on this matter (and your department head supports it), what choice do you have?

You must carry out the policy (at least until you get it changed). Otherwise, you'd be making an unsafe situation even more unsafe. And remember, if you're not acting exactly according to policy, you become legally liable.

All this doesn't mean you have to ignore your feeling that this could be an unsafe practice.

Your first step is to document why you think the practice is unsafe. Record facts and observations rather than opinions. Note whether the patients are moved out as soon as possible and whether staffing is adequate. Send your report through the proper nursing channels. Then try to set up a meeting of the staff with your department head and nursing supervisor. Together you may come up with an alternative to this "room for one more" policy.

CT scanning

What's the liability when patients have to be to transported a half hour away?

Q We don't have a computed tomography (CT) scanner at the small community hospital where I'm charge nurse. So whenever a doctor orders a CT scan, we send the patient to a radiology office about a half-hour ride away. A hospital van, not an ambulance, is used for the trip, and our security officer drives. The patient doesn't sign a leave-of-absence form before he leaves, and we don't send a nurse along.

Recently, we sent a child with significant neurologic symptoms. This really scared me—suppose he'd had a seizure while en route or the van was involved in an accident. I'm worried both about our patients and our liability. What's your opinion?

A You've been lucky so far. No question, every patient— especially a child—should be accompanied by a staff member who's prepared to handle an emergency. And an ambulance may sometimes be needed, depending on the patient's condition.

In your current situation, you have three things working against you legally: First, the patient hasn't been discharged when you send him to the radiology office, so he's still under the hospital's care. Second, the courts most likely would view any harmful incident as foreseeable, especially when the patient showed serious neurologic symptoms. And third, a patient like this probably wouldn't be judged responsible for contributing to the incident. But you, the doctors, or the hospital itself might be held liable.

Talk to your supervisors. If no changes are made, go up the line with your concerns—for the patients' sake and for yourself. And do it quickly, before that first accident happens.

Cytomegalovirus

Can a person have had it in the past without knowing it and now be immune?

Q We have many acquired immunodeficiency syndrome (AIDS) patients on our medical/surgical unit, so I always use gloves when necessary as well as good handwashing technique. However, many of these patients are infected with and excrete cytomegalovirus (CMV). Because I'm planning to become pregnant soon, I'm worried about contracting CMV and the risks of fetal exposure.

If I had CMV in the past without knowing it, would I now be immune? Is CMV spread only by secretions, or by airborne routes also?

A CMV is spread by direct contact with infected blood, urine, saliva, cervical secretions, breast milk, or donor organs. It's not spread by the airborne route. If you've been careful about handwashing and avoiding direct contact with potentially infectious materials, the risk of acquiring CMV infections through contact with AIDS patients is low.

Past infection with CMV doesn't ensure immunity because there are a number of different strains of CMV. In fact, about half the women of childbearing age have had a CMV infection; once the initial infection is over, the virus can become latent and be reactivated at any time. However, the effects on a fetus are usually less severe during a reactivation than during the primary CMV infection.

Of course, you could decrease your chances of contracting a CMV infection by transferring to a lower-risk area. If this isn't possible, you can have serologic screening before you try to become pregnant. Discuss this with your doctor.

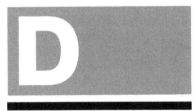

D & C

Is it routine to do one at the same time as a hysterectomy?

Q A surgeon at the hospital where I work usually does a diagnostic dilatation and curettage (D&C) at the same time he does a hysterectomy. Is this routine procedure?

A Performing the two procedures together isn't as common as it once was. Whether or not a previous D&C was performed, the surgeon may choose to do another one at the time of surgery if there's a question of pathology. And, if the D&C scrapings contain cancerous cells, this will influence the surgical procedure (removing lymph nodes or leaving staples as markers for future irradiation).

Deaf nurse

How can she be treated fairly?

Q I'm a charge nurse on the 11-to-7 shift of a 40-bed medical/surgical unit. My staff consists of a medication nurse and three nursing assistants, or a medication nurse, two nursing assistants, and an LPN. About 2 weeks ago, the nursing office sent me an LPN, competent in every way, except she's deaf. The very first night, her disability caused problems on the unit. For example, a patient was vomiting as this nurse passed his room, and she never heard him. Luckily, he didn't aspirate.

I don't want to hurt the nurse's feelings, but I'm concerned about the care she gives—especially in the subdued lighting in which we work.

Am I being unfair to her?

A That depends on how this nurse was assigned to your shift. If she was assigned to replace your regular LPN, then the nursing office was unfair in giving you a person with the same title but not the same capacity to do the job. On the other hand, if she was assigned with the understanding that she'd fill a limited role (such as taking temperatures and pulses), then you can't expect her to operate outside that role.

Express your concerns in a documented memo that you send through nursing channels. As one solution, you might suggest assigning this nurse to an area where patients are not as ill; for example, she could work in an ambulatory setting. Or suggest assigning this LPN to the day shift, when more nurses are around.

Either solution would be a lot fairer than giving her an assignment that would emphasize her deafness. Remember: You don't have to worry just about the LPN. You have to protect the patients and the staff, who will have the job of compensating.

What should be done about a nurse who has a hearing deficit?

Q I work nights on a busy medical/surgical unit, often with 10 or 11 patients to take care of. Another RN, who's worked on this unit for years, is a good nurse—except for one major problem. She has a hearing deficit. She can sit next to a beeping I.V. controller and not hear it.

As a newcomer to this hospital, I asked our unit coordinator about the situation. She said she knew about it, but the other nurse has only a year left before she retires, so everyone just "helps" her by doing her work. Frankly, we're just too busy to take on her responsibilities—and I'm worried about the patients. I'm caught between being cruel and being cautious.

A Your patients' interests come first—and you'll be kind, not cruel, to your co-worker if you can help her avoid a malpractice suit as a finale to her nursing career.

Before pursuing this with your supervisors, how about talking directly to the nurse herself? Perhaps she's been lulled into complacency by her co-workers' mistaken sense of loyalty. Find out whether she's seen a medical specialist recently; perhaps some new technology can help. Let her know that you don't mind pinch-hitting in an emergency, but you can't cover for anyone day after day.

You can temper your frankness with a sensitive blend of profes-sionalism and kindness. Your co-worker will hear your message. If she doesn't act on it, you'll have to speak up through channels.

Death

Any suggestions on what to tell visitors who arrive after the patient dies?

Q I work on a busy medical/surgical unit with cardiac patients, terminally ill cancer patients, and others who are equally ill but in different ways. In this setting, death confronts us daily. We handle our own reactions the best way we can and help the patient's family through their initial shock and grief.

But we're frequently faced with still another painful task: breaking the news of a patient's death to a friend who stops by for a visit *after* the body of the dead patient has been moved to the funeral home, and after the family's left the hospital.

Under these circumstances, the visitor can be shocked to learn that his friend has died. Naturally, we try to comfort him. Sometimes, though, we resist going through the shock and the grief again. Then there's the matter of time: We simply don't have enough.

On occasion, we've tried hedging—telling the visitor that the patient's been transferred to the intensive care unit and is doing too poorly for visitors. But we're embarrassed and uncomfortable about lying.

Any suggestions?

A Your question's not easy to answer. You shouldn't lie to the visitor who's come to see his friend and doesn't yet know he died. There's not much point in your lying or even hedging. The visitor's bound to sense by your reaction that something's wrong.

Escort him to a private area and, if you're familiar with the case, break the news gently. If you know only that the patient has died—and have no further details—call a colleague who *is* familiar with the case. Ask her if she'd talk with the visitor.

Whatever you do, don't leave the distraught visitor alone, and don't send him away without some transition time. Try to detain him at least until he regains his composure.

Make a courtesy telephone call to the family, telling them that the visitor came to the hospital and was informed of his friend's death.

The demands such posthumous visitors make must be difficult on your time and your emotions. But try to find the time and the inner resources to meet their needs. This is an integral part of true nursing.

Can you recommend a source for the names of support groups or any other information that might be helpful?

Q As an intensive care unit nurse, I wish I could do more for the grieving families of patients who die. Can you recommend a source for the names of support groups or any other information that might be helpful?

A Here's a gem of a book: Not a new book, but the expanded and revised 11th edition of *Dealing Creatively with Death: A Manual of Death Education and Simple Burial* edited by Jenifer Morgan (Burnsville, N.C.:Celo Press, 1988). This paperback contains directories of grief support groups; memorial societies in the United States and Canada; eye, organ, and tissue banks; plus an annotated bibliography of books, pamphlets, periodicals, and audiovisuals. The text explores practical and sensitive ways to deal with a number of death-related

problems—in many instances, using examples from actual experiences.

If a child dies at night, is it all right to wait and tell the parents in the morning?

Q As a night nurse in an intensive care nursery, I'm faced with a serious problem.

> *"The doctor instructed the night nurse to lie to parents who ask about an infant who is dead but not yet pronounced dead."*

Something like 90% of our infants are the patients of our only neonatologist. When one of his infant patients dies at night, he waits until morning to come and pronounce him dead. He has instructed the night nurse to lie to parents who ask about an infant who is dead but not yet pronounced dead.

One night, for example, when we called the neonatologist to inform him that an infant had just died, we told him the father was spending the night at the hospital and might ask to see the infant. The neonatologist told us to tell the father we were doing some procedure and that he couldn't see the infant for a while.

I talked to my supervisor, who said her hands are tied. I'd talk to the doctor, but I'm pretty sure I'd lose my job. He nearly controls the unit.

A Tough spot or not, your license makes you responsible to patients—not doctors. And the demands this doctor is making violate your state's nurse practice act and the American Nurses' Association's Code of Ethics, and more likely your own hospital's policy on the management of death. The demand also

involves cruelty to families by prolonging their false hopes.

Besides interfering with your ethical responsibility to the infants and their families, the doctor's demands also place you in legal jeopardy. What are your defenses if parents suspect their baby died long before they were notified and an autopsy confirms it? What if they blame poor nursing care for his death? What are you charting during those hours when the baby is dead but not yet pronounced dead? Do your notes indicate all significant changes in his condition and the time they took place? Do they show you notified the doctor and when?

You're right, you shouldn't approach the doctor alone because this problem involves the larger issue of who should determine standards of nursing practice at your hospital: this doctor or nursing administration?

Go back to your supervisor and tell her that you can't ethically or legally lie to the parents. Point out to her that any doctor—not just a neonatologist—can pronounce death. (Who pronounces death for the 10% of your patients not cared for by the neonatologist?) Tell her the decision about which doctor should pronounce death is the doctor's problem—not nursing's.

If your supervisor still shirks her responsibility, you'd better carry your refusal to collaborate up the ladder yourself. Good luck.

Is there any way to help a subordinate deal with her first encounter with death?

Q As charge nurse of a geriatric unit in a teaching hospital, I've cared for many dying patients. Possibly that's why I was caught off guard by this recent incident.

One of the nursing assistants asked if a patient I assigned to her might die soon. I told her all signs pointed to it, whereupon she burst into tears, sobbing loudly that she'd never seen a person die and that she would be sick if she had to do postmortem care. I quickly assigned another nursing assistant to care for the patient and tried to calm the weeping girl. Later that morning she went to personnel and asked for a transfer to another department.

The supervisor comforted me by saying the nursing assistant will get over this experience and, in fact, be better suited to working elsewhere. But I still feel terrible that death became so routine to me that I failed to help this nursing assistant deal with her first encounter with it. Any thoughts?

A Next time, you'll probably find out how a nursing assistant, or any staff member, feels about caring for a dying patient before making the assignment. (Remember, though, that some people, because of their emotional makeup, can *never* be assigned postmortem duty.)

Further suggestions for the next time you're faced with this situation: Ask a seasoned staff member to assume primary and *teaching* responsibility, with the inexperienced nursing assistant acting only as secondary assistant. Allow the *nursing assistant* to choose how she'll help the first time around. Have the experienced worker explain the physical changes taking place and why they're occurring: "The kidneys are shutting down, so the patient won't need a bedpan as often," "Hearing is the last sense to go; be careful what you say." Follow up closely with the nursing assistant after the patient's death. She handled this experience well, but there's no guarantee for next time. Schedule informal sessions to encourage staff members to talk openly about their feelings—especially on a unit like yours where death can become "routine." You may discover that seasoned nurses need guidance, too.

You may find helpful a new video, *Dealing with Death and Dying,* avail-

able from Springhouse Corporation, 1111 Bethlehem Pike, Springhouse, PA 19477. The video features Joy Ufema, RN, MSN, an internationally acclaimed thanatologist. It gives helpful advice on how to care for and talk with terminally ill patients.

Last but not least, don't be too hard on yourself. You will be disappointed in yourself at times. And you must learn to deal with that—and move forward.

Why can't doctors accept it?

Q Last week, my elderly uncle had a myocardial infarction and collapsed about a block from his home. Someone called an ambulance, and he was taken to the hospital. Although his doctor knew the prognosis was poor, he placed my uncle on a ventilator.

My uncle died the next day, but not before suffering needlessly at the hands of aggressive doctors who wouldn't accept his death. Why does this happen?

A Some people think dying is the worst thing that can happen. Your uncle's difficult death illustrates that belief. Unfortunately, his situation also reminds us that, sometimes, there *are* worse things than death.

The problem is emergency personnel didn't know your uncle's wishes. Nor did the emergency department (ED) staff. So they chose to be aggressive, just in case.

How are we to know what every unconscious person wants? Certainly carrying a living-will card in one's wallet helps, although the living will isn't legally recognized in all states.

Here's a suggestion for EDs: Instead of automatically placing an elderly patient on a ventilator, insert an endotracheal tube and manually bag him until a family member can be located to communicate his wishes. (Of course, that means peo-

ple must tell their kin what they want before a crisis occurs.)

This idea does create a staffing problem. A nurse or respiratory therapist must be present to squeeze the bag 16 times per minute. But it eliminates a problem that's far more troubling: when to unplug the ventilator. If the staff takes this suggestion, the machine is never plugged in.

Defibrillation

Does a crash course qualify anyone to use a defibrillator?

Q I'm the only person on duty at night in the infirmary of a large factory. Two nurses and a doctor work the day shift. For the 6 years I've worked here, a portable defibrillator has sat in a corner collecting dust. In all my years as a nurse, I've never been in a situation where one was needed. Yet the doctor in charge tells me that after "a few lessons" from him, I could skillfully defibrillate an employee if necessary.

I think an employee going into cardiac arrest would have a better chance of surviving if I used cardiopulmonary resuscitation until help arrived than he'd have if I tried to use an unfamiliar procedure alone.

I don't think a crash course qualifies anyone to use a defibrillator. Do you?

A No, and you're right to be concerned. Learning defibrillation technique may be easy; knowing when to do it and why is the difficult part. And the only way you'll know defibrillation is needed is by placing the patient on a monitor and interpreting his electrocardiogram. Even if you had proper training, carrying out these steps while on duty alone is still difficult.

Furthermore, you should be certified in basic life support and advanced cardiac life support. To be expected to perform alone something as vital as defibrillation after receiving only "a few lessons" from a doctor is to shortchange the employees and endanger their lives.

Additionally, any organization with a defibrillation policy should have specific written guidelines that are periodically reviewed against the American Heart Association's guidelines, which state "All defibrillators should be checked at regular, frequent intervals with suitable test equipment to determine the delivered energy." As it stands now, your "dusty" defibrillator is probably useless.

No way around it, a patient needing defibrillation has a better chance of survival if defibrillation is immediately available—and only if the equipment is in perfect condition and the operator confident and competent. Meet with the other nurses and the doctor to fill in the serious gaps in your factory's policy as soon as possible. And as though lives depended on it.

Degrees

What are the differences in education and philosophy of treatment among MDs, DOs, chiropractors, and naturopaths?

Q I'm curious about the difference in education and philosophy of treatment among various health care providers, say the "standard" medical doctor (MD), doctor of osteopathy (DO), chiropractor, and naturopath. When I asked my co-workers, no one seemed to actually know.

Can you give me some information to share with them?

A Generally, after earning a bachelor's degree, MD and DO candidates complete a 3- or 4-year MD or DO program. Then MDs spend 1 or 2 years in residency, and DOs serve a 1-year internship. MDs and DOs who specialize spend 2 to

5 more years in advanced residency training. About 85% of MDs and 11% of DOs specialize. Both the MD and DO use all accepted methods of treatment, but DOs put special emphasis on the musculoskeletal system and often perform therapy by manipulating with the hands. In the United States, there are approximately 430,000 MDs and 20,000 DOs.

Chiropractors finish at least 2 years of college, then enter a 4-year chiropractor program. They practice on the principle that health is largely determined by the nervous system and treat primarily by using the hands to manipulate muscles and bones, especially the spine. Chiropractors cannot prescribe drugs or perform surgery. About 25,000 chiropractors practice in the United States.

Naturopaths complete 3 years of college, then 4 years of naturopathic training. Emphasizing prevention, naturopaths rely solely on natural remedies such as light, heat, cold, water, and fruit. Naturopaths number about 2,000 in the United States.

Individual state licensing boards decide which medical practitioners can give orders to nurses. In Pennsylvania, for example, nurses can carry out orders given by MDs, DOs, and dentists only. Some states have ruled that a nurse can take orders for treatments from a chiropractor, but only if he's a member of the hospital staff.

Hope this helps.

What do the initials stand for?

Q Every time I read nursing journals or fliers for seminars, I feel as if I'm participating in a trivia quiz. Nurses have so many different initials after their names these days that I'm not sure what some of them stand for. Here are a few I've run across lately: DNS, CNS, TNS, FNP, FAAN, CGC, CNN, CNOR, COHN, CPNA. Talk about confusing. What's your reaction?

A Great! Not because you're confused, but because so many nurses are working to obtain advanced academic degrees and certifications. You'll soon start to sort out and recognize who's who in this alphabet soup.

For the record, here's a quick rundown of the titles behind the initials you listed: doctor of nursing science; clinical nurse specialist; trauma nurse specialist; family nurse practitioner; fellow, American Academy of Nursing; certified gastrointestinal clinician; certified nephrology nurse; certified nurse, operating room; certified occupational health nurse; certified pediatric nurse associate.

As the trend continues, many more nurses who head departments of nursing in hospitals will have a DNS, PhD, or EdD. Good for them—and for all of us—when the doctor in charge is a nurse.

What's the proper sequence for listing credentials?

Q In addition to my BSN, I recently received my rehabilitation nurse certification (CRRN). When signing my name, what is the proper sequence for listing my credentials?

A There's no universal rule, so you'll see a different order used from one textbook or journal to another. Most common: list your name, RN licensure, certification, and then your most advanced degree—thus RN, CRRN, BSN.

Departmental hierarchy

Who's responsible for whom?

Q At the small rural hospital where I work, hospital administrators have just placed the respiratory therapy department

D

"under the direct supervision of nursing." This department is staffed by unlicensed people who do treatments and administer aerosol medications.

We're concerned about our legal responsibility for these therapists. If one of them administers the wrong medication or gives the wrong treatment to a patient, would that patient's nurse be liable?

A In general, you needn't worry about liability because the hospital's new policy is administrative, not practice related. A staff nurse usually is liable only for her own actions (except when she's supervising a student nurse or serving as a preceptor for a new staff nurse). She isn't liable for the negligence of nonnursing personnel.

Many hospitals place departments under the administrative jurisdiction of others; for example, the critical care unit may operate under the control of the emergency department, anesthesia under surgery, and so on. But individuals employed in those departments aren't responsible for each other's actions.

You *could* run into liability when administering medications—for instance, if you pour a medication and give it to an unlicensed respiratory therapist to administer. State laws generally are specific about who may administer medications and under what circumstances.

Deposition

What does a deposition actually involve?

Q A few years ago, I was the witness to a medication error that led to a lawsuit against the hospital where I work. Now I've been asked to give a deposition about the incident. What does a deposition actually involve? Is there some way I can prepare for it?

A Before a lawsuit goes to trial, both parties in the suit are given the "right of discovery"—the right to question the witnesses about the matter in the suit. The witnesses' answers are called a deposition. This is given under oath, recorded, and used as evidence at the trial.

The purpose of a deposition is to diminish the possibility of surprise in a trial. It's a preview of the witnesses' versions of the story. That way, both parties are prepared to counter or corroborate those versions at the actual trial.

Many a nurse has been unnerved at the fast pace and unfamiliarity of the pretrial examination because she wasn't properly prepared. To make sure that doesn't happen to you, get the charts (and any other documents pertaining to the lawsuit) from your hospital's records. Go over these documents line by line to jog your memory of what happened and to help organize your thinking. Then get a lawyer. (If the hospital's lawyer or your malpractice insurance carrier's lawyer can't help you, get one on your own—it's worth it.)

Here are some other pointers to help you when giving your deposition:

• Don't be antagonistic toward the cross-examining lawyer, but don't let him intimidate you.

• Explain yourself simply and honestly without any dramatization. Be organized in your thinking and speaking.

• Never deny discussing your case with your lawyer.

• Ask the lawyers to repeat questions that you didn't hear or understand.

• Don't show any signs of displeasure at testimony with which you disagree.

Smart thinking to take the time *now* to prepare for your pretrial examination. Because when it comes to giving a deposition, the Boy Scouts got it right: be prepared.

Depressed nurse

How can a hospice nurse cope with her job?

Q My sister, a hospice nurse, once enjoyed the challenge of caring for dying patients. But now she seems depressed about her work. The other day, I heard her say that she's tired of seeing so much death. I love her and want to help—but how?

A You can begin by telling her that you love and care about her. But don't be upset if these wonderful words don't seem to make much of a difference at first. Her depression may prevent her from really hearing them.

Remember, depression is anger turned inward. Your sister may be feeling angry because death is snatching people away despite her efforts to save them.

The problem may be that she's now bottling up the emotions that accompany anger. A lot of people become so good at this that they aren't even aware of denying these feelings.

Suppose you say to your sister, "You don't seem like yourself. Is there anything you'd like to talk about?" She might respond, "Nothing's wrong; I'm fine."

If she does, just accept her statement. She may be denying her feelings, or she may just have difficulty appearing weak in front of you. Don't push her for more than she's ready to give. Even if she doesn't open up, your caring message still might have gotten through.

If she does open up to you, encourage her to discuss her feelings with other hospice nurses. They feel the same way.

If she continues to feel depressed, however, she may need a break from hospice nursing. Suggest that she find a nursing job that won't require her to care for dying patients every day.

But no job change can protect your sister from experiencing occasional periods of pain and stress. To guard against depression, she needs to know that she can talk openly about her feelings—to you, and to a few dear friends.

How can she be helped?

Q One of my staff, a terrific pediatric nurse, is professionally first-rate. Personally, however, she's unstable. She stays off from work at unpredictable times. Sometimes, she calls me at home in a depressed state and talks of committing suicide. She's been in and out of analysis for over 4 years. As a friend, I'd like to know how I can best help her. As a supervisor, I'd like to know if, because of her instability, she could ever pose a threat to the well-being of my patients?

A If you judge this nurse to be "professionally first-rate", it appears that she's got enough control to restrict her problems to her home life. If that's so, then it wouldn't seem you'd have any worry about her job performance.

As to your personal relationship, there seems to be a certain tone of overprotective ownership in your language that raises some questions: *my* staff, *my* patients, calls *me* at home, how *I* can best help her.

Is it possible you're being maneuvered into the role of "hovering mother hen?" Clearly the nurse's depressed phone calls and talk of suicide are cries for help. But did it ever occur to you that your continuing sympathetic responses could possibly be impeding her quest for emotional stability?

In terms of transactional analysis, your friend seems to be playing the "Ain't It Awful" game. In this, the player openly expresses distress because of his real suffering but is also secretly gratified at the satis-

factions wrought from his misfortune. As long as your friend can hang the rescue role on someone else, she's not going to take any responsibility for herself.

You're not qualified to give her the intensive, professional help she needs. So, the next time she calls with her problems, try responding in a kindly but no-nonsense manner. Tell her you understand her feelings, but that since she won't seek professional help, you're puzzled by the options open to you and her in this relationship. By maintaining a caring but constructive attitude, you may be able to motivate her to bring about change.

On the other hand, maybe it won't and she'll continue to call for help. If the relationship becomes too disturbing for you, you may have to protect yourself by withdrawing. That's an easy thing to say, much harder to do. Turning a deaf ear to a cry for help from a friend is difficult for anyone—especially for a nurse dedicated to a helping profession.

Sorry there's no pat answer to this second part of your question. It's a difficult decision. Just use your head as well as your heart.

Depression

How can a woman with postpartum depression be helped?

Q Working on an obstetric unit, we're so conscious of the physical and psychological implications of "postpartum blues" that we provide anticipatory teaching about this problem for each patient. Even so, two or three times a month, we'll get a patient who is unusually depressed around the third postpartum day.

These "blue" stages are short-lived and seldom represent ongoing psychopathology. But that's no help to the patient during her depressed

period. We just know that some nurse somewhere has met this problem and come up with a practical way to ease the patient's depression and help her cope. Suggestions?

A Beautiful! You really understand that we don't nurse *patients*—we nurse people. And how commendably aware you are of their individual needs. So, in answer to your question, forget about that tired truism, "Well, maybe if we all just smile a little more." If there's one thing the patient does *not* need at this point, it's the "cheer squad" bustling about, smiling, chirping, and emphasizing, by contrast, the patient's depression. Rather, consider the program of some innovative nurses at a hospital in Minneapolis.

Realizing that the patient's depression comes, in part, from feeling overwhelmed by awesome new responsibilities, the nurses set about to let the new mother know that she is *not* alone, that others *do* care. They had the administration reconsider some hospital policies. Now, in cooperation with the food services department, they invite the new mother and father to a special "Stork Dinner" on the evening of the patient's stay. This is a filet mignon dinner—with all the trimmings—served on special table linens, by candlelight and with a glass of wine or a cocktail. It really serves as an evening out and has been a highlight for both parents.

Then, with the support of administration and the medical staff, visiting hours were modified to permit the father to visit ad lib. He, in turn, is encouraged to bring any other children in the family to visit their mother and see the new baby through the nursery window. This involves the whole family and gives the mother something to look forward to.

If your hospital isn't prepared to implement all these changes, perhaps you could work on the special dinner first. Sometimes, it's just that little bit of extra attention that could turn the blues into a rainbow.

Dermatitis

How can a nurse keep her hands out of soap and water when they're dirty?

Q I'm a staff nurse working on a medical/surgical unit. About 6 months ago, my doctor told me I had chronic dermatitis and prescribed a topical steroid, which I apply frequently. He also told me to keep my hands out of soap and water. Sure—just try that when you're on duty.

There's got to be some solution to this problem, and I'd welcome any suggestions.

A Telling a nurse to avoid soap and water is like telling a painter to avoid turpentine. It just isn't practical.

Not to worry. Here are some ways you can avoid unnecessary contact with the three culprits that are most likely aggravating your chronic dermatitis:

> *"I have chronic dermatitis and the doctor told me to keep my hands out of soap and water—just try that when you're on duty."*

• Use tepid instead of hot water.
• Use a wide-spectrum antibacterial skin cleanser instead of soap. It won't irritate your hands when you use tepid water.
• Use cotton gloves inside surgeon's gloves when exposing your hands to solvents, such as alcohol, or during any procedure requiring gloved hands. (But don't routinely wear gloves.)

One final word: Follow your doctor's prescription carefully. The topical steroid you're applying "frequently" isn't a hand cream.

Diabetes educator

What's necessary to become one?

Q I've been working on a medical/surgical unit for 2 years now, but I want to be a diabetes educator someday—perhaps branching out to independent practice. You see, I have diabetes myself, and I already do a lot of patient teaching on this and other units. I also do volunteer work for the American Diabetes Association. What's the next step for me? And what do I need to know about private practice?

A To become a diabetes educator, you need to have 2 years or 2,000 hours of teaching diabetic patients. You also have to complete the certification examination given by the National Certification Board for Diabetes Educators (NCBDE). This certification will increase your chance of becoming eligible for third-party payment; having your education program recognized by the American Diabetes Association would also help.

As an independent practitioner, you could conduct group diabetes education classes in hospitals or in community programs, or you could teach individual patients in hospitals or homes. Some educators contract with doctors to do their patient teaching for a fee and so avoid the hassle of insurance paperwork or direct billing.

Of course, you should have malpractice insurance. And one caution: Whether you're working under contract or independently, always include a patient's "significant other" when you do any teaching in their home. This can save a lot

of grief for patients who become confused or forgetful—and for you.

For information about certification, contact NCBDE, Professional Testing Corp., Dept. N89, 1211 Avenue of the Americas, 15th Floor, New York, NY 10036, and ask for the *Handbook for Candidates*.

Diabetics

How many times can syringes be used?

Q I've heard that some diabetics reuse their syringes up to five times. Is this okay?

A Syringes may be reused, but five times seems excessive. The needle becomes duller after each use, and the risk of infection increases with each injection. Limit reuse to two or three times and recap and store the syringe in the refrigerator between uses.

A recent report in *Diabetes Care* supports this opinion. Investigators questioned 120 diabetic patients and found that 10 of them reused their syringes anywhere from 2 to 16 times. Local reactions were rare, although two patients experienced pain at the injection site after three injections with the same needle.

In a subsequent controlled study, 37 hospitalized diabetic patients received three consecutive injections reusing the same syringes and needles, with the series repeated from 2 to 20 times during the patients' hospital stays. No localized infection was observed at the injection site; however, 10 patients experienced pain at the injection site (four pain reports after the first injection, four after the second, and five after the third).

You might keep these statistics in mind. Diabetes is an expensive disease to have. So every savings that can be safely achieved will help your patients.

What can be done if she's refusing to follow even the most basic recommendations?

Q I'm having trouble with a patient in the nursing home where I work. She has diabetes, and her fasting blood sugar level has never dipped below 200 mg/dl (normal is 80 to 120 mg/dl). Yet she refuses to have routine blood samples drawn or to let us perform other diagnostic tests. She won't stick to her prescribed meal plan, which limits her to 1,800 calories a day. This woman eats two or three candy bars a day.

In short, she's refusing to follow our most basic recommendations.

What can we do?

A When you're confronted with a patient who refuses to accept sound medical and nursing care, you're in one of the toughest situations a nurse can face. You're sorely limited, but you *can* take these basic steps:
1. Try to find out why the patient isn't following recommendations.
2. Inform her family that she's refusing treatment. They might have information the patient's not sharing with you; and they may supply clues that will help you persuade the patient to comply.
3. Confer with all other health care personnel involved in her care. Maybe they've been giving the patient conflicting (and therefore confusing) information and advice.
4. Explain the purpose of the treatment and the consequences of noncompliance to her. Ask her to repeat what you've just told her to be sure she understood you.
5. Ask her to participate in developing her own care plan— one that she *and* the staff can accept and live with.
6. Document her refusal to follow treatment. If possible, have another nurse initial the chart as a witness.

Who knows? At some future time, you may find it useful to have someone back you up in this matter.
7. Keep trying to convince her that she's jeopardizing her health, and possibly her life, by ignoring the treatment plan.

You're free to do just about anything to persuade the patient to change her mind—short of issuing verbal threats or using physical force. But if she digs in her heels and holds her position, you cannot make her consent against her will.

Diarrhea

What will prevent it?

Q This summer, after we take the state board exams, three of my friends and I will be vacationing abroad. Money will be tight, so we'll be stopping at hostels and eating at places not mentioned in guidebooks.

We've heard lots of comedy routines about traveler's diarrhea. Do you have any tips that will help us avoid it?

A Traveler's diarrhea is no joke. Nothing can make you *homesick* faster than a severe attack of this malady.

You might escape it if you follow standard prevention tips: Don't drink tap water or reconstituted fruit juices. Instead, drink bottled carbonated drinks (the carbonation increases acidity and reduces the possibility of contamination). Avoid eating raw fruit and peeled vegetables, salads, or food from street vendors. Don't eat uncooked or undercooked meat or fish, and dairy products unless you know they've been pasteurized and kept chilled. Be vigilant. Don't decide after 10 days that you're impervious to the disease, or the next thing you eat or drink could prove you wrong—and ruin your trip.

A panel of medical experts recently gathered at the National Institutes of Health to discuss traveler's diarrhea. In contrast to the opinion of many doctors, the panel opposes taking any medications as a prophylaxis for diarrhea. Their rationale: Since drugs can cause adverse reactions, they're not worth the risk for all travelers (many wouldn't get diarrhea anyway, even without medication).

The panel does, however, suggest that certain medications can ease discomfort and shorten an attack of diarrhea. You'll probably want to have some on hand. So to be sure they're Food and Drug Administration-approved, buy them before you leave on your trip.

Among such medications are the antibiotics doxycycline (Vibramycin) and co-trimoxazole (Bactrim, Septra), obtainable by prescription only. Because these drugs act by killing the offending organism, taking them could reduce a diarrhea attack that might normally persist for 3 or more days to 30 hours or less. Over-the-counter drugs include kaolin-pectin mixtures (Kaopectate) and loperamide HCl (Imodium A-D). For a milder attack, take bismuth subsalicylate (Pepto-Bismol), but not if you're also taking aspirin. Both these products contain salicylate, so the combination could cause bleeding. According to recent studies, bismuth subsalicylate tablets are as effective as the liquid (although their onset of action is somewhat slower). They're also easier to pack.

Dictation

What will motivate the doctors to dictate their notes sooner?

Q At the busy family practice where I work, the doctors are 3 to 5 months behind in dictating their notes for patients' charts. This means that charts are stacked by the dictaphone; when we need one (to check phone requests for medication refills, or even for a patient making a return visit), the search begins. Can you imagine how frustrating and time-wasting this exercise becomes? And we nurses aren't the only ones hampered; the insurance clerk can't get her work done either.

> *"The doctors are 3 to 5 months behind in dictating their notes for patients' charts."*

We've complained to the office manager again and again. She claims the doctors always promise they'll do better—just to get her off their case—but they never change. Seems they just can't appreciate the bind we're in.

Do you have any workable ideas for us before we all quit?

A What you need stat is a session or two with an office management consultant who's familiar with medical practice. Someone who can streamline procedures, update forms, and recommend changes—dictation, filing, computer, and so forth—will help save your sanity and, incidentally, keep the malpractice lawyers away. (How good can notes be that are dictated even 3 months late?) A management consultant can also show your bosses the bottom line: how much in dollars and cents inefficency is actually costing *them*. This should grab their attention.

Plan ahead; use the consultant's time wisely. Know exactly what your problems are, avoid vague complaints, and be able to spell out how disorganization is affecting your job performance. Be ready with some suggestions, and keep your own documentation of proposals made during the meeting to be sure they're all included in the consultant's final report.

Difficult co-worker

Any tactics for dealing with an unpleasant nurse?

Q One of my co-workers is intelligent and skillful; she's also a manipulative know-it-all. If she's nice to us, we know she wants help getting her work done. No one on our unit can stand her.

I know that I have to get along with her—we're under enough strain trying to get our work done on our understaffed unit. But when I see her name on the schedule, I dread going to work. What do you suggest?

A You probably won't be able to change her basic personality, but you can identify and work on modifying those problem behaviors that really get to you. Keep your cool, and remind yourself often that all you want is a tolerable working relationship, not an enduring friendship.

Try using the same behavior modification techniques on your co-worker as you'd use with difficult patients: Reinforce her good points—there surely are some—by noticing them and complimenting her for them. Try to ignore the behaviors that make you mad (any attention, even anger, can be reinforcing).

When she's at her worst, note what events immediately preceded the incident. For some people, a precipitating factor triggers a particular behavior; knowing when to expect it can help you cope. Be creative: If she really "knows it all," encourage her to make a presentation at the next staff meeting. Is she lonely? Bite the bullet and ask her to have lunch with you.

Finally, try to take away the advantage she gains from her problem behavior. For instance, if there's no emergency, firmly and impersonally refuse to help with her patient care. How many days do you suppose she'll scramble at the end of the shift—getting her work done without your help—before she gets the message?

What can a newcomer do about a difficult nursing assistant?

Q We've just settled into a nice small town where my husband's taken a new job. I found a nursing job easily enough at the local hospital, but I've run into trouble already. The chief problem is one of the nursing assistants. She ridicules my Southern accent and complains to my supervisor that I don't "help" enough. She means I'm not helping her with *her* job—distributing pitchers of ice water and cleaning beds after they've been vacated.

As a newcomer, I don't feel in a position to make complaints. Besides, I'm not sure where I could turn in such a small hospital with established cliques.

Any advice?

A Why not deal with the assistant first?

Take a break with her in the cafeteria; share a cup of coffee and *some* of what's on your mind. Psychology suggests a wise way to handle such behavior is to ignore it; the theory is that any attention to the objectionable behavior can only reinforce it. Ignore her behavior, yes, but not the assistant. At this point, remember the old adage about catching more flies with honey than with vinegar. Tell her that you'd like to be friends and that you'd appreciate her help in adjusting to your new job.

If, after your best efforts, you're still meeting the nursing assistant's hostility, the situation swings from a primarily personal predicament to a professional responsibility.

You tried to work through the problem with an informal approach (taking your coffee break with her). Now the situation calls for a more formal approach: Take the problem to your unit manager.

You're not tattling; you're informing your supervisor of a situation that might threaten patient care.

Don't let this get you down. However, since yours is probably the only hospital in this "nice small town," you may have to bide your time, hold your temper—and call upon your personal and professional resources to help the situation evolve rather than erupt.

What can be done about a nursing assistant's poor performance?

Q I work part-time in a large teaching hospital. A girl who was a former nursing student here is currently working as a nursing assistant. She was suspended from the school for cheating but then, after sleeping with a male professor, was reinstated. Until the next semester starts, though, she's here as a nursing assistant.

Some nursing assistant! Just because she's made brownie points with the charge nurse and the nurse-manager, she's allowed to do catheterizations, tube feedings, and discontinue I.V.s. She takes doctors' orders over the phone and sometimes carries the narcotics keys when the nurses are off the floor. A lot of us resent this and question the legality of such practices.

Furthermore, she tries to tell everyone how to do their jobs and has said, behind my back, that I'm incompetent.

I'd like advice, but don't suggest that I find another job. The part-time I'm now on fits exactly with my home duties.

A First of all, we don't know how you know that this girl was dismissed for cheating. Such information is usually kept strictly between the covers of the student's file. And we don't know how you know this girl was sleeping with a professor. That kind of information is usually kept strictly between the

covers—period.

But, because it's *your* letter, we accept all this personal information as correct. Correct...but irrelevant.

The relevant part of your letter starts with this girl's working performance. We know that the scope of a nursing assistant's job will vary with the institution. We would very much question, however, a nursing assistant's transcribing doctors' telephone orders or carrying the narcotics key.

> *"I couldn't believe a former nursing student, who was suspended for cheating, was reinstated after sleeping with a male professor."*

We suggest you first check with your hospital policy manual for its description of a nursing assistant's job. Once you're sure of your ground, plan to take anecdotal notes on the duties assumed by this girl that are beyond the scope of a nursing assistant. For example: "April 15, Ms. X was given the narcotics keys from 1 p.m. to 3 p.m. On April 21, accepted two telephone orders from Drs. Y & Z."

This doesn't mean that you have to bird-dog the girl; it means that you should keep records as you see these things happen. When you have enough, take them to your nurse-manager. After all, she's the one who's legally responsible for delegating the authority—and for many mistakes that could occur from the misuse of that authority.

State the facts you've collected and *stick* to the facts. Make it clear that your primary concern is for patient safety. There are serious questions to be raised about an employee's functioning beyond her specified duties, and you are justified in having them answered.

Don't get into personalities. Let the documented facts speak for themselves.

What if there's been no response to complaints about a co-worker?

Q Over 3 months ago, I sent an anonymous letter to the director of nursing concerning the improper behavior of two of my co-workers.

Apparently my observations were disregarded because no changes have been made. Is there any other recourse I can take?

A Anonymous letters may be suitable means of communication for bank robbers and kidnappers. But highly unsuitable for a professional nurse.

If you had something sufficiently serious to report to someone in authority (not just gossip, or the like), then you should have done it in person or by signed notice.

Certainly you might not want face-to-face confrontation with co-workers you suspect of wrongdoing. But there must be someone in your organization to whom you could turn, knowing that she would strictly respect your request for anonymity.

A responsible person who asks for anonymity can still maintain her credibility. The author of an anonymous letter cannot.

As one administrator says, "The only anonymous letter I ever received concerning an employee was promptly shredded and 'filed' in the wastebasket."

Why should a nurse be expected to work overtime because of somebody else's irresponsibility?

Q I'm a 22-year-old charge nurse on a 42-bed medical/surgical unit. My problem is a 40-year-old nursing assistant. Her manner is loud and abrasive to patients and co-workers, and nobody likes her. We could endure her personality but her work performance is something else. She won't give postop care unless repeatedly pressed to do so. She frequently falsifies vital signs. She skips suctioning patients, and, when confronted, claims the patients didn't need it when she checked them.

I've tried to talk to her but it's always "somebody else's fault." I've had two supervisors speak to her—again without results.

The staff suspects the only reason she's lasted so long (6 years) is because she's the director of nursing's neighbor and they do a lot of socializing together.

I've been working behind this assistant, trying to give the care she neglects. But I'm sick of working overtime because of somebody else's irresponsibility. What can I do?

A The solution to your problem could very well lie in one word: documentation.

You and the two supervisors have verbally alerted the nursing assistant that her work is unsatisfactory. Now put it all in writing. You say she falsified vital signs. Call the supervisor immediately when you discover this, and get her to witness it. Aside from the moral irresponsibility toward the patients, falsification of records could present a legal liability for you, your supervisor, and the hospital.

Detail every incident (patient, room number, date, time, actions involved). Ask other nurses who work with the assistant for any evidence of patient neglect they observe. Again, get it in writing.

Once you have enough evidence (5 to 10 incidents), check your policy manual for procedure. If this isn't covered in your manual, bring duplicate copies of all your material to your supervisor.

If your supervisor doesn't act (and why she didn't take action against this nursing assistant long ago is a matter for speculation), then go to the director.

Perhaps others on the staff, wary of testing the director's professional responsibility against her personal friendship, have never told her about the nursing assistant. But your written documentation is something that cannot be ignored.

If the director chooses not to take action on it, however, then we suggest you ask for a transfer.

As a charge nurse, you're liable for any neglience that occurs on your unit. Why should you risk your career for this irresponsible worker? You've performed conscientiously toward your patients and your hospital. You must also be fair to yourself.

Difficult doctor

Any suggestions for dealing with him?

Q For 3 years, I worked for a general practitioner at a local clinic. We worked well together with no problems. He's now on a 1-year leave of absence, and I've been assigned to work for another doctor until he gets back.

This doctor is impossible to work with. For one thing, he's inconsistent about how he wants things done, and when he isn't satisfied with the way I drape a patient or set up the examining room, he launches into a long lecture, in front of the patient. This embarrasses me and the patient, and it wastes everybody's time.

Second, he expects me to order prescription refills when patients request them. He says he'll back me up if I make mistakes. I've told him that my ordering refills without first consulting him is illegal, but he's still insisting—very unpleasantly.

Third, when he's making hospital rounds, he wants me to see patients who come to the walk-in clinic with colds, sore throats, urinary tract infections, and so on, do what I can for their symptoms, and send them home.

So far, I've refused, but every time I call him to tell him a patient's in the clinic, he yells at me. Sometimes he refuses to come in. I've complained to my supervisor who says she can't relieve me because no one else will work with this nasty doctor. I don't want to leave the clinic because I know I'll get to work with the other doctor when he returns, but I'm at the end of my rope. What do you suggest?

A It's up to your supervisor and the clinic administrator to bail you out. If no one else will work with this doctor, how can they expect you to, without some help?

Document the occasions the doctor is verbally abusive and demands that you order prescriptions or diagnose illnesses. Give these to your supervisor, and tactfully, but firmly, insist on her help.

Your supervisor will probably have to consult the clinic administrator, who can deal with the doctor. You've given the clinic several years of competent nursing—now it's their turn to give you some support.

Should a nurse be expected to take verbal abuse?

Q I'm a 24-year-old team leader on a 36-bed medical/surgical unit. Recently I had to call a doctor because his patient had taken an unexpected turn for the worse with signs of impending ventricular fibrillation. The doctor ordered some medications, then suddenly launched into a lengthy, abusive tirade against me personally! He said I was getting upset over nothing (I was, in fact, completely calm) and that I needed treatment more than the patient. He continued on this personal level.

If I'd only been sure he was finished with his orders for the patient, I would have hung right up on him.

This doctor is known throughout the hospital as a loudmouth. And he's pulled this little number on other nurses, too. Our supervisor is sympathetic with us but says there's nothing she can do about it.

So where does that leave us nurses? Are we just expected to take this kind of verbal abuse?

A Congratulations on your professionalism in hanging on to your temper (and the phone) until you were certain you'd received all the orders for your failing patient.

This problem's not primarily the *supervisor's* responsibility. Since the conflict occurred between you and the doctor, *you* should take the *primary* step in settling it.

> *"The doctor suddenly launched into a lengthy, abusive tirade against me personally and said I needed treatment more than the patient."*

One way to deal with a "screamer" is on a one-to-one basis and in a private place (the supervisor's office). Make just such an appointment with this doctor. Without recrimination, explain that you welcome constructive criticism but his manner had precluded any possible learning experience for you. (For example, why had he judged you upset over nothing? Did he know something about the patient you didn't?)

This doctor's manner had also precluded any likely benefits for him. If he'd taken the time for an explanation, you might have been able to make more pertinent observations of his future patients and eliminate what he seems to consider unnecessary phone calls.

Even doctors admit that personal conflicts are gong to crop up (doctors take their lumps from nurses, too, you know) and these are best settled one-to-one.

If personal confrontation doesn't correct the situation, then you should pursue the matter through channels.

When a similar conflict occurred in one hospital, the complainant nurse and her supervisor followed it right up to the joint committee of medical staff and trustees where the problem was effectively settled.

The director of nursing related to the problem more personally: "When a team leader and her supervisor don't know where to turn for help in a case like this, it's an indictment of the entire nursing service leadership.

"If such an organization has a grievance procedure, it mustn't have been used in a long time. That shouldn't stop the nurse, however, from searching it out and reactivating it.

"One word of caution. As director of nursing, I have too often arranged to face down an offending physician only to have my complaisant nurse, at the last moment, desert me. If this nurse is serious about correcting the problem, she'd better convince her superiors that she has the courage and stamina to see it through. Perhaps that very action will generate a little backbone into their entire nursing service."

What can be done about a doctor's libelous remarks?

Q I work at a long-term care facility for the mentally retarded and physically disabled. Recently, our staff doctor castigated the night-shift nurses for failing to administer thyroid medication to several patients as ordered. Six nurses (myself included) had signed the patients' charts to indicate that we gave the medication— dessicated thyroid (Armour Thyroid), which normally increases serum thyroid hormone levels.

However, because the patients still had decreased thyroxine (T_4) levels, the doctor concluded that we couldn't have given the medication. Their triiodothyronine (T_3) levels were all within normal limits, but that didn't seem to matter to him. He ignored the fact that most of the patients were also receiving phenytoin (Dilantin), which can depress T_4 levels. He refused to order any further tests.

Instead, he changed the administration time from 6 a.m. (our shift) to 8 a.m. (next shift). He then wrote some caustic remarks about the night shift's competence right on the patients' charts, where other nurses and doctors could read them. We feel these remarks are libelous and may jeopardize our licenses.

The doctor won't talk to us about this matter. We did discuss it with our director of nursing, but she offered little support. We must do something to defend our professional reputations; otherwise, it looks as though we're admitting the doctor was right. What would you suggest?

A Take the offensive—all of you. Remember, there's strength in numbers. Get together and write a letter, pointing out that you gave the medication as ordered and that your signatures attesting to this fact are part of the patients' permanent records, as are the doctor's remarks.

The discrepancy between what you're saying and what the doctor's saying should ensure the administration's prompt attention, since such a discrepancy could put the facility in a vulnerable position in the event of a malpractice suit. Make sure you send a copy of the letter to the lawyer who represents the facility in court cases.

You're right to be concerned about how this incident might reflect on your reputations. But you're not about to lose your licenses over it. We sometimes overestimate a

D

doctor's influence when it comes to causing trouble for even one nurse—let alone an entire nursing shift, as in your case. Oh sure, a doctor may raise a ruckus and say disagreeable things about you, but he can't change your nurses' notes or jeopardize your licenses with an unsubstantiated accusation.

Whatever happened to the patient's advocate?

Q As a nursing student at a university hospital doing my first rotation in labor and delivery, I'm upset by what I see. Though the nursing care is superbly supportive, the attitude and behavior of many of the young doctors toward the patients is so uncaring that I'm appalled.

Yesterday, a resident and two medical students were talking about delivering porpoises at Sea World while a young woman was being prepared for her first delivery. Not one of the three men showed a mite of concern for this patient, who was so apprehensive she clutched my hand until the anesthetic took effect.

Here's another instance of the thoughtless care here: Today I witnessed a labor and delivery that was scheduled to be Lamaze. Both the wife and husband had attended classes for months in preparation. But the woman's doctor was out of town and another doctor took over. The stand-in doctor did not approve of the Lamaze approach. He refused to let the husband into the delivery room. When the patient was wheeled in for delivery, she needed only a few good contractions before the birth. But the anesthesiologist gave her nitrous oxide, which decreased her contractions. The doctor must have become impatient; he used forceps to hurry the delivery along, leaving a 2-inch-long mark on the baby's head.

Incidents like these make me furious. Some of my more cynical

friends tell me "this happens all the time." I don't think I'm dewy-eyed or naive enough to believe that everyone in the medical profession puts the patient's well-being first. But I'm wondering: Whatever happened to the patient's advocate?

A Your taking the time to write demonstrates admirable concern. In the situations you describe, the doctors sorely need some understanding of the feelings of women in labor and delivery.

The American College of Obstetrics and Gynecology has put out a position paper in which it joins with four other major medical and nursing organizations in advocating a humanistic approach to delivery and concerned care for the whole family unit. The father should not only be *allowed* but be *encouraged* to stay in the delivery room, the paper says.

Do *your* part in proving that the patient's advocate is alive, well, and at work.

Difficult nurse-manager

Should a letter of resignation blame her?

Q I love nursing and know I'm good at it. But after working for over a year in this hospital, I'm being driven to resignation by my nurse-manager. On several occasions I've tried to stand up to her; that just made her hostile toward me. I complained to the director of nursing; she just tried to soothe my ruffled feathers, saying the problem's a personality conflict.

In my letter of resignation, would it be appropriate to say I'm quitting because of this nurse-manager? And if I find out the director of nursing won't give me a good recommendation, can I omit this hos-

pital from my next application? (My other references are excellent.)

I feel frustrated and would appreciate your advice.

A Hold off taking any action immediately. Perhaps the nurse-manager has you so riled up you can't think straight. Try to separate your emotions from the facts while you consider your options.

Here are some of them. Quitting is only one of four options: (1) stick out the intolerable situation; (2) stick it out while trying to change it; (3) transfer to another unit; or (4) quit.

From what you say, you've had your fill of Option 1, and you're disillusioned with Option 2 because the director of nursing discounted your complaints. But what *are* your complaints? (You didn't mention a single example.) Did you give the director of nursing a list of specific incidents, with dates and witnesses? Without such documentation, she couldn't possibly evaluate the situation fairly.

If you're past giving it another try, how about transferring to another unit? Why let your anger at someone else drive you from your job? Finally, if quitting is the only option you can live with, naming names or listing grievances has no place in your letter of resignation. Just explain that you want to further your career and try nursing somewhere else. Then, if you want someone in personnel to know the details of your decision, mention your reasons during your exit interview. (Remember, your co-workers are bound to be curious. Avoid the temptation to discredit the nurse-manager.)

Can you omit this hospital's name in your next application? Better not. Most recruiters recommend listing all professional experience. During the interview, you can mention your reasons for leaving. If you stick to the facts, most interviewers will accept your version.

Difficult orderly

What can be done about him?

Q Since getting my license 18 months ago, I've worked nights on a medical/surgical unit in an urban hospital. Agency nurses usually make up the rest of the staff, so I'm in charge. We're all very busy and work well together—my only problem is with an orderly who's not doing his job.

> *"The orderly wears headphones and listens to rock music while on duty, and he hides out in patients' rooms eating or sleeping instead of working..."*

He wears headphones and listens to rock music while on duty, he hides out in patients' rooms eating or sleeping instead of working, and he doesn't take kindly to direction or criticism—especially from someone who's a few years younger than he is.

What should I do about him?

A You shouldn't be stuck dogging this orderly's behavior alone. Tip off the night supervisor that you're having problems; she can drop in during the shift and get on this orderly's case.

Here are other recommendations: Sit down with him and go over his job description. Spell out what's expected, such as helping to lift patients, emptying urine bags, running errands. Remain as neutral in tone as possible. When you're sure he understands his duties, give him a copy of his job description and let him know that all orderlies must meet these standards or risk being fired.

Document that you had this session, and continue to briefly document each time he's derelict, what's said, his response (just facts, not emotions), and any other staff complaints. Go back and share this documentation with him, so he can't say later that you never told him.

He should shape up—but don't wait too long for results. Annoyances like this can disrupt the whole unit. Meet with your manager, give her your documentation, and let her take it from there. Helping the orderly know what's expected is your job—reprimanding him if he doesn't follow through is hers.

Difficult patient

How should he be handled?

Q One of our patients makes lewd comments and obscene gestures to all the nurses—but to me especially, because I'm young and embarrass easily. The law protects against sexual harassment from a boss or co-worker in the workplace, but what am I supposed to do when a patient acts like this?

A You never have to tolerate outrageous behavior. Start by holding a conference with the nursing staff, and ask a psychiatric nurse clinician to attend. She can help identify your patient's underlying message. Actually, he may not be expressing sexual needs at all; he may be lonely or insecure. And feeling that he's lost control of his life, he might be acting out in ways that brought him control in the past. So your goal is to channel his energy away from his struggle for power toward more acceptable behavior.

Here are some suggestions: Let your patient know up front that you're reacting negatively to his *behavior,* not to him. Don't be afraid to let him know how you feel by saying something like, "I really don't like that kind of talk." And *you* set limits: "That kind of behavior makes it impossible for me to give you the care you need. I'll be back later; perhaps we can work together then." And when he acts appropriately, reinforce that behavior by rewarding him with added attention, perhaps a few extra minutes to chat. Allow him some control over his own care; that will focus his attention on his own care needs and increase his self-confidence. Last, but not least, don't be too hard on yourself. Sure, you may be embarrassed at first, but *you'll* gain confidence from coping professionally with this troublesome patient.

Difficult unit

What can be done to improve staff relationships?

Q I've recently been promoted from team leader to assistant unit manager on a 38-bed medical/surgical unit. In a way, as I'll explain presently, the unit manager is new to her job, too.

Together, we've inherited a unit with a reputation for disorganization and staff conflicts. Right now, being assigned to our unit's not too popular.

I'm sure the situation's not helped by the fact that our nurse-patient ratio is 9:1 (on the other floors, the ratio is 4:1). The nursing assistants seem to be doing a lot of the patient care while we nurses are saddled with an ever-increasing load of paperwork.

At the moment, our most troublesome problem is the inability to resolve the personality conflicts; in particular, the gap between nurses and nursing assistants seems to be widening. The staff conflict is intensified by the difference between the unit manager's leadership style and mine.

D

Here's some background: the unit manager, who's in her mid-forties, has recently returned to work after raising her family. She's an easygoing person, and takes a laissez-faire approach. She thinks if she stays out of the conflicts between staff members, the problems will take care of themselves. She counts on getting respect and cooperation from the staff because she's older and more experienced.

But things aren't working out that way: The staff (unit secretaries, nursing assistants, and nurses) keep their feelings to themselves until the unit manager's day off—then they come to me with their problems and complaints. They tell me it doesn't do any good to talk to the unit manager because "she never does anything."

But I don't think I'm handling this situation too well. I take a stern, authoritative approach—partly because I'm so much younger than the rest of the staff and I'm afraid they won't take me seriously otherwise, and partly because I just don't know what else to do.

Before I forget, I want to make an important point: I consider our staff members hard workers who care about our patients. And the truth is, I don't want to switch units. But neither do I want to continue coming home with a knot in my stomach every night.

I think our staff relationships need some intensive care. What can we do?

A Why not accentuate the positive? A difference in style between you and the unit manager could become a positive factor in your relationship—and a good thing for the unit. As unit manager, she has the responsibility for making decisions about nursing. But as her assistant, working closely with her, you can be effective in implementing those decisions—since this seems to be the area where she's weak.

However, there's an inherent risk in the situation you've described: By turning to you (and bypassing the unit manager), the staff could unwittingly be driving a wedge between you and the unit manager—and be adding to the existing conflict.

If your unit manager is serenely unaware of all this, as she seems to be, you should point out to her that the staff's making a habit of coming to *you* with their complaints and problems. Your unit manager will soon figure out that something's awry—that *she's* the unit mnager and the staff should be coming to her.

Why not step back and assess the problem as a whole? Examine the possibility that the underlying difficulty is an unreasonable work load. When a staff's overworked and disgruntled, you have a natural breeding ground for conflict. But you'll need facts and figures to determine whether the work load *is* excessive and *is* provoking problems. If you find evidence that the nurse-patient ratio on your unit is burdensomely high, send a documented memo about this through nursing channels. As always, be careful to include only facts and firsthand observations—*not* opinions, hearsay, and impressions.

Discharge

Are there guidelines on how long a sedated patient should stay on the unit before discharge?

Q In my work on an outpatient short procedure unit, I frequently evaluate patients for discharge. Many of them have had the drugs morphine, meperidine (Demerol), diazepam (Valium), or midazolam (Versed). Are there any guidelines on how long a patient who received these drugs should

stay on the unit before discharge—particularly someone who intends to drive home?

A You can't base your decision on time alone. Before discharging any outpatient who has received sedatives, be certain:
• his vital signs (blood pressure, pulse rate, and respirations) are stable for at least 30 minutes
• he has been out of bed for 15 minutes or more
• he shows no signs or symptoms of complications, such as hypotension, pain, bleeding, diaphoresis, or vomiting
• he understands your verbal and written instructions on how to manage his care at home.

So far, so good. But you still can't discharge him if he intends to drive himself home—a patient who receives any of the drugs you mentioned shouldn't drive for at least 12 hours. The Joint Commission on Accreditation of Healthcare Organizations addresses this point in its 1988 accreditation manual. It recommends that outpatients who receive sedatives be accompanied at discharge by another adult who can take them home.

So save yourself the hassle, and find out before the procedure begins whether the patient has a driver coming for him. If he doesn't, let him telephone for someone to come get him, or if he has no one to call, ask his doctor if he'll write an order for the patient to go home in a taxicab. If neither works out, you'll have to reschedule the procedure.

Should an RN certified in advanced cardiac life support have transported her father?

Q A few weeks ago, we were arranging for an ambulance to take a patient to a larger metropolitan hospital for a cardiac consultation. (This patient had been admitted for observation after syncope.) But he wanted his daughter—an RN certified in advanced cardiac life support—to drive him there right away. He'd had no further episodes of syncope, so the doctor agreed to this plan, as did the daughter. I charted the patient's request in my nurse's notes. The transfer occurred without incident.

A few days later, the director of medical records asked me to write on the patient's chart "Cancel ambulance. May transfer with daughter by car." And she wanted me to backdate the entry to the day the patient was discharged. When I asked why, she said she wanted to protect the hospital from possible liability.

I refused to do what she asked, but now I'm wondering if she was right. What do you think? (By the way, the original order never specified the mode of transportation.)

A Why had the ambulance been requested in the first place? If ambulance transport was medically indicated, releasing this patient into the care of a relative—no matter how skilled—was inappropriate.

Suppose the patient had had a myocardial infarction or an episode of syncope on the way to the hospital. What would the daughter have done—stopped and performed one-person cardiopulmonary resuscitation? Or rushed her father to the nearest hospital, endangering them and others on the road? If the patient had died or been injured, you and the hospital could have been liable for an inappropriate release and transfer. (Of course, you wouldn't have been at fault if the patient had signed an against-medical-advice form.)

As for the second issue, you were right not to adjust the chart; you could have been charged with fraud. Legally, you can't backdate, tamper

with, or add to notes that were previously written. You may, however, safely add late entries, as long as you label them as such (for example, dating your entry so it's clear you didn't write the note on the same day the patient was discharged).

You might talk with the hospital risk manager about what happened. He may want to find out if other nurses have altered charts in the past. Although the director of medical records meant well, her request could have caused legal problems if the hospital had been sued.

You weren't the person who should have canceled the order anyway. That was the responsibility of the doctor who wrote the original order. However, because his order was ambiguous—it should have specified the mode of transport—you should have clarified it when it was written.

Should a nurse allow an agitated husband to wheel his wife to the car?

Q Recently, I was transferring one of my patients from the bed to a wheelchair for discharge. As soon as she was settled, her husband—who'd been hovering in the background—pushed me aside, grabbed the handles of the wheelchair, and took off for the elevator. I went after him and explained that someone from the hospital had to wheel her to the car. He said that he was tired of all our rules and that he was perfectly capable of taking his wife to the car himself. Because he was so agitated, I let him go. But if my patient had been injured, could I have gotten in trouble for not stopping him?

A No one expects you to confront a patient's agitated or angry spouse—you or the patient might have been injured. But you should have notified your manager and the

security department right away. That's your only responsibility in a situation like this.

You wouldn't be accountable if the patient were injured; you were taken off-guard and couldn't have anticipated the husband's actions.

Should patients be allowed to go home on pass without a written order?

Q I'm an RN on a rehabilitation unit. I've been working here only a few months, but our policy for sending patients home on pass has me worried.

I don't question the benefit of this policy to the patients; I just question the casual way we handle it.

Patients on the unit are allowed to go home at their request without a written order, yet the hospital has no *written* policy stating that this is part of our rehabilitation program. And, since most of the patients need medication, the nurses give them the medication they'll need while they're gone.

Both of these practices worry me. What if something happens to the patient while he's at home? Am I liable for sending him without an order? And am I liable for giving him drugs—even if they've been ordered by his doctor? Everyone else seems to accept our way of handling things—they're even a little irritated at my concern. Am I worrying about nothing?

A You're exposing yourself to potential civil liability for malpractice when you allow patients to leave without written orders. You're also exposing yourself to criminal liability when you dispense dangerous drugs in violation of the law. In short, you have plenty to worry about.

To protect yourself against liability for patients on pass, prior written orders are best. If this isn't practical, you should record the order as a verbal order when the patient leaves, then have the doctor countersign the order as soon as possible.

To protect yourself against liability for dispensing drugs, never dispense any amount of drug greater than the next dose from the nursing station's supply. Any greater amount must be given by the doctor or ordered by him and dispensed by a licensed pharmacist.

You can be sure that you won't win any popularity contests when you insist on these procedures. But—better unpopular than hauled off to court.

Would a nurse be held liable for failing to teach a patient everything about his drugs?

Q I work on a very busy medical/surgical unit. Sometimes I worry that my co-workers and I don't do enough discharge teaching—especially about drugs the patients will be taking at home. Nursing administrators have developed drug cards and information sheets that we give to patients before discharge, but I don't think that's any substitute for one-to-one teaching. Would I be held liable for failing to teach a patient everything he needs to know about his drugs?

A You could be, if he were harmed. Your discharge-teaching duties include instructing your patient about his medications and possible adverse reactions. The drug cards and information sheets you mention may be adequate, as long as you believe he can understand written instructions. But if you feel he can't, you must do more teaching.

In any event, remember to document all patient teaching you do. If a legal problem arises someday, this information would be valuable evidence that you'd performed your duty.

Discharge orders

Should full care be continued while the patient awaits discharge instructions, insurance paperwork, or his ride home?

Q Our medical director says that once he writes discharge orders for a patient, these orders cancel all previous standing medication and treatment orders, and we shouldn't call him about the patient or provide any more care. This is fine for a patient who leaves on schedule. But sometimes a patient must wait several hours for discharge instructions, to finalize insurance paperwork, or for his ride home. We nurses feel we should continue to give full care while he waits—checking vital signs and blood glucose and administering medications—but we have no written policy to support our actions. What do you think of this?

A Discharge orders are only one part of the discharge process and not the end of your responsibility or the hospital's liability for the patient who's leaving. You must maintain a reasonable standard of nursing care for the entire time the patient is under your supervision and until the patient leaves the hospital building. In fact, departing patients are usually escorted to the door.

> *"The medical director says once he writes discharge orders we shouldn't call him about the patient or provide any more care."*

Discuss the issue with your supervisor, and ask nursing administration for written guidelines. The hospital's lawyer will probably sit up, take notice, and act to rescind any order that so flagrantly invites legal liability for the hospital.

Discharge planning

How can a patient accept her doctor's decision?

Q One of my elderly patients has been hospitalized for 2 weeks with a fractured left hip. She can't go back to her apartment because she doesn't have anyone to look after her. The doctor wants her to go to a nursing home, but she's resisting. When I ask why, she just says, "I know that nursing homes are terrible places."

I'm not sure a nursing home is the best alternative for her, but I don't know what else to suggest. I tried to explain that nursing homes aren't as bad as she imagines, but her mind's made up. How can I help her accept her doctor's decision?

A Your patient undoubtedly resents having this major decision thrust upon her—and rightly so. Assuming she's competent, she should participate in the decision making, too. And you can help her by presenting all the options.

First, find out whether her nursing home admission is likely to be temporary or permanent. If it will be temporary, tell her how long she can expect to be there. Then, address her short-term concerns. For instance, she may worry about protecting her belongings, paying her rent, and caring for pets or plants. The hospital's discharge planner can help find relatives or neighbors willing to manage those temporary problems.

Even if her doctor is recommending that she move to a nursing home permanently, she still has options. Perhaps she could stay in her apartment if she had a visiting nurse or a homemaker-companion. Or maybe she could enter an adult family home, a foster care arrangement that's available in many areas. Contact the hospital's social services department to discuss alternatives.

For your patient, entering a nursing home probably represents a permanent loss of control over her life. Help her maintain as much control as possible by giving her all the options and encouraging her to make her own choices.

Is it okay to do a discharge assessment 12 or more hours before discharge?

Q I work on the evening shift in the newborn nursery of a community hospital. Lately, to help the day shift nurses, both the evening and night nurses have been asked to do discharge assessment on some of the babies scheduled for discharge in the morning.

We nurses are concerned about doing a discharge assessment 12 or more hours before discharge. How does this practice sound to you?

A Sounds as reasonable as wearing your clothes to bed to save dressing in the morning. *Come on.* The discharge assessment should be done a maximum of 1 hour before discharge—for a brand-new baby or any patient on any unit.

Obviously babies can't speak up for themselves. You'll have to do the talking for them.

Discouraged nurse

Any advice for a neophyte who's not holding up well under baptism by fire?

Q I'm a recent nursing school graduate and the "new kid on the block" at the hospital where I work. The other nurses tell me it takes time to adjust to the real world of nursing. But after my first few hectic months, I'm beginning to wonder if I'm cut out for this profession.

A big part of the problem is that I'm moved from unit to unit and from shift to shift. One week I might be in the nursery working days; the next week, I'll be working nights in the intensive care unit. I can't seem to work in one unit long enough to learn the ropes and develop any kind of routine.

As a result, my work is becoming more and more disorganized. I'm getting careless—and sometimes fail to double-check things. I can't seem to troubleshoot the way a good nurse should. And when I'm the charge nurse, I'm not sure which jobs to delegate and which jobs to do myself.

Every day I go to work thinking: "Today I'm going to be organized and stay on top of things." And every day I come home frustrated. What advice do you have for a neophyte who's not holding up too well under this baptism by fire?

A Your first few months on a job can be trying, so here are some practical points to help you through this difficult time.
• Meet with your supervisor or nurse-manager and share your concerns with her. Tell her that you don't feel comfortable with floating and you'd like to work in just one unit on a consistent shift schedule for a while. (If you need some backup, cite the studies that have shown that any worker on a variable schedule is likely to become somewhat disoriented and less effective on the job.)
• Get into the habit of attending the staff development sessions offered by your hospital covering areas where you lack knowledge and confidence. If none are scheduled, tell your supervisors how much they're needed.
• Choose an experienced colleague you admire and respect—confide in her—and make her the role model for the nurse you'd like to be. Working closely with an example of nursing competence can be worth all the books on the subject.

• Don't be too hard on yourself. You've successfully completed your nursing school program and passed your state board exams. That means you've worked to reach these goals. Don't give up now.

You certainly have what it takes to become a good nurse. What you need now is some support and some consistent on-the-job training to reinforce your firm foundation.

How much orientation is usual for a nurse with limited experience?

Q After 1 year's experience on a medical/surgical unit, I started a new job last week. My orientation consisted of following a staff nurse around for 2 days as a gofer. She didn't explain techniques, equipment, or unit policy. On my third day, one nurse called in sick, and I was assigned full responsibility for 10 patients. I felt very depressed by the end of that shift.

How much orientation is usual for someone with my limited experience, and what should it include? I'm surviving, but nervous.

A No wonder. Two days' orientation isn't enough for anyone. And caring for 10 patients is too much to expect, especially for someone not familiar with the unit. (Actually, it's a heavy patient load for anyone.) Perhaps you were unlucky enough to be caught in an especially bad bind.

What should you expect of orientation? Depending on size, location, and patient care focus, most hospitals offer a fixed period: 2 weeks, 6 weeks, 3 months. Others gear orientation to an individualized checklist of tasks for new employees to complete. Two weeks is the minimum for orienting someone with limited experience—and not 2 weeks spent just following someone around as a gofer. Each day should be spent on gradually caring for more patients.

Bravo. You've survived your baptism by fire. And you've learned a lesson for next time. Before accepting any job, ask for specifics about the orientation program. Don't be afraid to speak up if your preceptor doesn't help you or if the program isn't all it's cracked up to be.

You can help yourself settle in better now by attending staff development sessions; if none are scheduled, tell your supervisors how much they're needed. Choose an experienced colleague you can turn to for help in answering questions. You may feel nervous now, but before long, you won't be the new kid on the block.

Is being a nursing assistant similar to being a nurse?

Q I worked for a year and a half as a unit secretary in a large hospital. The job took me to all units—from the emergency department to the nursery. I loved the work and decided I'd like to be a nurse.

Having finished my first year of nursing school, I got a summer job as a nursing assistant at the same hospital where I'd previously worked. Not only was the experience unrewarding—I hated every day of it.

Originally, I was attracted to nursing because I'm interested in medicine and like to work with people. But if the work of a nursing assistant is very much like that of a registered nurse, I'd like to know now because I could never be happy at it.

I'd appreciate hearing your thoughts.

A As a unit secretary, you got a certain amount of "psychic income" from knowing that you were part of a helping, humanitarian agency. You enjoyed clean desk work in a role that was highly visible to the public. Your rotation schedule provided you with a stimulating change of surroundings. Your chief contact was not with sick and helpless patients, but with active, competent professionals.

However, with the exception of the first point (working for a humanitarian agency), none of these work experiences was very much related to the role of a nurse. That work experience had to wait until you took a job as a nurse's assistant

Having done so, you now really understand what nursing is basically about. *A nurse cares for the sick.* In so doing, she performs tasks that at times may be offensive (emptying drainage bags, changing foul-smelling dressings). And she deals with difficult people. More than any other member of the hospital staff, the nurse sees the patient at his very worst.

This isn't to minimize the rewards of the profession—helping a new life into this world, easing a failing life out of it. But before you make a lifetime commitment, you owe it to yourself to fully understand the responsibilities, rewards, and frustrations you can look forward to.

First discuss your feelings with your school counselor—or whatever professor you feel most comfortable with. Then—this is important—turn to nurses who are working at the bedside. Watch them in their work and *talk to them.*

You can be perfectly honest about your feelings (that's one of the psychic rewards of nursing—a sense of sisterhood). The nurses you talk to will know of some nurse who really wasn't cut out for the profession and isn't happy in her work. Most of these nurses are students who went along with a trade they weren't really committed to. But, unlike you, they didn't have the foresight and courage to ask the right questions themselves and of experienced counselors. Think again. And good luck whatever your decision.

Is it normal to feel inadequate?

Q Since passing my boards, I've been working on a medical/surgical unit. I wish it were different, but I frankly feel inadequate and scared.

> *"Being new in the field, I feel inadequate, scared, and like a fraud...I'd be satisfied if I could even feel like a good nurse."*

My patients love me and think I'm a great nurse. But I'd be satisfied if I could even feel like a good nurse. Right now, I feel like a fraud, there's so much I don't know. Am I expecting too much too soon?

A Pick any one of the "great" nurses you work with and ask about her early days on the job. Most certainly she, too, felt "frankly inadequate and scared."

Honestly, all you need is practice, practice, practice. You can't expect to soar with the eagles when you're just taking wing.

Is nursing the right profession?

Q I'm 22 and have my BSN from a highly respected university. I started out with energy and high hopes, but now I'm one unhappy nurse, wondering if I'm in the right profession.

In a little more than a year, I've had two jobs. My first was in a coronary care unit, where I felt altogether unprepared for the overwhelming responsibility thrust upon me. My second job was in psychiatric nursing. I enjoyed the work thoroughly and felt comfortable in this milieu. But there was no way of enjoying the disorganization of the staff or of bearing the brunt of a severe nursing shortage.

I'm seriously considering changing fields. But first I think I should try to find some career counseling in nursing. Where can I get the guidance I sorely need?

A There *are* organizations—fledgling organizations—set up to counsel nurses who are disenchanted and thinking of leaving nursing. One of the first ones in the country was started 4 years ago at the University of Texas M.D. Anderson Hospital and Tumor Institute at Houston. As a result of this program, the average tenure of a nurse at M.D. Anderson has increased from 8 to 17 months. (The national average is reportedly only 6 months.)

If you can't locate a comparable counseling service near you, call your school of nursing. Ask if a faculty member (perhaps one you remember with special respect) would talk with you.

Inquire about a career counselor in your area who's *not* solely involved with nursing. Use his services to explore other options and other careers open to you.

Consider having your own psychotherapy. If you continue in a psychiatric area, therapy will be important both for your insight into everyday dealings with patients and for your increased knowledge of yourself.

Even within your present setting, there *are* things you can try. For example, hold regular weekly staff meetings with small groups rather than with the whole staff. The group meetings give everybody a chance to talk about the frustrations of handling the work load and the scheduling, of dealing with patients, and of working with each other. In a small group, staff members seem able to give each other support and positive feedback. What can make or break your job in nursing is the staff with whom you work and the relationships that develop.

Is there any place to go for aptitude tests and career counseling?

Q I had 6 years of general duty in big city hospitals. I wasn't getting anywhere, so I decided to try a smaller setting.

I went to a 40-bed hospital in Maryland where my first year was a crash course in obstetrics. I hadn't had obstetric experience since training but I thought I was doing well. Then nursing administration claimed I was too strong with the people in my charge, so I left.

My next assignment was a 60-bed hospital in Montana. I was disappointed because I couldn't get into obstetrics but I was learning good I.V. and respiratory therapy. After 6 months, the director called me to her office and criticized me for being too strong with my co-workers. She said an LPN resigned because of me.

Now I'm in the state of Washington, and I'm having trouble with electrocardiogram (ECG) monitoring. Staff development is planning a great coronary care course for next month but I don't know if I'll still be here. My supervisor has warned me that doctors have complained that I don't know how to interpret ECGs; my co-workers have complained that I'm hard to work with.

I'm so discouraged. Could you suggest a place I can go for aptitude tests and career counseling? Or should I just give up nursing?

A Look at what you said: In Maryland you were charged with being "too strong" with people. Ditto in Montana and Washington.

Aren't you really saying that your interpersonal relationships—not your nursing performance—need evaluating?

Why not seek psychological counseling in your town? If you don't find anything suitable, contact the nearest large university. It probably has good counseling programs.

As to giving up nursing, don't make any major changes in your life—until you get some professional guidance.

Should someone give up nursing because of the rise in the number of liability suits?

Q I've been nursing for 10 years; the last 5 in intensive care. Our department has a good staff and pleasant working conditions. However, the more I read about the appalling rise in the number of liability suits, the more seriously I'm considering giving up nursing altogether—before the law of averages catches up with me. In my opinion, the present court system encourages suits from almost every patient entering the hospital; and huge settlements cause some people to sue for minor, sometimes unavoidable occurrences.

I can't be the only one who feels this way. Am I?

A No, you're not—and small wonder when nurses are reminded so frequently by the media about the increase in successful malpractice litigation. It's easy to forget the vast majority of "reasonably prudent" nurses working day in and day out, year after year, without ever being sued.

Not everybody feels pressured by statistics, however. If your practice is solid—your clinical skills and documentation skills are sharp and if you stay within your scope of practice, you shouldn't be worried about being sued. Should you carry malpractice insurance? Of course, for the same reasons drivers carry automobile insurance. No one goes out expecting to have a collision—but having coverage just in case an incident occurs is smart and sensible.

Discretion

Why aren't some people more discreet in saying unfavorable things in front of patients?

Q Last week, one of our patients fell in the bathroom. Fortunately, his sister was visiting at the time and summoned help. Unfortunately, the unit secretary called out in a loud voice to a nurse at the end of the corridor, "We need help in 501. Ann left the patient alone in the bathroom and he fell."

> *"This is just one of many examples I could give of personnel saying the worst things possible about our care right in front of patients and visitors."*

Indiscreet? This is just one of many examples I could give of department personnel—from secretaries to nurses— saying the worst things possible about our care right in front of patients and visitors. Usually the talk involves some other staff member and causes a lot of disharmony.

I've warned them about this more than once. Don't people realize there's a right time and place to discuss potentially slanderous situations?

A Right time and right place...not to mention, to the right person in the right way.

And as for your efforts to stamp out this demoralizing and legally hazardous conduct—right on.

Discrimination

Can an RN be turned down for a job because she's childless or because of her religion?

Q I recently applied for a job as office nurse and operating room assistant to two general surgeons. The application asked for my education, experience, age, marital status, and number of children. In answer, I stated that I'm a diploma RN; 2 years, operating room experience; 25 years old; married, with no children.

In the personal interview, the doctors told me that I had the ideal background for the job, then they asked me my religion and my plans for raising a family. I answered honestly, stating that we have no intention of starting a family for a minimum of 5 years.

Several days later, I got a turn-down letter stating that my "qualifications were ideal," but they prefer a nurse who already has a family past preschool age.

I feel that I've been discriminated against because of my childlessness and would like to know if they had a right to ask me such questions. I also wonder if I shouldn't have lied about my religion and about my plans to have children eventually.

A There are four federal acts and endless state laws designed to prevent the kind of discrimination you've just experienced. While federal laws do not expressly forbid an employer to ask an applicant *any* question, the Equal Employment Opportunity Commission (EEOC), which oversees the enforcement of these laws, looks with "extreme disfavor" on questions regarding race, color, religion, age, or national origin. (State laws differ in that some states *do* expressly forbid the employer to ask certain questions that might be discriminatory.)

This doesn't mean that the federal laws are toothless watchdogs. The EEOC and the courts have determined that many preemployment questions are probably illegal. Such questions are not primarily job-related and are really being used to screen out minorities and women. Some of these suspect questions are the very ones you were asked.

The EEOC, for example, does not expect an applicant to be asked her marital status or child-care problems unless those questions are asked of both men and women. (Asking the applicant to fill in "Mr., Mrs., or Miss/Ms" is okay if it's not for a discriminatory purpose.)

The EEOC is very suspicious of the motives of an employer who questions an applicant on her contraceptive practices or plans for motherhood.

If you feel strongly enough about this experience to want to make an issue of it, contact your state's Fair Employment Practices Commission and the federal government's EEOC office in your area.

You realize, of course that such proceedings progress very slowly. So, in the meantime, you'd do well to start looking for another job. But for heaven's sake, don't lie. The least the world expects of a nurse is that she be honest. That's not a selective condition—you'll be honest on your medicine count, but dishonest on your job application. Honest is honest. You be honest.

Can a supervisor exclude male nurses from certain nursing procedures just because they're male?

Q I've got a problem that many male RNs must deal with: I'm not permitted to assist with patients' gynecological examinations. The nursing supervisor in my county clinic is so adamant about this policy that she's sometimes used female, *non*medical personnel to assist, instead of me.

I feel discriminated against—and isolated. Can my supervisor exclude me from certain nursing procedures because I'm a man?

A In theory, reverse discrimination against male nurses shouldn't be a problem. After all, male doctors perform gynecological exams, and female nurses can perform any exam on male patients. But in reality, institutional policies on male nurses vary greatly. Most institutions protect male personnel from suits by requiring that either two health professionals or at least one woman be present at gynecological exams. Some institutional policies specifically exclude male nurses.

In that case, you have three options: (1) accept your clinic's policy and live with it; (2) challenge the policy within the clinic; or (3) find a medical setting with a more liberal policy.

Keep in mind that the patient's right to privacy is the controlling factor in *any* medical situation—and that female patients will usually resist having an unknown male present just for the gynecological exam.

You can lower this resistance by introducing yourself to female patients and talking them through preliminary tests. Then, if you're in a clinic or hospital that allows you to be present during gynecological exams, *these* patients may accept your presence more readily.

You could also do a little PR work. If your employer has a patient admission booklet, it should state that male nurses serve on the clinic staff and attend the patient in much the same way that female nurses do.

Can't male nurses perform female catheterizations or physical assessments without a chaperon?

Q Because I'm a male nursing student, my obstetrics clinical instructor says I can't perform female catheterization at all, and can

perform physical assessments of female patients only in her presence. Most of the time, however, my instructor's too busy to chaperon me; as a result, my assessments can be hours late.

When I complained, she snapped, "That's the law. And I can't always arrange my schedule to suit your time."

Is this really a law?

A Surely no state prohibits male nurses from assessing, planning, or implementing care for female patients. What your instructor's probably referring to is the hospital's own policy.

Many times the reasoning behind such a hospital ruling is twofold: the patient's right to privacy and comfort, and protection for you, the nurse. Catheterization requires intimate touching and can be embarrassing to the patient. Whenever possible, a female colleague should catheterize a female patient—to save the patient from possible embarrassment. But you should at least know *how* to catheterize a female for an emergency situation in which necessity would overrule nicety.

Time now for a heart to heart with your instructor. Any teacher worth her salt respects assignment deadlines. If your instructor can't accommodate yours, the least she should do is arrange for a substitute chaperon to help you complete your assessments on time.

Is it fair to favor a private patient over one on medical assistance?

Q Last week, we had to move a patient off the critical care unit (CCU) to make room for an emergency patient. We had two stable patients: Mr. Warner, who'd been off the ventilator for 2 days without any problems, and Mr. Sykes, who'd been off the ventilator for less than a day. I felt safer moving Mr. Warner,

so I called his doctor, got an order to move him to the step-down unit, and transferred him.

Later, the evening supervisor told me to move Mr. Warner back to the CCU and to move Mr. Sykes out. The reason: Mr. Warner was a private patient and Mr. Sykes was on medical assistance. The CCU's medical director was insisting on the change.

> *"I couldn't believe the CCU's medical director insisted that I should favor a private patient over a patient on medical assistance."*

I politely explained that I couldn't follow the order because I didn't think it was ethical to favor a private patient. The evening supervisor made the change herself and said she'd write an incident report.

I don't feel so sure of myself now. What should I have done?

A You did the right thing. Ideally, you'd like the hospital to treat all patients fairly on the basis of medical need. Realistically, that doesn't always happen, but that shouldn't stop you from trying to promote justice in nursing care.

To protect future patients, consider these actions:
• Talk to other nurses on your unit and ask how they feel about the treatment of patients on medical assistance. If they agree that these patients are often treated unfairly, put your objections in a memo and send it to nursing and hospital administration.
• Discuss the problem with the manager of your unit. Ask for a meeting to discuss a nursing and hospital policy that would address the problem.
• Research the hospital's mission statement or policy about discrimination (limitation of services) against indigent, elderly, minority, or disabled patients.

D

- Present the situation to the hospital's ethics committee for more discussion.

Dismissal

Should a nurse have been terminated for documenting missed medication?

Q I've been an LPN for 11 years and, for the past 8 months, I worked in a nursing home. Although I had some general duty, too, my principal responsibility was as meds nurse.

Six weeks ago, after a review from the Medicare examiners, I was complimented on my charting and summaries. Two weeks ago while getting ready to turn in the medication sheets at the end of the month, I discovered that my initials had been repeatedly forged. For example, if a patient had received his medicine from the first to the eighth of the month, the sheet was initialed properly. If his medicine then ran out and was not administered again until the sixteenth of the month, we would have sent an incident report to the nursing office, and placed a zero on the medication sheet for those days. Instead, I saw on every chart that every zero had been written over with my initials.

I immediately called the director of nursing who confounded me by admitting that she had signed my initials and would continue to do so because "Medicare does not like to see zeros showing that medications have been missed."

The next week, I continued placing zeros where appropriate and also made out two incident reports on medications that were missing or not being dispensed as ordered. Because the director was out and her office locked, I sealed the incident reports in an envelope and taped them to her door. The next day, I was terminated because "my services were no longer needed."

Everyone I've talked with tells me that this could be a blessing in disguise because it takes me out of a sticky situation. They also say that if I make an issue of this, I could get myself in trouble and jeopardize my license. As for me, I'm still in shock and don't know what to think. What do you think?

A This kind of high-handed dishonesty by your director of nursing is not to be tolerated. What might be a blessing for you could someday turn out to be a life-threatening situation for a patient. Nurses who respect the profession and are licensed by the state have an accountability to both the profession and the state. Bring this situation to the attention of your state board of nurse examiners.

Will anyone hire a nurse if she's filed suit against a hospital?

Q Last week, my director of nursing summoned me to her office and fired me—without warning and, in my opinion, without cause. In those few minutes, 8 years of accrued benefits and the good feelings I had about myself as a nurse went down the drain. Shocked and angry, I called my lawyer. He said I have an open-and-shut case of unlawful firing, so I should sue.

My first reaction was to go for it. Now my friends are saying if I sue the hospital, I can kiss my future in nursing good-bye because no one will hire me.

Is this true? Will you find out from someone who's "been there"?

A A nurse who sued her hospital for unlawful firing several years ago says:

"Any nurse who wins a suit for unlawful firing will have little, if any, problem finding another job. You'll probably continue to work steadily and be in excellent standing with several nursing agencies and hospitals."

What's the verdict? Listen to your lawyer, not to your friends. They may mean well, but they have nothing at stake. And don't feel guilty about standing up for your rights. Remember, whether you win or lose the suit, you have the same nursing skills now as before.

Would an anonymous letter warrant dismissal?

Q I worked for 9 years in the same hospital. Eighteen months ago, I suspected one of my fellow nurses of giving patients substitutes instead of their prescribed narcotics. For example, after end-of-shift drug count, she'd chart that she'd given patients meperidine (Demerol) before she left for home. Also, on weekends, when we were short of meperidine, she would just write patients' names on the charts to cover up the missing narcotics.

I decided to report her, but since I had no confidence in the nurse-manager on our unit, I called the pharmacist. When I couldn't get him in, I sent him an anonymous letter outlining my suspicions.

Many months later, the director of personnel called me to his office. Two of the hospital's security guards were also present. They showed me the letter and asked me if I had written it. I said no.

They said that, based on the accusations in the letter, they had conducted a lengthy and expensive investigation and found nothing irregular. They said that they were now going to call for an official police investigation and, if I had written the letter, I'd lose my license.

I then admitted to sending the letter. They asked me to resign and, foolishly, I did. Now, because I resigned, I can't get unemployment compensation. And, after 2 months of looking, I can't get another job because of the bad references the hospital has sent.

Is it fair for the hospital to blacken my reputation? I was only doing my duty as a nurse.

A As a nurse, your duty is to provide the *proper* authorities with *documented* accounts of a co-worker's questionable behavior. You seem to have overlooked some of the finer points of this procedure.

First, if you couldn't trust your immediate superior, you should have gone to *her* supervisor or, if need be, right up to the director of nursing. After all, the problem was initially a departmental matter, so action should have been initiated within the department.

Second, if for some unforeseeable reason you could only confide in the pharmacist, you should have identified yourself. You trusted his judgment enough to choose him as your confidante: you should have trusted his discretion enough to go to him in person—or at least sign your name.

Third, and most important, you should have documented all your suspicions about your co-worker. You shouldn't have been forced to resign if you had documented the times this nurse falsified the records by just listing patients' names to cover missing narcotics.

Lying to the personnel director when he first presented you with the evidence didn't help things, either.

So you see, you used very poor judgment all around. But when this one incident of poor judgment is weighed against your 9 years of satisfactory service (and it must have been satisfactory or why would they have kept you on?), you don't deserve to lose your livelihood.

You resigned hastily and under pressure. Perhaps the administration was acting similarly. Now, in the time that's passed, perhaps they've had time to reconsider.

Why not go back to them, acknowledge your error and ask for reemployment on a trial or probation period. If you're not granted this second chance, ask for a reference that at least acknowledges your 9 years of satisfactory service.

If you don't receive this, seek legal advice.

Dispensing

How can administration be convinced that we need a *real* pharmacist?

Q A few months ago our hospital pharmacist left. Our hospital administrator didn't replace him, but instead assigned a nurse to dispense drugs and fill the medication cart for daily rounds. This nurse has no special background in pharmacology. In fact, she hasn't even passed her state board exam.

For the most part, our hospital uses prepackaged, unit-dose medications. But we also use some drugs that must be dispensed from the manufacturers' large bottles into our smaller bottles. These must then be accurately labeled with the drug's name, dose, and expiration date.

I'm worried that this nurse could mislabel a bottle and cause a medication error. When I expressed my concern to our director of nursing, she just said, "Your complaint has been noted."

I feel the administration is putting an unfair responsibility on the nurse who's "playing" pharmacist and on the rest of us who administer the drugs she's dispensing.

Our former pharmacist gave 6 months notice. I can't see why a replacement hasn't been hired. How do I convince the administration that we need a "real" pharmacist?

A Most nurses would refuse to give drugs in this situation. So your concern is genuine. Also, in most states, a nurse *can't* legally assume the responsibilities of a pharmacist. In the situation you describe, the nurse and the hospital could be subject to legal action. Possibly even the nurses who know about the situation (and know it's illegal) would be liable.

If your hospital administrator doesn't wish to hire a replacement pharmacist, why doesn't he order properly dispensed and currently labeled drugs from a nearby hospital which *does* have qualified pharmaceutical services?

You obviously want to protect yourself *and* change the situation. Then document your complaints and ask the administration to change this risky procedure. Allow enough time for a new system to be established or a pharmacist to be hired—perhaps a week or so. Then, if nothing's been changed, refuse to administer the drugs this nurse dispenses.

Your administration sorely needs an attitude as professional and responsible as yours.

Is it legal for "medicine technicians" to administer medication?

Q Our hospital is planning to introduce medicine technicians to dispense medications to patients. These technicians will be given a 2-month course in anatomy, physiology, medications, and dosages. (They will not, however, be allowed to administer I.V. medications or drugs requiring special precautions, such as heparin.)

Before administering p.r.n. medicines, the technician will first ask the RN to assess the patient's needs and then get the RN's permission to administer the medicine. The technician will then record that the medication was given with the permission of the RN and specify the RN by name. The technician then signs the chart.

Is this procedure legal? What if the technician makes a mistake?

Wouldn't the RN be liable? I'm willing to be responsible for my own acts, but I don't want to be responsible for someone else administering medications. Could I be fired for refusing to participate in such a plan?

A The system, such as you've described, depends on who your people report to—pharmacy or nursing. Certainly if the nurse is paid, she'll stand responsible but, on the whole, the technician'd stand responsible for his own skills.

The RN could either countersign the medicine technician's statement that such permission was given or else show this in the nurses' notes.

Divorce

Isn't it unethical for one nurse to testify against another in a divorce hearing?

Q After spending 17 years at home raising five children, I took a refresher course and got a part-time nursing job. Going back wasn't all that easy—I still have two teenagers.

Now, my husband and I are going through a bitter divorce. His lawyer's fighting hard against giving me enough financial support—which doesn't surprise me. But you can imagine my surprise when a nurse-friend of his testified against me, citing the various jobs that are open because of the nursing shortage and how much I could earn if I worked full-time. I couldn't believe she'd use information like this to hurt a fellow RN; it seems unethical or even illegal if she was paid for her testimony. What's your opinion?

A Sure, it would be great if nurses would support each other unconditionally across the board. But the nurse's testimony wasn't really illegal or unethical—and it probably wasn't very conclusive either. The statistics on jobs and salaries are available in any library, and judges know that most statistics can be manipulated to suit any perspective.

> *"My husband and I are going through a bitter divorce...I couldn't believe it when a fellow RN testified against me in court."*

So, save your emotional and physical strength. In the days ahead, you'll need every ounce you can muster to work your way through this crisis. Ruminating over reasons to be angry, or searching for people to blame, won't help.

Doctor-patient relations

How can a nurse help a patient change doctors without creating an uncomfortable situation?

Q One of my patients is dissatisfied with her doctor. I've never worked with him before, but I've heard some of my colleagues question his competence and professionalism. How can I help my patient change doctors without creating an uncomfortable situation?

A The issue here isn't what you've heard about the doctor; it's how the patient feels about him. Explore her concerns, then tell her she may want to discuss the situation with the doctor. Advise her that she has a right to request a second opinion or even a new doctor if that's what she wants. Just make sure she understands that *she* must tell the doctor how she feels.

A doctor who's sure of himself won't feel threatened by her decision. But if you suspect that this doctor won't handle the news well, warn your patient that he may become angry. Reassure her that as her advocate, you'll support her right to decide who will handle her care.

The advocate role isn't without risk, of course. You must speak up for your patient and her decisions, setting aside your own beliefs and opinions. You may also have to stand up to a colleague who thinks he knows best for the patient. So be prepared to deal with conflict. Only you can decide how tall you wish to stand.

Doctor's behavior

What can be done about an irresponsible doctor who's jeopardizing lives?

Q One of our in-house anesthesiologists has been behaving in such a totally unprofessional way we're beginning to fear for our patients' lives.

Here's a sampling of his behavior:

He leaves the delivery room in the middle of deliveries and cesarean sections; swears at nurses and patients; and resuscitates newborns *very* vigorously. He doesn't check the oxygen or nitrous oxide tank levels and doesn't check the equipment to make sure it's working properly.

And as if these things weren't bad enough, one day he gave a patient the wrong anesthetic. If another doctor hadn't intervened, the patient might have died.

For the past 3 months, we've documented each of these incidents and sent the reports to the director of nursing. Our unit manager has also reported the problem to the director. And now I call the nursing supervisor whenever a new incident occurs.

We nurses have lost all faith in "proper channels." So far, absolutely nothing's been done about this doctor. Do we have to wait until a patient dies before someone takes us seriously?

A This problem calls for alerting two department heads—the doctor's and yours. Take a double-barreled approach: Talk to the department heads *and* send a thoroughly documented report through the proper channels.

If after a week or two you've had no word and no action, then it's time to move up to the next level of authority: Take the matter up with those who are *over* the department heads who've failed to act. (Professional courtesy requires that you let your department head and the doctor's *know* that you're now going over their heads.)

You can, if you have to, go a step further, to the hospital's board of directors. If you can get no response within the hospital, you can even go to an outside authority. Call your state's Office of Complaints in the Bureau of Professional and Occupational Affairs. Request an official complaint form. Fill out the form; and if you wish, request that your name be withheld. You'll be notified by mail about the action taken by this state agency.

No obstetric or gynecologic procedure should be started when the dangerous situation you describe exists. For example, if the proper equipment checks have not been made, as you report, the surgeon and the unit manager should be told. They have to know that a dangerous situation exists in the delivery room. Until that situation is remedied, the procedure should not *begin*.

Be prepared: There's obviously going to be a confrontation. But be sure the patient's not present (or at least not conscious of the confrontation going on).

If you conduct yourself knowledgeably and with conviction, both the nursing and medical staffs will recognize that you and your co-workers mean business when it comes to safe and effective patient care.

Aside from the safety of the patient, there is another danger here: If you cooperate with this anesthesiologist *knowing* that he's set up a dangerous situation for the patient, you could be legally liable.

Before the matter's settled, there may be a lot of sound and fury. But when calm's restored, the entire medical team will have avoided serious trouble—and you will have earned new respect from your colleagues.

Doctor's orders

Can a doctor's order supersede the hospital's written policy?

Q Hospital policy says that when we administer certain drugs I.V.—insulin, for example—we must use an infusion pump. Last week, a doctor wrote an order for I.V. insulin and included in his order "don't use pump." I immediately questioned this, reminding him of the policy. He verbally abused me and told me I'd better follow his order. I called my manager, who also told me to "obey the doctor's order."

Concerned about my patient's safety, I hung the I.V. on the pump anyway. Later, my manager saw what I'd done and told me to "either take that I.V. off the pump or lose your job." I reluctantly complied. Legally, can a doctor's written order supersede the hospital's written policy?

A Yes it can, because the doctor is the final authority on his patient's care.

In a situation like this, you have two choices: carry out the order as

written or, if you believe it's dangerous, refuse to carry it out. But you can't simply disregard the order and take another action, as you did by using a pump.

Because your primary concern was your patient's safety, you were right to question the order. When the doctor refused to change it, you should have told your manager why you felt you couldn't carry it out. And you shouldn't have been swayed by verbal abuse. If your patient were injured, you wouldn't be immune from liability just because someone threatened you.

Finally, to protect yourself in a case like this, you might want to document the facts in an objective, nonaccusatory memo. Send a copy to nursing administration and keep a copy for your records.

Can a nurse legally conform to the patient's or relative's wishes, or must she follow the doctor's orders?

Q Last night, a 74-year-old woman was transferred to our intensive care unit (ICU) from a medical/surgical unit. The patient had been admitted to the hospital 11 weeks ago with chronic obstructive pulmonary disease complicated by pneumonia and diabetes. Twice during the 11 weeks, she was sent to the ICU in respiratory distress; each time, she required mechanical ventilation.

When I saw her last night, her blood pressure was 78/50 mmHg, her respirations were shallow, and she was unresponsive to verbal stimuli. We checked her arterial blood gases, and the results warranted her being placed on mechanical ventilation once again. However, her son, the closest living relative, objected.

He told me that after one of his mother's stays in the ICU, she'd written her doctor a letter requesting that she never be placed on a ventilator again. The son had promised her wishes would be followed.

I didn't see this patient's note, but the son was willing to sign a paper refusing mechanical ventilation for his mother—even after I explained that failure to use the ventilator might hasten her death.

In spite of the son's wishes, the doctor ordered the patient placed on the ventilator.

I followed the doctor's orders, but I was *not* following my conscience. If this situation should come up again, can I legally conform to the patient's or relative's wishes—or must I follow the doctor's orders?

A There doesn't seem to be any easy solution. When it comes to a confrontation between doctor and patient, or between hospital and family, a court order's the only answer.

Obviously, you'd want to avoid open conflict. Consider these questions before it comes to a confrontation: Did the doctor and the patient's son ever meet face to face? Did anyone ever see the letter the patient supposedly wrote? Was the letter documented? And if not, why not? Ask your supervisor what existing hospital policy covers such a situation. If none exists, *you* must take the responsibility for documenting the facts—if you should face a similar situation another time.

If there *is* a next time, call in your supervisor. Let *her* talk to the patient or relative. But you must document the request for refusing treatment; also note all conferences involving patient, relatives, the supervisor, and you.

Refusal to place a patient on a ventilator is risky. Without proper documentation to support your actions, you could be sued.

Document your facts; it's still your best protection. At the same time, work toward a clear, written hospital policy that will convert the sensitive gray area into black and white.

Can a nurse on the unit accept a verbal order from a doctor's office nurse?

Q The nursing staff on our maternity unit is at odds over a recent incident. A doctor asked his office nurse to call our unit with an order to change the medication for one of his patients. Our unit manager refused to accept the order, and the doctor was incensed.

> *"How can a nurse on the unit accept a verbal order from a doctor's office nurse?"*

The doctor contends that since we allow telephone orders in other instances, we should have accepted *his* order—even when called in by his nurse. (He pointed out that he'd promised to get in the next morning to sign the order sheet.)

Can a nurse on the floor accept a telephone order from a doctor's office nurse?

A Any question about telephone orders opens a can of worms. The whole matter remains highly controversial—but the law clearly backs your refusal to accept orders from the office nurse. The nurse practice act in some states says nursing includes "executing medical regimen as prescribed by a *licensed or otherwise legally authorized physician or dentist.*" In the incident you cite, it *could* be claimed that the office nurse, not the doctor, was prescribing the medical regimen. According to law, she's not qualified to prescribe. However, to be safe, you should check your hospital policy.

Remember: The doctor has the option of calling a resident on his service and having *him* write the order. Doctor-to-doctor communication is better in this instance, if only because the nurse is not covered for telephone orders.

As an overall policy, restrict telephone orders to emergency situations—when you can't reach a doctor. Once you relax this restriction, the privilege of telephone orders can easily be abused. Then you'll have to insist that *no* telephone orders will be accepted at any time.

Can the medication nurse renew expired medication orders before the doctor signs them?

Q I've recently moved to a new state and got a job as a unit manager in a small hospital. At this hospital, standard practice is for the medication nurse, without first checking with the doctor, to write a verbal order on all narcotics and antibiotics that are on the 72-hour stop list. The doctor eventually signs the order—but sometimes that's not until 1 or 2 days after it was written.

Tell me, what's your opinion on this practice?

A It's a violation of the law to allow *any* nurse to renew expired narcotics and antibiotics orders without a written order for the narcotics and at least a verbal order for the antibiotics—even though the doctor does eventually sign the order.

If these medications ever caused some untoward effect on a patient, the nurse who wrote the unauthorized order and the nurse who knowingly carried it out would be excellent targets for a malpractice suit. The hospital and the doctor would be held vicariously liable, too.

The medication nurse could be in violation of your state's medical practice act for practicing medicine without a license, and in violation of its nurse practice act for prescribing medications.

Is a nurse legally obligated to carry out a written order?

Q Yesterday, a doctor wrote an order to have his postoperative patient walk for 10 minutes each day. The patient told me she felt dizzy, but she didn't refuse to get out of bed. As we were walking, she fell and broke her wrist.

When the doctor found out, he told me I shouldn't have had her walk if she wasn't ready. I'm confused. Aren't I legally obligated to carry out a doctor's written order?

A As a rule, yes—unless, in your professional judgment, the order is dangerous or inappropriate. In this case, you should have assessed whether your patient was ready to get out of bed. If you believed she was still too weak to walk safely, you should have charted that, then called the doctor and discussed your findings. In other words, you should never blindly follow a doctor's order if doing so might harm your patient.

Suppose, for example, the doctor orders an unusually large drug dose. Rather than giving the drug without question, you'd discuss your concerns with the doctor. He may simply have made a mistake. Or his explanation may clear up your doubts.

But what if he won't change his order and you still believe it's inappropriate or dangerous? Tell him why you object—and why you won't carry it out. Also explain the situation to your nurse-manager and ask for advice. She may want the doctor to administer the drug himself. That way, he'd be solely responsible for the outcome. Of course, you should thoroughly document the facts and the steps you take.

The bottom line is that you're responsible for the consequences of every order you carry out. Better to challenge the doctor now than to defend your actions later—in court.

Is diagnosing and prescribing considered using "standing orders"?

Q I'm a school nurse for a small private college. Once a month a doctor comes on campus to teach a class and see patients. He leaves "standing orders" for me to follow when he's not here. These generally involve routine prescription medications, because our dispensary doesn't stock any narcotics, tranquilizers, or other controlled substances.

I enjoy my work but sometimes wonder if I'm not really diagnosing and prescribing by using these "standing orders." The doctor almost never sees any of the patients. And although I can and do talk to the doctor frequently by phone, I can't send patients to his office—150 miles (240 km) away. I do, of course, refer any patients I'm in doubt about to local doctors.

Several doctors have assured me that what I'm doing is perfectly legal and standard procedure for small schools, but I'd appreciate your opinion.

A Unfortunately, in medicine, long distance isn't "the next best thing to being there." By adapting the doctor's standing orders for patients he "almost never sees," you *are* diagnosing and prescribing.

True, standing orders have been routine procedure in many small schools. But lately, because the standing orders won't "stand up" in malpractice actions, these orders have been disappearing from college campuses.

Were you to misdiagnose and treat a student with a medication that caused a reaction, the student could sue you and the college. And although most institutions *say* they'll stand behind a nurse unless she errs grossly, such support is shaky at best. When confronted with an actual lawsuit, the school could claim *any* error resulted from your gross neglect.

To be on firmer ground, insist that the school hire a doctor at least part-time. Until a doctor's found, refer students to area doctors, and fill their prescriptions from your dispensary supply. The students will probably get tired of spending time (and money!) for outside medical care and will pressure the college to provide care on campus. With the students' support, your efforts should lead to improved campus health services—and reduced long-distance bills.

Is it fair to be reprimanded for following a written order?

Q Last Wednesday, during shift report, the evening nurse told me that a new patient had been admitted at 9 p.m. with a 3-day history of bloody stools. His blood pressure had been dropping steadily from his admission reading of 124/68 mm Hg. She then showed me the doctor's orders she'd written on the Kardex: Vital signs every 15 minutes, complete blood count, type and crossmatch two units of blood tonight. And she told me that the laboratory would call when the blood was ready.

Shortly after midnight, I checked the patient and found his blood pressure had continued to drop; his pulse was weak and hard to obtain. A few minutes later, the lab called to say the blood was ready. I administered both units during the night.

The next day, I was called on the carpet by my supervisor. She said the doctor was furious because I had not checked with him before administering the blood.

My question is, why should I be reprimanded? The evening nurse recorded the order, and the lab got the blood ready. All I did was carry out the order as written.

A Ah, but you didn't carry out the order. It said, "type and crossmatch two units," not "type, crossmatch, and *give* two units." The laboratory told you that the blood was ready for you, when and *if* you got the order to give it.

Your nursing instincts were right, and no harm was done. But next time, you'll be sure to remember this lesson and read the order carefully.

Is it legal to transcribe a doctor's order as a verbal order?

Q As an RN employed by a physician in private practice, I not only work in the office but also make hospital rounds as needed.

If, while making rounds at the various hospitals, I find a patient in need of further care, I phone the physician with my findings. If he then dictates an order, I transcribe it as a verbal order from him and sign my name on the patient's order sheet. The physician, in accordance with hospital policy, countersigns the order sheet within 24 hours.

Recently, this arrangement was challenged by the administrator of one hospital. He feels that what I'm doing amounts to "third-party gossip"—meaning that the orders come from the doctor to me and then to the unit nurse. I say that the arrangement is analogous to a doctor's giving phone orders to an evening nurse for medications to be given by the day nurse. The administrator also said that I could be violating our nurse practice act.

Will you set me straight on this?

A What you're doing doesn't quite add up to "third-party gossip," but it is *not* analogous to a physician's giving verbal orders to a *hospital* nurse to carry out. In the latter instance, both nurses are hospital employees for whom the hospital is legally responsible. You are not a hospital employee. You are, in this situation, an interloper over whom the hospital has no control.

If ever a patient were injured because your reports to your physician were inaccurate and his response in terms of orders were correspondingly incorrect, the hospital could eventually be held responsible. Your physician employer, in sponsoring such practices, is not living up to his responsibility to his patients (under his physician-patient relationship) nor to the hospital.

In many states an RN does not have the right to make independent judgment about diagnosis and treatment. Although, in fact, hospital nurses frequently do just that, they are acting legally as a "lent servant" of the hospital to the physician. Under these circumstances the nurse is the agent of both the hospital and the physician and is considered to be merely exercising nursing functions. You, having no relationship to the hospital, could be considered to be exercising medical functions in violation of both medical and nurse practice acts.

Now all this may appear to you to add up to no *real* difference at all. But the law is tremendously complex and this is how the practice acts have been interpreted.

It's time to sit down with your employer and the administrators of the hospitals where you visit and discuss possible changes in your role that will enable you to perform within the particularities of the law.

Shouldn't a nurse question a drug dosage?

Q I work on the night shift in the orthopedic unit of a teaching hospital. Last week, a multiple sclerosis patient was admitted for bone splitting, and his doctor left orders to give 80 units of adrenocorticotropic hormone (ACTH) in 500 ml dextrose 5% in water I.V. over 8 hours.

Because I wasn't familiar with this regimen, I looked in three different drug books. None of them recommended an I.V. dosage of ACTH higher than 25 units. My supervisor told me to check with the on-call doctor, who reacted angrily. "If you're not comfortable with the order, give 25 units if that's what you want." (Later, he claimed I had harassed him to change the order.)

The patient's doctor was furious when he heard about this the next day; he said I had no right to withhold the prescribed dose.

I don't understand what happened. Wasn't I right to question this dosage? What do you say?

A Bravo for you. You were 100% correct. What happened here is a classic example of the confusion caused by a doctor who orders an investigational dosage without sharing his rationale with the staff—including the on-call doctor, evidently. This entire situation could have been avoided if the doctor had simply attached a drug reference to the patient's chart.

For diseases with no cure, like multiple sclerosis, you'll find doctors at teaching hospitals trying new drugs or high doses of currently available drugs, or using drugs in ways that aren't correct in the package insert. Most investigational dosages aren't listed in standard drug references. (Besides the dosage, the order you questioned is unusual because ACTH is rarely administered intravenously for treatment of multiple sclerosis except for a patient whose disease is advancing rapidly.)

Does this mean you can throw caution to the wind the next time you receive an unusual order like this? By no means. You must protect your patient and yourself by checking it out. In the meantime, why don't *you* write an appropriate protocol for the staff to follow on unusual orders and submit it to administration? Clearly, it's needed.

What can be done if verbal orders cause a problem?

Q In the respiratory unit of our hospital, medical residents give us verbal orders in person or orders over the telephone.

Until recently, we nurses had no problem with the system: We'd write down the resident's order, initial the entry in a log, then carry out the order.

But last week, when a resident was questioned by a senior staff member on one particular verbal order, the resident flatly denied ever giving it to us. That left us looking as though we'd acted without any authority.

Of course we were angry. But that's secondary. Our primary concern is to avoid another such incident.

But we're in a quandary: We don't want to refuse verbal orders. We're aware that our residents are under a lot of pressure; at the same time, we don't want our patients to suffer any delay in getting pain medications, transfusions, ventilator setting changes, or other urgent attention.

What's the best way to handle the problem? We could use a word of wisdom.

A The wisest word is "don't." Don't accept verbal orders, except in a life-threatening emergency. In case of an error that resulted in an injury to the patient, the ensuing lawsuit would center around the responsibility for the verbal order. But how could you *prove* who said what, or that you

were in the right? Even a record of the verbal order could be questioned.

The Arizona State Nurses' Association has issued a statement saying that verbal orders will be accepted only in a life-threatening situation. They point out that "the greater danger for negligence is created by the doctor's failure to take the time to enter the order..." while "the nurse's liability is increased by accepting the verbal order."

The association makes a distinction between verbal orders and telephone orders: "The verbal orders imply the doctor's presence; telephone orders, the doctor's absence."

If you *must* have a telephone order, here are their recommendations:

• Identify the person relaying the order. If the person is not the doctor himself, get the name and title of the speaker.
• Record the order. Include the names of the doctor (or other speaker relaying the order) and the nurse taking the order.
• Read the order back to the person who gave it, as an extra check for accuracy.
• Record the date and time the order is received.

Have another person listen in on the conversation and initial your record of the order. Since the regulations in this critical matter can differ, readers who do not live in Arizona should check with the board of nursing in their own state.

The association strongly recommends that each health care facility have its own written policy on verbal orders, telephone orders, and telephone orders given by a third party.

If your hospital doesn't have written policies on these three issues, work with other nurses to have such a policy formulated.

In a nutshell, get it in writing whenever possible, for both your own and the patient's protection.

What if a doctor writes an order out of spite?

Q While reviewing orders for a terminally ill cancer patient, I noticed one written during the previous shift that made absolutely no sense. It read: "Vital signs q15min. Up in chair q2h." There had been no change in the patient's condition that would warrant an increase in vital signs, and getting him into a chair every 2 hours would exhaust him and require assistance from four people. When I asked a co-worker about the order, she said the doctor who wrote it was annoyed with a nurse who was too busy to make rounds with him. So he wrote the order out of spite! The nurse just laughed and ignored the order. But the doctor didn't write a cancellation, and no documentation appeared in the nurses' notes.

Our unit supervisor (away on vacation at the time) agrees that something should have been done to cover us for not following the order. Moreover, we're both appalled that a doctor could be so immature and would use a legal document for a personal vendetta. Since then, I've heard this is nothing new for him; he's written similar orders before for various "annoyances."

How do you feel about this?

A How sad for the patients who are unwitting pawns in this game playing.

Call a staff meeting stat, discuss the problem, and decide on what approach the nurses will follow (and follow consistently) if the doctor pulls this stunt again. Ask a psychiatric nurse clinician to attend the meeting and make suggestions— there could be more to this than immaturity.

Your supervisor should then meet privately with the doctor to define the problem, to tell him what the nurses see as their approach, and

D

to ask how everyone can work together to end this conflict. Give him time to change. If his game playing continues, document and report the situation to his medical supervisor and hospital administration. The hospital's lawyer would gladly explain the appropriate use of legal records to this doctor.

What if following them leads to a reprimand?

Q Yesterday, my nurse-manager called me into her office and gave me a written reprimand. She said that one of my patients had no bowel sounds when she checked him in the morning, that I'd failed to assess him properly, and that I'd discontinued his I.V. fluids too soon after his exploratory laparotomy surgery.

She angrily asked me what I had to say for myself. I told her was following doctor's orders, which said the I.V. could be discontinued when the patient tolerated liquids. He tolerated both water and a clear liquid supper without complaint shortly after he returned to our unit at 4 p.m., so I removed his I.V. at 9 p.m.

I'm still smarting from that experience. This is my first nursing job, and it bothers me to have a reprimand in my file, especially when I followed the orders as written. My co-workers said they would have done the same as I did; what would you say?

A Nobody's perfect, and in this instance, nobody's right. Your nurse-manager vented her frustration on you, wounded your feelings, and lost her opportunity to teach you and to set a positive tone on the unit. The doctor failed to write clear, complete orders. And, because of inexperience, you didn't assess your patient properly.

In the future, remember that an exploratory laparotomy always involves manipulation of the bowel,

so checking for the presence of bowel sounds should be a crucial part of your assessment. Always continue I.V. therapy until you're sure the patient hasn't developed an ileus (4 to 5 hours isn't usually long enough).

Do something constructive rather than dwelling on your hurt feelings. Go back to your nurse-manager; tell her that you have a better perspective now and are hoping she'll reconsider the reprimand. Ask for a staff development session on the early care of abdominal surgery patients. From what you say, everyone on staff could benefit from the review.

What is a nurse's professional and legal responsibility if she writes medication renewals herself?

Q The nurses at our acute care community hospital disagree with the doctors about what constitutes a correct medication renewal order. The doctors don't want to take the time to rewrite the name, dose, frequency, and route in each renewal order. They propose the following as acceptable:
• "renew meds"
• "renew Demerol"
• "same I.V.s"
• "add to daily I.V.s—500 cc D₅S¼, all in by 9 a.m."

With this method of abbreviated notation, the nurses and the secretarial personnel on our unit would have to find the original order each time, and then write it themselves.

This alternate method would save time for the doctors— but that's not our nursing concern: Our job is to be sure the patient's medication is accurate.

Thus far, the hospital's pharmacy and therapeutics committee has been skirting the issue. And no one has bothered to call the hospital's lawyer for advice.

To protect ourselves, the nurses in our hospital want to know what our professional and legal responsibilities are if we write the medication renewals ourselves.

A It's the responsibility of the doctor to write all I.V. and medication orders completely and accurately. Any shortcuts, including the notations and abbreviations your doctors suggested, are not allowable. In the words of malpractice law, they do not promote "reasonable patient care."

Point out to the doctors that the 3 or 4 minutes it might take to write the patient orders each day would protect not only the patient but also the doctors themselves. If a lawsuit developed over a patient's care and the chart revealed abbreviations and shortcuts for the patient's medication renewals, the lawyer might claim that his client received inferior care.

To make your position even stronger, a spokesperson at the national office of the Joint Commission on Accreditation of Healthcare Organizations says unequivocally that a system for notifying the medical staff of all drug renewals is needed in every hospital. Yes, it's time to get your hospital on the right track.

What should a nurse do if she disagrees?

Q For the past several weeks, our intensive care unit (ICU) has been caring for a patient who's had massive intracranial bleeding. He's relatively unresponsive and has little or no rehabilitation potential.

Besides his other problems, he has copious pulmonary secretions that require suctioning every 30 to 45 minutes. A neurosurgeon filling in for the patient's regular doctor (who's on vacation) took one look at the patient and wrote an order to suction the patient *no more* than once every 4 hours.

I feel that carrying out such an order would be negligent on my part, especially in the ICU where, by definition, we provide *intensive* care. What do you think?

A Determining when to suction—or not to—is a *nursing assessment* based on throat and breath sounds, respiratory rate, and significant signs.

> *"I feel that carrying out such an order would be negligent on my part, especially in the ICU where we provide intensive care."*

Also, from a physiologic viewpoint, an order for suctioning every 4 hours (or even every 3 or 2 hours) is a poor one, because secretions may not peak within any specific time frame.

Discuss your concerns with the doctor immediately, but *continue to suction the patient as necessary.*

If the doctor disagrees with you, let him know, as a professional courtesy, that you intend to pursue the matter through channels with an incident report or memo. (You'll get quicker results with an incident report.) In either case, mark your correspondence "for *immediate* attention."

What should a nurse have done when she disagreed with the doctor?

Q One morning last week, a 75-year-old patient with chronic obstructive pulmonary disease became tachycardic and flushed; his theophylline (Slo-Phyllin) level was well above the therapeutic range of 10 to 20 μg/ml used by our hospital laboratory. He was receiving an aminophylline (Aminophyllin) drip at 80 mg/hour throughout the night, as well as respiratory therapy with

metaproterenol sulfate (Alupent).

I telephoned his doctor at once, expecting him to discontinue the drip. He caught me off guard when he replied, "It's okay." Four hours went by before the doctor finally ordered the aminophylline drip discontinued.

The patient was fine, but I felt ineffectual and frustrated. What do you say?

A Join the club. Most nurses have found themselves staring at the phone receiver in disbelief and talking to the dial tone at least once. In the future, *before* you report a problem, think about what you expect the doctor will or should do, and plan what to say if he doesn't.

For instance, you could tell him what you're thinking: "This patient's already in distress; I'm worried about how long his heart can take that rate. Do you want me to slow the drip and see what happens to the heart rate? Do you want the laboratory to recheck?"

Suppose he doesn't change the orders. Take 10 minutes to organize your thoughts, then call back. "I've taken the pulse again; it's still up. Do you want the drip slowed or the aminophylline discontinued? Do you want the laboratory to recheck?"

Again, suppose he doesn't take either cue. Document your actions; ask your supervisor to contact him or, if need be, the chief of medicine. (If your supervisor doesn't, you'll have to call.)

Gutsy? Yes. But for your patient's sake, persistence—not keeping your mouth shut and hoping—is the key to getting the action you need.

What should be done when a doctor routinely ignores hospital policy?

Q One of our consulting doctors routinely ignores hospital policy by writing orders on patients' charts instead of writing them on

the consultant's report. This same doctor also assumes certain patients will be referred to him "anyway," so he takes charge of them and (again) writes on their charts—without the attending doctor's knowledge.

Can I be held liable for following his orders? Someone should talk to him, but who?

A These really sound like problems for the medical staff members to settle among themselves. But for now, yes, you can be held liable under certain circumstances. For instance, if this doctor's orders endangered a patient's life, the court could find him in violation of hospital policy and conclude that you, too, were negligent for the same reason.

Next time, remind the doctor about hospital policy, or have your supervisor talk to him.

Why should children be subjected to painful intramuscular injections when oral medication might work just as well?

Q I work nights on a pediatric unit. While checking charts on my first night back after vacation, I came across a culture report showing *Staphylococcus aureus* resistant to ampicillin. Then I noticed that the patient (a 10-month-old infant) had been receiving ampicillin intramuscularly every 6 hours for 5 days, although the lab report had been on the chart for 3 days. I flagged the chart so the doctor would change the medication order.

When I came on duty the next night, the infant's medication order still hadn't been changed. I asked the evening nurse about it, and she said, "The doctor wants it given anyway." The next day, the infant was discharged on oral erythromycin stearate (Erythrocin Stearate Filmtab).

This particular doctor orders intramuscular ampicillin for almost all his patients. Most other doctors, however, order oral medication, even for children who *seem* more ill.

My questions are these: Why should children be subjected to painful intramuscular injections when oral medication might work just as well? Why would a doctor continue to order a medication that wasn't effective? And how can we get this doctor to change an order when the medication is clearly ineffective, or when we think an alternate route would be more comfortable for the patient?

A Medication injected intramuscularly is absorbed into the blood more rapidly, achieving higher serum levels than medications given orally. Faster absorption still doesn't explain why the doctor continued to order ampicillin when the culture report showed the causative organism was resistant to ampicillin.

> *"Why should children be subjected to painful intramuscular injections when oral medication might work just as well?"*

Is it possible that the problem started with a failure in communication? Are you sure the doctor was aware of the culture report? Do your lab technologists routinely notify the doctor when a culture report shows an organism resistant to the medication ordered? If the lab didn't notify the doctor, and if this particular doctor is one who tends to overlook the patient's chart, then he may simply not have been aware that the medication *needed* to be changed.

A personal approach, then, would certainly be a more effective way of getting his attention than flagging a chart. Since you're not on duty when he makes his rounds, you'd have to tell the day and evening nurses during report that you have a question for this doctor and ask that he give the answer in writing.

If, after you've considered all the possibilities, you find that the doctor *has* read the culture report, that he *has* read your notes on the chart, how do you "persuade" him to change his orders? Give the doctor every chance to save face. Remember—he's human, too. If a pharmacist at the hospital is assigned to monitor antibiotic therapy, why couldn't *he* approach the doctor and suggest an alternate medication or an alternate method of administering the medication?

As a last resort, turn your information over to the charge nurse on the day shift. If other nurses share your concern about the doctor's practice of prescribing intramuscular injections when oral medication would be at least as effective, then a group of you should talk to your supervisor. (Remember that you'll need thorough documentation of the problem.

Yes, accomplishing change means working through channels. But, if you're convinced the doctor's practice is causing a child undue trauma, change is in order.

Bravo for being sharp enough to pick up the problem in the first place.

Documentation

Are full signatures required every time?

Q At a recent seminar I attended, a medical records consultant from another state made one statement that I question. She said that we, as nurses, must sign our complete signature every time we make an entry into the nurses' notes. For example, if we note something at 9:15 and again at 9:20, we must sign our full signature each time. This is now official policy in the hospital and I think it's a nuisance.

In other hospitals where I've worked (all in California), the accepted practice was to sign our full signature once on the first page; then, after that, use our initials.

What's the current thinking on this?

A According to the *Guinness Book of World Records,* the longest name in the world belongs to a man who signs himself "Hubert Blaine Wolfe + 590, Sr., because there are actually 590 more letters in his last name.

Unless you're related to this gentleman, go along with the expert's testimony.

The multiplicity of health care regulations now makes it all but impossible for anyone (except records experts) to keep up with the latest interpretations. And even the experts admit they have to work hard just to stay in place.

Remember, the point of signatures on medical records is to determine unshakably the responsibility for the actions recorded therein. So when you get annoyed with signing the additional letters of your name, think of each push-pull of your pen as an additional protection from ever being charged with somebody else's mistakes.

Maybe it will make the new rules less onerous.

Aren't nurses responsible for documenting oxygen used by a patient?

Q As a charge auditor, I double-check that every patient is billed for all items and services documented in his medical record. Several times lately, I couldn't justify a charge for oxygen use because the amount of oxygen the patient used wasn't documented in his record.

When I called the nursing administrator, she said the respiratory care department should supply this information.

I always thought that nurses were responsible for documenting oxygen used by the patient. After all, nurses are the ones accountable for round-the-clock care of the patient, including monitoring his oxygen use.

What do you say?

A A distinction must be made between nurses documenting that patients received oxygen on the appropriate form and their becoming involved in the billing process. Documenting and keeping track of the amount for billing purposes is the responsibility of the department receiving revenues for the oxygen—in most hospitals, respiratory care. However, if the respiratory care department wants to "hire" nursing to get involved in billing, okay. Then nursing time for this service should be charged to respiratory care.

In the good old days before cost cutting and diagnosis-related groups, it didn't matter much who spent time working on interdepartmental services. But now that administrators are equating the value of services with the revenues they generate, nursing can't afford to give away valuable time doing other departments' work "for free." A tough-minded attitude? Sure. But when nursing's called upon to share another department's responsibility, it should get credit for it on the books.

Can a nurse get into legal trouble by charting a patient discharged 2 or 3 months earlier?

Q I'm frequently asked to complete charts on patients who've already been discharged. Sometimes I'm expected to write notes on a patient who was discharged 2 or 3 months earlier.

Can't I get into legal trouble by charting a patient I don't even remember? How can I avoid this situation?

A Head off trouble by doing a patient's chart as soon as possible after you've treated him. If all charts are checked for completeness each day the problem of back-dating won't come up. But if deficiencies do occur—as they will—have them cleared up *within the week.*

In a malpractice suit against you, charts filled in from memory months after the fact would offer you poor protection. But notes written while the patient is fresh in your mind could prove that your care met the standards required by law.

Refuse to do any more backdated charting. If the administration pressures you to take part in this questionable practice, try looking for a hospital with a more professional—and more defensible—policy.

Could sketchy details hurt a nurse in court?

Q Last week, a patient at our nursing home took a turn for the worse. As he rapidly deteriorated, a co-worker called his doctor and asked him to come in. But the doctor didn't think he needed to get here immediately. When she called again, about an hour later, he said he'd arrive in a couple of hours. Meanwhile, the patient died.

Now his family is suing us for negligence. The doctor claims my co-worker didn't tell him the seriousness of the situation. Unfortunately, her charting was sketchy and she didn't fully document her conversations with the doctor. Will that hurt her in court?

A It could. In this case, the court may conclude that your colleague didn't give the doctor all the details, so he had no way of knowing the seriousness of his patient's illness. For that reason, she may be found guilty of negligence.

If this situation happens in the future, carefully document the time of your call and the content of your conversation. Don't let a doctor's failure to respond go unnoticed. Tell your manager immediately, and record what you've done in the patient's chart.

How should a medication error be corrected?

Q We recently had a question on the proper documentation for a medication error. Here's what happened: One of our doctors ordered epinephrine 0.05 mg subcutaneously for a pediatric patient. The nurse meant to give 0.05 mg; she charted that she gave that correct dose, but later she realized that she had administered 0.5 mg by mistake. The patient was treated for the symptoms caused by the overdose. How should she have documented this mix-up on the chart? We'd appreciate your comments on the best way to handle this.

A She should have written "see nurses' notes" on the medication Kardex and on the doctor's order sheet where she signed off the time and person administering the medication. In the nurses' notes, she should have written the dose that was actually given and the follow-up nursing actions—including her assessment and her plans for monitoring ("will take vital signs every 5 minutes," and so forth). In other words, the record should show that the wrong dose was administered but should also include what actions the nurse took after the error.

For the future, any nurse who's administering such potentially life-threatening medications to a child should check her calculations with another nurse *before* administering the medication.

How should patients be referred to in charts?

Q Where I currently work, the staff frequently uses terms like "Peter," "Mr. Black," or "patient" when charting nurses' notes. Is such terminology necessary? Are any legal implications involved here?

A There doesn't seem to be any legal implications using any of these ways of referring to patients. Common practice usually follows the hospital policy.

Some administrations prefer that adult patients always be addressed as Mr., Mrs., or Ms. They consider it a more professional and respectful approach. Other administrations state no preference. Most nurses say that if an adult patient prefers to be called by his first name and the nurse is comfortable in doing so, it's not disrespectful.

You *could* get through a patient's entire chart without once using his name—that's usually the policy.

If an order isn't signed the day it's written, how can the charts be ready for inspection?

Q After a maternity leave, I returned to my job at a dialysis center that serves 55 patients. I couldn't believe my first assignment—to check and make sure that all charts were ready for inspection by signing off doctors' orders that, in some instances, had been written as long as 2 years before! My supervisor didn't see any problem. She told me to use the daily record sheets for documenting when the medications were given.

I began signing off orders using the current date. Later, my supervisor said to cross out the current date, write "error," and note the original date of administration on

the charts. Fortunately, when she saw my hesitation, she put the job on hold.

We all realize any order should be signed the day it's written. But because this wasn't the case, how can we now get the charts ready for inspection? The supervisor doesn't want to look bad at inspection, but neither do I want to lose my license.

A Who wouldn't want all charts in perfect shape for inspection? But, too bad. What's blank should be left blank; what's wrong, left wrong. Any supervisor who lets charts go unchecked for 2 years will just have to face the music.

Hard words? Maybe. But don't put yourself in jeopardy by updating charts. Remember the charting rule no hospital can change: Don't backdate, tamper with, or add to notes previously written.

By choosing to speak up now, you may be saving yourself a lengthy discussion about this later in court.

If one patient reports that another one is suicidal, should the name of the "reporter" be documented?

Q On the psychiatric unit where I work, patients socialize and interact with each other constantly.

At times, we receive a report from one patient about another that might be pertinent to our nursing care. For instance, one patient reported that another talked about committing suicide. But the "reporter" in this instance is unreliable and often makes up stories like this.

When we chart this information, would it be appropriate to mention the name of the reporter? I've been told that to mention one patient's name in another's chart is an invasion of privacy. Yet we could be charting false information and causing the allegedly suicidal patient to be unfairly scrutinized.

What do you think?

A You were given the right information: You would be guilty of invading the reporting patient's privacy by mentioning his name in another's chart. You can, however, identify him by oblique reference, such as "another male patient," "a frequent patient companion," "a peer."

Another word of warning here. When it comes to suicide, better to err on the side of caution. Observe the allegedly suicidal patient more carefully than usual, and mark his chart so that oncoming shifts will do the same. If you can prevent a tragedy by heeding the usually unreliable reporter, you'll come to see the "unfair" scrutiny as extra care and dedication.

If some important information is omitted, can it be added later?

Q If I inadvertently omit some important information when charting in the nurses' notes, can I add the missing information later? Or would such "after the fact" charting undermine confidence in the records?

A By all means, write the entry when you discover the omission. Write next to the time of the entry, "late note." For example: *3:30 p.m. late note. At 2 p.m. small amount of drainage noted....*

Never, never try to squeeze the information in where it *should* have been recorded chronologically. In a malpractice suit, nothing makes a plaintiff's attorney happier than finding such information squeezed in—obviously added after the fact.

Is it legal for a nurse-manager to alter nurse's notes?

Q The nurse-manager at the small clinic where I work often alters my nurse's notes without telling me. I'm concerned about the legality of this practice. If changes need to be made, shouldn't she ask me to make the entry—or at least write a note indicating a possible error? In either case, shouldn't I be told?

A You're right to be concerned. One of the first rules of charting is, "Don't backdate, tamper with, or add to notes that were previously written."

Whether you're told or not isn't the issue; your manager simply shouldn't be doing it. When she edits your notes, she's tampering with their integrity. What if they were needed as evidence in a lawsuit? Her changes could cast doubt on your honesty and your notes' accuracy. Would the jury believe you if they thought your manager had to correct your notes?

You shouldn't be altering earlier observations either. But you can safely add late entries, as long as you label them as such.

How can you change your manager's behavior? Try explaining that the changes she makes compromise your notes. If that doesn't get results, write a memo describing your concerns and send it through channels to the director of the clinic. You might ask to meet with the director, your nurse-manager, and the clinic's lawyer to discuss the legal ramifications of tampering with nurses' notes. Keep a copy of the memo for yourself.

A final thought: Do any of your colleagues have the same problem? If so, ask them to sign the memo, too.

Is it legal to backdate the plans?

Q The state department of health recently gave the nursing home where I work a provisional license, citing it for inadequate care plans. According to the inspector, our plans don't cover all problems that we chart. Administrators now want us to go through 6 months worth of charts and complete our care plans. What's more, they want us to backdate the plans. We've been told that this is legal and that if we want to keep our jobs, we'll do it. What do you think?

A You should never backdate or otherwise tamper with an official record. You may add documentation later, but these entries must reflect the date and time they were actually written.

So going through the charts, extracting information on patients' problems, and writing care plans is legal, as long as your documentation is dated accurately. But backdating is a different matter because it involves altering the record. That could put you in a delicate legal position if those records were ever needed in a lawsuit.

Take your concerns to your administrators and try to negotiate. For example, you could agree to write the care plans, but you should refuse to backdate them.

Is it legal to document something as a "late entry"?

Q The lawyer at the hospital where I work tells us that if we've forgotten to document something on a patient's chart, we can add it later—even after the patient has gone home. She says we should document the information as a "late entry." Couldn't this practice affect the chart's credibility if it's ever needed in court?

A The lawyer's advice is correct. Just make sure you record the date of the late entry and the reason why you're including it (for example, "Forgot to record this information when patient was in hospital, but have now remembered it").

You could create problems if you add information to a patient's chart *after* he sues the hospital or *after* you receive a request to see his records. Although you can still make a late entry under these circumstances, doing so invites the patient's lawyer—and later, the jury—to wonder if someone's hiding something. And that could turn a "winnable" case into a loser.

Is it legal to leave a chart incomplete?

Q Recently, an anesthesiologist broke a patient's front tooth during a difficult intubation. I documented this in the patient's chart, then filled out an incident report.

Later, a nurse I work with said I shouldn't have charted what happened. She said that if the patient sues the hospital, her lawyer could use this information against us. Is she right?

A Incomplete charting just invites a lawyer to wonder what you've left out—and why. So you did the right thing.

When you fill out incident reports, always chart what happened in the patient's medical record, too. Briefly describe the incident, record your assessment, indicate whether you called the patient's doctor or family, and note what treatment was given, if any. In this case, you might also have included a statement that the patient's vital signs remained stable to show that she wasn't in danger after the incident.

One more thing: You *wouldn't* chart that you'd filed an incident report. That's an administrative report only; information about it doesn't belong in the patient's medical record.

Is it legal to reconstruct nurse's notes?

Q Several months ago, emergency medical technicians brought a severely intoxicated man found in an alley to our emergency department. After an hour of I.V. therapy, he became agitated, ripped out his I.V., and urinated on the floor. We called the police, who dragged him away in handcuffs. In the confusion, our nurses' notes were lost.

Now hospital administrators want me to reconstruct my notes. I'm uncomfortable with this because I don't remember much about the patient's vital signs and other clinical information. Are they asking me to do something illegal?

A Although reconstructing notes isn't the ideal way to document patient care, it's not illegal. Just make sure you state that you're documenting from memory; then, chart only what you can recall. Equally important, date your entry so it's clear that you didn't write the notes on the same day you gave care.

Take pains to avoid the appearance of a cover-up. To a plaintiff's attorney, ambiguous notes suggest the possibility of fraud. If you later wind up in court, he'd use them to undermine your credibility.

Is it legal to sign nurse's notes only once each shift?

Q Instead of signing her name after each entry, a nurse on our unit signs her notes only once—after making her last entry for the shift. Each entry before that contains only the time and her note. Is this legal?

A Although not exactly illegal, it's certainly inappropriate. A nurse's notes should be consistent with the standards of nursing practice, and they must conform to the hospital's policies, procedures, and protocols. Each entry should at least be initialed so it can be easily distinguished from the others. If the notes are computerized, each entry should be identified with a code.

Clearly and accurately documenting nursing care protects you, the hospital, *and* the patient.

Is it legal to sign off all the medications to be given during the shift?

Q A new nurse on our unit has a practice that disturbs me: At the beginning of her shift, she signs off all the medications that are scheduled to be given during the shift. What's more, other nurses are starting to copy her. I don't know how they can accurately keep track of the medications they've administered plus the ones they've yet to give. Is this nurse's unusual charting method legally sound?

A You're right to be concerned—it isn't legal. What's more, it breaches nursing practice standards. And because hospital policies and procedures are based on the law and prevailing standards, the practice surely violates hospital guidelines.

Discuss your concerns with your new colleague, who may not realize the ramifications of her charting method. She's still on probation, so make sure you explain hospital policy to her. Those nurses who've picked up her bad habit may also need to be reeducated on proper charting procedures through a staff development workshop.

Is it okay to abbreviate "and" as "&" and "et?"

Q Some of our nurses are concerned because "and" is written in the charts as "&" and "et." The hospital has no policy on this large matter, and the staff development department refuses to address such a trivial point.

But I have to ask you: Which form would be appropriate and legally safe if a chart were used as evidence in court proceedings?

A Use either "and" or "&," but draw the line at "et," since it's quite possible not everybody will know what "et" means. Your hospital should have its own list of accepted abbreviations.

The disagreement among the staff is probably just healthy difference of opinion, and not rancor in disguise.

Is it okay to transfer notes onto the designated form after a code?

Q I work in the intensive care unit (ICU) of a small hospital. When a code's called anywhere in the hospital (except in the emergency department), a nurse from ICU is expected to respond and become a code leader until the doctor arrives. During the code, one of the floor nurses will usually write down the code notes.

We *try* to keep a clipboard (and the proper forms) on each of the crash carts. But if the clipboard and forms are missing at the time of a code, the nurse delegated to take notes will use any handy piece of paper. After the code, she transfers her notes onto the designated form.

My main concern is that this practice might be construed as altering the original record. What's your opinion?

A You've probably arrived at the best way to handle the situation. The clipboard and forms should *be* on each cart, but unfortunately "in the real world" everything isn't where it belongs.

The procedure you describe seems okay—particularly if the nurse who jots down the notes is the same one who transfers them, and if she does this as soon after the code as possible. (Also, she should ask the nurses who took part in the code to review the notes for accuracy.)

Be careful though, not to let this become routine. If you really want to get it together—and avoid the problem of missing clipboards—why not attach the clipboard and its forms to the cart?

Is the patient's chart a place to register disagreement?

Q As a charge nurse in a nursing home, I've gotten into hot water with my supervisors over a charting issue. The trouble started when I noted on a patient's chart that I couldn't assess him adequately because he wasn't receiving the proper treatment. The doctor had ordered a nebulizer treatment, which I always thought should produce a visible mist. Because the nebulizer wasn't producing such a mist, I made a note of this on the chart. Later, the day supervisor checked the equipment, said it was fine, then upbraided me for "inappropriate documentation."

A second incident involved a patient with a pressure sore that was being aggravated, I felt, by improper positioning. I said so in the patient's chart—time after time. This went on for more than 3 months. At one point I even offered, in my notes, to show the staff how to position the patient correctly.

The response? The nursing office accused me of "waging war" in the patient's chart. What's your opinion?

A You may not have been waging war, but you're certainly not going to win any peace prizes with that kind of documentation. Working with supervisors who seem more concerned with regulations than with patient welfare can be frustrating, but the nurses' notes in a patient's chart should concern *only* the patient and his problems—not problems involving the staff, such as you were addressing in your notes.

If you don't like the way a patient is being cared for, tell your supervisor about it or write a memo or incident report. Criticizing treatments or procedures in a patient's chart, which doctors and other hospital personnel also read, violates both professional standards and common courtesy.

Certainly, continue to try to change things that you feel are detrimental to your patients. Just make sure you stay in the proper channels and stay out of hot water.

Must an RN who's a BSN student sign "SN"?

Q One policy of the baccalaureate program I'm attending has me peeved. It requires all students to sign "SN" after their names on patients' charts. As an associate degree nurse I resent not being able to chart "RN" after my name. Can you blame me?

A No, you can't be blamed for protecting your RN status. And you'll be pleased to hear that the school probably can't force you to sign SN. Some states have specifically ruled that students within a baccalaureate program who are licensed registered nurses should use the initials RN after their name.

> *"I resent not being able to chart 'RN' after my name. I am required to sign 'SN' instead."*

If the school insists that you identify your student status, suggest these alternatives: RN, SN; RN, student; or RN, BSN student. Any of these options should protect your legal status, observe safe documentation practice—and allow for the RN you've already earned.

Must nurses' notes be charted on the doctors' progress notes?

Q My hospital recently changed its charting system: Nurses and other health care providers are now required to chart their notes on the doctors' progress notes. We've already had some problems with the new system.

For one thing, a doctor will often leave blank lines between his notes and those of the nurse or health care provider. Isn't this a dangerous practice?

A second problem is that some nurses don't chart *anything* when they see the doctor's already written a note adequately covering the patient's condition and care. Is this good nursing practice?

A First things first. Leaving blank lines between entries on a patient's chart is inviting legal trouble. Someone could add an entry out of chronological order, or pad the notes' content.

If, for some reason, the notes are used as evidence in court, a lawyer would be likely to zero in on any suspicious entries. Therefore, you (or preferably your hospital administrator) must establish a protocol that clearly states *no one* can leave blank lines.

Your second problem is just as serious. Nurses aren't relieved of their responsibilities in charting when a doctor writes a note, even if his note *more* than adequately describes the patient's condition and care. Medical care is not nursing care.

The nurse must still document her *own* observations, interactions with the patient, and nursing care provided. When the question of care provided comes up in court, the rule of thumb is documentation means *done,* and no documentation means *not done.*

D

D

Just keep in mind that careful charting:
• helps ensure quality and continuity of care.
• tells supervisors about the patient's condition and the care he's receiving.
• protects you legally in case something goes wrong.

Should a blood transfusion be recorded as fluid intake?

Q Should we consider a blood transfusion as intake—and record it on the intake and output sheet?

A Blood is indeed considered intake and must be charted as such. Remember that every time you infuse *any* solution you must be concerned about fluid overload.

Blood components (packed red cells, platelets, white cells, deglycerolized red cells, fresh frozen plasma, washed red cells, and cryoprecipitate) are also considered intake and should be charted.

By the same token, gross bleeding is considered output. If such bleeding should occur, be sure to record it on the intake and output sheet.

Should an unsafe nurse-patient ratio be documented?

Q Certain nurses on our unit have been writing on the patients' charts that "primary nursing care could not be given because nurse-patient ratio was 1:20."

To me, charting that primary nursing care wasn't done implies the patients didn't receive *any* nursing care. But we have nurses here who see the situation differently: What they're charting, they say, is the fact that although an unsafe nurse-patient ratio exists, they're giving what care they can. (And they *do* chart what care's been given.)

Does the negative "nursing" information belong on the patients' charts?

A Staffing information does *not* belong on a patient's chart. A nurse's charting "primary care not given" could be risky if the chart were to be used as evidence in a negligence suit against her. Legally you can protect yourself better by avoiding generalized statements and by charting *exactly* what care you could and did give.

But your question raises a far larger issue: How can nurses deal with staffing shortages and unsafe nurse-patient ratios? This one's tough to answer, in part because the definition of primary nursing differs from hospital to hospital. In the opinion of a vice-president for nursing at a large hospital who did some of the early groundwork in primary nursing, a primary nurse can care for 6 to 10 patients—providing she has help. "In my definition of primary nursing," this distinguished nurse said, "the nurse is accountable and responsible for the care of her patient—this does not necessarily mean carrying it all out herself. However, in other hospitals primary nursing does mean the nurse handles all aspects of the patient's nursing care *herself*. This is obviously an impossibility when the nurse-patient ratio is 1:20."

When inadequate staffing prevents you from doing primary nursing, what can you do besides your best under the circumstances?

Work closely with your immediate supervisors and your director of nursing on the issue of providing quality care. As the shortages persist, nurses must work with nursing leadership in the search for feasible solutions.

Here's a small example of a possible solution: Take a good look at the hospital's support system, and determine whether you, as a nurse, are doing duties that other departments should handle.

Should a nurse sign notes that contain information she hasn't observed firsthand?

Q A suggestion by the day shift in our long-term care facility has those of us on the night shift upset. We're being asked to write the monthly notes on the general condition of our patients and to include the nursing notes from the day shift.

Though the day shift nursing supervisor says this is legal, we're not sure. Can we sign notes that contain information we haven't observed firsthand?

A Certainly, one can appreciate your reluctance to sign secondhand information, since you don't want to be held responsible for observations you haven't made yourself. Still, you *can* write the monthly notes—provided they're a summary of *all* the nurses' notes (day, evening, and night shifts) and are *clearly labeled* as a summary.

Your signature would then indicate only that you've read and summarized the notes from all the shifts, not that you're personally attesting to everything the summary contains.

Present the suggestion (for the exact labeling of the notes) to the nursing supervisor. She'll probably agree this approach is correct and appreciate your effort to *improve* a nursing procedure, rather than *criticize* it.

Should medication errors be documented in the progress notes?

Q Our hospital has a new and radically different policy on documenting medication errors. We still must file an incident report, but now we must also document in the patient's progress notes that we made a medication error. We include the medication given, the dose, route of administration, and the time we notified the doctor.

In the past, we were told *not* to document medication errors in the progress notes, that it would be a "red flag" for lawyers. We're wondering why administration would change that policy now. Won't we be making it easier for a malpractice lawyer to find evidence against us?

A Your concern is understandable—any change in accepted practice is unsettling at first. But your hospital policy reflects a changing attitude toward documentation, a change that could prove beneficial to you. For example, if you're ever sued, documentation will be the key to your defense. What's documented, what's *not* documented, and the inferences the jury draws can weigh heavily on your case's outcome. So you'll be in a much better position with the error clearly documented in the patient's record.

The old hide-and-hope-the-lawyer-won't-seek approach to medication errors is outdated. In today's world, a malpractice lawyer handles more and more cases involving nurses, so he's more experienced in reviewing progress notes and picking up an error, whether you "flag" it or not. He knows what to look for—and he knows what questions to ask during legal discovery proceedings. He'll surely ask whether you filed an incident report, and he can subpoena the patient's hospital record, including a copy of any incident report, from the hospital's risk management department.

The extra documentation simply protects you more. That alone makes it worth doing.

Should vulgar words be documented?

Q After our nursing school class reunion, we talked about things we never learned in school. One of my friends, a prison nurse,

mentioned a dilemma with charting. We were taught to be specific in charting behavior and to use quotes, but in the prison infirmary where she works, the patients' language is often quite vulgar. Her manager called her in and told her not to use specific words in the record.

What's your opinion?

A No matter what the setting, the purpose of charting remains the same: to properly record and communicate the patient's condition and needs, and to document your actions.

So, generally speaking, your manager's right. Your friend should chart what relates to her patients' health status—and delete the expletives. However, if the vulgar language is directed as a personal attack, she should chart that the patient is yelling angrily and give examples of what he said. Or, if a patient who never uses this type language suddenly begins to, she should record some examples. This new behavior could indicate a change in his coping patterns (drinking, drugs) or a deterioration in his neurologic condition.

What are the legal implications of charting "charge nurse notified"?

Q A new policy on our labor and delivery unit prohibits writing "charge nurse notified" in our nurses' notes. The reason? The charge nurse might disagree with our assessment that a·patient care problem exists. If she were to decide that no action is needed, our report would still be on record and could implicate her in a future liability action. Now we're worried about our own liability. The patient's chart will show that we identified a problem without doing anything about it.

What's your opinion?

Q Recently, I started working as nursing supervisor in a long-term care facility. Early on, I urged the nurses to write care plans and improve their documentation, even though they have very little time for this. When I audited the patients' charts this week, I found notations such as, "Treatments not done—no time—notified nursing supervisor," and they included my name.

Comments like that put all responsibility on my shoulders, and I don't want to be implicated legally. Yet I'm the one who encouraged the nurses to improve their documentation, and I don't want to be on bad terms with them. How would you handle this?

A At first glance, these problems seem the same but just from opposite sides. What's different, though, is the type of information being charted.

Whenever you identify a *care* problem or *symptom* that requires the attention of the charge nurse (or, possibly, more senior nursing or medical personnel), you should note the problem in the patient's chart. And you should also write the name of the person you notified, her title, the date and time. If the chart's taken to court and there isn't any record that you notified the proper person, that person may allege that she wasn't notified. Or she may have forgotten—she's only human, after all.

However, any information about staffing, patient census, or other administrative matters doesn't belong in a patient's chart. It should be documented in either an incident report or other appropriate administrative form.

The best course in either case is to call a staff meeting. Air your concerns openly; discuss the legal implications of charting—what's appropriate and what isn't—and how to communicate staffing needs and grievances. When you disagree about writing for the record, talking it out may help.

What are the legal risks of an RN signing assistants' notes as if they are her own?

Q I work in a small hospital where, on the 3-to-11 and 11-to-7 shifts, the nursery is staffed only by a nursing assistant. The assistant makes notes on the babies' charts and takes the charts to an RN in the labor and delivery area. The RN then signs these notes as if they were her own.

What are the legal risks of this practice?

A The practice you describe doesn't meet minimum guidelines of good charting. For legal protection, your hospital should require that notes be charted and signed by the person doing or seeing the events being recorded. In most cases, that person should be an RN.

> *"Is it legal for an RN to sign the assistant's notes as if they were her own?"*

The nursing assistant should be charting only routine functions—feedings, temperature readings, and stools. Then the RN could check the charts and cosign them.

But if an RN in the labor and delivery area is signing charts on babies in the nursery, she can't legally or morally attest to the care these babies were actually given. The RN and the hospital are taking grave legal risks by continuing the practice you describe.

We think you should *suggest* a change in the nursery staffing pattern, and *urge* a change in the charting policy, too.

What can a nurse do about the "gumming up" of mistakes?

Q The legal office at my hospital insists that we simply line out and then cover any errors on a patient's chart with white, gummed labels. The long list of errors includes stamping the chart with the wrong patient's plate, making mistakes on the temperature, pulse, and respiration graph, writing notes on the wrong patient's chart, and so on.

I've refused to cover up mistakes because it contradicts everything I've learned in nursing. I still think what I was taught is right: Draw a single line through the error, initial it, and write in the correction. I'm always warning my colleagues about the legal problems they could face if they "gum up" mistakes, and I've complained to my supervisor about the covering procedure. But I feel like I'm beating my head against a wall.

Although the legal staff can't prove that the labeling practice *is* legal, they say I have to *prove* it's illegal before the situation can be changed. Please help—I don't want to leave this job.

By the way, this is a military hospital. Does that change the situation?

A Your hospital's charting strategy is a mess. Gumming over the faulty entries will cripple any legal defense for the hospital or its personnel in a court action. The believability of the charts and of the records will be suspect. In fact, the charts with labels may not even be legally admissible. Your best plan, says our consultant, is to mark an error as soon as you discover it, then refer the reader to the recorded correction.

The rules are different in a military setting. A military hospital can't be sued without its consent.

Visit the hospital's legal office again. Get more information about your liability and the hospital's under the Federal Torts Claims Act.

Remember, taking the effort to clean your hospital's poor charting practice now may save you and your hospital from trouble later.

What can be done about a nurse's incorrect documentation?

Q At the small hospital where I work as a recovery room nurse, anesthesia is usually induced by certified registered nurse-anesthetists (CRNAs).

One of them routinely charts that the patient's state of anesthesia lasts for 5 to 15 minutes longer than it actually does. Of course she's paid for this added time, at the patient's expense, even though she's usually on her way home by then. Worse still, the unit manager wants all the charts to jibe and told us to use the CRNA's notation as the patient's transfer time to the recovery room. This means the CRNA is on record as being responsible for the patient during that interval, but in actuality we are.

I refuse to go along with this; I chart the time the recovery room clock reads, whether or not it agrees with the CRNA's notation. I complained more than once to the CRNA. Her excuse: "Our clocks don't agree." I don't buy this answer. What's your opinion?

A Sounds like more than the clocks are out of sync here. Keep charting the exact time the patient arrives in the recovery room according to the clock on your wall. If a patient gets into trouble in the time overlap, you want the protection of unchallengeable records. As a matter of fact, ethics aside, why would anyone—given the exorbitant insurance rates for anesthetists—risk falsifying a medical record just to round out a quarter hour's pay?

How curious that any unit manager worth her salt would let this discrepancy slide. Document both the problem and the implications through channels. And ask for a written policy. It's about time.

What can be done when a doctor "edits" nurses' notes?

Q Several weeks ago, a woman with the diagnosis of acute myocardial infarction was admitted to our critical care unit from a doctor's office. The nurse performing the initial nursing assessment wrote in the nurses' notes, "2 + pitting edema of hands and feet" and "bilateral basilar crackles in the lungs." But when the patient's doctor came in later that evening, he circled these two items in the nurses' notes and wrote "no" and "not true" in the margin.

The nurse was upset at this "editing"—not only because of the insult but also because of the possible legal implications of a doctor's writing on nurses' notes.

Our unit manager asked the doctor to confine his comments or criticisms to his progress notes. He replied that the nurses' notes were sometimes incorrect; for example, that the patient in this case had had fat ankles—not edema. The doctor said he didn't want the chart to imply that the patient was in congestive heart failure when she wasn't.

As a final comment, the doctor said he *frequently* corrects nurses' notes—when they're "wrong"—because it's his duty.

We think the *doctor's* wrong. What do you think of his "editing"?

A Not much. Maybe the doctor deserves some credit for *reading* the nurses' notes—a sign of professional respect many doctors omit.

Perhaps this doctor doesn't realize that by adding his comments to the nurses' notes, he's tampering with their integrity (even when he feels he has a sound medical reason for his editing). As you know, even nurses shouldn't change their earlier observations on the notes. Any pertinent information should be added on later pages.

Since your unit manager has already discussed the problem with the doctor without success, why don't you write a documented memo describing your concerns? Ask your co-workers to sign the memo, then send it up through nursing channels to nursing administration.

In the memo, request a meeting with a member of nursing administration, other staff members, the doctor involved, and the hospital's lawyer.

If the nursing administration sees your determination and realizes the legal ramifications of any tampering with the nurses' notes, perhaps they'll take your complaints to the hospital administration.

As a show of good faith, mention in your memo that the staff nurses would welcome a separate meeting with the doctor to review the nursing assessments he feels duty-bound to change. Perhaps this review will promote learning on both sides—and persuade the doctor to restrict his editorial comments to his *own* progress notes.

What's the best way to correct a charting mistake?

Q I'm usually supercareful about charting, but the other day I goofed—and I can't stop worrying about it. I'm probably extra sensitive because I've just returned to nursing after 8 years at home raising my children.

Here's what happened: After giving one of my patients flurazepam (Dalmane), 30 mg, as ordered, I

mistakenly charted that I'd given her acetaminophen (Tylenol). (Another patient had just asked me for Tylenol, so it must have been on my mind.) As soon as I realized my mistake, I erased the word *Tylenol* and wrote *Dalmane*. On the advice of my manager, I then filled out an incident report.

Would this erasure suggest "foul play" if the chart were to be reviewed in court? And for the next time, what is the best way to correct a charting mistake?

A Usually, the *best* way to correct a charting error is to draw a line through the incorrect word or words and write: *Error—wrong notation*. Then put the name of the right drug on the *following* line. A note written out of chronological order might indicate chart manipulation or some other wrong doing. Erasure *is* suspicious and a definite "no-no."

Because you had already erased your error, filing an incident report, as you did, is the second best way to handling your mistake and your erasure. If the chart, with its correction, should ever come into court, the incident report would dispel any intention of "foul play."

You're wise to be concerned about protecting yourself legally. But now stop worrying about past mistakes, and focus on not making new ones.

Welcome back to nursing—and good luck.

Who should document a code?

Q Just as I arrived for duty in the surgical intensive care unit, a code was called, and I was told to take charge of documentation.

I did as best I could and the code team's efforts were successful, but I felt uncomfortable throughout the procedure. You see, the patient was admitted during the night shift, so I knew nothing about him.

Do you think I should've been pulled in cold like that to perform such an important job?

A No. Ideally, the nurse documenting the code (the recorder nurse) should be the same person who was first on the scene. After starting cardiopulmonary resuscitation, calling in the code, and giving details to the code team, *she* stands back and assumes the role of recorder nurse.

As recorder nurse you have many responsibilities, such as:
• documenting the highlights of the resuscitation efforts
• detecting problems not seen by other members of the team (such as noting that a team member is tiring and should be relieved, or asking gathering onlookers to leave)
• summarizing the resuscitation efforts by writing a postarrest progress note (best if done by the person who was there from the beginning)
• providing the patient with emotional support afterward or, if he didn't survive, guiding the patient's family through the grieving process.

Before the situation you describe happens again, discuss your concerns with your supervisor. It sounds like hospital protocol was pushed aside. That should not happen during a code, but you deserve praise for the way you handled yourself under the circumstances.

Who's responsible for cosignatures?

Q Nursing students from a nearby college get their clinical experience at the hospital where I work. Recently, a doctor—who also sits on our board of directors—was outraged when a student charted that she'd palpated a mass in his patient's abdomen. He said she was "diagnosing." And he wanted to know which RN was responsible for that student's work.

To appease him, hospital administrators have come up with a new policy: Staff nurses must cosign students' chart entries. I have enough to do just caring for my patients. Should I be held responsible for students' charting, too?

A No. Responsibility rightfully belongs to nursing school instructors, not staff nurses. If you agree to cosign charts, you're assuming legal responsibility for directly supervising the students. That means *you* could be held liable if a student acts negligently.

Ideally, you would communicate closely with the student and her instructor, but you wouldn't cosign her entries—you'd leave that for her instructor.

But if you must comply with this new policy, protect yourself by adding a statement that clarifies the situation. For example, if you didn't see the student perform the care she charted, say so. In case of litigation, you want the facts to be perfectly clear.

Your best bet, though, would be to share your concerns with your manager, then request a meeting with hospital and nursing administration and the nursing school faculty. If you put your heads together, surely you can come up with an amicable solution.

Would bedside charting pose legal risks?

Q Our hospital has just introduced primary nursing—and the staff's delighted. But now we want to try bedside charting. What we have in mind is keeping nurses' notes and a flow sheet (but not the *entire* chart) at the patient's bedside.

Our administration has balked at the idea. The hospital lawyer tells us that bedside charting could cause too many legal problems. Yet

other hospitals in our area have accepted bedside charting. Why won't ours?

A Your hospital could use a second legal opinion. Bedside charting doesn't necessarily pose undue legal dangers.

The touchy legal issues here revolve around possible damage to the patient's right to privacy through the release of his records to sources *outside* the hospital. But while the patient's still in the hospital and his record's still being kept, a release of information to the outside doesn't seem a major threat.

What about the patient's seeing his own chart? In certain hospitals, a patient is allowed to see the entire chart—simply for the asking. But if your hospital doesn't allow this, you might have a problem. Obviously, bedside charting *would* make it possible for a patient to read his record.

If a patient wants to see his record, he should see it. (*After* his discharge, he does have the legal right to see his entire medical record—although he may have to obtain signed hospital authorization or a subpoena first.) But the truth is, most patients simply won't bother to read their charts—with or without permission. So your administration may be making much ado about nothing.

Bolster your arguments for bedside charting by checking with local hospitals that are already using it. Find out what kind of problems they've run into. With your argument carefully supported, why not approach your administration with a "try-it-you'll-like-it" proposal?

Wouldn't a universal symbol for a mistaken entry be quicker, readily recognized, and legal?

Q At our hospital, we've recently changed from writing "error" next to an incorrect entry to "mistaken entry." I've found that "mistaken entry" followed by the nurse's initials is space consuming and time consuming, too. Wouldn't a universal symbol for mistaken entry be quicker, readily recognizable, and legal? Perhaps something as simple as an M in black ink encircled by red ink. It would stand out in the chart without taking up space. I don't know where to take this suggestion, because the symbol would have to be officially accepted and used nationwide as a legal abbreviation, wouldn't it? Perhaps you can help.

A Getting a symbol recognized isn't a matter of licensing or national distribution by some central bureau. Mostly, these symbols and abbreviations start in medical schools. Fledgling doctors bring them to different parts of the country; after time and use, the symbols may become part of that area's medical language. If enough doctors use the same symbols in enough places, sometimes national recognition results. (Sometimes the abbreviation of a polysyllabic medical term in a scientific paper sticks and becomes popular usage.)

You'd be wise to give up on the notion of introducing an M—large, small, encircled, or whatever. M's of various shapes and sizes already have 90 meanings. Another reason: When a plaintiff's attorney introduces a chart as evidence, interpreting abbreviations becomes crucial. But for court purposes, the chart will be photocopied; the black M encircled with red ink will then become a black M encircled with black.

If you really want an abbreviated form of "mistaken entry" accepted where you work, you'd need both words indicated (M.E.). And this wouldn't be clear unless every page of nurses' notes carried the footnote, "M.E. = mistaken entry." And think of the possible implication here: An observer might take this

to mean that numerous mistakes are *expected!*

Whatever happened to the word "error" followed by the nurse's initials?

Draft

Will nurses ever be drafted into military service?

Q One day after class, several of us students got into a discussion about war, and someone said that nurses will be drafted.

Honestly, it scares me enough to think of war, but it's even worse to worry that as a nurse I'd be drafted.

What do you say about this?

A Put your worries on the back burner. In this country, no women have ever been drafted—not even nurses—and the likelihood that they ever will be is remote.

Your primary concerns right now are to finish your nursing program, do well in your state boards, find a nursing job you like, and become as good a nurse as you can for your patients' sake and your own self-satisfaction.

Drainage tubes

How can infection be prevented?

Q Many of our patients come back from surgery with very long drainage tubes. These tubes are often resting on the floor beside and under the patient's bed. I was taught that pathogens are capable of ascending the outside of any tubes (chest tubes, gastric lavage tubes, or indwelling urinary catheters) and possibly causing infection. Is this a legitimate concern?

A Yes, microorganisms can migrate upward, creating a potential for infection. To prevent long tubing from resting on the floor

while the patient's in bed or when he walks around, simply slipknot a rubber band around the tubing and attach it to the patient's gown with a safety pin. Be careful not to pull the tube when its pinned to the gown.

Dress code

What are nurses wearing today?

Q We're developing a dress code on the unit where I work, and I need information. What can you tell us about what nurses are wearing today?

A Dress codes vary by department in most hospitals—all white isn't what all nurses are wearing. On medical/surgical units, most nurses do wear all white, but in intensive care units, emergency departments, and obstetrics/gynecology and pediatric units, about half the nurses are allowed to wear scrubs or colored tops.

Most nurses say they have some voice in deciding the dress code where they work. Interestingly enough, however, the majority say that white uniforms seem to project professionalism and command respect from doctors, patients, and administrators.

Before you develop a dress code for your unit, find out what your colleagues *want* to wear, and check on the availability of their preferences in your area. This will help you compile a list of workable dress code options to choose from.

What if nurses oppose it?

Q Our new director of nursing just told us, "Wear a cap or resign." Yet at least 80% of us don't want to wear caps. This order is wrong.

D

Q At the hospital where I work, we must wear white nurses' shoes—sneakers and athletic shoes with white leather uppers are taboo. When I wear regulation nurses' shoes, my feet hurt all day.

Q Nursing administration tells us we must now wear white pantsuits with tunic tops or standard uniforms. Many of us put together our own uniforms from conventional women's clothing that not only look professional but also are more comfortable, durable, and less expensive than standard uniforms. No one bothered to ask us what *we* thought about this change.

A And so it goes. If you were one of the many who thought strict uniform codes were history, remember that history tends to repeat itself. The people who interpreted the looser codes of the 1960s and 1970s as "sloppy attire" just may have spoiled things for the rest of us. Whatever the impetus, dress codes throughout the nation seem to be returning to conservatism, with the Midwest having the strictest codes (in some places, white for uniforms, shoes, laces, stockings, and caps). Besides the clothing issue, hairstyles, makeup, jewelry, and facial hair (on men) are also being regulated.

Can you do anything about changing a dress code you dislike? Yes. Begin by calling a general meeting of all nurses, and be prepared to present your ideas *objectively*. After this group meeting, establish a committee of all those concerned—which might include the director of nursing, unit manager, supervisor, and a member of administration—to review the dress code policy. Ask a nurse who's the "best on her feet" to represent the nurses and present your views. Remember, objectivity is the key word; personal and emotional attacks should be avoided, or they'll defeat your purpose.

In the meantime, do your own public relations by adhering to the current dress code until changes occur.

What should it be for nurses at an extended care facility?

Q At the extended care facility where I work, the printed and practiced dress codes are far apart. For example, some staff members wear dangling loop earrings, chain necklaces, brightly colored nail polish, and flamboyant makeup. As staff development director, I have the job of coming up with a new dress code.

> *"Some staff members wear dangling loop earrings, chain necklaces, brightly colored nail polish and flamboyant makeup."*

Of course, I'm concerned with safety, infection control, and a presentable image for nursing professionals. But I don't want to present an unrealistic or outdated picture. Do you have any suggestions?

A Dress codes have long been a tricky question in extended care facilities—with as many answers as there are institutions.

Begin by setting up a brainstorming session for everyone involved. Let the staff tell you what *they* feel are reasonable guidelines.

And why not ask the residents to be "fashion consultants"? They'll probably offer a mixture of the practical and the impractical.

Obviously, long loop earrings, chain necklaces, and high-heeled sandals are dangerously out of place in a nursing setting—and have to be on the verboten list.

Perhaps a staff development meeting on cosmetics could subtly discourage inappropriate makeup. In drawing up your dress code, start with the prospective employee. Es-

tablishing ground rules on what's appropriate to wear on the job before hiring an applicant is the best way to avoid hassles afterward.

Dressings

How often should transparent nonocclusive dressings be changed?

Q Our hospital policy manual needs updating, and we can't agree on how often we should change transparent nonocclusive dressings on central lines. Our previous policy required routine changes of all dressings every 48 hours. Do you have any information on how often the transparent nonocclusive dressings should be changed?

A The tendency is to leave them on longer than gauze dressings. Nonocclusive dressings can be left on up to 7 days if there's no evidence of tenderness or exudate. Because the dressing's transparent, you can see what's happening at the insertion site—as long as you don't place an occlusive pad under the dressing.

Isn't initialing them and dating them a bit much?

Q I recently took a job in a nursing home, and I'm finding some of the rules confusing. For instance, last week we were told to put our initials and the date on all dressings.

In my opinion, writing on a dressing is sloppy and could contaminate a wound. What do you think?

A The instructions weren't clear. It's common practice to note the exact time of a dressing change on a *tape* attached to the dressing (you'd never write on the dressing itself). This way, you can check the condition of the dressing during the time that's elapsed.

Drug abuse

How can a patient be helped if he denies there's a problem?

Q One of my patients was recently admitted with hepatitis. His family gave us a history of heavy drug abuse and several arrests for selling narcotics. But when I began my patient teaching, he denied any drug use. How can I help him if he won't admit his problem?

A First, make sure you've got the right information. Although he may have a history of drug abuse, he may be truthfully denying any *current* use. Talk to him in a nonjudgmental manner, and show him that you respect him by listening to his side of the story.

Then, if you believe that he's still actively using drugs, you could take one of three approaches:
• Ask a psychiatric nurse clinical specialist, who's prepared to deal with drug problems, to talk with the patient.
• Speak to the doctor about a psychiatric consultation.
• Refer the patient to a drug abuse treatment program.

If you take the third option, focus your patient teaching on the program, and be prepared to answer his questions about length of stay and cost of treatment.

Should nurses have to watch a suspected orderly?

Q Some of us who work in a busy emergency department suspect an orderly is abusing drugs. Twice recently he asked our nurses to obtain I.V. drugs for him (they thought he was kidding). But that same week, one of the nurses saw him pocketing a 10-mg ampule of diazepam (Valium) from our floor stock. Naturally, she notified the unit manager, and statements documenting the incident were filed.

At that time, the unit manager said the orderly could either choose to be treated for chemical dependency or be terminated. He attended a meeting with her, the division coordinator, and the vice-president for nursing service. The next thing we know, he's back at work!

We nurses feel that administration is wrong; the orderly should be suspended so we won't have the extra burden of watching him. What are your thoughts on this?

A In a busy emergency department, you have enough sick people coming in through the door without having to watch over one of your co-workers, too. Certainly there's merit in that thinking.

On the other hand, the new philosophy of dealing with drug abusers is to keep them in a supportive environment (same jobs, friends, and so forth) while they receive help. There's merit in that, too. But the least you should expect from administration is direction on what's now expected of the orderly, what's expected of the rest of you in relation to him, and what procedure to follow for determining whether he's cooperating with the drug program and competent to remain on the job. Talk to your unit manager about this now.

And remember, being supportive does not mean covering up. If you see that the orderly is not functioning competently, then by all means, speak up right away.

What if nothing's done after reporting a co-worker for pilfering narcotics?

Q Another nurse and I staff the evening shift in the emergency department of a medium-sized hospital. A lot of the patients on our shift do not have true emergencies, but we treat them upon contacting either their family doctor or our doctor on call.

I'm convinced that my co-worker is taking almost all of the prescribed narcotics for her own use. She doesn't give a placebo, but substitutes a milder type of drug that's not on the signout list at our hospital. A number of patients have reported no relief or some strange sensitivity from her "shots." I also find her mood changes very evident. I've indirectly pointed this out to my unit manager, supervisor, and the director of nursing. But nothing has been done. Now what?

A You say you have indirectly pointed this out to your unit manager, supervisor, and director of nursing. Doesn't it seem unlikely that three different people in such responsible positions have simply chosen to ignore this problem? Is it possible that they didn't understand the point you were trying to make? Maybe what you consider "indirect" is simply "obscure" to others. Discuss your suspicions clearly and *directly* with the three people. Once you've done that, be patient. Things aren't going to happen overnight. Drug addiction is such a serious charge that all other possibilities have to be ruled out. Diagnosis of drug addiction can only be made by medical evaluation, including laboratory testing of blood levels. Your director of nursing can, however, ask the staff doctor to visit the nurse on duty and make a cursory evaluation. Most doctors are reluctant to be involved in such matters, though, especially if the person involved isn't their own patient.

Wait a reasonable length of time after directly discussing this with your unit manager. If, after that time, you feel that no internal investigation has been made, contact your state board of licensure and recount your experience. They will investigate the matter while keeping your part completely anonymous.

D

What should a "suspected" nurse do?

Q Two weeks ago, one of my best friends on our unit resigned. Before leaving, she took me aside and warned me to watch my step. She'd heard that my name came up at a management meeting as one of several nurses suspected of drug abuse. I thought she was joking, but she wasn't.

After analyzing my behavior over and over, looking for any reason I'd be suspect, I can't find one. I don't even smoke or drink alcohol.

So far, I haven't heard one word about this from anyone else, but for all I know, documentation of this suspicion could show up in my personnel file. If I bring up the question, "Do you suspect me of drug abuse?" I'm in effect giving credence to this outlandish accusation.

I'm quaking and don't know what to do.

A First, get hold of yourself. Self-torture is pointless; you're not guilty, and you haven't been accused of anything yet. Your friend, as well meaning as she may be, could be mistaken.

Request a meeting with your unit manager and supervisor (better to involve upper management), and ask if there's any truth to the report you received. If so, find out who brought up your name, who was present at the meeting, what documentation exists, and how it's being used. Keep calm and take notes. Then request a follow-up meeting, this time to include the nurse who accused you so that you can resolve this conflict quickly.

If you're satisfied with the outcome of the second meeting, let the matter drop. Because (as you yourself agreed) if "the lady doth protest too much," you'll call more attention to this incident than it deserves.

Drug-addicted nurse

Will past problems interfere with reciprocity in licensing?

Q Over a period of years, I developed a serious problem with drug addiction. I voluntarily committed myself to a residential drug-treatment center from which I "graduated" after 2 years.

During my period of treatment, my license was suspended. I have since been completely reinstated, however, and now have an excellent work record for the past 3 years.

Within the next year, my husband will be transferred to California and I'd like to apply for license reciprocity there. I know that my present board of nursing is required to inform any other state licensing board of my past history. I accept that fact, but I'd like some idea on the chances of my receiving reciprocity. If I'm sure to be turned down, I'd prefer to save myself the trouble and embarrassment and just not bother to apply.

> *"I'm a former drug addict but I've had an excellent work record for the past 3 years. Will I have trouble getting license reciprocity?"*

My current board of nursing has responded to my letters on this subject with what I consider vague non-answers. Can you give me some straight information?

A A consultant from the California State Board of Nursing was unable to supply figures on applicants who have been refused licensure because of past drug addiction. She did say, however, that each case

is judged on an individual basis. When you consider the effort you put into getting a nursing education—and the even greater struggle you must have gone through to cure your addiction—surely the application is worth a try.

The application form will ask if you have been involved in any criminal violation of the law—other than traffic violations. In your answer, honestly discuss your drug problem but also stress your successful return to nursing and your excellent work record over the last 3 years.

If your application *is* turned down, you still have the right to petition the board for a private hearing. And do it. After all, your career is at stake.

Good luck.

Drug addiction

What if a hospital caters to a patient's drug addiction?

Q One of the patients who frequents our small community hospital emergency department (ED) has been receiving meperidine (Demerol) injections for the past 10 years—both as an outpatient and inpatient. She's had multiple surgeries, suffered a myocardial infarction, and developed severe angina. She's been advised to have open-heart surgery but has refused. Last year she totaled 60 visits to the ED and 11 hospital admissions.

When she walks into the ED, she asks, "Has the doctor called in my shot?" We're almost sure she's addicted to the drug but her doctor always backs up her request for an injection. After her shot, she hangs around the ED visiting and buying coffee for everyone. Does *that* sound like a patient in pain?

As unit manager, I've tried every route I know of to put a halt to the injections. I have:
• presented the nurses' concerns at our supervisor meetings.

• recommended to the patient care committee that the injections be discontinued.

• recommended to the nurse-doctor committee that they be discontinued.

• approached the individual doctor and asked him to explain his reason for ordering the injections. He said he didn't want to be responsible for the patient's pain—and seemed amused that we were so concerned.

• attended medical staff meetings and presented our complaints. (The doctors refused to take any action.)

• approached the hospital administrator, who, by the way, supports the doctors' inaction.

I think we're caught between a rock and a hard place—can you help?

A The situation you describe is an abuse of your ED. Doesn't your department have guidelines for what is and is not acceptable in administering drugs? If you don't, you *should* have written guidelines, which would help to resolve future problems.

Guidelines would be a basic resolution, but there are other suggestions you might try:

• Enlist the support of the doctor who's head of the ED, and ask *him* to present your reservations to the attending doctor. Perhaps this doctor won't reject his colleague's appeal as easily as he rejects the nurses'.

• Talk to your director of nursing—ask her to support you. She may carry more clout.

• If you exhaust all means *within* the hospital, look *outside* for a solution. Call your state board of nursing and ask for the address and phone number of your state's professional standards review organization (PSRO). If you have to go as far as the PSRO, make sure you document your case. Include a list of the means you've already exhausted.

These suggestions may not work. But they're worth trying. While

you're working on the problem, try to keep your cool. This *is* an emergency of sorts.

What's the best way to avoid giving drugs to a suspected drug abuser in the ED?

Q I'm sure any nurse who's worked in an emergency department (ED) is familiar with the drug abuser who makes the rounds of the EDs, complaining of questionable ailments in order to obtain a prescription for a medication. Well, these abusers, who are sometimes hostilely referred to as "crocks," seem to be swarming into our ED lately.

Do I *have to* give a suspected drug abuser the medication he's attempting to obtain in this devious way? Or can I withhold it? These abusers need long-term drug counseling, not another pill or needle.

A There's no clear-cut yes or no answer about your giving pills or injections to a suspected drug abuser. But we *can* tell you it's unfair to the patient to determine whether to give him these *without* your having the whole picture and calling on the hospital's support system to help him.

If you think you have grounds, you *do* have the right to refuse to administer medication. But this has two potential traps: (1) Your seemingly well-founded suspicions could prove wrong. (2) Cutting a drug abuser "cold turkey" from his drug supply could do more harm than good—if the process isn't properly supervised.

So the next time a suspected drug abuser shows up in your ED, discuss your suspicion with the doctor. If you all agree there is indeed an abuse problem, use the system to help him. Call for the hospital's drug abuse counselor, if there is one, or for a staff psychiatrist or psychologist. That way, you'd be pointing the patient in the right direction—toward kicking the habit.

Drug administration

What should be done about unclear orders?

D

Q One of our patients who had a transurethral resection (TUR) of the prostate has been diagnosed as having leukemia. For the past 2 weeks, he's been bleeding through his indwelling urinary catheter. His doctor's orders are written: aminocaproic acid (Amicar) 4 grams every 6 hours. Pharmacy has been mixing the medication in 50 ml of dextrose 5% in water, then labeling the flow rate on the bottle as they do on piggybacks.

On previous shifts, the nurses hung the aminocaproic acid as a piggyback at the flow rate of 100 ml/hr. Before I hung a bottle, I questioned pharmacy about the rate typed on the label—8.3 ml/hr. They said that aminocaproic acid should be run as a continuous drip to keep the patient's blood level up and stop the bleeding. The piggyback flow rate is too fast; the aminocaproic acid would be excreted without effect.

I called the doctor, who said it really didn't make that much difference how the medication was run because the bleeding isn't the patient's main problem. I could go ahead and run it as a continuous drip.

What troubles me is that the doctor didn't write the order as a continuous drip. Then the nurses were confused by what "looked like" a piggyback instead of checking the rate on the label. Who's wrong in this situation?

A A general review of medication administration could help all around.

For starters, the doctor's responsible for writing clear and complete orders. He should've included how he wanted the aminocaproic acid administered—either writing "run as a continuous drip" or "piggyback every 6 hrs." His laissez-faire attitude, in effect, sanctions carelessness. His rationale, too, seems both callous and wrong.

Rapid piggyback-like infusion of aminocaproic acid could cause hypotension, bradycardia, or arrhythmias. The maximum rate is 4 to 5 g over 1 hour, and this is prescribed only in cases of severe, acute bleeding. Your pharmacy assumed the doctor wanted the drug given as a continuous infusion, a natural assumption since aminocaproic acid is usually administered that way. They calculated the proper rate of 8.3 ml/hr and labeled the bag. "Working by the book," though, pharmacy should've double-checked with the doctor; a few such calls could remind him to write complete and proper orders.

Now for the nurses' part in this mix-up. If all of them read the label, as you did, they wouldn't be confused over the "look-alike" piggyback. *Read the label* is a basic rule of medication administration.

Drug incompatibilities

If literature advises against a combination of drugs, yet the doctor demands them, should they be given?

Q When ordering medication, doctors in our hospital sometimes disregard the official literature on drug incompatibilities. They explain that they've never had a patient adversely affected by such orders.

But where does this leave us, the nurses? If the literature, for example, advises against a combination of drugs yet the doctor demands that they be combined in a single injection, should we administer it or not?

A At one time, the nurse functioned exclusively under the direction, supervision, and control of the doctor. This meant "hers not to reason why, hers but to do...and not disagree." Such a role put all the responsibility on the doctor, freeing the nurse of legal and professional worries.

This is no longer the case. The law now considers the nurse a primary health care provider. As such, you must know all about the medications you administer—their dosages, indications, contraindications, and interactions with other drugs. If you administer a combination of medications that may produce adverse interactions, you do so at your legal peril.

Yes, the doctor is also liable. But that still doesn't excuse you from your duty to refuse to administer a drug that's incorrectly prescribed.

Now comes the hard part. How do you execute your duty in the face of the doctor's superior role in the management of his patient?

First, have all the pertinent information on hand to reinforce your position. Second, present this to the doctor in the manner of one concerned professional to another. The doctor should reexamine his orders and change them accordingly.

> *"The doctors in our hospital ignore the official literature on drug incompatibilities. Should we administer the drugs or not?"*

If he doesn't, however, you should advise him that you're professionally and legally unable to give the medications. *You must then immediately report this to your supervisor.*

Obviously, this type of confrontation can cause considerable uproar. Any nurse who takes this stand will undoubtedly be unpopular with the doctor in question—and possibly with many of his

medical colleagues. But this is the price of professionalism.

Nursing service, then, must stand together. The director of nursing must confer with the hospital administrator, reminding him that if a nurse administers incompatible medication that harms the patient, the hospital would be vicariously liable, too.

It's from just such confrontations and subsequent conferences that new—and better—hospital procedures evolve. Let's trust that this will be the outcome of your action.

Drug samples

Would giving a sample to a co-worker be risking a nurse's license?

Q We frequently get free drug samples from the drug company salespeople who stop in at the clinic where I work. I see other nurses in the clinic giving these samples to office workers who've complained about their various ailments. I'm talking about prescription drugs that have *not* been ordered by a doctor for that particular person. Antihistamines seem to be especially popular.

Just what *is* the law governing these circumstances? For example, can I give a drug sample to a receptionist if she asks for one? Could I risk my license by this act?

A You most certainly could. The law is clear: Nurses are not licensed to prescribe or dispense medication in your state. And it sounds like some of your co-workers are doing exactly that.

Discuss this matter with the director of the clinic as soon as possible. Does he know what's going on? What if one of the office workers on "free" medication should develop an adverse reaction? The nurses and your clinic could be in costly trouble

Drug screening

Can a nurse be required to witness a urine specimen collection?

Q We do many preemployment physicals at the hospital clinic where I work. Lately, our clients have been asking us to witness applicants' urine specimens for drug testing. That means a nurse must go into the bathroom with the applicant to make sure he's giving us his own urine.

Naturally, most applicants are offended by this procedure. I've refused to participate because I believe it's unethical. I'm a nurse, not a spy. What should I do?

A Before making a decision, consider changes that the clinic could make in the testing procedure. For instance, a job applicant could be asked to disrobe and put on a gown in the examination room, then use a bathroom that isn't connected to that room. That way, he couldn't easily take a sample with him to substitute for his own urine. When he returns with the specimen, you could feel the cup: A fresh specimen will be warm.

But if your clients still insist on witnessed specimens, don't participate unless the applicant has signed a consent form that spells out what's required. Make sure the form contains a statement like this: "I understand that I will be observed during the urination process to assure that the urine tested is my own. I consent to direct observation of urination by a licensed health care professional." The clinic should keep copies of those forms on file.

Also, you should observe only applicants of your sex. During testing hours, the clinic should provide male and female nurses.

Finally, check to make sure the clinic's policies and procedures for drug testing comply with federal and state laws regarding individual privacy. Union regulations may also affect how you and the clinic conduct preemployment drug testing.

How can tests come up positive when a person has never done drugs?

Q My husband applied for a job at a company where all applicants must take a drug-screening urine test. The laboratory that processes the test reported my husband's results as positive for cocaine and marijuana.

This was incredible. Neither my husband nor I have ever used drugs, so we immediately asked our doctor to order another test conducted at a different laboratory. The results came back negative. Still, the company doctor says his recommendation against hiring must be based on the original test result. Period.

We all know that tests can show a false positive, or the laboratory itself can mix up the specimens or reports. You can imagine how frustrated and angry we are—especially because my husband is out of work and really wanted that job.

We'd appreciate your opinion.

A Drug testing on employees (or prospective employees) is a hot topic still being debated and delineated. As you point out, the procedure isn't fail-safe. Test results are about 90% accurate if the tests are done by a certified laboratory.

Unfortunately, an employer can reject any applicant based on a urine screen without stating all the conditions for which the screen was performed or why the applicant was rejected. An applicant has no inherent *right* to be hired and can be rejected even for a bad reason, such as incorrect test results, as long as the reason does not demonstrate illegal discrimination based on age, sex, race, union activity, and so forth.

Your husband should write a memo detailing his treatment as an applicant and his objections; include a copy of the privately obtained test results; have the memo notarized; and send it to the president of the company, return receipt requested. Also ask that this memo be kept on file with his application.

Then good luck to your husband in his job search—elsewhere. Handling this situation as intelligently as he did suggests that he'd be a good prospect for any employer.

DTP vaccines

Is it okay to administer DT boosters instead of DTP?

Q At the large doctors' office where I work, diphtheria-tetanus-pertussis (DTP) vaccinations cost so much that some young parents complained. After this, two of the doctors started administering diphtheria-tetanus (DT) boosters to children 18 months and older who had had the series of three DTP shots as infants.

Is this okay? And what's behind the drastic jump in price?

A The price of DTP vaccine soared from $4.29 per dose to $11.40 because the new price includes $8 to cover the manufacturer against product liability. Here's what happened: Lederle Laboratories' insurance coverage for vaccine-related claims expired earlier this year with no replacement coverage available. To continue offering the vaccine at all, the company had to self-insure against future liability exposure for DTP-associated injury. And the new price takes into account the continued escalation of liability claims in both number and size of awards. (Lederle reports 100 vaccine-related lawsuits filed last year, more than the total number of claims for the previous 3 years combined.)

But the U.S. Public Health Service still recommends the five-dose regimen of DTP, high priced or not. And with plenty of vaccine available to fill the demand, the health service says that practitioners shouldn't administer partial doses of DTP vaccine (the degree of protection afforded by such partial doses is not certain). Nor should they substitute DT vaccine in the routine DTP schedule for 18-month-old and 4- to 6-year-old children.

Here's where you can help—by educating parents about this highly contagious and debilitating disease. When you think about it, pertussis (or whooping cough, or the hundred days' cough, as it's known in Japan) even *sounds* old fashioned; it's rarely seen in the United States today thanks to the widespread use of vaccines. So young parents (and young doctors, too) could well underestimate the need for full protection. Until a better vaccine comes along, or we're able to put a cap on liability claims, the five-dose regimen of DTP offers the best protection.

Dying patient

Any suggestions to help a fearful nurse communicate with her patients?

Q I'm a nursing student, and I know I may eventually have to tell a patient he's dying. I want to be a good nurse, but I'm frightened by this aspect of my job. Could you offer some suggestions?

A First of all, your honesty is refreshing. Many nurses have the same fear but won't acknowledge it.

You must understand that death is a taboo subject in our society. So you can expect to have some difficulty, simply because you're a product of society. You don't want to be blamed for upsetting patients with bad news or for not being able to treat them. You may have to admit that you don't know all the answers to a patient's questions. Plus, talking about death can remind you of your own.

In short, the whole thing can be quite upsetting.

The issue isn't whether you should or shouldn't tell a patient he's dying. He'll probably tell *you*. Instead, it's about listening to his concerns.

So you might sit down with your patient, hold his hand, and tell him that you'll stick by him as he dies, making sure you keep his pain under control. Patients often fear that they'll be abandoned by their caregivers and that they'll be in excruciating, unmanaged pain.

Encourage him to ask questions and assure him that you'll always answer him honestly. Don't say, "We can't do anything more for you." Shift your focus from "cure" to "care." Develop the skills to keep a terminally ill patient's pain and other symptoms under control.

You have plenty of work ahead. And the reward of many good feelings.

How can a nurse break through a patient's denial?

Q One of my terminally ill patients refuses to admit that he's dying. He believes his lung cancer is just an infection and that he'll soon be back at his farm. He's even talking about the next planting season and the new tractor he's going to buy. How do you get patients to face reality?

A Don't force them. Let *them* decide when they're ready.

You're witnessing your patient's defense mechanism in action. He's come up with a reason for his illness, and that's sustaining him. When he's ready, he'll deal with death in his own way.

A patient who's desperately denying his illness is vulnerable. Even if you could convince him that he's dying, you shouldn't; he's not ready.

Remain supportive and nonjudgmental. Your patient might eventually work through his fears and share his feelings. But he might not. That's okay, too, because that's what he wants. And isn't that what *you* want for him?

How can a nurse help her patient face it?

Q One of my patients is dying of liver cancer. He's a warm, funny man—even when he's in pain—and I enjoy talking with him about his family and hobbies.

One thing bothers me though: Whenever his wife or daughter mentions his illness, he makes a joke and changes the subject. Should I be concerned that he isn't facing his death?

A He is facing his death, in his own way. We're all fairly predictable in the way we cope with crises. Your patient has probably laughed off past disasters to protect his family from pain.

The next time you have a quiet moment alone with him, try asking him how he got through other painful times in his life. As he recalls the way he handled past crises, he may find another way to deal with this one.

How can a nurse objectively communicate with someone she knows?

Q My best friend's terminally ill father was recently admitted to the unit where I work. Although we've been close for years, I'm having trouble talking with him now. I don't want to abandon him, but I feel uncomfortable discussing death.

A Your last statement could be the crux of this problem. Perhaps *you've* created an obstacle because you feel obligated to sit down and have a "death session." But that's not necessary—your patient knows he's dying. All he wants is for you to listen and to answer his questions honestly.

If he senses that his questions make you uncomfortable, though, he may try to protect you by changing the subject. Then you both lose. He'll die without ever knowing how his dying has affected you.

Next time you're in his room, sit down and have a chat. Don't force the conversation—start by asking him how things are going. If he begins to talk about being seriously ill, don't pull back and hide behind trite responses or technical language. Be honest, affectionate, and respectful. In other words, be yourself. Let him know that you care about him and will stand by him throughout the entire dying process.

Finally, don't be too hard on yourself. Acknowledge your humanness. And trust your heart—it won't lead you astray.

How do you get patients to make their last requests in time?

Q I've cared for only a few dying patients. But I noticed that each of them had something in common—a special last request. Unfortunately, several of them waited too long to tell anyone what they wanted. How can I get future patients to talk about their last requests?

A Don't wait for them to ask. In most cases, you'll have to make the first move. There are three universal questions you should ask a dying patient:

• *What do you want now?* "Now" is different than 6 weeks ago, when he was still hoping for a remission. "Now" is different, because radiation treatments haven't helped. So ask this question often. As his con-

dition worsens, his needs may change dramatically.

• *From whom do you want it?* Your patient may want to talk to someone besides you. Don't take that personally. After all, you may not be the best person to help him. Find out, from him, who is.

• *When do you want it?* Timing is important. For example, your patient may want you to locate a loved one by next week for his birthday.

Ask your patient what he wants. Don't rely on his doctor, spouse, or social worker to tell you. You need to hear the answers from him.

Should a patient be allowed to say good-bye to a pet?

Q A terminally ill patient on my unit asked to see her dog one last time. When my manager said no, the patient was crushed. Do you think we should do this favor for her?

A Yes, because she's making a legitimate request. First, find out why seeing her dog is so important. Take that information to your manager and explain the situation. Then, you and she should get together with other people at the hospital, including the infection-control nurse, and see how you can grant your patient's request. The point here is if you believe in helping her, put your beliefs into action.

When is the right time to call the family?

Q Although my terminally ill patient has some good days, I know he won't last much longer. Most of his family is here with him, but one son lives out in Wyoming. When is the right time for the family to call him? They don't want him to come here too soon. But they don't want to wait until it's too late either.

A There's rarely a time that's *precisely* right. But most people would prefer to come early and have a few last days with their loved one, rather than arrive only in time for the funeral.

In your situation, what's the worst thing that can happen? The son comes to see his father, returns to Wyoming, then a day later finds out his father has died? He'll probably be grateful for those last few days that he had with his father.

So, call your patient's son and give him all the information you have. Then let him make his own decision.

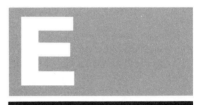

Education

Is there any way to get better scores on multiple-choice tests?

Q After working for 20 years as an LPN, I've returned to school to get my associate's degree. Although I'm doing well enough, I'm having trouble with multiple-choice tests. Often it seems that more than one answer is correct, and I'm not sure which type of response is best—clinical, psychological, or social. So even though I know my material, I don't score as high as I should, and I'm becoming discouraged. Can you help me?

A Many LPNs in associate degree programs have the same problem—so don't panic. You bring a lot of practical knowledge with you that the other students don't have; naturally, your reaction to these questions is influenced by your experience. But all you're supposed to know about the patient is given in the question, so focus on that information, analyze what's really being asked, and connect it with the choices given. (As a rule of thumb, whenever a question presents an emergency situation, the appropriate clinical action will be the best answer.) Remember, too, that each teacher favors a special area of nursing. After taking several of her tests, you'll know the area she's most likely to stress.

Practice helps. Buy a state-board exam review; do a lot of questions and look up the answers. You'll soon become adept at this kind of test and be reviewing for state boards at the same time—and that can't hurt.

Look for *American Nursing Review for NCLEX-RN* by Carol J. Bininger, et al. (Springhouse, Pa.: Springhouse Corporation, 1989).

Should an experienced nurse seek a BS or a BSN?

Q As an RN, I can enroll in a college BS program that will give me 30 semester hours of credit for my nursing experience. Doesn't this make more sense than enrolling in the BSN program and having to challenge courses or repeat many of the things I've already learned?

A Here's the National League for Nursing's (NLN) appraisal of college degree programs that have no major in nursing:

"The programs in question (which promise large blocks of credit for previous nursing education) lead to associate or baccalaureate degrees in such fields as applied science, biology, education, health science, occupational therapy, psychology, and sociology. Such collegiate programs may provide the student with increased knowledge in the area of the major, but they do *not* offer additional preparation in nursing.

"Students are misguided by the publicity about these programs which:
1. Implies that a major in another field is the equal of the major in nursing as preparation for nursing practice—when it is not.
2. Implies that they are acceptable as a base for further education in nursing—when they are not.
3. Implies that they lead to advancement in employment—which in many instances they do not.
4. Implies that because only graduates of NLN-accredited nursing programs are awarded credit, the degree programs are therefore approved by NLN—which they are not."

Now to amplify point 2 of the statement for those who are interested in advanced degrees: Be forewarned that the basic requirement in most MSN programs is that you be a graduate of an NLN-accredited baccalaureate program or a baccalaureate program with an upper division major in nursing.

Elder abuse

What should a nurse do if she suspects it?

Q Months ago, I noticed several bruises on an elderly woman who'd been admitted to the emergency department (ED) with the flu. She was vague about how she got them—"I fall a lot," was all she'd say. Yesterday, she came to the ED again, this time with a fractured arm and more bruises. As I was questioning her about the fracture, she broke down and admitted that her nephew had been abusing her since he moved in with her a year ago.

Besides being horrified that this happened, I'm concerned about the fact that I'd missed signs of abuse. Could I be held liable for the injuries she suffered afterward?

A Not likely, unless you hadn't adequately assessed and documented her condition the first time—or if you had a good reason to suspect abuse but didn't report it. (Abuse is reportable in all states.)

"As I was questioning her about the fracture, she broke down and admitted that her nephew had been abusing her."

Suppose this patient decided to sue you. In deciding negligence, the court would ask whether another reasonably prudent nurse in a similar situation would have acted as you did. The answer in this case is probably yes. You had no reason to suspect that the patient was hiding something, so you didn't breach the standard of nursing care.

Electrocardiograms

Can you recommend a workbook that will help me brush up?

Q Back in 1980, I took a course in electrocardiogram (ECG) interpretation but didn't get a chance to use the skill. Recently, I landed my dream job in the emergency department, and true to the old saying "Use it or lose it," I've forgotten most of what I learned about rhythm interpretation.

Can you recommend a workbook that will help me brush up?

A *Clinical Electrocardiography: A Self-Study Course,* by Emanuel Stein (Philadelphia: Lea & Febiger, 1987), explains interpretations of normal and abnormal ECGs and includes practice ECGs.

Or, for a video demonstration, try *Reading ECGs,* one of eight videocassette titles in a new low-cost video skills series. You can order by writing to Springhouse Corporation

Book Division, 1111 Bethlehem Pike, Springhouse, PA 19477; call 1-215-646-8700 for prices.

Emergency department

Is it legal to give narcotics to patients with standing orders?

Q Several patients have become emergency department (ED) regulars in the rural hospital where I work. When they come in complaining of headaches, backaches, abdominal pain, or other discomforts, they bring with them standing orders for narcotics from their private doctors. These patients never see an ED doctor. We're expected to evaluate them and give them the medications named in the standing orders.

We don't feel comfortable about this. What can we do?

A You shouldn't be participating in this practice. Essentially, you're evaluating patients and prescribing (as opposed to administering) medication, so you're practicing medicine. True, some nurses are taking on expanded roles in certain circumstances. But what you describe isn't one of those.

Remember, you aren't obligated to blindly follow a standing order. The courts expect you to know why a drug is being used, how it interacts with other drugs, and what adverse reactions it can cause. In this case, you may be giving medications that are inappropriate for the patients' ailments.

Insist that the ED doctors evaluate these patients and prescribe appropriate medication. If they resist, and nursing administration doesn't support you, detail your concerns in a memo and send it through channels. Make sure the hospital's lawyer and risk manager get a copy.

Is there a liability in detaining a patient because beds aren't available on other units?

Q In my hospital, patients often have to wait in the emergency department (ED) until beds become available on other units. Several times I've been unable to monitor these patients as closely as I should. I'm concerned about my liability if one of them develops a serious complication. What should I do the next time I'm asked to keep a patient in the ED?

A You're facing a common problem. Staffing shortages have forced hospitals to close beds temporarily, which may back up the ED. Patients can end up waiting hours— even days—for an open bed.

Although in limbo, these patients have essentially been admitted to the hospital, so both you and the hospital are obligated to provide quality care. You can't shrug off that responsibility. You're expected to maintain the usual standard of care and perform routine nursing duties, including monitoring. In recent court cases, patients have won verdicts because the ED staff failed to monitor them properly.

As always, documentation is critical. Record not only the patient's signs and symptoms but also staffing patterns and needs. Of course, you shouldn't put staffing information in the patient's chart; instead, use the appropriate administrative form and send it through channels. If an injured patient names you in a negligence lawsuit, you'd have to prove that you requested—but didn't receive—extra staff to handle the crunch. You'd also have to show that you frequently assessed and recorded his vital signs, and that you left him only to care for others with greater needs.

If short staffing is a chronic problem, your manager should suggest that administration beef up the ED staff. Failing that, administrators may have to divert ambulances to other hospitals.

Shouldn't parents be allowed in?

Q After the mother of a 3-year-old fainted and hit her head during her son's treatment, our emergency department (ED) director issued a new policy: No family members allowed in the treatment rooms. I'm concerned that our young patients will miss the emotional support their parents can give. I'm also wondering if we can really bar parents from the treatment rooms. And what if I disregard policy and let parents in anyway? Could I be liable if one of them were injured?

A You bet you could. And because you'd violated a hospital policy, your employer might not have to share liability with you if a parent were injured. Even if a court did allow a parent to recover damages from the hospital, administrators could turn around and sue *you*.

Remember, although parents usually must consent to treatment for their minor children, they don't have a legal right to be in the treatment room. That's a courtesy health care practitioners sometimes grant for two reasons: so the parents can help control the child and so they can provide emotional support during treatment.

But if parents are becoming troublesome, a policy like the one handed down by your ED director makes sense.

What can be done about understaffing?

Q The pediatric unit where I work is minimally staffed at night. We have all we can do to care for our patients, make phone calls, and

E

E

get the paperwork done. But we're also expected to be on call for our emergency department (ED).

Last night, as often happens, I got tied up for hours helping with a multiple trauma patient in the ED. This left my co-worker in pediatrics with all her work—and all of mine, too. When we complained to the administrator, he shrugged his shoulders and said we should call the coordinator when we're in a bind.

Let's be realistic—when you're caught up in an emergency, you can't waste time on the telephone. Besides, who will the coordinator call? Nurses in other departments don't know where to find anything in the ED. And I wouldn't dream of trusting a very sick infant to someone inexperienced.

Sure, hospitals everywhere are cutting costs. But our licenses go on the line when we leave our pediatric patients and again when we give less than optimal care to patients in the ED because we're in a hurry to get back.

Do you see why we're worried?

A What you have is double trouble. Emergency and pediatrics are two hospital departments where the public least accepts mediocre care. In fact, the largest lawsuit settlements involve children. Any administrator worth his salt should know this. And you should know by now that you'll continue to be dumped on—until you say *enough,* loud and clear.

But say it in *writing,* through channels that include the medical chiefs of both departments. Send statistics on how often and for how long you're called to the ED. And offer solutions. The best one, of course, would be a full-time nurse in the ED. But if this is out of the question, nurses from other departments, once properly oriented, could safely answer calls to the ED. After all, you're not the only ones capable of taking on this responsibility.

Also, contact the nurses at your local chapter of the Emergency Nurses Association; they'll be interested in your plight and may offer further suggestions.

What if an ED nurse can't work in an overseas ED?

Q I am, or maybe I should say I *was,* an emergency department (ED) nurse. Several months ago I signed up to work in a hospital overseas for a year. I accepted a job in the ED offered by a recruiter.

But when I arrived at the hospital, I was assigned to a medical/surgical unit. They told me the ED was already overstaffed.

I hate floor nursing and would never have come if I had all the facts. Belatedly, I studied my contract and found it did *not* specify that I was to work in the ED.

To take this job, I gave up an ED position I loved, surrendered the lease on my apartment, stored my furniture, and sold my car. I tried to explain all this to the director of nursing as calmly and tactfully as I could, but I got nowhere. Now I've written an official letter requesting a transfer to the ED as soon as there's an opening.

Have I overlooked any other options? Should I consult a lawyer? I not only want your opinion, but I also want to warn other nurses to read the fine print in their contracts before signing up for a great adventure.

A The legal route will probably not prove useful since your contract doesn't guarantee you an ED position. But don't give up yet. If you don't hear from the director of nursing soon, send her another polite transfer request. Send copies of your request to the hospital administration and to the American office where your recruiter is stationed.

You're caught in a situation that could have happened here on the home front. That's not to belittle

your problem, which is magnified by your distance from home.

Since you're already there, thousands of miles from home, keep trying to remedy the situation. There's always the possibility that when they get to know you and your nursing strengths, they'll transfer you to a position where you'll be happier.

You're undoubtedly going through a period of adjustment—and a normal bit of homesickness. (That's part of foreign employment, although not the alluring part.) Your year in a foreign country still comes under the heading of a new experience, although it's not exactly the experience you had in mind. The year sounds like a time to grow and learn. Try it—you may like it.

Where should ED patients wait for their private doctor until he arrives?

Q One of our staff doctors frequently instructs private patients having problems after office hours to meet him at the emergency department (ED) as soon as possible. The patient can arrive in as little as 15 minutes; the doctor frequently takes an hour or more.

As an ED nurse, what are my responsibilities to these private patients? The patients expect their doctor, and they're reluctant to see anyone else.

Where should they wait for their doctor? In the waiting room? If so, are we responsible for them if anything happens?

A The ED is *not* the doctor's office. No sick or injured person should go unchecked and left in the waiting room marking time until his private doctor arrives.

Anyone meeting a private doctor in the ED should be registered as an ED patient and taken to the treatment area. You should record his vital signs; evaluate him and call in the ED doctor if you find signs that warrant immediate attention. Of course, the patient can refuse examination by the ED doctor. If this happens, carefully document it in the patient's chart.

Chances are, any jury would question why a person with complaints signaling an emergency would be left untreated—right in the ED. The ED personnel should get together and decide on a policy—both for handling the patients and raising the consciousness of the dawdling doctor.

Who's liable for agency nurses?

Q When we're short-staffed in the emergency department (ED)—particularly on weekends and holidays—we're often forced to call in agency nurses to fill the gaps. We've been concerned about liability in these situations. If a patient were injured by a negligent agency nurse, would the staff nurses working with her be held responsible, too?

A They could be, if they'd participated in the patient's care. Or, a court could find them liable if they knew, or should have known, that an error was being made, or if they knew the agency nurse was incompetent.

Incidentally, both the hospital and agency could be held responsible for an agency nurse's negligence. Because of this, the hospital may have what's known as a "hold harmless" agreement with the agency. Basically, this type of agreement requires the agency to defend the hospital in a negligence lawsuit and pay any damages awarded to an injured patient.

Who's responsible for the patient's treatment?

Q Last week, a patient's private doctor telephoned our emergency department (ED), arguing loud and long against the ED doctor's care of his patient. He claimed that what he says, goes. We say that while a patient is in the ED, we're responsible for his treatment. What do you say?

A While a patient's in the ED, you're responsible for his treatment, and you don't have to follow directions given over the phone by his private doctor. However, if the patient's doctor is in the ED, then *he* should decide how his patient will be treated. When this happens, the ED doctor should document his own findings in your department's record and note that he transferred responsibility to the patient's doctor.

Your ED needs a written policy covering this. Until then, call in the department's medical chief to act as mediator.

Would a nurse be helping to perpetuate fraud if a patient said he was faking an injury?

Q A 32-year-old man recently came to our emergency department (ED) for a return-to-work certificate. He told me he'd faked a wrist injury so he wouldn't have to work during a heat wave. I wasn't sure if he was telling the truth, so I let him see the doctor.

But he gave the doctor a different story—he said he really had injured his wrist. I took the doctor aside and told him what the man had said to me, but the doctor decided to order an X-ray and an elastic bandage for the wrist anyway. Then he wrote the certificate.

I've been concerned ever since that the doctor and I may have helped this man commit fraud. Should we have called this man's bluff, or did we act correctly?

A Legally, you can't go wrong by referring an ED patient for treatment. That's because the law gives the patient the benefit of the doubt, even if there's only a slight possibility that he needs treatment. Besides, you couldn't be sure he was telling the truth when he said his wrist was all right.

For the same reason, the doctor was legally correct when he ordered the X-ray. But he shouldn't have ordered the elastic bandage unless he believed the patient really had an injury. Otherwise, the extra treatment could be construed as unnecessary work that the patient's employer must pay for.

As for granting the certificate, the patient was fit to return to work, wasn't he? So that, too, was legally correct, regardless of whether he'd been unable to work for legitimate reasons.

If you and the doctor had been *absolutely* sure that the man was malingering, your actions might be construed as helping to perpetuate a fraud against the man's employer. But in the situation you describe, that doesn't seem to be the case.

Emotional involvement

Is caring for a patient for a long time good for a nurse?

Q For many years, I was a private-duty nurse to an elderly woman in her own apartment. Two months ago, her family placed her in a nursing home.

Although I found a new job quickly enough, it was hard for me to let go of this patient. She became a good friend over the years, and she often told me how much she dreaded leaving her own home. When I visit her in the evenings, she seems content as long as she knows I'll be back. Maybe she's adjusting to the change better than I am.

Having this experience makes me wonder if caring for a patient for a long time is good for a nurse. Should I just try not to get involved?

A How intensely you get emotionally involved with another person depends more on your capacity for caring than on the calendar. And getting emotionally involved with a patient presents the same risks as any other relationship. When a warm relationship of long standing is altered or ended, you're bound to feel it.

What you're going through now seems to be a form of the grief-loss process we experience with the death of someone dear to us. Only, in your case, that person is still very much alive. So, look at the good side of the situation: The contact you maintain is extremely good for you both. And surely you can take comfort in knowing that the patient is starting to adjust to her new life—once again, thanks to your faithful caring.

Emotional support

Isn't it as important as physical care?

Q My manager says I spend too much time talking with my patients. I know I'm sometimes late with treatments and baths, but isn't my emotional support as important as my physical care? I don't want to rush around, cutting off patients in midsentence, just to complete my charting.

A You raise an important issue: Nurses must make ethical choices when deciding how to set priorities. Which patient has the greatest need? Should one patient have a nurse all to himself while others see very little of her during the shift? Is physical or psychological care more important for this patient at this time? These are quality-of-life choices, especially for very sick or very anxious patients.

To answer your question, physical and emotional interventions are equally important. Instead of seeing them as opposites competing for your time, you should find ways to integrate them. For example, you could use such techniques as therapeutic touch, relaxation therapy, meditation, or prayer while you bathe or reposition your patients or when you change their dressings.

The key is to clarify your patient-care goals and to stay focused on them. That way, you'll spend quality time with your patients and your conversations will be more meaningful. Patient teaching, for example, could be part of your dialogue. Use active listening skills and ask open-ended questions that require more than yes-or-no answers. Chart your conversations so you can identify and evaluate the psychological interventions you've included in your care plan.

By planning ahead, you can perform routine tasks efficiently without sacrificing your patients' emotional needs. That should satisfy your manager as well as your patients.

Employee problems

Must an RN work where she's assigned?

Q I'm director of nursing in a small hospital. I try to take my nurses' preferences into account, but I expect them to take orientation wherever I assign them.

Recently I asked a part-time RN to take orientation in two specific units. In both cases she flatly refused, saying that she hated those units and wouldn't even prepare to work on either.

But the units where she preferred to work were already adequately staffed. I followed hospital policy and suspended her. Naturally, she was angry. Can I insist that she work where I assign her?

A Yes, you can insist. Now, about the nurse who refused an assignment: Unless she's contracted to work on a specific unit, a quality nurse must work where you assign her. You were justified in suspending her.

If you must make an unpopular assignment, it's your job to do it—and the nurse's obligation to comply.

Employment

Can't a retired nurse work without being considered a nurse?

Q Several months ago, I started working in an adult day-care center as an activities coordinator—not as a *nurse*. I haven't worked as a nurse for many years. I'm past 60, and I don't want the responsibility anymore—although I still have my license.

Unfortunately, the managers noted this on my application. And while they agreed in principle that I wouldn't be expected to nurse, they've told the staff and clients that I'm an RN, implying that I'm available for consultation.

Now I'm worried about liability. Can't a nurse retire?

A Quite simply, once you become an RN, you remain an RN unless your license is revoked for cause by your state board of nursing. You're responsible for any *nursing* action you decide to perform. But you can make a conscious decision to avoid performing nursing duties where you work and on your own time if that's what you want.

Let your employer know, in writing, that you won't be performing nursing duties as part of your job and that you want this stipulated in your personnel file. After all, no law forces you to assume a nurse-patient relationship.

If a nurse is *needed* in the day-care center, management is responsible for hiring one. You, on the other hand, should feel valued for performing well in the job you were hired to do—not for any extras management hoped your nursing license would provide.

How can a director of nursing be overqualified?

Q I can't make sense out of a recent administrative decision at the 80-bed, acute-care hospital where I work. Here's a brief account, as I understand it: The position of director of nursing opened up at the same time that an experienced and respected nursing supervisor with a master's degree in nursing administration moved here from out of state. When she applied for the job, she was turned down. I'm not questioning the rejection itself, since there may have been factors I knew nothing about. But I was nonplussed by the reason the committee gave for turning her down. They told the applicant she was "overqualified" for the job and therefore would not fit into their management structure.

How can a nurse be overqualified to direct the nursing care of 80 human beings? The hospital serves an inner-city population of patients: about 75% are black, and 95% are in a low-income bracket. Is the committee implying that patients without money or clout do not warrant a director of nursing with first-class credentials?

A Your hospital—the interviewing committee in particular—needs to move into the 1990s. Excellence should be the basic nursing goal. You might tell the members of the committee that many inner-city hospitals throughout the country consider a doctoral degree a requisite for the position of director of nursing. Some hospitals even require that the director of surgical nursing or the director of operating room nursing have a doctorate.

You're right in questioning how the applicant you describe could be "overqualified." Perhaps it will help to send a photocopy of this to each committee member for enlightenment.

How should a nurse express her complaints effectively?

Q After 9 years as a part-time RN in a hospital, I got a letter yesterday telling me my workdays were being cut from 3 days a week to every-other weekend. All part-time nurses are getting the same cut. Today, I got a form letter from the hospital asking me to will part of my estate to the hospital in the event of my death. Talk about nerve!

The cut will drastically decrease my salary and will also eliminate my 10-day paid vacation every year. It just isn't fair. Is there any way I can fight back?

A Not really. As you've no doubt found out, part-time workers miss out on many of the benefits full-time workers take for granted.

Still, after 9 years of faithful service, you should rate an appointment with your director of nursing or administrator. You don't have anything to lose, and you might find them receptive to your argument that loyal, permanent employees, albeit part-timers, are too valuable to be treated so uncaringly.

As for the form letter about leaving part of your estate to the hospital: Don't pay any attention to it—it's just a form letter that probably went out to everyone who's contributed to the hospital or connected to it in any way.

What if a job offer sounds too good to be true?

Q Last week, I received a letter from a nursing agency in California with a job offer that sounds too good to be true. For instance,

if I contract for 1 to 5 years for a steady hospital assignment or as a float-pool nurse, I'd be guaranteed a 48-hour workweek at a salary of $50,000 to $65,000 a year. The agency would pay for my round-trip airfare plus my rent and utilities in a studio apartment (luxury accommodations with swimming pool, Jacuzzi whirlpool, and tennis courts) while I work for them. They promise quick licensing reciprocity so that I could start working almost immediately.

> *"The nursing agency would pay for my airfare plus rent and utilities in a studio apartment (luxury accommodations with swimming pool, Jacuzzi and tennis courts)."*

I'm tempted because I could save toward buying a house. But I'd hate to be miserable for a whole year. Any advice for a skeptic?

A The offering could be perfectly legitimate. If you know what you want and make sure your requirements are written into the contract before you sign on, you could have a great and profitable time. Others do.

Here are some questions to ask: Is there an "escape" clause with airfare home if the housing or other arrangements don't live up to your expectations? If you'd rather move up to a one-bedroom apartment, how much would you have to "co-pay"? Can they give you the names and phone numbers of nurses (preferably from Canada) who are currently working for the agency so you can call them? And can they tell you in advance which hospitals you could be working in, the terms of employment, nurse-patient ratio, commuting distance (you may need a car), and security arrangements in case you'd be working at night?

Who would pay for your malpractice insurance? Are health benefits included? Is the cost of living prohibitive? What about taxes? Any agency on the up and up should welcome your scrutiny. And if you're still skeptical, you can phone the chamber of commerce or Better Business Bureau in the city where the agency's headquartered and ask whether there's any information available.

Whenever you make a drastic life change, even for a limited time, you're bound to be happy on some days and down on others. A year or two passes quickly. And nursing in a new environment can expand your professional and personal horizons—which is especially nice to look back on, from home.

Endoscopy

Doesn't Versed cause respiratory distress?

Q We do a lot of endoscopy procedures at this small hospital; all are performed by a general surgeon under what he calls "local" I.V. sedation of 4 to 8 mg of Stadol and 5 to 20 mg of Versed by I.V. titration.

I've heard that Versed is a dangerous drug. But the surgeon insists that we nurses administer it and monitor these patients. Twice when I sedated patients slowly with a minimum titration of Versed, they went into respiratory distress. That scared me and the other nurses, but the surgeon shrugged and laughed at our fears.

Please give your comments and advice. Are we making too much of this?

A On the contrary, you're not making enough of it. Intravenous Versed (midazolam) must be used very cautiously. For you to determine the amount of Versed to be titrated is beyond your scope of practice. The doctor should inject the initial dose; then (if your hospital policy permits) you could follow his orders to inject specific amounts of additional Versed needed during the procedure. Document it as a verbal order. However, if the doctor wants a dosage higher than the manufacturer recommends, he should give it himself.

The high dosage of Versed you mention could cause respiratory depression and arrest, especially when combined with Stadol (butorphanol tartrate). The usual dosage range is 1 to 3 mg when given with I.V. meperidine (pethidine, Demerol), and the Versed is diluted with saline or dextrose 5% in water to a concentration of 1 mg/ml (diluting the drug gives a larger volume to work with and facilitates slower injection). The doctor starts with an initial dose of 1 mg and slowly titrates additional doses after 2- to 3-minute intervals, stopping as soon as the patient's speech becomes slurred, because the sedative effect continues to increase after the injection. During and after the injection, nurses monitor the patient with an oximeter to provide a continuous recording of his oxygen saturation and pulse rate. And, as the manufacturer suggests, resuscitative equipment is kept readily available.

A citizens' group asked the Food and Drug Administration (FDA) to ban the use of Versed for conscious sedation, claiming that the FDA's authorization invites its use in settings where patients aren't closely supervised. In reply, the FDA reported that the manufacturer, Hoffman-LaRoche, made several labeling changes to give cautions and clarify dosing recommendations. Why not contact their representative and ask for literature and a presentation? Then pass this information, along with your concerns, to the chief of surgery, the director of anesthesia, and the hospital lawyer. They should be as interested as you are in changing this dangerous practice.

Endotracheal intubation

Can a nurse refuse to intubate newborns?

Q In the small hospital nursery where I work, a new policy says that we must learn how to intubate a newborn in case of emergency.

The prospect makes me very uncomfortable. Learning to intubate newborns is one thing, but if I don't practice it on a routine basis, I'll hardly be proficient in an emergency. I'd like to refuse this responsibility. Do you agree?

A No, and we'll tell you why. A newborn's delicate tissues can be severely damaged by intubation performed by an inexperienced person. But the trend these days *is* to train nurses, such as yourself, to do this procedure in an emergency.

According to the standards published by the Nurses' Association of the American College of Obstetrics and Gynecology, you'd be wise to follow your hospital's policy and the current trend. Legally, any nurse can refuse to intubate only if she's *not* trained.

Should EMTs be doing intubation in the ICU?

Q Our hospital's emergency medical technicians (EMTs) help with patient care whenever they're not needed for ambulance service. The EMTs in the coronary intensive care unit (ICU)—where I'm the charge nurse—start I.V. lines, give medications, and perform other duties. All these are done under nursing supervision.

My problem is that the EMTs are now doing endotracheal intubations (frequently with just a telephone order, because no doctor's available). Neither the other nurses nor I are trained in intubation, because the doctors have turned down our requests for this training: They said the procedure wouldn't be used frequently enough to provide us with sufficient practice.

But if I'm being held responsible for supervising intubations done by the EMTs, does this make sense?

A No, it doesn't. EMTs should *not* be doing endotracheal intubations in the hospital without adequate supervision.

Patients enter a hospital expecting skilled and knowledgeable care, and they shouldn't be put in jeopardy by having a technician who is not properly supervised perform this sophisticated and potentially dangerous procedure. Unless—and until—the doctors agree to train you in endotracheal intubation or provide someone qualified to supervise the EMTs, your responsibility to your patients requires that this procedure be off limits to EMTs working in your unit.

Should nurses be expected to intubate a patient whenever they're called upon?

Q The head of the intensive care unit (ICU) where I work wants all the nurses in the unit to learn how to intubate patients with an endotracheal (ET) tube. Once we've acquired this skill, should we restrict our practice of it to the ICU? Or, when a doctor isn't available, should we be expected to intubate a patient whenever we're called upon?

A Insertion of an ET tube is a sophisticated and potentially dangerous procedure. To intubate smoothly, without traumatizing the patient, requires consistent practice.

Why should nurses have to shoulder this responsibility? More and more hospitals have nurse anesthetists and anesthesiologists available on a 24-hour basis to conform with Joint Commission on Accreditation of Healthcare Organizations' standards. As an interim emergency measure, nurses could be trained to insert an esophageal obturator airway. If they take on the responsibility for intubation, they should be paid for it and thoroughly trained.

Incidentally, you might want to check with your malpractice insurance carrier to see whether your policy covers intubation.

What drugs can be given through an ET tube?

Q We have no hospital policy listing drugs that can be given through an endotracheal (ET) tube in an emergency. I remember from my Advanced Cardiac Life Support (ACLS) course that naloxone HCI (Narcan), stropine, epinephinre, lidocaine (lignocaine), and sodium bicarbonate may be given in this manner. My co-workers disagree.

What do you say?

A Sodium bicarbonate should *never* be given through an ET tube.

To help you remember the drugs that are suitable, according to ACLS standards, think of the acronym NAVEL: *N*arcan, *A*tropine, *V*alium, *E*pinephrine, and *L*idocaine.

What should a nurse do if she's aware that interns and medical students are doing a procedure without consent?

Q I'm a charge nurse on the 7-to-11 shift in a teaching hospital. I've only been here 4 months, having just moved from another state.

Last night, a patient went into cardiac arrest and died. Later, several interns and medical students arrived to practice intubation on the corpse. This was without the patient's or family's consent. (Later, the family even refused to allow an autopsy.)

I was very upset. I know I'm the patient's advocate while he's alive and I assumed that the responsibility continued until the family claimed the body.

When I tried to discuss this with my supervisor, she simply said I should look the other way when this happens because "after all, how are the doctors going to learn?"

I never heard of this in my home state where I trained and practiced. Is this legal? What are my responsibilities?

A No matter where you train or practice in the United States, a person's right to the privacy of his own body does not cease with his death. The intubation of a dead patient without a premortem consent (or a postmortem consent of his next of kin) is morally and ethically indefensible. It also legally constitutes malpractice. The persons performing this procedure, the physicians supervising it, and the hospital allowing it are all legally culpable.

As to *your* responsibilities, go through channels until you're satisfied that the administration knows your concerns about the legalities of the situation. Ask that they consult with their counsel on this.

If this action does not end the practice, you are then duty bound to report it to the appropriate state agency responsible for hospital care; the Joint Commission on Accreditation of Healthcare Organizations; and the medical licensing board. Allowing this practice to continue could subject *you* to civil liability for malpractice and disciplinary action by the nurse licensing board.

This could place you in a difficult position with your employers. Still, each nurse is responsible for her own practice, and you are quite right in your feeling that your patient advocacy doesn't cease with the patient's death.

If, for whatever reason, you are not willing to report these illegal procedures, you should resign your position to protect yourself.

E

Why can't nurses do it?

Q I work the night shift in the recovery room of a community hospital where the following situation is common: A patient needs emergency endotracheal intubation, but because current policy doesn't allow nurses to intubate, I must waste time locating an anesthesiologist or other doctor. To me, that's ridiculous. With my years of experience and with proper training, I guarantee I could intubate as well as any doctor.

What do you think?

A You've already answered your own question—hospital policy mandates against it. Administration's probably thinking of the insurance coverage the hospital would need. You should consider your increased liability, too.

> *"I guarantee I could do emergency endotracheal intubation as well as any doctor, but instead, I must waste time finding one."*

Nurses *are* being trained (supervised theory and practice with periodic reviews) to intubate, but why would you want to take on this added responsibility? Learning to do smooth intubation takes a lot of time and practice, which is why anesthetists or anesthesiologists are adept at it. Even if you were trained,

they'd still have to be right there in case of complications, so why not let them perform the intubation in the first place?

Enemas

What's a reasonable time interval between them?

Q Nursing texts I've consulted recommend limiting the number of consecutive tap water enemas to three. However, if enemas are ordered until clear and the results remain unsatisfactory, how soon could I safely begin administering the second series? Or would another series be safe at all?

A You should never start a second series of tap water enemas without reassessing the purpose of the enemas and consulting the patient's doctor. In fact, even one series of tap water enemas can be too fatiguing for some elderly patients. And for those with decreased kidney function or acute heart failure, tap water enemas can cause water toxicity, circulatory overload, and hyponatremia because of water absorption by the colon.

As an alternative to tap water enemas, the doctor might consider ordering an oral gastrointestinal lavage solution (GoLytely) that acts as an osmotic agent. This drug, a powder of polyethylene glycol and sodium salts with potassium chloride, is dissolved in 4 liters of water, and the patient drinks 8 ounces every 10 minutes until rectal effluent is clear or the 4 liters are consumed. A bowel movement usually occurs within the first hour; bowel cleansing can take 4 hours without affecting the patient's water and electrolyte balance. This method is used for bowel cleansing before colonoscopy, barium enema for radiologic examination, and colon surgery.

Enteral feedings

Is it appropriate to add food coloring to all tube feedings?

Q At the hospital where I work, we're reviewing our policies on enteral feedings. We've heard that many hospitals add food coloring to all tube feedings, and we're wondering whether this is appropriate. What do you say?

A You should add food coloring only to the tube feedings of tracheostomy patients who are at high risk for pulmonary aspiration. The coloring helps distinguish gastric from tracheal contents.

What color should you use? Green is the best choice. Blue is less desirable because it can cause false-positive guaiac stool tests. Also, some blue food colorings contain an ingredient (FD&C Yellow No. 5) that may cause rare allergic reactions; you could be held liable for any injury caused by allergic reactions. The colors red and yellow are out because of their similarity to blood and pus.

One final note: If you decide to add food coloring to tube feedings, use 1.5 ml of food coloring per liter of enteral solution.

Should methylene blue coloring be added?

Q At the hospital where I work, we add methylene blue to our enteral feedings as a safeguard against aspiration. At my previous job, we used blue food coloring. I wonder if methylene blue is better than blue food coloring or if either is really necessary.

Q We had a patient on our ICU who turned bluish green from head to toe while receiving enteral feedings with methylene blue coloring added. Once we stopped adding the coloring, his skin tone returned to normal, so we can only conclude the coloring caused his condition. What's your opinion?

A Adding coloring to enteral feedings is one topic that never makes headlines but keeps surfacing—and opinions keep changing. The latest word is that you needn't add coloring to any enteral feedings. A better way to distinguish gastric secretions in tracheal contents is to test the aspirate for glucose concentration with a reagent strip. If the concentration is over 200 mg/dl (or over 150, depending on serum glucose levels), the patient has probably aspirated enteral solution while vomiting.

If your hospital policy calls for adding coloring to the feedings besides using the reagent strip for a few selected patients (known aspirators, tracheostomy patients who are at high risk for pulmonary aspiration), use no more than 1.5 ml of food coloring per liter of enteral solution. And don't use methylene blue. It can be absorbed systemically and cause urine, lips, and skin to take on a bluish tint, which can alarm the patient, his family—and the staff. It doesn't dissolve in enteral feedings, and it's almost impossible to keep evenly distributed in the solution.

Epidural catheters

Should nurses be expected to administer medication?

Q On our medical/surgical unit, several patients with chronic low back pain or intractable cancer pain have permanent or temporary epidural catheters.

In the past, we were told to call a resident to administer their epidural medications, such as bupivacaine (Marcaine) or fentanyl (Sublimaze), because these medi-

cations are too dangerous for nurses to administer. Last week, however, policy changed—and after a staff development program on this new procedure, we'll start administering medications through an epidural catheter.

Several of us feel uncomfortable about this sudden change. If administering medications epidurally was too dangerous for nursing personnel before, what's changed?

A Nothing's changed—except that your hospital policy's been updated to allow you to administer certain medications for analgesia through an epidural catheter. And after you've learned how, you'll have no more reason to fear using an epidural catheter than an I.V. catheter; all routes of administration have potential adverse effects. However, note exactly what medications your policy says you can administer: In some states, certified nurse anesthetists are still the only nurses permitted to administer anesthetics epidurally, which includes the bupivacaine you mentioned.

In others, registered nurses may administer narcotics such as fentanyl, morphine, and meperidine, and such anesthetics as bupivacaine through an epidural catheter for analgesia, providing: X-rays have been taken to determine catheter placement; the catheter is sutured in place; a doctor administers the initial dose; the nurse has preparation, supervised practice, and the required skill; and she knows the risks and complications.

In some states, nurses aren't allowed to administer narcotics epidurally at all—even when these same nurses are expected to teach their patients with chronic cancer pain how to administer boluses for themselves via patient-controlled analgesia devices. So any confusion about what's permitted and what's prohibited in a particular state is understandable. When in doubt, check with the state board of nursing.

Epileptic nurse

Must she inform her supervisor of her physical problem?

Q One of our staff nurses in the emergency department (ED) told me confidentially that she's just started treatment for epilepsy. She's taking phenytoin (Dilantin) and phenobarbital (Barbita), but still has a rare seizure and sometimes becomes groggy from the medications. So far, none of this has interfered with her working in the ED. Nonetheless, I worry about her making a mistake.

We're close friends. And she made me promise to keep her condition a secret because she's afraid she'll lose her job. The situation has me worried. Does she have an obligation to inform her supervisor of her physical problem? And where do I stand: Do I have some responsibility, too?

I don't want to be disloyal or hurtful, but I have to think of my responsibility to the patients.

A Certainly your colleague might *think* she'd lose her job once word gets out that she has epilepsy. The old myths and prejudices about epilepsy are hard to root out. But nurses with epilepsy are now routinely doing professional jobs without special attention or concern, once medications protect them from seizures. Your colleague should reach this point herself once the correct dosage has been established for her. During the period of adjustment to her medications, however, she should be open and aboveboard and accept the special measures that will protect everybody. Having another RN check her calculations for patient medications is one such protective measure. But she needs to protect everyone—including herself—by telling the su-

E

pervisor about the seizures and about the possible adverse reactions the drugs could produce.

If you can't encourage your colleague to do this, then you don't have much choice. *You* must explain the situation to the supervisor.

Paradoxically, you'll be protecting your friend by revealing the problem. If she were to make an error because of a seizure or the impact of the drugs she's taking, think of the legal and professional consequences she'd face.

> *"I worry that my epileptic friend will have a seizure or become groggy from her medication and will make a mistake."*

Epilepsy's going to be a long-term challenge for this nurse. Even after she's adjusted to her medications, she could have a bad day, for one reason or another. When a bad day comes, she must know how to ask for and accept help. Then the staff won't be put in the untenable position of shielding her from her mistakes. She won't be forcing everyone to pretend the problem doesn't exist.

Equipment bag

Is bag technique old hat?

Q At the home health agency where I work, few of the nurses follow written policy on handling the equipment bag during house calls. Present policy calls for putting down a piece of newspaper and placing the bag on top, spreading wax paper for supplies taken from the bag, closing the bag and leaving it on the newspaper until the visit's completed. This technique was developed for working in homes with poor sanitation and with insect infestation.

Most of the nurses feel this is unnecessary, even insulting to the pa-

tients and their families. Instead, they leave their bags in the car and bring only essential assessment tools into the homes.

What do you think—is bag technique old hat?

A Bag technique has been around since the inception of public health nursing, and many professionals to this day frown on any modification in this longstanding ritual. Others, like the nurses at your agency, agree that in this age of disposables, you can leave your bag in the car and bring in only those supplies you'll need during the visit. In another agency the admitting nurse sets up a corner on her first visit for most of the supplies (such as dressings) that will be used during future calls. Thereafter, the visiting nurse carries in one or two additional items, perhaps a disposable syringe or an otoscope (cleaned in the car between visits).

No matter whether you use the bag technique—or on which side of the tracks the patient lives—the one absolutely essential ritual is to thoroughly wash your hands both before and after examining the patient.

Euthanasia

What if a dying patient requests it?

Q A patient who's dying of cancer has asked me to help him commit suicide painlessly. He talked about death with dignity, and he told me I was the only one he could trust. How do I handle this?

A Assure him that you won't abandon him, no matter what happens; that's what most dying patients fear the most.

But explain that you can't do what he's asking because it's both illegal and unethical. Although some people say that mercy killing or assisted

suicide is humane or dignified, it still means deliberately taking a human life.

Encourage him to speak honestly about his fears of dying. Then plan your care and patient teaching to help him cope with those fears at all levels—physical, emotional, and spiritual. And make sure he receives adequate pain relief. In the final stages of his illness, he shouldn't have to suffer.

Exhibitionism

What can be done about a patient's exhibitionistic conduct?

Q Since we don't always have orderlies available in our small community hospital, we female RNs sometimes catheterize men and change their perineal dressings. We accept this as part of our job. Recently, however, we had a patient develop a postvasectomy scrotal hemorrhage. Almost immediately, the younger nurses became aware of this patient's exhibitionistic conduct: He often uncovered his genitals whenever a young woman—nurse, nursing assistant, visitor—appeared. Since he did not act this way with the older women, we younger nurses felt that his dressings should be changed only by the older nurses, or he should wait until an orderly arrived for the next shift. The patient suspected what was happening and reported the three of us younger nurses to the doctor. The doctor gave us a stiff reprimand, and our unit manager did not back us up at all. Isn't there some charter in nursing to protect the nurse from having to do something that is morally or ethically distasteful to her?

A The real question here seems to be can nurses neglect patient care? Granted, the patient's behavior was upsetting and his care had to be unpleasant. But caring for him *was* a duty. A professional does not walk away from responsibility.

Did you report the patient's exhibitionism to your supervisor and ask for help from older nurses or orderlies? In many hospitals, the supervisor simply reports a case like this to the attending doctor and he talks to the patient about it.

If (for whatever reason) none of this help was available on your shift, however, you shouldn't have neglected your tasks. You should have dealt directly with the problem. Because of your inexperience in this kind of situation, it probably would have been easier if you worked in pairs. If the patient seemed to be knowingly uncovering himself, you and the other nurse should have said, "Look, Mr. A., we'd very much like to take care of you, but you are making us uncomfortable by your actions. We think we can treat you better if we can be more at ease with you." The patient would likely have acted surprised (feigned, if not real) and asked what you meant. Then you should have told him what he was doing that made you uncomfortable.

Although this man's behavior was not acceptable, you might have weighed some possibly mitigating circumstances. Because a vasectomy is expected to produce an irreversible change in a man's biological function, it has a profound psychological implication for him and his self-image of masculinity. Perhaps this patient still harbored feelings of ambivalence about the operation. Perhaps unexpected complications of the hemorrhage further shook his confidence in the advisability of the operation. Certainly exhibitionism is the act of a person who feels sexually insecure.

Increasing numbers of vasectomies are projected for the future. Your experience with this patient will serve you well in preparing you emotionally—as well as techni-cally—for possible problems that could arise with other vasectomy patients.

Expiration dates

How should they be interpreted?

Q I work in a doctor's office where I'm responsible for restocking the medicine cabinet. Some of our drugs have expiration dates with no exact day—just a month and year ("Aug./1990," for example). What does this mean? Is the drug only good until the first day of the month? Or is it good until the last day? Or maybe somewhere in between?

A A drug company guarantees the full potency of its drugs with month-year expiration dates until midnight on the last day of that month. In other words, you can use a drug with the expiration date of Aug./1990 until midnight on August 31, 1990 under full guarantee of the manufacturer.

However, the expiration dates are usually conservative, and a drug may be potent for a while after it has officially expired.

If antimicrobial skin cleanser must be disposed of after 30 days, why doesn't the manufacturer say so?

Q I work in a military hospital. Recently our infection control department instructed us that *any* open bottle of chlorhexidine gluconate antimicrobial skin cleanser must be disposed of after 30 days.

This seems like a tremendous waste to me, but if it is appropriate, why doesn't the manufacturer use an expiration date? Can you give me guidelines?

A If you're using full-strength, commercially available chlorhexidine gluconate cleanser, you shouldn't have to worry about environmental contamination of opened bottles, says the manufacturer. In fact, a study published in the *Journal of Pharmaceutical Sciences* reports no contamination in the product even after 6 months of environmental exposure.

A few cases of contamination *were* reported outside the United States, however. On investigation, the contaminated products proved to be diluted, aqueous-based chlorhexidine gluconate.

So find out whether your hospital is using a diluted skin cleanser. If so, cost-effectiveness may be going down the drain.

Externs

Can a charge nurse be held responsible for the actions of an extern?

Q I'm uneasy about an extern program recently established at the small county hospital where I work. The externs are student nurses who've completed 1 year of a 2-year AD program, or 3 years of a 4-year BSN program. The student externs work on the unit as team leaders, responsible for as many as eight patients. On duty they give out all medications, including narcotics.

I'm so uneasy giving the externs this much responsibility that I've refused to be the charge nurse when the externs are working on the unit. But my unit manager assures me the program's covered by our hospital insurance policy, so I have no reason to worry.

I still have my doubts, no matter what the unit manager says. What I'm asking you is: Do other hospitals assign so much responsibility to externs? And can a charge nurse be held responsible for the actions of an extern in case of an error or injury to a patient?

E

A Other hospitals will use externs—*but only* with faculty supervision. Your feeling is right, and the situation you describe is wrong. Giving externs so much responsibility is irresponsible. Being a team leader requires experience and know-how that an extern doesn't have yet.

At least one state board of nursing says it's *illegal* for externs to dispense medications or to act as team leaders without faculty supervision. Assigning unqualified personnel to perform nursing functions, which is what you'd be doing as the charge nurse in this situation, could be grounds for disciplinary action.

Take all the facts to your supervisor. Stress that if a patient were to sue the hospital, everyone could be involved in the ensuing litigation: the hospital administrators, the charge nurse, the doctor, and even the extern. For your protection, keep a record of your discussion with your supervisor.

If she still holds to her original position—that you *can* safely delegate these responsibilities to externs—take your case to the state board of nursing. Give them a dispassionate statement of the facts, and ask for a review of your hospital's extern program.

Your willingness to take a stand and to put your personal stamp of responsibility on nursing in your hospital is commendable.

Eye patch

Could a nurse be held liable for any accidents the patient's involved in?

Q When I first started working in the emergency department, our orders were to not allow a patient who'd been given an eye patch to drive himself home. Lately, one of the doctors says it makes no difference; the patient can drive with a patch on.

I feel uneasy about this—both for the patient and myself. Could I be held liable for any accidents the patient's involved in? What's your advice?

A Don't go along with this doctor's laissez-faire attitude. Driving is risky business under the best of circumstances. And any patient who's just received emergency care *and* an eye patch has two strikes against him before he slips behind the wheel. An eye patch blocks peripheral vision and, until the patient learns to compensate for this, two eyes are needed for depth perception.

Your first responsibility is to assess whether the patient's vision is sharp enough for driving after the emergency treatment. If so, he could drive home and then put the eye patch in place. But if his vision is impaired, or if he must start wearing the eye patch right away, have him arrange for someone else to drive him home.

Be sure to document your instructions. The patient should listen to your reasoning. But if not and an accident occurred, at least you'd be in the clear.

Eye trouble

Is using a needle safe?

Q At the clinic where I work, a patient recently came in with a foreign object embedded in his eye. The attending doctor has his own method of removing foreign objects. He applies a few drops of a topical anesthetic to the eye, then the object is removed with a sterile cotton-tipped applicator. If this doesn't work, he uses a metal spud. With this patient, the spud wasn't successful, so the doctor used the side of a large-gauge needle to scrape the object off.

Is using a needle safe?

A When swabbing doesn't work, most ophthalmologists prefer to use a needle rather than a spud. A needle is sharp, disposable, and sterile, whereas spuds tend to become blunt after extended use.

One caution: Using either a spud or needle in the eye isn't recognized practice for a nurse.

False accusation

Can a nurse have a doctor's accusation removed from her record?

Q I am an RN who's worked at the same hospital for 6 years. For the last 2 years, I've been charge nurse on the 11-to-7 shift in a 6-bed intensive care unit (ICU). A doctor came in at two o'clock one morning and found no one in the unit. I was sitting in the anteroom where we keep the coffee and sodas, and the technician had just gone to the bathroom. I admit I had my eyes closed, but the minute the doctor said "good morning," I got up and accompanied him to his patient.

Several days later, I was called to the nursing office and read a statement which the doctor had dictated and signed, stating that I had been asleep on duty and he'd had to say "good morning" twice before I awoke. I was asked to sign this, but I refused.

Two months later, there was an opening for night supervisor in a different unit. I applied and was turned down on the basis of the doctor's report.

Can I have this doctor's statement removed from my record? Should I take this doctor to court?

A Before you start thinking of courtroom scenes, review the circumstances as you relate them. They do not, quite frankly, place you in a good light. Grant that you weren't sleeping on duty (or napping, dozing, nodding, or anything approximating sleep), but were just sitting with your eyes closed. Why was the unit unattended? The ICU is for the *constant* monitoring of patients. It was your responsibility to make sure you and the technician weren't out of the unit at the same time. The fact that you *were* represents poor management on your part, and you must keep that in mind.

Poor management, however, is different from dereliction of duty, which is what you should be charged with if you were sleeping on the job. You say you weren't sleeping, however, so you were right to refuse to sign the doctor's statement. But you were wrong to let it end there. This is a serious charge against you. Why didn't you take it to your grievance committee? If your hospital doesn't have a setup to handle such situations, then you should have demanded a confrontation with the doctor. You must get your side of the story on record. Your integrity is as valid as the doctor's, and you have much more at stake—your job future.

Doctors are human. Perhaps when he hears your explanation, he'll realize that he's misjudged the situation, and will withdraw his statement from your records. If not, you will at least get your position on file. If you feel need of further action on this problem, contact your state nurses' association. Explain the whole picture and ask what further options are open to you under the nursing laws of your particular state.

Do not jump into court action precipitously. Lawsuits take a lot out of you financially—and emotionally. Before you think "court," think "last resort."

Falsifying records

Can an administrator ask a nurse to change information on forms?

Q As director of nursing in a nursing home, I prepare all the forms for our monthly utilization review committee meetings.

Last week, the administrator asked me to change the date on all the forms the doctors had signed at the last meeting because *we* had exceeded the 30-, 60-, or 90-day review period.

I changed the dates as asked.

Now, the administrator has asked me to change the minutes of all our meetings, to show that one of the nurses was present at the meetings as the utilization review secretary. She wasn't there, of course, because we don't have a secretary, but our nursing home policy requires one.

"The administrator asked me to change the date on all the forms and to change the minutes of all our meetings to show that one of the nurses was present."

What can I do to protect myself? I feel so guilty and also afraid—afraid that I might be liable for this action.

A "Oh, what a tangled web we weave when first we practice to deceive." That observation is as true today as it was when it was first quoted in the 19th century. You can see now that changing the dates was just the beginning—unless you summon up the courage to say *no*.

Your hesitation was a step in the right direction, but the harder step is to talk with the administrator. Obviously, you must tell him that you can't falsify any more records,

that you know he's in a tough position but that you won't break the law for him. And if he appeals to your concern for the nursing home, remember that you are responsible for your own actions, orders or not. If legal action is taken, the person who makes the changes bears the guilt.

Family members

Is it risky to get them involved in a patient's care?

Q Recently, one of my patients returned to his room after surgical repair of a hernia. His postoperative orders allowed bathroom privileges with assistance. So I told his son to call me if his father needed to use the bathroom. About an hour later, I walked into the room just in time to see the son helping his father back into bed. He said he didn't want to disturb me just to take his father to the bathroom. I repeated my warning, but now I'm wondering: *Is* there any reason not to get family members involved in a patient's care if they want to help out?

A You bet there is: The hospital is legally responsible for every patient's safety. Family members don't have the preparation that you do to fulfill this obligation.

Suppose the patient had fallen because his son didn't know how to support his weight properly. If he or his son had been injured, they could sue you and the hospital for negligence—and stand a good chance of winning.

That doesn't mean you should exclude family members from a loved one's care. They could give back rubs, assist with meals and bathing, and even walk up and down the hall with ambulatory patients. But only a nurse should give even routine care to a recently postoperative patient.

Check your hospital's policy and procedure manuals for information about involving family members in a patient's care. If you don't find anything, talk with your manager or the hospital's risk manager.

In this case, reinforcing your instructions was the right thing to do. The next step would have been to document your conversation in your nurse's notes, to show that the patient and his son had previously disregarded your caution. Your notes would be important evidence if they continued to ignore your warning, the patient was injured, and you wound up in court.

Family questions

Should they be told the truth?

Q Last week, a cancer patient's brother stopped me in the hall and asked, "Is he going to be all right?" The patient is dying, so I said, "No." I guess I sounded abrupt, because the brother got very upset and wouldn't let me explain.

Later, my manager reprimanded me for being too blunt. When I asked what I should have said, she replied, "It doesn't hurt to offer hope. You could have said, 'He's having a good day.'"

I disagree, but I know a lot of nurses who would agree with her. How do you feel about this?

A Your manager is right about the importance of hope, but that doesn't mean you should mislead people or offer *false* hope. Holding out hope for recovery when you know the patient is dying would be deceptive. And if you say, "He's having a good day," you're ducking the question and perhaps trivializing a family member's concerns.

But bluntness doesn't help either. Instead of answering so quickly, you should have responded to the brother's obvious anxiety. You could have assessed what he knew and how he felt by asking him something like this: "You look worried. What has

your brother told you?" or "You sound uncertain. What did the doctor say?" By listening to his answers, you might have discovered the feelings behind his question—confusion, desire for reassurance, fear that someone is keeping something from him, denial, or anger. Then you could have responded more appropriately.

Your quick answer may also have revealed more about your patient's illness than he wanted his brother to know. Remember, you have an ethical duty to protect his privacy.

To help this patient and his family in the future, find out how much he knows about his condition and how much he wants others to know. Then, if he and his doctor approve, set up a family conference. Use it to teach the family about the patient's cancer, prognosis, and treatment—and to find out what support they want for the difficult period ahead.

FDA

Are nurses justified in refusing to enlist patients for questionable studies?

Q We are 7 RNs employed in a private hematology clinic. Our doctors routinely conduct drug studies of various new medications pending Food and Drug Administration (FDA) approval. Part of our job is to obtain informed consents, present the protocols, reinforce positive aspects of the studies, and dispense medications (topical and P.O.) to be taken by the patients at future dates. Under the doctors' supervision, we also monitor the effects of such medications.

We are, however, concerned about participating in a new study that requires unusually careful selection of patients, extensive workups, and monitoring of these patients. According to published

literature, the drug has produced potentially hazardous internal (thromboembolic) effects in 17% of a trial group of 500.

Are we justified in refusing to enlist patients for such studies if we judge the usual office care and monitoring not sufficient for safety? If we do refuse to participate in a specific study, do the doctors have the right to fire us? Would we have any legal redress? Any advice you can give will be much appreciated.

A Your concerns are justified professionally and legally. One of the FDA requirements for investigators of new drugs is that the investigator conduct the study *personally.* Ancillary personnel, including nurses, are to assist only. Furthermore, when investigation studies are being pursued, it is contrary to accepted medical practice to have the nurse obtain the informed consent, dispense the investigational medication, and monitor the effects of the medication given under direct supervision. It's questionable whether a nurse should present the protocols and reinforce positive aspects.

You most certainly have a legal right to refuse to participate in such studies. Not only is your employer subjecting himself to legal hazards involving the FDA, but also subjecting himself and you to potential malpractice problems.

Obviously legal rights and a right to a job are two different things. However, your employers will likely agree to modify the present setup when the legal hazards to them and to you are properly explained.

Feeding tubes

What can be done about clogging?

Q As a home health nurse, I often receive calls from patients who say their feeding tubes are clogged only a week or two after hospital discharge. When I ask if they irrigate the tube before and after feedings, they say absolutely yes. Any ideas?

A Here's one. Perhaps they weren't instructed to irrigate before and after administering *medication* through the tube. If this isn't being done, coarsely crushed pills can mix with feeding solutions to form a frustrating type of cement known only to nurses. So tell your patients *before* the problem occurs.

When the bed is lowered for various procedures, should the pump be turned off?

Q Several of our patients have feeding tubes connected to enteral pumps, and the feeding solution is infused over 24 hours. Our policy calls for keeping the head of the bed elevated about 35 degrees at all times during infusion to prevent aspiration. But when we have to lower the bed for various treatments or procedures, should we turn the pump off?

A The answer to your question depends on where the tip of the feeding tube is located. If it's in the *duodenum,* leave the pump *on* when the patient's head is lowered. If it's in the *stomach,* turn the pump *off* while the patient's head is down to prevent regurgitation and aspiration. If you're not sure where the tip is positioned, play it safe and turn the pump off.

Why did the doctor insist on exposing the patient to an unnecessary X-ray?

Q On our pediatric unit, we sometimes use metal-weighted pliable plastic feeding tubes. Recently, after a surgeon inserted one of these tubes into an 8-month-old

child, he ordered a stat flat plate of the child's abdomen to check the tube's placement. When we told him that hospital policy doesn't require an abdominal X-ray when the tube isn't advanced out of the stomach, he still wanted the X-ray he'd ordered.

We usually confirm tube placement by auscultating over the gastric area while air is injected into the tube and by aspirating gastric contents. Why did this doctor insist on exposing the patient to an unnecessary X-ray?

A He knew that not ordering a stat flat plate might have been unsafe practice. Pliable plastic feeding tubes have small lumens and are very flexible; they may kink on insertion or may be passed into a patient's trachea without causing obvious symptoms. Your auscultating-for-air method isn't foolproof either. Gas in the stomach could be mistaken for air. Conversely, even if you can't aspirate gastric contents, the tube could actually be in the right place. Sometimes the tube's wall collapses from the negative pressure caused by aspiration and nothing passes through. So checking placement with an X-ray makes sense. The doctor should have explained this to you.

Felony

Will a past felony jeopardize nursing licensure in a different state?

Q Two years ago I was convicted on a felony charge for "possession of a controlled substance." The court placed me on probation, but I received an early discharge and enrolled in a drug-abuse program.

I've straightened out my life and am now ready to get on with my nursing career. But I'm not sure I'll be able to.

From the time of my conviction until recently, I heard nothing from my state board of nursing. I deliberately stayed in the same area in order to "live down" my reputation. I worked in a nonnursing job at first, but for the past 6 months I've held a nursing post—successfully.

Now I'm ready to start over somewhere else. So I applied for licensure in another state. In the meantime, I received a notice from my *present* state announcing a hearing for possible suspension or revocation of my license.

This news was followed by a letter from the board of nursing in the state I'm hoping to move to. That board decided to grant my license (even though I'd informed them of my conviction when I applied).

I'm confused and worried. If my *present* state board of nursing takes any action against my license at the hearing I'm about to have, will it affect my license in the *new* state automatically? Or do state boards act independently?

A Certainly you're puzzled—and worried—but generally, in the matter of licensure suspension or revocation, you're innocent until proven guilty. If a nurse's license is under consideration for suspension or revocation in another state, most state boards will still endorse the license—*at least until the case has been decided.* That's probably why you received your license from the second state.

But unfortunately your worries aren't over. If your current state board of nursing rules against you, the second state board may also impose strictures. For example, the second state board might suspend your license if the first state board does so. Or the second state may rule that your practice be limited to working in areas not involving access to medications.

Obtain legal counsel. Then get in touch with both state boards and report on how well you've been doing (backed by statements from your employers), in the hope they'll feel you're ready to return to nursing. You've fought your way back, and you have an impressive story to tell.

Fetal monitoring

What's the correct way to perform electronic fetal monitoring of twins?

Q I'd appreciate an expert's opinion on the correct way to perform electronic fetal monitoring of twins when the mother's membranes are intact. Will using two external monitors with an ultrasound transducer on each fetus give an accurate tracing of each twin? Or will the sound be bounced from one fetus to the other, causing the fetal heart rate tracing of one twin to be picked up and printed on both monitors? What are the legal implications of using this procedure?

A In twin gestations, there's a higher incidence of premature labor. Under these circumstances, fetal monitoring is essential, and standard practice is to monitor both fetuses using the external ultrasound mode. If you know the position of the fetuses (by ultrasonography or palpation), you can usually get tracings of both of them if you're careful about transducer placement. The twins probably wouldn't have identical fetal heart patterns and rates at any given time.

From the legal standpoint, your performance would be judged by the national standards expected of nurses in your specialty. Specifically, for electronic fetal monitoring, the Nurses Association of the American College of Obstetrics and Gynecology (NAACOG) says you must know how to operate the equipment, how to interpret fetal heart rate patterns, and what ac-

tions to take when monitoring indicates a change in the status of the fetuses. Also, you must follow your hospital policy, make sure that your documentation is complete, and use your skill and good judgment to protect the mother and twins from harm.

Fibrosis

If a fibrotic area is used as an injection site, will the medication be absorbed effectively?

Q I work for a family practitioner who sees several patients with chronic pain. A few of these patients have developed severe fibrosis from meperidine (pethidine, Demerol) injections over the years. If a fibrotic area is used as an injection site, will the medication be absorbed effectively?

A Scarred areas usually have poor blood supply, so for effective absorption, avoid injecting the meperidine in the fibrotic tissue whenever possible.

Fingernail polish

Would clear, pale nail polish be a source of infection?

Q A recent policy on the medical/surgical unit where I work says that nurses can't wear fingernail polish. We all know the importance of keeping our nails short and clean. But I have a special problem with psoriasis of my nails; believe me, polish certainly helps their appearance.

Would clear, pale nail polish be a source of infection?

A Cracks, even tiny ones, in the smooth surface of fingernail polish can provide a site for micro-

organisms to hide. (The shade makes no difference—bacteria aren't color selective.) And the same rationale for short, clean nails applies to the ban on nail polish: to reduce the bacteria on the hands to the lowest possible number.

In your case, though, polish could be helpful. The psoriasis must be kept under control to avoid shedding excessive amounts of organisms such as *Staphylococcus aureus.* You may actually have more success keeping the nail surface smooth and clean with a coat of nail polish over the pitting and cracking caused by the psoriasis.

Why not check with your nursing supervisor and the infection control nurse for an evaluation? And if you do wear nail polish, examine it daily for cracks and be prepared to correct this problem immediately.

Fingernails

Are there infection hazards with artificial nails?

Q At the hospital where I work, many of the nurses wear artificial fingernails. They say the nails hold up through our frequent scrubbings in hot water.

Before I get these nails for myself, I'd like to hear what you have to say.

A Your fingernails should be short, clean, unpolished—and real. Nurses need clean hands, and wearing artificial nails can cause health problems. For example, frequent handwashing can promote fungal growth between the real and artificial nail. And nail compounds that include methyl and polymethyl methacrylates have caused serious reactions, including loss of nails. Also, artificial nails can be sharp enough to hurt patients or to puncture surgical gloves, leaving the wearer unprotected.

Fire drills

Should bedridden patients be evacuated?

Q A new fire drill policy's been put into effect at the nursing home where I work. This policy requires the nurses to evacuate patients—*real* patients, not stand-ins—during routine fire drills. We're expected to evacuate even bedridden patients. How? By dragging them out of their rooms and down the halls on blankets.

In past fire drills, we didn't evacuate actual patients from the facility. During a practice drill, the staff members would pose as patients.

I consider the new policy unnecessary, unprofessional, and unsafe. It entails considerable risk to the seriously ill bedridden patients and could place us in legal jeopardy for contributing to the risk.

What do *you* think of this new policy?

A Not much. A fire drill is supposed to help *save* lives, not endanger them needlessly. During a genuine emergency, dragging sick patients out on blankets is risky but necessary. But endangering your patients for the sake of staging a realistic drill violates common sense and your patients' rights. Talk with the nursing home administration about going back to the old method of having stand-in staff members pose as patients.

Flexion deformity

Is it advisable to place an object in the hand of a brain-damaged patient with contracted fingers?

Q Recently a lecturer cautioned against placing an object in the hand of any brain-damaged patient with contracted fingers. He says this only encourages a flexion deformity, which can become permanent.

Yet when I was nursing an auto crash victim whose fingers curled inward, the physiotherapist made a cone-shaped device for the patient to hold.

Will you comment on this?

A First of all, "brain damaged" is too indefinite a description. If the brain-damaged patient is also comatose, placing an object in his hand for purposes of exercise is pointless.

A splint, however, may be used to maintain functional position, then removed for regularly scheduled range-of-motion exercises.

If the brain-damaged patient is not comatose and maintains some motion in his hand, a cone or splint may help somewhat with passive stretching, but either must be removed several times a day to allow for range-of-motion exercises.

The point to remember here is that any patient with a flexion contracture of the hand has a problem with *extension* of the fingers, and a splint or a cone can be used to maintain *functional* position of the hand and prevent full flexion contractures. Be careful, however, not to use a ball or an object like a rolled washcloth or ill-fitting hand roll; these won't increase extension of the fingers and will only encourage further flexion.

Flirting

Who should tell a director she's ruining her image as a nursing professional?

Q The director of nursing where I work is well-credentialed, innovative, and fair to the nursing staff. However, she's flirtatious to the point of embarrassment for all those around. She comes to the hospital parties stag and becomes the life of the party. At hospital seminars, she always parks herself next to a doctor or two and flirts openly and outrageously. Already a visitor from another hospital remarked to me, "This is your *director*?"

In case you think that I don't like her, you're wrong. But who should tell her she's ruining her image (and ours by association) as a nursing professional?

A Probably no one. Look at it this way: To get where she is today, your director must be considerably smarter and more on the ball than you give her credit for.

If she hasn't realized the effect she's creating, she will someday. Meanwhile, keep quiet. You'll only seem impertinent by talking to her about her behavior.

Floating

How can it be avoided?

Q I just quit my job because I was forced to float to the intensive care unit (ICU) and obstetrics. I'd protested to the unit managers that I wasn't prepared to work on these units and that I was concerned about patient safety. But they just seemed to want bodies to staff their units. They told me I'd probably end up floating every week because I was a new nurse without much seniority.

I want to avoid this kind of problem in my next job. What would you recommend?

A First, clarify your rights *before* you're put in this difficult situation again. Ask if you might be floated and, if so, how you'll be oriented and what responsibilities you'll be expected to assume. Obtain a copy of the hospital's policy on floating and find out if you can say no if you feel you're unprepared to work on a certain unit.

You should also make sure you'll be oriented to other units before you're actually assigned there. Make a list of what you need to learn, and refer to it during the orientation. Have all of your questions been answered? If not, speak up.

What if you're asked to float without adequate preparation? Legally, you can't refuse unless you're permitted to do so by hospital policy or a collective-bargaining agreement. But most managers will agree to a trade-off: You can handle the tasks you're competent to perform while other nurses cover those that are unfamiliar to you. Just make sure you tell the manager you don't have the specialized skills you need to give safe care. And document your conversation in your personal records. Then get the necessary preparation before being floated to the unit again.

What's the best way to reduce the stress of being pulled to another unit?

Q I work on a cardiac intensive care unit (ICU). When our patient census is low, we have to float to other units. Because we come from the ICU, we're dumped on—given the most critical patients to care for and assigned *more* patients than the regular nurses. We get no time to read charts and don't learn enough from report. Is that any way to care for patients?

> *"Because we come from the ICU, we're dumped on—given the most critical patients to care for and assigned more patients than the regular nurses."*

How can we reduce the problems and stress of being pulled to another unit?

A First, by accepting the fact that floating is here to stay. Thanks to diagnosis-related groups, decreased staff patterns are becoming more common. So remember, you're not the only ones having to float.

Now, for the specific problems you mention, here are other suggestions.
• Ask to rotate to the other units at nonbusy hours so you can familiarize yourself with the routines.
• Socialize with the staff: It's hard to "dump on" a friend.
• Trade with another nurse if you feel uncomfortable doing a certain task.
• Speak up through proper channels if you feel patient care is unsafe or there's *really* a difference between the regular unit nurses' assignments and yours.

Also, try suggesting to administration some incentives that would make floating more tolerable. For example, a nurse who floats could get a free cafeteria meal, 2 days off in a row for 2 weeks, or an extra weekend off a month. Or you might suggest that nurses who float be paid a higher hourly wage. This incentive could attract enough nurses to relieve the pressure on those who'd rather not float. (And faced with paying extra money, administration may be more likely to base staffing on real rather than anticipated need.)

By persuading administration that you're all in this together, you can accomplish more—and float with ease.

Would a nurse be liable for making mistakes on an unfamiliar unit?

Q During slack periods, operating room nurses are asked to float to understaffed units. We've told our manager that we don't feel competent caring for patients on other units, but she says we shouldn't worry.

Well, we *are* worried. We're afraid we'll be liable for our mistakes. What should we do?

A Unfortunately, you have a common problem: The nursing shortage has made floating a fact of life in many hospitals. Legally, you can't refuse to float simply because you think your skills are rusty or because you're worried about liability risks. But you *can* decline an assigned task that you've never been taught to do.

If you're assigned to a unit where you feel uncomfortable, immediately tell the unit's manager that your work may not meet accepted nursing practice standards and explain why. Also, send a memo through channels to administration. Your voiced and written concern will notify managers and the hospital of a potentially dangerous situation and encourages them to act *before* a crisis occurs.

Even in difficult circumstances, you're expected to give competent nursing care. But your employer is responsible for maintaining adequate staffing. Your documentation will help ensure that the hospital shares liability if one of your patients is injured because of a staffing problem.

In the meantime, look for ways to minimize problems when you float. For example, if you feel poorly oriented for duty on unfamiliar units, suggest that each unit prepare a simple outline of its procedures and a unit floor plan. Or take a quick tour of an unfamiliar unit before you start work. If nothing else, you'll know where to find the crash cart, medication cabinet, and treatment rooms.

Florence Nightingale

Did she really die of syphilis?

Q Over the years, I've attended nursing meetings from one end of the country to the other, and I've noticed that whenever Florence

Nightingale is mentioned, someone is likely to ask, "Did you ever hear that she died of syphilis?"

Until now, I've dismissed the question as nonsense, but now it's time to ask you.

Is this *just* a rumor?

A Boyoboy. Next thing you know, they'll say she had acquired immunodeficiency syndrome.

Go to the library. You'll find a shelfful of books written about Florence Nightingale. One biography in particular, by Cecil Woodham-Smith (published by Atheneum), chronicles every detail of her long life. As the author describes Nightingale, the hard-driving, often difficult—but ever courageous and steadfast—young woman mellowed with age. She lived into her early 90s, and toward the end suffered the predictable effects of great age—failing eyesight, hearing, and so on—but syphilis was never once hinted as the cause of her failing health and death. Nor was it mentioned in any of the other books about her.

Let's put that rumor to rest.

Fluid intake

Is it okay to "frighten" a child into drinking?

Q I've worked 11 years in pediatrics. Last week, we had an 8-year-old tonsillectomy-adenoidectomy patient who absolutely refused to drink postoperatively. The doctor told her in the presence of her parents that if she didn't drink, he'd have to start an I.V. (This child had previous hospital experience, including I.V.s.) In private, I asked the doctor and the child's parents if I could just wheel an I.V. stand in the child's room. The doctor, foreseeing the ordeal of an I.V., agreed. The mother said, "Do anything, as long as it makes her drink." I put an I.V. stand at the foot of the child's bed. She immediately sat up,

grabbed the water glass, and downed it. She did well with liquids throughout the night and was discharged in the morning well-hydrated.

The pediatric instructor later severely chastised me for "frightening" and "threatening" the patient. Was she correct or was I?

A Most people would have to condemn the use of fear as a way to control a child. And its use raises a lot of questions.

Why was the child refusing to drink? Hadn't she been prepared for this in her preoperative teaching? Was she afraid to swallow because her throat was sore? Had you tried sodas, ice pops, or slushes?

Assuming all these points had been covered and the child still wouldn't drink, couldn't you have tried to reason with her on a level she'd be more familiar with? For example, you might have told her that her parents could visit with her for 15 minutes as long as she drank "this much" (marking a line on the glass). Then return in 15 minutes and mark another line, and so on. These are the "trade-offs" children use at their own level and your patient might have been more amenable to the exchange.

Deliberate use of scare tactics on a patient is never permissible. But when an automatic fear reaction in a patient brings about desirable results—there's no sense in your feeling guilty.

Flunking

Any suggestions on what a nurse's next step should be after she flunks her state boards?

Q I'm so ashamed and feel so stupid. You see, I just flunked my state nursing boards—for the second time. I even paid $250 for a review course. My co-workers on the maternity unit where I work

must wonder how I ever got a BSN degree.

Can you give me any advice on what my next step should be? I don't know what I'll do if I flunk again.

A First of all, you're not stupid. Getting through a 4-year nursing program certainly proves that. People fail exams for many reasons, such as getting no sleep the night before or suffering from anxiety. Although you can't avoid thinking about it, you already seem overly anxious about failing again. That won't help anything, so calm down and try these suggestions.

> *"I feel so ashamed and stupid because I just flunked my state nursing boards for the second time. I even paid $250 for a review course."*

Go back to your nursing school and ask the faculty for some study guidelines. If one area—for example, cardiac nursing—is causing you problems, talk to the cardiac nursing instructor and ask her to recommend review material. Then, contact the people who ran the review course. Do they have a follow-up course? Do they offer a money-back guarantee if you fail? At your job, observe nursing procedures and try to make up test questions that apply to them. Ask the staff to assign you to routine procedures—board questions usually concentrate on common problems.

When you study, are you focusing only on review questions, expecting to see them in the test? Instead, focus on theory and practice you've had; get out notes you've taken and books you've used, then test yourself with questions from the review book on the content you've gone over.

Take comfort—you're not alone. Some nurses throughout the country must retake their state boards.

To you and anyone else facing the same situation, remember: Don't lose heart. You *can* pass the boards.

Foot care

Should nurses perform foot care in a nursing home?

Q I'm an LPN working at a nursing home. Until recently, a podiatrist routinely performed foot care for our residents. Now, because of budget cutbacks, administration has discontinued this service and says we nurses must perform foot care for all patients—including diabetics, who need special care.

Am I right to be concerned?

A Yes, but not overly so. Most likely you can perform routine foot care for a diabetic patient. But just as a refresher, here are some special considerations.

Because a diabetic is vulnerable to infection and gangrene, be sure to observe his feet for redness, drying, cracking, blisters, or discoloration—these conditions require immediate treatment.

To trim a diabetic patient's toenails, cut straight across, clipping small sections of the nail at a time. Be sure to file trimmed toenails with an emery board to smooth rough edges. But don't try to cut back calluses or corns, or to trim thick, tough, or ingrown nails. If your patient needs such a procedure—or you see any signs of infection—notify your supervisor so she can contact a podiatrist.

Forced absence

Should it be without pay?

Q A few days after a family picnic, I learned that two of the children had come down with chicken pox. Because I'd never had the vi-

rus, I reported this exposure to the supervisor on the medical/surgical unit where I work. She referred me to the nurse epidemiologist, who ordered a varicella titer drawn. I was then sent home and told to stay there until either the incubation period (13 to 17 days) was over or my varicella antibody titer proved satisfactory.

Naturally, I accept that I couldn't be around my patients at that time—that's why I reported the exposure in the first place. What I do not accept is not getting paid for this forced absence from work.

As it turned out, the titer results came back high, and I returned to work within one week. Still, I'm out a week's pay for being honest. Don't get me wrong. I don't expect to be rewarded for honesty—I just don't want to be penalized. Where do you stand?

A Any administration that fails to encourage employees' honesty is myopic to the point of needing a white cane. You should've received sick pay during your absence. Or barring that, you could've been paid for work you could do at home—such as reviewing and revising procedure policies.

Write a memo to administration asking them to review their stand and to reconsider paying you for the lost time.

In the meantime, one small consolation for you and other nurses who have never had chicken pox is news from Children's Hospital of Philadelphia, where researchers have successfully tested a vaccine to immunize against this disease. Officials of Merck Sharpe & Dohme, the pharmaceutical company that will manufacture the vaccine, estimate that the vaccine will be ready and approved for general use in about 2 years.

So here's a cheer for progress—and while we're at it, a special cheer for you and your old-fashioned virtues of honesty and concern.

Forced labor

What should be done?

Q About 9 months ago, I started working on the obstetric unit of a small rural hospital. I enjoy my work, but I can't get something that happened a few months ago out of my mind.

During the 2 or 3 weeks before one obstetrician left on his overseas vacation, he induced labor in many of his patients. Some had delivery dates of up to a month later, and a few babies were born marginally premature.

At that time, I was working in the postpartum unit. And the nurses who were in the labor and delivery units didn't question the doctor's actions. But I do. I'm concerned that history may repeat itself when vacation time rolls around. If so, what should I do?

A As you probably know, inducing labor is common practice that's considered safe as long as the baby is fully developed. Delivering premature babies to suit a doctor's convenience *isn't* safe. If this situation occurs again, gather the proof you'll need to file a complaint.

Record information on each baby delivered over the 3 to 4 week period before the doctor goes on vacation. Ask questions, too. For instance, you might say to the doctor, "Mrs. Jones isn't due for a month; why is she coming in early?" Record his answer. Ask the mother, "Is there a reason why you're here a month early?" By asking this question, you're alerting her to assume some responsibility for the decision to induce labor. And you can compare the patient's answer to the doctor's. If they don't agree, your index of suspicion should rise.

If your information leads you to conclude that the doctor is deliberately delivering premature babies, pass it along to your nursing supervisor. Ask her to review the information, then pass it through formal channels to the doctor's supervisor.

He should handle the problem from there.

Forcing treatment

What are the legal implications of forcing treatment on a patient who seems lucid?

Q A recent incident on the medical/surgical unit where I've been working for 5 years has left me puzzled.

An 80-year-old woman was admitted for a pinning of a fractured hip. She had occasional moments of confusion, but on the whole seemed oriented to time and place.

Her laboratory tests before surgery showed a low potassium level of 3.3 mEq/liter (normal is 3.5 to 5 mEq/ liter), so the orthopedic surgeon ordered I.V. fluids with 20 ml KCl added to each liter to be administered over a 12-hour period.

We couldn't start the I.V. because the patient wouldn't allow it. Her family tried to persuade her to agree to the I.V., but she said no.

The surgeon was angry and told us to "get it started even if you have to tie her down." He added that this patient was not equipped to decide for herself because she had organic brain syndrome. We found no mention of this in the patient's chart.

Our staff nurses got together and came up with an alternative: oral administration of potassium. The surgeon agreed, and the patient consented. All ended well.

But I'm still wondering: What are the legal implications of forcing treatment on a patient who *seems* lucid?

A This patient, like any other patient, has the right to refuse treatment *until* she's been declared legally incompetent in a court of law. Nothing in your account indicates that had been done. Therefore, in the situation you describe, when a patient's clearheaded most of the time and refuses the I.V., she should not be restrained in order to administer it. Any competent patient has the right to refuse treatment. For the patient who's usually lucid, the diagnosis of organic brain syndrome alone cannot be used as the basis for denying her the right to give or withhold consent for her own care.

By the way, here's a bouquet for coming up with the suggestion for *oral* potassium. You and your colleagues thus offered a sensible and satisfactory solution that allowed everybody to go beyond the impasse.

Formula feedings

Should supplementary formula feedings be given to healthy infants who don't seem satisfied after breast-feeding?

Q Until a mother's milk supply is well-established, should we give supplementary formula feedings to healthy infants who don't seem satisfied after breast-feeding? My co-workers on the obstetrics unit say absolutely *no* formula, not even for infants who are large at birth. Why not?

A Supplemental formula feedings aren't necessary to prevent elevated bilirubin levels, jaundice, or weight loss. And by satisfying the infant's hunger, these feedings can diminish the mother's milk production, which depends on stimulation by her baby's vigorous sucking and frequent feedings. During this taking-hold period, the mother's self-image is fragile, and she may feel confused and easily discouraged if her early attempts to breast-feed aren't successful. She may think her baby doesn't like the breast, her milk, or even her.

Supplemental bottles can also create nipple confusion. To breast-feed, the infant thrusts his tongue under the areola, pulling the breast so that the nipple is in the back of his mouth and his jaws are on the areola. He curves his tongue and thrusts it back to create enough suction to milk the breast. With a rubber nipple, the infant must thrust his tongue forward and press upward at intervals to stop the easy flow of milk. He'll usually discover that sucking on a rubber nipple is easier, and he may fuss and cry when faced with the more difficult process of sucking on his mother's breast.

So remember: Offering early formula supplements can interfere with the establishment of breast-feeding—and undermine a mother's confidence. Her success in breast-feeding when she's at home may depend on your support when she's in the hospital.

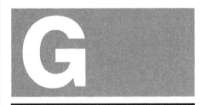

Gastrostomy tubes

Which type of catheter is better to use as replacements?

Q At our facility for severely developmentally disabled children, several residents are fed exclusively by gastrostomy tube. Frequently, these tubes become dislodged during handling. In the past, we noted that only mushroom-type catheters were used to replace them, but now balloon-tip catheters are being used. Which is better?

A The mushroom catheter is more expensive but much more reliable for long-term gastrostomy placement. A balloon

G

catheter is really useful in a temporary situation only; it has a tendency to dislodge and obstruct the duodenum via the pylorus. In fact, an incident occured when the balloon tip of the catheter became displaced in the duodenum and was mistakenly identified on X-ray as a duodenal polyp.

Before a mushroom catheter can be inserted, the patient's GI tract must be mature enough (at least 6 to 8 weeks old), then correct placement should be confirmed by X-ray. For this reason, some doctors choose a balloon-tip catheter initially and then replace it at a later date with the mushroom type.

Generic substitutes

How can confusion be avoided?

Q Substituting generic drugs for trade drugs is legal in our state—and encouraged at the nursing home where we work, to keep down costs. So the pharmacy routinely makes substitutions when the doctor orders a drug by its trade name.

But that policy causes problems for us nurses because we're unfamiliar with many generic drug names. If a prescription label lists only the generic name, we have to spend time checking a drug reference book to match it with a trade name.

Also, we don't know what many of these generic medications look like. If we can't identify a drug by sight, we're not sure that the prescription label accurately reflects what's in the container.

To make substitutions safer for residents and easier on us, shouldn't the pharmacist put *both* names on labels?

A Ideally, yes. But in some states, it's illegal for a pharmacist to label a generic drug with a corresponding trade name, even when

he's substituting. Some pharmacists get around this by using label statements (for example, "diazepam substituted for Valium" or "same as Valium"), but some states forbid that, too. So depending on where you work, you may have to continue using reference books to double-check unfamiliar generic names.

But your pharmacist could help you by:
• using the commercial unit-dose packaging provided by many generic drug manufacturers. Each dose is individually labeled, significantly reducing the chance for a mistake.
• limiting the number of manufacturers who supply generic drugs to your nursing home. Then you could identify the drugs he dispenses by consulting posters or loose-leaf notebooks supplied by the manufacturers.
• doing business only with manufacturers that emboss codes on their tablets or capsules. With the right charts, you can quickly and accurately "decode" those drugs.

Geriatric nursing

Should a nurse ask for a raise in recognition of her certification?

Q As a career-oriented nurse, I've recently become certified in my specialty, geriatric nursing. The hospital where I work offers a pay increase to nurses earning a BSN degree, but doesn't compensate for certification. Should I ask for a raise in recognition of my certification?

A No harm in trying! However, you should know that yours isn't the only hospital not automatically giving a pay increase for certification. Many hospitals don't provide a salary increase. But for some nurses, being recognized among the staff is enough reward.

This shouldn't stop you from trying to get a raise in recognition of your certification. First, have all pertinent information photocopied and placed in your personnel file. Since certification is an expensive process, include the expenses and time involved in getting it. Then approach your director of nursing and your personnel manager. You may have to try more than once. But even if you *don't* make headway with the raise, you'll still have the satisfaction of your expertise in your specialty. You can't put a price on that.

Gift giving

Where should the line be drawn?

Q Mike, a 10-year-old with leukemia, is frequently readmitted to our unit for treatment. After Mike's first hospitalization, his parents sent flowers and candy to thank us for his care. Since then, they've given several of us personal gifts. I didn't see anything wrong with that practice, because the gifts were always little things, like homemade cookies or a box of candy.

But a week ago, I overheard one of the nurses thanking Mike's mother for a leather purse. I also found out that Mike's mother had given another nurse a gift certificate to a department store. As nurse-manager, I know that I have to draw the line. But where?

A Ideally, the hospital should have a policy about gifts (some hospitals won't allow employees to accept *anything*). But if it doesn't, work with your staff to draft a policy for your unit. It should specify the type of gifts that nurses may accept; for example, gifts intended for the whole unit rather than an individual nurse. If you permit nurses to accept cash gifts, the money could go into a fund to buy items for the unit—say, a coffee machine, extra stethoscopes, even a Doppler stethoscope.

By adopting a policy that everyone agrees on, you emphasize that patient care is a team effort; sharing gifts rewards every nurse for her contribution. And no one can be accused of reserving her best efforts for patients who shower her with gifts.

Chances are, other managers at your hospital have similar problems. So why not approach hospital and nursing administration about establishing a hospitalwide policy? Offer your unit's policy as a model.

Of course, no policy should *encourage* gift giving; it should simply set ground rules for families who want to thank the nursing staff in a tangible way. Consistently applied, a clear gift policy lets everyone—patients, families, and nurses—feel good about gestures of appreciation.

Gloves

Are vinyl gloves as effective as latex ones in protecting against infection?

Q In response to recent precautions from the Centers for Disease Control, the hospital where I work provides us with vinyl gloves to use when we come in contact with patients' blood or body fluids. Yet last week, I heard that the company that does all of our dialysis told its nurses to use latex, not vinyl gloves.

Are vinyl gloves as effective as latex gloves in protecting us against pathogens such as the human immunodeficiency virus (HIV)?

A A rumor has been circulating for several months that vinyl gloves (or sometimes latex gloves, depending on which rumor you hear) aren't effective protection against HIV. No published study to date has indicated any difference between vinyl and latex gloves in their effectiveness

as barriers against HIV— as long as they're *intact*. So if you're using good quality, intact gloves, it shouldn't make any difference whether they're latex or vinyl.

Should gloves or forceps be used for each transfer of instruments?

Q In the dermatology office where I work, we're concerned (for ourselves) about our method of handling and cleaning surgical instruments. We don't usually glove to handle the instruments. Now because of acquired immunodeficiency syndrome (AIDS), we're wondering if we should be using gloves or forceps for each transfer of instruments.

A Always wear gloves while you're cleaning and processing dirty instruments. The threat of AIDS is not the only thing to worry about. According to the Association of Operating Room Nurses' standards, using transfer forceps for this procedure is *not* acceptable.

If you have the proper equipment, here's the sequence to follow: Wash and sterilize the instruments using a detergent recommended by the machine's manufacturer. Next, clean the instruments ultrasonically; milk them (soak them in an antirust solution); then dry and bag for final sterilization.

Why are some hospitals requiring that the staff wear gloves during CPR?

Q I can understand the necessity if we're inserting a chest tube or a subclavian line during a traumatic (and bloody) code. However, I can't understand why we need to wear gloves for performing cardiopulmonary resuscitation (CPR) on someone who has had a heart attack. Any advice?

A Gloves should be worn during any procedure when the patient's body fluids can't be confined and contained, and CPR fits this criteria. So, even though you're performing CPR because the patient has had a heart attack, you have no way of knowing what underlying diseases he may have. Wearing gloves will protect you.

Glucose levels

What levels require emergency treatment?

Q Our hospital's unit managers think that our standards for glucose levels requiring emergency treatment (below 50 mg/dl or above 350 mg/dl) are off target. After checking around, however, we found these "panic values" to be the standard for this area.

What is your opinion?

A What you're doing is unsafe. Treatment should start if values go below 60 mg/dl or if they go above 240 mg/dl.

But blood glucose levels are just one part of the picture. When the glucose value is elevated, check for ketonuria and ketonemia. Look for electrolyte depletion, and check pH and sodium bicarbonate values. Also, observe for physical signs and symptoms such as hypotension, tachycardia, confusion, vomiting, and Kussmaul's respirations.

Good Samaritan

Is it legal to administer drugs while off duty?

Q Recently, a friend and I were at a local dance club when another patron collapsed. Because we're both RNs certified in advanced cardiac life support, we performed cardiopulmonary resuscitation until the emergency medical technicians arrived. They set up

G

an electrocardiogram (ECG) monitor, but didn't start administering drugs because they couldn't establish contact with the doctor at their medical base. So my friend read the ECG strip and administered the drugs on her own. Was she taking a risk by giving these drugs without an order? Or was she covered by the Good Samaritan act? (By the way, the man recovered.)

A Good Samaritan acts usually grant immunity from liability only when emergency care is given *within the scope of your practice.* Your friend exceeded that scope. By prescribing and treating—actions reserved for doctors—she was essentially practicing medicine without a license. Although she has specialized knowledge and skills, she may use them only under the direction of a licensed doctor.

> *"My friend read the ECG strip and administered the drugs on her own...but I wondered if she was taking a risk."*

Luckily, this man wasn't injured by your friend's actions, so she wouldn't be liable for malpractice. But if she were reported to the board of nursing, her nursing license would be in jeopardy.

Should a nurse do CPR on a victim out on the streets?

Q What is my liability as a critical care nurse if I don't stop to do cardiopulmonary resuscitation (CPR) on a victim out on the streets? I know it sounds terrible, but I'm afraid of getting a disease, being mugged, or being sued.

A The law says most people don't have a "duty to rescue." Only those who perform rescues as a

regular part of their job, such as fire fighters and emergency medical technicians, have this legal duty. In your state, unless you're responsible for the victim's condition, you have two choices: to help in an emergency or to decide not to help. When you help an accident victim, the Good Samaritan law offers you immunity from lawsuits as long as you don't intentionally or recklessly cause injury.

A recent article in JAMA by the American Heart Association says the risk of contracting hepatitis B or acquired immunodeficiency syndrome infection during mouth-to-mouth rescuscitation is "minimal". No cases of such transmission have been reported. Even so, use of a barrier device to prevent direct contact is recommended.

Should a student nurse help at the scene?

Q I'm a student nurse (I'll have my associate degree in 4 months) who needs advice about helping out in an emergency.

At church one Sunday a woman of about 70 in the pew in front of us became ill. From where I was sitting, I could see that her color was ashen, her breathing seemed somewhat labored, and her behavior was confused. Of course, I thought of transient ischemic attack or myocardial infarction.

I had a debate with myself: Should I or shouldn't I offer to help? I held back because so many solicitous people had quickly gathered around the woman, and because I'd learned that one of the ushers had already called for an ambulance.

Luckily, the woman didn't seem to be getting worse, and nobody was taking inappropriate action, so I did nothing. But I was mightily relieved when the ambulance arrived quickly. I no longer had a decision to make.

Perhaps the incident still rankles because one of my sons asked on

the way home, "Mommy, why didn't you help that lady? You're a nurse."

Should I have helped?

A You probably made a sensible decision, so try to tamp down the guilt. Your impulse to help was right and natural, but under the circumstances, your help might just have overloaded the poor woman with attention.

Your student status wasn't as much an issue as you seemed to think. An alert student nurse— 4 months from graduation—would be in a much better position to help—if help were needed—than most laypeople.

About answering your son's question: Why not explain the situation to him without being either defensive or apologetic? *His* reaction's bound to reflect your own attitude toward the incident.

Before you find yourself in another student Samaritan situation, bone up on the legal and ethical implications of "helping" in an emergency.

Gossip

Should a nurse do anything about a co-worker's gossip?

Q Another nurse and I often attend the same parties. She loves to entertain the crowd with stories about her patients. She even mentions their names. I doubt her stories will spread, but I still think she's wrong. Should I do anything?

A Yes. Your co-worker's gossiping is unprofessional and destructive. Besides destroying the trusting relationships she should have with her patients, it undermines public confidence in the nursing profession.

Remember, the American Nurses' Association Code for Nurses says nurses have a duty to protect their patients' privacy by not disclosing personal, medical, or psychological information. Many hospitals strictly discipline employees who breach patient confidentiality, so this nurse could be jeopardizing her job. She might even face a lawsuit from a patient who resents being cocktail party entertainment.

For everybody's sake, talk to your co-worker. She needs to understand that gossiping about patients is no joking matter. Avoid preaching, but be clear, straightforward, and firm.

If insensitivity to patient privacy seems widespread at your hospital, talk to the head of staff development about starting an in-house program on protecting confidential information.

Graduate nurses

Can the night nurses refuse to let graduate nurses with temporary permits give medications?

Q I'm having problems with the night RNs at the small hospital where I'm director of nursing. The night nurses won't let any graduate nurse or practical nurse who hasn't yet passed her state boards give medications—even if she's met our hospital performance objectives.

But our graduates and practicals who haven't yet passed their exams *do* have temporary permits issued by the state board of nursing. The permits allows them to give medications under the supervision of a fully qualified RN.

Under the circumstances, can the night RNs refuse to cooperate?

A If the state board says graduate and practical nurses can give medications under supervision, and that's also part of your hospital policy, the night RNs *cannot* refuse to cooperate. But to avoid unnecessary confrontation, be sure your RNs understand that the graduates

are capable, that they are licensed and completely covered by state law. Besides, the new nurses need the experience—in order to become good night nurses themselves. You're not being high-handed—you're just being the boss.

Incidentally, in answer to what might be your next question: The board interprets "supervision" to mean having the qualified RN available—not necessarily having her check each medication as it's administered.

Could a nurse who failed her state board exam cause other nurses to be liable for her mistakes?

Q One of the graduate nurses on our medical/surgical unit just told us that she failed her state board exam. If we cosign her chart entries, are we responsible for her patient care and any errors she may make?

A In some states, graduate nurses who fail the state boards can function only as nursing assistants until they pass the exam. So this graduate nurse probably shouldn't be charting at all. But you should check with your state board on its policy.

Working as an assistant may frustrate her; after all, she has many nursing skills that she'll be tempted to use. But working strictly as a nursing assistant will greatly reduce her risk of being sued—and eliminate the risk that you, your colleagues, and hospital administration would face if you were party to illegal nursing practice.

Would a nurse-manager be responsible for their mistakes?

Q As the nurse-manager on a medical/surgical unit, I'm responsible for overseeing the work of our new graduate nurses. Legally,

am I also responsible for mistakes they make?

A Yes. Until a graduate demonstrates her skills and judgment to your satisfaction, *you're* responsible for her patients' care. So continue to double-check her work until you're sure she's competent to work more independently. That may take a few days to a few months, depending on the kind of work she's doing.

No matter how busy you are, you can't neglect your supervisory responsibilities. Even when you're overworked and understaffed, the law can hold you responsible for a new graduate's mistakes.

G

Grief

Why wouldn't a twin want to attend her sister's funeral?

Q After a 2-year battle with leukemia, our daughter died. Her twin sister, who I'll call Jenny, refuses to attend the funeral, which is in a few days. I'm surprised by her reaction. She often visited her sister during her lengthy hospitalization, and we kept her informed of her sister's condition. I don't want to force her to attend the funeral. What should I do?

A Because twins share a deep emotional bond, Jenny was identifying with her sister. So a large part of her "self" not only was hospitalized but actually died. She may be feeling responsible for the illness, suffering, and pain her sister felt. And she may be afraid the same thing could happen to her.

Try taking Jenny into her room, sit with her on her bed, and hold her tightly. Then, ask her if she feels like talking about what happened to her sister. If she says no, don't worry. She's vulnerable now, and she wants life to be steady and predictable. She needs to talk, but you shouldn't force her.

You can help her open up by talking about your own sadness. Crying is quite acceptable. When she sees you talking freely about your pain, she'll probably join in. You can set the tone and pace.

You will also need to explain what she can expect to happen at the funeral. Encourage her to ask questions. If she asks something you can't answer, don't be afraid to say, "I don't know."

After she has all this information, she still may choose to remain at home. That's okay. Just make sure she stays with someone who loves her while you go.

But if she doesn't attend the funeral, she still needs to see her sister's body—to confirm that she really died and can't return. You might ask Jenny if she would like to write a letter to her sister, which she could place in the casket. Or, find out if she has a special gift that she'd like to have buried with her.

You're both hurting right now. Hold on tight to each other.

Guardianship

Is there a difference between being a patient's legal guardian and having power of attorney?

Q "Legal guardian" and "power of attorney"—everyone on our critical care unit uses these terms interchangeably. But I'd feel a lot more comfortable next time we have an unconscious patient if I knew the legal definitions. Can you set the record straight?

A We went right to the source: In *Black's Law Dictionary,* these terms are defined as follows:

Legal guardian—One who is lawfully invested with the power, and charged with the duty, of taking care of the *person* and managing the property and rights of another person who for some peculiarity of status or defect of age, understand-

ing, or self-control is considered incapable of administering his own affairs.

Power of attorney—The instrument authorizing another to act as one's agent or attorney.

To clarify, the power of attorney is usually freely conferred on someone for a specific time and purpose by a competent, conscious person. This might be done to manage property, bank accounts, checks, and so forth. A legal guardian, however, is appointed by the court to manage the rights and property of an incompetent or unconscious person. Legal guardianship also includes power of attorney.

> *"I'd sure feel a lot more comfortable next time we have an unconscious patient if I knew the legal definitions of 'legal guardian' and 'power of attorney'."*

How does this relate to unconscious patients? Well, unless the patient was mentally ill or developmentally disabled *before* he became unconscious, he probably won't have a legal guardian. In most such cases, the court will appoint a relative to assume responsibility temporarily and consent to treatment. Or, if no relative can be found, the state can authorize treatment. Of course, the doctor must explain the nature, purpose, and risks of the treatment to the relative or the court so they can give their informed consent. Failure to do so can result in legal action.

One last point: If someone says he's the legal guardian of an unconscious patient, ask for some identification, such as a letter from a lawyer. If he has no proof, use your judgment. Question him further or insist he bring in proof if you have any doubts. Of course, always document all conversations. Then, if litigation should result, you'll have some protection.

Guest-patient

Are there legal implications for not charting their care?

Q The hospital where I work is religiously affiliated. From time to time, clergymen, with no admitting papers, are checked into rooms on our unit. According to the unit supervisor, the clergy are just "guests" of the hospital. So, okay.

Last week, however, one of the guests was unable to take his prescribed medications (cephalexin [Keflex], ibuprofen [Motrin], furosemide [Lasix], and pentazocine [Talwin]) by himself. We were told to give them to him, but not to chart this information on the medications record. In fact, we were told not to do any charting for this patient-guest.

I'm concerned about the irregularities here. After all, this is a hospital, not a hotel. Are we taking legal risks in caring for people without charting that care?

A The hospital is probably acting with some charitable intent in mind. But charity begins at home and that means with you, the staff. You should not be asked to follow such irregular practices. If these guests have no charts, apparently there are no signed consent forms and no doctors' orders for the drugs—all of which could lead to big trouble for you.

Explain your concerns to administration and ask your hospital's legal department its opinion too. In the meantime, if any more "guests" with no charts arrive on the scene, remember: As a nurse, you have the right to refuse to do something you're not comfortable with. This situation is one that would make any reasonable nurse—who values her license, freedom from legal liability, and patients' safety—most uncomfortable.

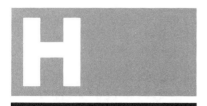

Handiwork

What's wrong with doing it when patients are sleeping?

Q In the past, the night staff at the nursing home where I work was always allowed to knit or embroider during quiet time between tasks. Now the supervisor decreed that we must stop making handicrafts on paid time.

Most of us always do more than expected, and heaven knows we're underpaid, considering the work we do. If all our work is done and the residents are asleep, what's wrong with spending a few minutes doing some quiet activity?

What do you hear from other facilities about this?

A More nurses are concerned about protecting their jobs in the face of cost cutting and corporate takeovers than how they're allowed to fill downtime. As one nurse put it, "If our administrator came across a nurse on any shift with enough time to knit or embroider, he'd take that as his cue to cut back staff."

Another nurse says, "What downtime? When caring for the sick and elderly, there's never time to sit. At our facility, the staff initiated a round-the-clock preventive toileting program—when rounds are finished, it's time to start over. Also, we use nursing measures such as back rubs and one-on-one talking time for those residents having trouble falling asleep. This requires nursing time."

In most facilities the night shift nurses are expected to use any quiet time for paperwork (tallying intakes and outputs, preparing lab slips, treatment sheets, and so forth) plus numerous other jobs such as checking linens and supplies. Many sharp night supervisors schedule staff development sessions to help the staff keep their skills current—good for the facility and even better for the nurses as a way to keep confident and prepared for job changes if they come.

Harsh treatment

Should a nurse speak up against it?

Q One night, emergency medical technicians brought in a young woman who'd overdosed on drugs for the third time. I was assisting another nurse and a doctor as they passed a tube to pump her stomach. They seemed too rough—almost as if they were angry—and several times the other nurse said to the patient, "Now Karen, you aren't going to do this again, are you?" I felt they were trying to punish her, so I spoke up. They finished the process more gently, but now they're giving *me* the cold shoulder. Did I handle this situation correctly?

A Absolutely. As the patient's advocate, you have an ethical duty to question any treatment that seems harsh or abusive, whether it's physical roughness, rudeness, verbal pressure, or manipulative behavior.

When your colleagues behave this way, ask yourself why. In the situation you described, the reason could have been frustration, prejudice, or fear of failure. Other times, insecurity or anxiety may cause a co-worker to abuse a patient. These feelings aren't easy to admit, but they're somewhat common among health care workers who deal with difficult patients—including those who use drugs, attempt suicide, or refuse to comply with treatment.

Approach your co-workers and initiate an honest discussion about personal feelings and how they can interfere with professional responsibilities. Talk about how you all can protect the quality of care by finding ways to cope with these feelings.

Perhaps a workshop on burnout would help. A psychiatric clinical nurse specialist or a counselor could identify the stresses that can lead to burnout—for instance, having to deal with patients (like this young woman) who are repeatedly in the emergency department despite your best interventions. Pressure to perform or to meet deadlines, constant tension or conflict among co-workers, or an atmosphere that's cold and uncaring can also contribute to burnout. A mental health professional can shed some light on how burnout translates into problems in patient care and how you and your co-workers can take steps toward positive change.

Heel sticks

Do other hospitals screen all newborns and should we be expected to perform the venipuncture if indicated?

Q In the small hospital nursery where I work, we have a new policy calling for a heel-stick hematocrit (capillary blood sample) on all newborns 4 hours after birth. If the results are 65% or greater, a central hematocrit (venous blood sample) is drawn to diagnose polycythemia.

Are other hospitals screening all newborns? And should we nurses be expected to perform the venipuncture if indicated?

A Opinions vary. Some hospital policies call for screening *all* newborns. Others favor screening only those in a high-risk category for polycythemia—newborns who were hypoxic during delivery because they were small or large for gestational age or who were postmature. Although protocols differ on who is screened and when, all agree on follow-up with a venous sample and close monitoring if heel-stick results are 65% or greater.

Standards of the Nurses Association of the American College of Obstetrics and Gynecology say it's inappropriate for nurses without proper preparation to draw venous samples from a newborn. And preparation in this technique may be practical in a small hospital like your own.

Hematoma

If the I.V. infiltrates, should warm or cold packs be applied?

Q On our pediatric unit, 13-year-old Johnny was receiving I.V. heparin and the I.V. infiltrated. The nurses discontinued the I.V. and applied warm packs. Naturally, the nurses were alarmed when a hematoma the size of a small apple developed on the boy's wrist. I was called in at this point, as the shift supervisor.

We conferred on what should be done. I suggested that the effects of cold packs would be more desirable than the vasodilating action of the warm packs we'd been applying.

Dr. A., the orthopedist who'd performed Johnny's knee surgery, agreed with using the cold packs.

Dr. B., Johnny's pediatrician, discontinued this treatment when he came the next morning. Dr. B. ordered warm packs, not cold, and indicated angrily that the original warm packs should have been continued.

I'm still trying to determine what *was* the right treatment in this situation: the application of heat or cold?

Luckily, Johnny's swelling subsided and he's had no permanent aftereffects.

Because we have no written policy if a comparable situation should occur again, we've requested one. Our request has gotten as far as the hospital's policy and procedure committee, where it's been mired for months without a reply.

What can you tell me?

A You're puzzled and frustrated by the medical contradictions, and understandably so—especially if there's no hospital policy forthcoming.

The right procedure is the procedure that works, whether it's hot or cold.

> *"Naturally, the nurses were alarmed when a hematoma the size of a small apple developed on the boy's wrist."*

Here's why: At one time, the directions for applying heat or cold were very clear. But with our increasing understanding of the pathophysiology of pain and infiltrate absorption, the tidy distinctions have been blurred. The tendency now is to do what gets results in reducing swelling, relieving pain, and promoting healing.

But here are some general guidelines: For the first 8 to 24 hours, apply ice; this will constrict blood vessels, reducing blood flow to the area and inhibiting the release of injury agents (bradykinin, histamine, and so on). Ice, which works as a local anesthetic, will also help reduce pain.

After the acute stage has passed, heat can be applied to bring healing agents (for example, lymphocytes) to the area and get rid of debris. These actions will be increased by vasodilation.

You'll find plenty of valuable background information on the application of heat and cold in your nursing library. But the books, like the doctors, don't always agree with one another.

Heparin injections

Is there a therapeutic reason for administering heparin by the I.M. route?

Q A member of our medical staff insists on ordering heparin given I.M., despite the protests from our pharmacists and other hospital personnel.

I administered it once, as he ordered, but I regretted doing it. When I returned after my weekend off, I could see large hematomas on the patient's buttocks resulting from the injections.

I'd like to refuse to give heparin I.M. the next time—but my action won't be taken lightly in the small community hospital where I work.

Before I take my stand, I'd like to know: *Is* there a therapeutic reason for administering heparin by the I.M. route?

A Heparin should not be routinely administered intramuscularly.

The I.M. route should not be used because of the likelihood of producing tissue irritation, local bleeding, or hematoma; in addition, absorption is unpredictable after I.M. administration.

When you returned and noted the hematomas, you should have filed an incident report: "Hematomas noted on same sites as I.M. heparin injections"—and included the hematomas' measurements as well as the patient's complaints about pain. But that's *after* the fact.

Before the fact, you have the right and the responsibility to tell the doctor that you're uncomfortable administering heparin intramuscularly. But ask first if he has a special reason for choosing the I.M. route in this particular case—or if he has new information on the subject that you're not yet familiar with.

If he has neither a sound medical reason nor new information, call in your pharmacist. He's the expert in this matter. When you've done your groundwork, you can feel comfortable telling the doctor you'll administer the drug by any *recommended* route. But if the doctor insists on I.M., give him the option of administering the heparin himself. Document fully as you go. If you're knowledgeable and confident, if you handle the matter discreetly and privately (so the doctor isn't put on the defensive publicly), he surely won't pursue the issue.

However, if he *still* insists on ordering the heparin to be given I.M., you must now present your documentation to your supervisor. Keep going up the administrative ladder until you get results.

This includes seeking support for your position from other doctors (this could mean a letter of complaint to the chief of medicine). Keep a file of all your efforts: You'll have written proof as well as the knowledge within yourself that you did your professional best to be your patient's advocate.

Heparin locks

How long does it take before blood clots the line?

Q We use many heparin locks on our busy medical/surgical unit. However, we frequently don't flush the locks *immediately* after the I.V. infusion's finished.

How long can we put off flushing before blood clots the line?

A How long you wait depends on whether blood flows back into the cannula when the infusion is finished.

Here's the principle: When you allow an I.V. infusion to run dry, it stops running at the point where the head pressure of the fluid and the pressure in the patient's venous system are equal. If the patient's venous pressure increases for any reason (say through contraction of arm muscles or rise in blood pressure), blood is forced back into the cannula and will clot.

However, if you turn the infusion off just before it runs dry, the I.V. fluid remaining in the cannula will keep the line patent and prevent blood from flowing back. For most patients, the I.V. line can be safely turned off for as long as an hour without clotting. Within that hour, you should find time to flush the lock.

Hepatitis B

Can a nurse be a danger to patients?

Q I was recently appointed nurse coordinator for a continuous ambulatory peritoneal dialysis unit.

Ten years ago, while working for a kidney transplantation service, I contracted an active case of hepatitis B.

Routine blood work required for the dialysis unit shows I'm HBsAg-positive (surface antigen positive, surface antibody negative with positive core antibodies) with all normal liver functions.

Opinion here at the hospital is sharply divided on whether the HBsAg-positive means that I'm a chronic carrier of hepatitis B. Some people say I should stay away from hands-on nursing altogether because I'm a danger to patients.

What would you do?

A Listen to the opinion of an authority: the Centers for Disease Control (CDC).

Recent guidelines from the CDC say that a carrier is defined as a

person who is HBsAg-positive on two or more occasions at least 6 months apart. So first have your blood work repeated to confirm that you actually are a chronic carrier.

The CDC guidelines then go on to say that persons with hepatitis B or chronic carriers *may* continue to have patient contact. Gloves should be worn for procedures that cause trauma to tissue or involve contact with mucous membranes or open wounds.

Transmission of hepatitis B takes place through direct inoculation from the carrier's blood or mucosal secretions. In a few documented instances, hepatitis B was transmitted by gynecologists performing complex pelvic surgery and by dentists performing oral surgery. In the dialysis unit, you'll have minimal contact with the patient's blood (again, your blood has to be present for transmission) and gloves will decrease any likelihood of that occurring.

Now that you've the go-ahead to stay in hands-on nursing, you can be positive about your ability and eligibility for your new job. Good luck.

Should a carrier give CPR?

Q Several years ago, while working in a rural emergency department, I contracted hepatitis B. A recent screening test showed that I'm a carrier.

I'm now 57 and work as the only live-in nurse in a small retirement home. The 60 residents, most of whom are well or have varying degrees of chronic illnesses, have become like family to me.

In checking over past records, I noticed that every year one or two residents needed cardiopulmonary resuscitation (CPR). As a hepatitis carrier, should I give CPR—or do you think I should join the ranks of retirees?

H

A The answer to both your questions is a simple no. As a hepatitis carrier, you can't perform CPR safely as the rescuer at the mouth—but you don't have to retire just because of this.

Instead, you can make arrangements for other employees (nursing assistant, manager, security guard, cook) to take a CPR course so they'll be able to help. Then, if your worst fear happens and a resident needs CPR, one of them can be the rescuer at the mouth while you do chest compressions and make sure that the code is organized and running smoothly.

Discuss the situation with your manager and ask her to buy you a new airway with a one-way valve that you could use in an emergency. The cost of this equipment is a small price to pay to keep someone like you on the job at "home."

What is the risk of getting it?

Q I'm a nurse at a day treatment-training program for developmentally disabled adults. We have 100 clients who range in age from 21 to 70 years old; their functioning levels range from profound to moderate mental retardation, and their hygiene skills leave much to be desired. Furthermore, some of them act out by biting and scratching.

Given the setting, none of these circumstances would be too worrisome except that four of our clients are known hepatitis B carriers. Their families know this and have all been vaccinated. But what about our staff?

Aren't they at risk for contracting hepatitis B? Should they undergo hepatitis screening? Should they receive hepatitis vaccine? (The agency won't pay for the screening and vaccine.)

Right now all I'm recommending to them is good hygiene techniques, especially careful handwashing and

using gloves when in contact with a known carrier's blood.

I'd like comments on this from you.

A Working with hepatitis B carriers can be risky business anytime, and more so under the circumstances you describe. You're certainly on track recommending good hygiene techniques for the staff—especially wearing gloves—but these precautions may not be enough.

What the staff needs first is screening with an anti-HBs antibody test. Those with positive results won't need the vaccine. Those who do need the vaccine can be assured that the vaccine is about 95% effective, and of the 400,000 or more Americans who have received it, very few reported adverse reactions.

But now the money. These protective measures cost money—quite a lot when the expense is out of pocket. Screening costs about $50; vaccine, $100; and hepatitis B immune globulin for those *not* vaccinated, $150 any time blood contact occurs. But contracting hepatitis B would be by far the most costly.

Try to convince the administration that even if they won't pay for the staff's expenses, all newly admitted clients should be screened to identify the carriers and the population at risk. We hope they would agree this is one policy when spending dollars makes good sense.

Will hepatitis B vaccine affect a pregnant nurse?

Q Several months ago, I began working on a dialysis unit and was advised to have the hepatitis B vaccine. Now, after receiving two of the three required doses, I found out that I'm pregnant.

The *Physicians' Desk Reference* says that no animal reproduction studies were conducted with

Heptavax-B, it isn't known whether the vaccine can cause fetal harm, and it should be given to a pregnant woman only if clearly needed.

My doctor says that everything should be okay, but I'm still uneasy. What can you tell me?

A Pregnant women aren't usually asked to test drugs just to find out what the risks are, so data isn't available on the safety of the vaccine for the developing fetus. However, during a clinical trial of Heptavax-B among medical staff members of dialysis units, eight pregnancies occurred among women who received the vaccine; all eight women had healthy babies. Nineteen pregnancies occurred among women receiving placebos: Twelve had healthy infants, five had induced abortions, one miscarried, and one had an ectopic pregnancy.

The Centers for Disease Control stated in a recent report: "Because the vaccine contains only noninfectious HBsAg (hepatitis B surface antigen) particles, there should be no risk to the fetus. In contrast, hepatitis B infection in a pregnant woman can result in severe disease for the mother and chronic infection for the newborn. Pregnancy should not be considered a contraindication to the use of this vaccine for persons who are otherwise eligible." As a dialysis nurse, you're certainly among those at increased risk for infection.

According to the manufacturer, Merck Sharp & Dohme, any woman who's received two doses of Heptavax-B before learning she's pregnant can reasonably assume she's developed an adequate antibody level. This means you can defer taking the third dose until after your baby is born, just as long as you receive it within 12 months after the first dose. And although the number of women receiving the vaccine while pregnant is unknown, no serious adverse reactions among them have been reported to date.

So rest assured. Good luck!

HIV antibody test

Can administration force a nurse to be tested?

Q A rumor is going around that a nurse on our unit has acquired immunodeficiency syndrome (AIDS). A couple of my coworkers think hospital administrators should force her to have an human immunodeficiency virus (HIV)-antibody test so we'll know for sure. They're also claiming they'll refuse to work with her if the test is positive. What do you think? Should she be forced to have the test?

A Definitely not—if she's only suspected of having AIDS. But if she were obviously ill, hospital administrators could require testing or a physical examination, according to the American Hospital Association's *AIDS and the Law: Responding to the Special Concerns of Hospitals.*

Even if she tested positive, administrators couldn't reassign her unless she were ill, couldn't do her job, or wouldn't use proper infection-control technique. But if they determined that she threatened the health and safety of her co-workers or patients, they could find her another job in the hospital.

They'd better have plenty of documentation, though. Otherwise, they could be accused of discrimination.

How should a nurse tell patients they've tested positive?

Q Another nurse practitioner and I work in a clinic. Recently, we counseled an I.V. drug user who came in for an human immunodeficiency virus (HIV) antibody test. After drawing blood, we arranged for her to come back for the results. She told us she planned to commit suicide if the results were positive.

She broke her follow-up appointment. A week later, she called and asked me to tell her the results over the phone. When I refused, she said she wouldn't return to the clinic. So we're at a standoff. But she needs to know that she's HIV-positive. What should we do?

A You were right to refuse; you should always give HIV-test results in person so you can provide support for the patient.

Because she won't come to you, you'll have to go to her. As soon as possible, make an appointment for a home visit so you can explain the meaning of her test results and arrange for counseling and medical treatment. When you call her, just make sure you don't say anything that will make her assume she's HIV-positive. You could tell her you're following clinic policy to give test results in person.

Until you get more information, you also have to take her suicide threat seriously. Assess her risk. Then, if you believe she might carry out her threat, document your assessment and seek a consultation with a psychiatrist or psychiatric clinical nurse specialist.

You and your co-worker shouldn't assume responsibility for this woman's actions. But you should let her know that you're concerned, that you care, and that you'll be consulting with a mental health professional.

Finally, evaluate her support system. Whom does she turn to for assistance? With her approval, enlist these people to help her cope with the test results.

Is it legal for hospitals to test their employees?

Q Hospital administrators have announced that we'll all be tested for human immunodeficiency virus (HIV) at our annual physicals. Is that legal?

A In most states, yes. According to the American Hospital Association's *AIDS and the Law: Responding to the Special Concerns of Hospitals,* an employer may seek information to determine whether employees are fit to work without endangering themselves or others. So unless local law prohibits large-scale HIV testing, the policy is legal.

But it still raises plenty of questions, both legal and practical. For example, what will administrators do about the positive test results? They can't fire HIV-positive employees—now *that* would be illegal. Unless they can offer jobs that don't involve patient care to each of these employees, they open themselves up to legal problems.

They should also consider the practical problems common to large-scale testing efforts: Are they prepared to deal with false positives and false negatives? Will they provide pre-test and post-test counseling? Can they ensure confidentiality?

In light of all the headaches this policy could cause, hospital administrators would be wise to think twice before going ahead with it.

Is it legal to fire someone for refusing to disclose test results?

Q One of my co-workers was recently fired because he wouldn't disclose the results of his human immunodeficiency virus (HIV) test. Aren't these results personal and confidential?

A Usually they are, although the U.S. Supreme Court has said employers may investigate the health of an employee suspected of having a contagious disease.

In a similar case, a U.S. District Court in Louisiana recently ruled that hospital administrators are entitled to information about the HIV status of an employee who they believe is infected. The judge relied on guidelines from the Centers for Disease Control that are intended to help employers decide which job assignments the employee may safely undertake. So while your hospital's policy is controversial, legal precedent to support it does exist.

Who should know the results?

Q At the hospital where I work, only a patient's primary doctor is told the results of a human immunodeficiency virus (HIV) antibody test if one is run. He doesn't share this information with the nurses or other staff, and nothing appears in the patient's chart. Frankly, we want to protect ourselves. Any advice?

A child with hemophilia was admitted to our pediatric unit. While reading through his complex medical history, I came across a positive HIV antibody test report from an independent laboratory. When I spoke to his doctor about this, he forbade me to mention it to anyone or chart it because of medical confidentiality. But shouldn't the direct caregivers be informed?

Yesterday, one of the doctors told us that he's currently giving prenatal care to three patients with acquired immunodeficiency syndrome (AIDS). But he won't say who they are because they have a right to confidentiality. Don't we have a right to know who these patients are so we can protect ourselves?

A Some states (California, for one) currently have laws prohibiting doctors from telling staff members which of their patients have AIDS or positive HIV antibody tests. Others, including Pennsylvania, have no such laws on the books, but you might find a doctor here and there who refuses to identify a patient with AIDS—to protect himself. He's probably afraid the patient will sue him, even though

there's every good clinical reason for telling you. Knowing this information, you could take extra care to protect yourself.

But in a way, such disclosure could be dangerous, too. If doctors were to routinely tell you which patients have AIDS, you might develop a false sense of security. And you might let your defenses down—even though other patients haven't been tested.

So, resolve not to take any chances. Treat all patients as potential AIDS victims. This means wearing gloves for all I.V. starts, tubing changes, and venipunctures.

If you're likely to come in contact with a patient's blood or body fluids, take full precautions. Gloves, always. But when blood might spatter, wear a gown, a mask, and even protective eye wear when appropriate. Those working in the high-risk areas of emergency and obstetrics should be particularly careful. Incidentally, labor and delivery nurses are among the last to fully adopt self-protective measures.

Remember, be careful out there.

Home health care

How can a nurse make more money?

Q As a home health nurse, I've become increasingly frustrated: I love my patients, but the money is terrible. At the agency where I work, nurses are paid a flat rate for each visit to the patient's home, whether it takes 1 or 2 hours. Not included at all is the time spent phoning (patients, family members, doctors), completing forms, updating patient records, or traveling home when a patient lives a good distance away.

More in truth than in jest, my colleagues and I frequently declare, "Yes, we work for free 2 days a week."

Are we wrong to expect more?

A When you accept a flat rate for a visit, it's understood that it includes office time, phone calls, and paperwork. (You should, however, get mileage from the office to the patient's home and back. Mileage to and from your home is not reimbursable.) Obviously, if the flat rate is high enough, you'll be paid a fair wage.

Why not canvass several agencies where you live to find out what they're paying? If your rate's at the low end of the scale, negotiate for a raise or investigate registering with other agencies. Where's it written that you can't be paid well for doing a job you enjoy?

Is it risky to take a patient for a car ride?

Q I manage a home health agency in a small town. We have a wonderful staff including one nurse who visits a terminally ill, housebound patient after work. She even takes her out for a ride several times a week because the woman wouldn't get out otherwise. I see nothing wrong with this, but my administrator advised me to take the nurse off this case because she could be increasing the agency's liability. What do you think about this?

A Exaggerated fears about liability are clouding your administrator's judgment. Legally, a nurse working in any setting—home health or otherwise—is liable for her own actions on and off the job. Her agency and its insurance company could share in this liability only during the hours she's paid for. (Of course, for her own sake, she should be covered by personal malpractice and auto insurance policies.)

The patient would be the loser if this nurse were discouraged from doing what she thinks best on her own time. And this certainly would send the wrong signals to the other nurses. Here's a message you can pass along to your supervisor from one agency owner: Home health nurses have high visibility in the community because they're going into patients' homes. And far from a liability, the little extras they do after hours are great public relations for the agency—the kind that mere money can't buy.

Is there a good book for laypersons who are caring for the chronically disabled or terminally ill at home?

Q I work for a county home health agency. Do you know of a practical guide I can recommend to laypersons who choose to take care of the chronically disabled or terminally ill at home?

A Florine Du Fresne's book, *Home Care: An Alternative to the Nursing Home,* (Elgin, Ill.: Brethren Press, 1983) is just what you need. As the book's foreword promises, the particulars of home nursing care are covered in a commonsense, A-to-Z fashion, while the author's personal thoughts and feelings are quietly shared. Anyone seeking straightforward, practical information in easy-to-understand outline form, an honest appraisal of the weariness of carrying through, and encouragement to share this "adventure in love" will benefit from reading this book.

Should a nurse report a patient who's incapable of driving?

Q I'm a home health care nurse. I recently learned that one of my physically disabled, supposedly homebound patients has been driving a car—and he admits to doing it more than once. He's a hazard to himself and others on the road because he's partially deaf and visu-

ally impaired. I've also noticed that he's becoming increasingly forgetful. I'm concerned about my legal responsibilities in this situation. Should I report him to the department of motor vehicles?

A You ask a difficult question that's been grappled with—often unsuccessfully—by state motor vehicle departments and other state officials.

Technically, the state is responsible for regulating licensees. However, the trend is to place more responsibility on individuals who may know about a potentially dangerous situation. For example, bar owners, bartenders, and even hosts of parties where alcohol is served are expected to prevent intoxicated people from driving home. In some states, these individuals could be liable if they fail to intervene and a drunk driver subsequently has an accident.

> *"My physically disabled patient is a hazard to himself and others on the road because he's partially deaf, visually impaired, and forgetful."*

Where does that leave you? Although you have no more legal responsibility than anyone else, in this case you have a moral and ethical responsibility to talk with your patient and tell him that he must stop driving. If you can't reason with him, inform him that you're going to report him to his doctor and to other appropriate authorities.

You should also explore *why* your patient is driving. Perhaps he still needs help after you've left—to pick up a prescription, to go to the doctor, or to do his grocery shopping. If so, he may feel he must take the risk. As an alternative, discuss how family, friends, or neighbors can help him out. Developing a reliable

support network will be a positive step toward preventing a tragedy.

What are the RN's responsibilities?

Q I'm an RN working for a home health care agency. I understand that LPNs have different responsibilities in different areas and institutions. The LPNs working for this agency are caring for patients who have triple-lumen central venous catheters or tracheostomies and those who are ventilator-dependent. I'm worried that I may be responsible for their actions if something goes wrong. Because I insisted, the agency's administrator wrote a letter saying I'm responsible for my 12-hour shifts only. Still, I'm wondering if that's enough protection. Would I be held liable for the actions of the LPN on the other shift?

A You might be. The LPN's preparation, scope of practice, and the agency's policies and procedures determine her responsibilities. Of course an LPN, like any health care professional, is also responsible for her actions.

If you're supervising her or if you know (or should have known) that she hasn't been prepared to give competent care, you could share liability for her errors. So, you must find out whether the LPN who takes over for you has been adequately prepared to perform her assignments correctly.

What if an employee wants to moonlight for an agency's patient?

Q My sister and I run a home health care agency. We recently discovered that one of our nursing assistants is caring for a patient when she's off duty. She said he requested extra help and pays her directly. If she injures him and he sues, would we be liable?

A That depends on how the court balances two questions: Was your employee acting beyond the scope of her employment contract? Did the patient hire her only because of your agency's reputation?

If you can prove this nursing assistant wasn't acting as your employee when she was moonlighting, you might avoid liability. Even so, the patient could prevail if he proves that he hired your employee because he believed she had your stamp of approval; in other words, because he believed your agency guarantees the competency of its employees.

The court would also want to know if you've allowed other employees to moonlight or if you prohibit it in your employment contract or written job description. So, to avoid this kind of worry in the future, take these precautions:

• add a paragraph to your employment contract that prohibits moonlighting, at least with your agency's current patients. If you don't have an employment contract, put the prohibition in a handbook or written job description

• amend your standard contract with patients to state that you aren't responsible for employees' actions when they're off duty.

Who can assume responsibility for a patient at the end of shift time?

Q I recently began working for a home care agency. My first client, a 20-year-old with muscular dystrophy, is alert and able to use a bed control and call bell—but not much more. He has a tracheostomy and is on a ventilator, which he can be off for up to 2 hours at a time. His parents contracted for nursing care 8 hours a day, 7 days a week.

When my shift ended today, only his teenage sister was at home with us. She said it was okay for me to leave, that she'd taken care of her brother, including suctioning his

trach, lots of times before I came on the scene. While I didn't feel right leaving until the parents returned, there was no telling when that would be. And my own kids were waiting for me at the baby-sitter's, so I had to go.

I called my agency supervisor and offered to bring my kids back to wait with me for the patient's parents. She told me just to make sure the sister knew the agency phone number in case of any problems, and then to go home.

I felt very guilty leaving and angry at the parents. Any thoughts to share?

A Common courtesy says the parents should have at least checked in with you by phone. However, many teenage siblings fill in as temporary caregivers. And they can do a good job of it. If you're guilty of anything, it's leaving your patient out of your decision making. You should have asked *him* first if it was appropriate for you to go. After all, he's legally competent. Giving him some control over his care would have been courteous as well as practical.

Of course, you were right to alert the agency supervisor. If the patient was leery about having his sister fill in, the supervisor would have had to arrange for another nurse to relieve you (and bill the parents accordingly). And bringing your children into the patient's home wouldn't have been appropriate. When you're on the job, your kids should ideally neither be seen nor heard.

Homicide

Is it legal to obtain a blood specimen from the suspect without consent?

Q I've been working in the emergency department (ED) of a large metropolitan hospital, where we frequently treat victims of as-

sault and battery, rape, alcohol-related accidents, and other violence. We're sometimes asked to cooperate with investigating police officers by obtaining blood specimens to be used as legal evidence.

Just last month I was asked to obtain a blood smear from a patient allegedly involved in a murder, whose arm was streaked with blood. I did what I was asked to do, but I was unsure of how legal my action was.

Since the man was fully conscious, should I have obtained his consent before I took the blood sample? Since the procedure was noninvasive, was his verbal or written consent necessary at all? And how about informing the man of his rights before I took the specimen as legal evidence?

Our ED has no established policy or procedure for incidents like this. I'd like to devise one to prevent possible legal difficulties and confusion for our nursing staff in the future.

Can you help me out?

A There aren't any reported cases of hospitals or health care providers being held liable for doing a nonconsensual procedure as part of a police request. Your best protection against liability is an informed consent signed by the patient. Ideally, the consent form should describe *what* the procedure is, *why* it's being done, and *how* the results will be used. When you get all this straightened out beforehand, there can be no question of the patient having been misled.

A U.S. Supreme Court decision handed down in 1966 in the case of *Schmerber vs. California* held that a health care provider could obtain a blood sample against the patient's wishes *only if he was under arrest and the test was likely to produce evidence.* If these criteria are met, a noninvasive procedure such as taking a blood smear sample would be permissible. As an added precaution, the arresting officer should read the patient his legal rights.

To ensure *your* legal protection, ask for a hospital policy in writing to cover such circumstances in the future. That is the best way to deal with your uncertainty and your possible legal liability.

Homosexuality

Should a patient's sexual preference be documented?

Q While I was taking the history of an alcoholic patient at the detoxification unit where I work, he told me he was homosexual. Because he didn't seem comfortable with his homosexuality, I made a note of it on his chart. But my supervisor reprimanded me; she said "homosexual" was an inappropriate entry on a patient's chart, that it could incriminate the patient if the chart were introduced in court.

Is she right? Should I have ignored the patient's sexual identity—even though it appeared to be a matter of some discomfort to him?

A You're on dangerous ground when you document a patient's sexual preference (note that homosexual is his sexual *preference,* not his sexual identity), unless the information's pertinent to his case. In this instance, the information *might* be pertinent if the patient's homosexuality and drinking were clearly related. Otherwise, remember that taking a sexual history is not routine—particularly in a detoxification unit where the chief objective is to clear the patient's system of drugs, not to psychoanalyze him.

Also, why did you feel the patient found his homosexuality disturbing? He did not *say* this; you surmised it. Therefore, beware and be wary. Subjective reporting is risky business. You're safer to stick to the facts and to the patient's own words when charting controversial material.

If you feel strongly enough that something should be said or done

for this patient, go to the doctor, give him the information verbally, and discuss your concerns.

As far as the legal issue: The chart could not possibly be used to incriminate the patient, because homosexuality is not a crime. Nevertheless, when you write homosexual on the chart, you could create enormous difficulties for the patient. People from other departments have access to the patient's chart; some of these other "readers" could take a negative, hostile attitude toward the patient's sexual preference.

You'd be a lot safer if you were discreet—and documented only the facts called for in this case.

Hospital manual

Should it be detailed and should standard nursing procedures be addressed?

Q I'm a member of the policy and procedure committee at the hospital where I work. At yesterday's meeting, we had a heated discussion on how detailed the procedure manual should be. One school of thought says that if the manual is too detailed, there's no room left for nursing judgment. The flip side says that if the statements aren't detailed enough, the hospital could be held liable for an injury caused by loosely defined procedures.

Do you have any guidelines? And what benefit do you think there would be to addressing standard nursing procedures in the manual?

A Before any other decisions are made, your committee must identify your goals for the procedure manual. Do you want it to be a reference for complex, rare procedures *and* an instructional tool for new and temporary nurses? Should it identify standards by which staff nurses will be evaluated in-house? In a court situation, should this manual demonstrate the

nursing staff's consensus on what constitutes "safe practices?" In many hospitals, the policy and procedure committee wants its manuals to include all of these goals.

If your committee wants the manual to act as a ready reference—a hospital yardstick, if you will—by all means, include detailed basic procedures such as inserting an indwelling urinary catheter. Probably even the most experienced nurse has tense moments when her brain draws a blank. That's when a detailed procedure manual is really valuable.

Hypnosis

Are there any legal risks in teaching self-hypnosis while practicing nursing?

Q I've become more and more concerned with the interplay between a patient's mind and his state of health. This, in turn, has led to my intense interest in self-hypnosis. I did some reading, learned the techniques, and eventually became an instructor.

> *"I've developed an interest in self-hypnosis and have been offered an instructor's job, but I don't know what the legalities are."*

At present, I work full-time as an intensive care unit nurse at an acute care hospital. As part of my job, I teach the patients relaxation exercises to help them control pain and reduce anxiety.

I've now been offered a part-time instructor's job at a local hypnosis center, where I'd be teaching paying clients the techniques of self-hypnosis. I'd like to take this job, but I'm concerned about the legality of the situation.

Naturally, I'd present myself only as a self-hypnosis *instructor*—not as a therapist who hypnotizes others. And I'd never solicit clients at the hospital. Do you think I can safely and legally juggle the two jobs?

A Check first with your state board of nursing. Is teaching self-hypnosis covered under the state's nurse practice act? Chances are, there'll be no specific legislation either permitting *or* prohibiting you from teaching self-hypnosis. If you teach self-hypnosis as a registered nurse (for example, if you were to list your RN licensure in your job qualifications), then your actions *are* considered nursing actions, and you must be accountable for them. As a fundamental protection, you must have the necessary education to teach self-hypnosis competently.

Here's the key: Whether or not you can safely take the instructor's job depends on your qualifications for teaching self-hypnosis. If you feel both your education and competence are solid, you should be able to accept the job at the hypnosis center without jeopardizing your RN status.

Hypochondria

Do other nurses become hopeless wrecks over family sickness?

Q I'm 34 years old and recently quit my unit manager position to stay home with my baby. On the job, I never doubted my nursing skills for a minute. But now that I'm a full-time mother, it's another story.

For example, when my baby had a rash on her neck and torso, I was so convinced she had the measles that I panicked about possible complications. Our doctor finally reassured me the rash was from the heat.

Another time, I developed a constant pain in my knee. After some

research, I decided I had a sarcoma and became too tense to eat or sleep. I cried when I thought of dying and leaving my baby. Once again, our doctor convinced me that I was wrong.

Am I a little crazy? Do other nurses become hopeless wrecks over family sickness?

A You've probably heard the adage: "A doctor who treats himself has a fool for a patient." The same could be said for a nurse and her family. Most of us are just too involved to assess and treat illnesses in our families objectively.

Your problem is common—especially for nurses who are new mothers. So, be assured that your panic doesn't indicate that you're crazy, only that you're concerned.

When someone in your family gets sick, call your doctor for reassurance and guidance, give lots of tender loving care, and take each day as it comes. Oh, and brace yourself, too. You'll hear from lots of people that these are the best days of your life.

Hypothermia blankets

What should the initial minimum setting be?

Q At our large medical center, we frequently use hypothermia blankets to decrease the elevated temperature of our febrile patients.

We nurses disagree about what the initial minimum setting of the blankets should be. I say the minimum setting should be no lower than 50° F (10° C), to avoid reducing the patient's temperature too rapidly.

We have no set protocol to refer to, and I'd like your opinion.

A You need a written protocol, certainly. But what your department also needs is a staff development session on the pre-

cautions and related care necessary for using this potentially risky treatment.

To answer your specific question, one widely accepted protocol calls for initially setting the control on the thermal pad at 40° F (4.4° C) for approximately 5 minutes. Then reset the control to 1° F above the desired patient temperature. (Using one thermal pad, count on 3 to 4 hours to bring a patient's temperature to the desired range.) For safety's sake, be sure to use the automatic mode with the rectal probe in place.

ICCU

What can be done about understaffing?

Q I recently joined the staff on the night shift of an intensive coronary care unit (ICCU) in a small-town community hospital. The hospital is remarkably new and bright, yet I feel I'm having a wide-awake nightmare.

The ICCU has eight beds and is *supposedly* staffed throughout the night shift with two RNs. "Throughout the night" is subject to the clause in our job description that says one of us must make an ambulance run in case of a cardiac emergency. If one of us goes on an ambulance run, the other nurse is left alone on the unit, responsible for the care of eight potentially critical patients. An 8:1 patient-nurse ratio in an ICCU? Does that sound safe to you? What would happen if two patients required having a code called at the same time—with only one nurse on duty?

There's more for us to worry about: The nurse who takes the ambulance run may be asked to start an I.V. line, administer lidocaine (lignocaine, xylocaine) or atropine, or defibrillate if necessary. Although these tasks are covered by standing orders, I'm not comfortable. Are we performing these tasks legally?

A No wonder you're shaken up. This new job puts you in an untenable position on two scores.

First, the staffing pattern you describe is unsafe—even an 8:2 ratio given there are no "nights and days" in an ICCU. No one nurse could give eight patients in an ICCU the required care. And no matter how great the odds against two codes being called simultaneously, even the slimmest possibility is frightening.

Second, an ambulance run should not be part of an ICCU nurse's duty. Just because you work in critical care doesn't mean you're qualified to do what's needed on an ambulance run. In fact, there's no such thing anymore as the old simple "ambulance run"; the job's now a specialty unto itself. Even emergency department nurses won't take ambulance duty unless they've been specially prepared.

This job can also make you legally vulnerable. You're part of a staffing setup that's so inadequate the patients' safety is in jeopardy, and you're doing a job in the ambulance that calls for special qualifications. (You haven't indicated whether you *have* these qualifications.) In an ensuing lawsuit, your lack of preparation and skills could make you legally liable.

Thorough documentation is your best protection. So express your concerns and propose alternatives in writing; send copies through channels; and, of course, keep copies for yourself. Continue to report and record *each* incident that puts you or a patient in jeopardy. Do this as long as you're on the job.

A good critical care nurse needs a good critical care setting to do

justice to herself and her patients. While you're doing your best to improve the scene, remember how much these patients need you—a nurse who refuses to lower her sights.

ICU

Because patients are being monitored, don't they need constant assessment?

Q I work on the medical/surgical unit of a small community hospital. We've got 27 beds on our unit; the intensive care unit (ICU) has four. Here's the problem: If the ICU gets a new admission at a time when all its beds are occupied, the ICU nurses transfer one of their patients—a patient on a portable cardiac monitor—to our floor. The most recent transfer patient was on a monitor *and* had a lidocaine drip going during the night.

> *"We wouldn't even hear the alarm on the cardiac monitor unless we happen to be walking by the patient's room."*

Most of the nurses on our floor don't know how to use a cardiac monitor and can't recognize arrhythmias. Because our nurses' station is at the far end of the hall, we probably wouldn't even hear the alarm on the monitor unless we happened to be walking by the patient's room.

Because these patients are being monitored, don't they need constant assessment? And if a fatal arrhythmia occurs while the patient's unattended, could we be held legally responsible? I've documented the problem and sent a memo to the director of nursing for consideration. But what should we do *until* we get an official decision?

A Unfortunately, you're caught between an overworked ICU staff and a foot-dragging administration. But in the meantime, you're in a dangerous position.

What good is it to have a patient hooked to a monitor that no one on your unit knows how to use?

In the short term, nursing service should have someone assigned to your unit who knows how to use the monitor.

But in the long run, the problem begs a more thorough solution. You'll find sicker and sicker patients being transferred from ICU to your unit—what with the trends toward economy and cutbacks. Therefore, your staff must be better prepared to work with these patients. That means at least one nurse on any shift knowing how to use a monitor.

There's another solution: Get telemetry set up with the monitor screen in the ICU.

In the meantime, if another patient on a monitor is transferred to your unit before a short- or long-term solution has been put into place, take the following steps for your protection:
• Report to your supervisor as soon as a patient on a monitor is transferred to your unit.
• With another nurse present and serving as a witness, inform the supervisor that your unit staff can't take responsibility for this patient. Explain that no one on your staff is qualified to use the monitor. Ask to have a nurse who *is* qualified assigned to your unit.
• Document what you said to the supervisor and how the supervisor responded. Ask the nurse who served as a witness to sign the document.
• Check your malpractice insurance; be sure it covers you in this kind of situation.

Such documentation should support your case in the event of a malpractice suit. But you and your colleagues should keep pressing for a fundamental resolution to the problem. You owe it to the patients who are transferred from the ICU—and to yourselves.

Could we be held responsible for a less experienced nurse's mistake?

Q In the intensive care unit (ICU) of the small community hospital where I work, the administration has been hiring nurses right out of school. I know these new nurses have passed their state boards and have their RN licenses, but they don't seem to have the experience and knowledge needed to work in the ICU.

We're worried about our patients. And we're worried about *our* responsibility. Could we, because we're more experienced, be held responsible for a less experienced nurse's mistake?

A No, you wouldn't be responsible. But there's more to this answer. All nursing programs prepare *beginning* practitioners, and critical care nursing is not an area for beginners. (In fact, many hospitals now require a minimum of a year's medical/surgical experience before an RN can work in critical care.)

If a hospital's forced to put new graduates into critical care units, then the hospital has two obligations: to provide the beginning nurse with a well-defined learning program that combines theory and practice, and moves from the basic to the complex; and *not* to assign her to roles for which she's not prepared, for example, to a charge position or on an evening or night shift with other inexperienced nurses.

The new graduate has her responsibility: She's expected to ask for information whenever she's unsure or confronted with unfamiliar situations.

In turn, the experienced nurse has *her* obligation: to make the new nurse feel comfortable so she *can* ask questions and *can* come for help when she needs it.

In short, communication between the inexperienced nurse and the senior staff members must be kept in good working order.

About the legal aspects: The new nurse *is* an RN, so she stands responsible for those nursing actions for which she's been prepared. If she were called upon to do a procedure new to her and *didn't* seek help, she'd be on her own legally and could be held liable.

But if her supervisor were to knowingly assign this inexperienced nurse to a task she wasn't qualified for, then the supervisor could share in any legal liability resulting from possible error or injury to the patient.

How can a nurse prevent being caught in the middle of professional jousting?

Q A new medical department policy at our small community hospital says that doctors admitting patients to the intensive care unit (ICU) must be certified in advanced cardiac life support (ACLS). Any doctor who isn't ACLS-certified must immediately order a consultation from a doctor who is. And he can't write orders for his patient without the consultant's approval. We're told this policy was designed to "weed out the less competent, older doctors and prevent them from admitting patients to the ICU."

The nursing problem begins when we're caught in the middle of this professional jousting. Our department head told us to quietly bend the policy for some doctors (although they aren't certified in ACLS) because these doctors are influential in the community. We're supposed to follow any orders they write. Other doctors aren't treated so respectfully.

What should we do?

A Nurses, fasten your seat belts for a bumpy ride. The doctors may well destroy their working relationships because of this policy, and you'll be caught in the middle—unless you act quickly on your own behalf.

> *"We're told this policy was designed to 'weed out the less competent, older doctors and prevent them from admitting patients to the ICU.'"*

Go through channels and ask for a *written* policy on how the new system will work, plus a protocol for the *nurses* to follow. Then follow the protocol to a T, with no exceptions. If any doctor questions your actions, you can reply, "Here's the policy I must follow. If you disagree with it, please contact administration." When you step out of the picture, the doctors will have to confront one another and work out the problem themselves. (The truth is that ACLS certification is hardly the criterion for judging a doctor's competency for critical care practice.)

What can be done about a paraplegic who's lived on the unit for 2½ years?

Q We have a 67-year-old paraplegic patient on a ventilator who's been literally living on our ICU for 2½ years. Frankly, it seems much longer because he's uncooperative, obnoxious, and abusive. His doctor allows him to manage his own care, so he won't try weaning from the ventilator even though he's been stable for 2 years. In fact, the patient has chosen do-not-resuscitate (DNR) status for himself, so we can do little for him other than giving routine care, bringing meals, and lifting him into a chair once a day.

The way we see it, the patient's miserable, his doctor's indifferent, we're frustrated, and the ICU is short one bed for a critically ill patient—all because the hospital's making too much money ($10,000 per month) to order this patient's transfer to our skilled nursing facility.

What are your thoughts on this?

A You're caught in a classic situation: Nobody's right, everybody's wronged. You need help before you burn out; even more so, the patient needs a new approach to his care. After all, as you pointed out, the hospital's his home—maybe his last.

Start by separating fact from fallacy. You can rule out the profit motive. $10,000 per month (about $333 per day) is way below average daily ICU rates; in fact, patients who have DNR status are seldom allowed to remain on the ICU. So this patient's insurance company must have contracted with the hospital for his custodial care—most likely because no other facility in your area can provide care for a ventilator-dependent patient. This inability to change the situation probably accounts for his doctor's attitude as well. But your administrators should have told you the facts.

If you haven't done so already, talk to your unit manager about your frustration and confirm the facts. Then, have all the ICU nurses and a member of nursing administration meet with a psychiatric nurse consultant and vent your feelings; she can suggest some personal coping strategies and ways to modify your patient's behavior. Think about diversionary activities for your patient—physical therapy sessions, visits from the clergy or a hospital volunteer, or changes in his room (flowers, pictures, clock, calendar). Discuss with the psychiatric nurse how to resolve the patient's demands versus your needs.

Talk, too, with the nursing administrator. Could nurses from the medical/surgical unit learn to handle a ventilator-dependent patient? This patient could then be transferred out of the ICU—if only temporarily—to a whole new scene where he hasn't worn out his welcome.

What can be done about floating and understaffing?

Q On the intensive care unit (ICU) where I'm charge nurse, we usually have four ICU nurses to care for 11 patients and do an occasional recovery watch.

Lately, though, the supervisor started routinely pulling one of our nurses for assignment to the medical/surgical unit and replacing her with a medical/surgical nurse. Believe me, I'm not trying to put down the medical/surgical nurses, but this, in effect, reduces our ICU staffing to 3½ nurses.

Our complaints to the supervisor have been answered with the explanation that she wants the medical/surgical nurses to get ICU experience.

What do you think about this?

A ICU nurses have been floated to other units, rarely without griping. Now, however, with rising patient acuity levels on the medical/surgical unit, this new floating arrangement serves several purposes. Medical/surgical nurses learn ICU procedures that soon may appear on medical/surgial units, and after working ICU often enough, medical/surgical nurses can safely take on more than recovery watch duty there.

No matter how laudable the supervisor's goal, however, floating should never be done unless it's necessary and the ICU can function effectively with a medical/surgical nurse. Your immediate priorities on ICU remain unchanged—making sure the patients are well taken care of, and keeping your staff from overwork and burnout. Double-check that nursing assignments are as equitable as possible, so that no one ICU nurse gets all patients needing complex care. (If this can't be done, alert your supervisor—by phone with a witness on another line—that you need your full complement of ICU nurses that day.)

Truth to tell, ICU nurses will probably never *welcome* floating. Why should they? But with today's trend toward hospitals becoming acute care facilities, medical/surgical nurses will certainly need all the critical care experience they can get.

ID badges

What can be done about badges that only have pictures and first names on them?

Q Recently, our hospital administrator ordered new ID badges with only our pictures and first names on them. Several of us wrote him letters objecting to these new badges, but he told us to start wearing them, period. He said, "The public isn't concerned about who provides them with care as long as they get it."

We think this attitude is a real put-down—of us and the public. What's your reaction?

A Your full name, credentials, and department should appear on your ID badge. You deserve such professional recognition and, contrary to what your administrator says, patients have become very consumer-oriented and want to know who's at their bedside. (In fact, not being able to identify the caregiver was part of a recent successful lawsuit against a large hospital.) Maybe your administrator has a hidden agenda: If you're as short-staffed as most hospitals, he might want to "disguise" caregivers so patients and their families just can't tell how many (or how few) RNs are actually taking care of them.

Go back to the administrator with your objections, but first enlist the support of the hospital lawyer and your director of nursing. She knows that to handle some patients, you must establish a strictly professional relationship, and you don't want to be on a first-name basis—unless you choose to be.

ID bracelet

Should a baby's footprint also be recorded?

Q In the birthing unit of the community hospital where I work, each newborn gets one identification (ID) bracelet on the wrist and another on the ankle, before being taken to the nursery. (The baby's ID bracelets match the mother's.)

What concerns me is something we *don't* do: We don't record the baby's footprint. At present, we're the only hospital in our area that doesn't use footprint identification. Are we overlooking some essential protection for the baby? Can you straighten me out on the facts of the matter?

A Of course every baby should be properly identified before being transferred to the nursery. The ID bracelets you describe, which are widely used, carry information about the baby's sex, surname, date and time of birth, as well as the mother's given name. The bracelets can be easily checked each time the baby's taken from the nursery for any reason. The baby should still be wearing the bracelets when he's discharged.

A footprint is required identification (and part of the permanent records) in many hospitals. In fact, it's mandatory in some states. A footprint would certainly prove valuable in one of those dramatic mix-ups of babies, which all moth-

ers (and all nurses on the maternity unit) dread. But footprints are difficult to get. The head of one maternity unit told us they'd even called in the local police department to help the staff learn how to take footprints properly. But even with professional "troops," it didn't work out.

A footprint must be made with great care in order to be legible; heavy inking or smudging can make the print useless, although a *clear* footprint becomes a permanent means of identification. The imprint of the toes and soles (like that of the fingers and palms) is unique to each individual. The ridges in the foot present at birth do not change during a lifetime.

You may be interested to learn that photographing the baby's ear is being studied as permanent identification; the size, form, and configuration of the ear are unique to each individual and change only minutely during growth.

Even though the footprint's hard to get and isn't mandatory, you may still wish to try it on your birthing unit. The more foolproof an infant's identification, the better. Good luck!

I.M. injections

Is the deltoid muscle a proper site?

Q Is the deltoid muscle a proper site for I.M. injections? Our nursing preceptor contends that the deltoid muscle is rarely used as an injection site—and then only as a site of last resort. But others on that unit—some of our most seasoned nurses—disagree: They say the deltoid muscle can be used to administer small doses of medication.

A The deltoid muscle should rarely be used because of its small size and its proximity to the radial nerve.

However, agreement is universal that the deltoid muscle should never be used as the site for delivering large doses of medication, antibiotics, or certain other medications, such as iron dextran (Imferon).

Also, you should find out whether your hospital has a written policy on deltoid injections.

Should a small amount of air be drawn into the syringe after measuring the medications?

Q We're in the process of rewriting our procedures for giving I.M. and S.C. injections—but we can't agree on one point. Should we draw a small amount of air into the syringe after measuring the medication? Some of us were taught that this helps prevent leakage of medication back into the subcutaneous tissue. But the rest of us were taught that we *shouldn't* draw air into the syringe because this might cause us to deliver an inaccurate dose of medication. What do the experts say?

A You *should* draw air into the syringe after measuring the medication. The air will force all the medication out of the needle—thus clearing it.

Of course, the amount of air you draw up depends on the size of the needle and the type of medication. For instance, if you're injecting an antibiotic, you can safely draw up 0.2 cc of air with a 1½″ needle.

Incident report

Does one need to be filled out if the medication error didn't cause any harm?

Q After I made a medication error, I told my manager that I was going to call the patient's doctor and fill out an incident report. I was surprised when she told me I shouldn't bother because no harm was done. I decided against following her advice and went ahead anyway. Although she cosigned the incident report, she's been giving me the cold shoulder ever since. Did I do something wrong?

A No. She may simply be embarrassed because she realizes she was wrong. But maybe you should have let her know (politely but firmly) that you still planned to report the error. She may feel you stepped on her toes by disregarding her advice.

Check your hospital policy. It probably requires you to do exactly what you did: Notify the doctor and fill out an incident report. Even if it doesn't, you acted correctly. You had a duty to report what had happened.

What's more, the *doctor* needed to assess the effect—if any—that the medication error had on his patient. This is a medical, not a nursing, judgment. So you were right to call him promptly with the facts.

An incident report doesn't cast blame or determine negligence. It helps administrators maintain patient-care standards and develop quality-assurance measures. In this case, for example, they could use the incident report to design medication procedures that are less likely to cause mistakes in the future.

Is there any risk of reports disappearing from employee health files?

Q Hospital policy says that we should fill out an incident report when a needle stick occurs. Maybe I'm paranoid, but how can I be sure the report won't disappear from employee health files?

A Removing an incident report from a hospital's file wouldn't serve any purpose. If you have any reason to distrust the system where

you work, keep personal anecdotal notes of an incident when warranted. The incident report filed in a patient's medical records must be factual and objective, but a nurse's own anecdotal notes can address other aspects of the incident—including personal, political, and personnel concerns.

Of greater concern is whether you know how to avoid sticks when you're disposing of used needles. Don't recap, bend, or break needles; don't remove them from disposable syringes or otherwise manipulate them by hand. Keep a puncture-resistant container close by for used needles to avoid walking any distance with an exposed needle.

Ask your unit manager to check with someone from central supply. Find out whether they plan to order needles that are especially designed to prevent needle sticks.

Should an incident report have been filled out?

Q I just started working at a children's hospital. The policy here is for the charge nurse to check the narcotics administered by all newly hired nurses. At the end of my first week, the narcotics count on my unit was off—we were short one morphine and had one extra meperidine (pethidine, Demerol). Because all of my medications had been double-checked, I was sure I hadn't made the error. But the charge nurse and unit manager insisted that I fill out the incident report. When I refused, the unit manager reminded me that I was still on probation and I could be fired if I didn't comply. So against my better judgment, I filled out the form. Now I'm wondering if I really want a job at a hospital that would treat me so badly—and would act so unethically. What should I have done?

A Unless *you* discovered the error, you shouldn't have filled out the incident report.

As you know, an incident report documents any nonroutine occur-

rence. When you fill one out, you should indicate only what you saw, heard, or did—not what you suppose, assume, or conclude. The report doesn't become part of the patient's medical record, nor does it necessarily say what caused the incident or who was at fault.

So, you should never worry that filing an incident report implies an admission of guilt. But in this case, you *should* worry about the psychological coercion you experienced. Have a frank talk with your charge nurse about your concerns. You and she need to build a more trusting relationship.

Incompetent colleague

Should suspicions be taken to the manager?

Q I think one of my colleagues is incompetent. I've been noticing little things: Her I.V.s often aren't hung on time, her postoperative patients look as if they haven't been turned for hours, and she lets newer nurses start her I.V.s and insert nasogastric tubes "so they'll get experience." I've also found her checking a drug handbook for information she should already know. I realize this all sounds vague, but I'm concerned about her patients' safety. Should I take my suspicions to our manager?

A Not yet. First, you have to separate facts from suspicions. You might want to start by getting to know this nurse better. Observe her strengths and weaknesses in patient care. Then, perhaps you could say something like this: "I wish I had your ability to comfort patients. I'm much more confident with technical procedures like starting I.V.s. But I feel awkward talking with a patient who's dying or family members who are grieving. Maybe we could work more closely together and help each other." This approach might open the door to a positive, trusting relationship that could strengthen the entire staff.

But what if she rejects your offer? If you're still concerned about patient safety, talk with your manager. Make sure you have specific examples of problems, and be ready to explore ways she can help your colleague improve her skills—for example, by providing continuing education for the unit or developing a preceptor program.

Incompetent patient

How can a person sign a check when she's not aware of what she's doing?

Q I work on a medical/surgical unit in a community hospital. Although my supervisor told me point-blank to mind my own business, I'm concerned about what could be funny business going on in our unit. Here's what happened:

About 2 months ago, an alert 90-year-old woman was admitted with unstable angina. Shortly thereafter, she suffered a stroke and her condition worsened considerably. She remains partially paralyzed, has difficulty speaking, and exhibits periods of confusion when she doesn't know where she is or who we are.

I suspect that her grandson, her only relative, is taking and cashing her Social Security checks. Yesterday, accompanied by a nursing supervisor and administrator, he came in to have the check "signed." He put a pen in his grandmother's hand and guided her hand with his to make an X on the back of the check. Then the supervisor and administrator both signed the check as witnesses.

How can a person sign a check when she's not aware of what she's doing? Should Social Security be alerted to investigate?

A Before jumping to any sinister conclusions, you'll be relieved to learn that what you witnessed is legal and aboveboard: Social Security has set up a process so an incapacitated person won't miss payments that may be needed for immediate expenses (apartment rent and such) during the interim it takes to appoint a payee. (Social Security uses the term payee, not power of attorney.)

The grandson, in this case, seems a likely person for appointment as payee—but this takes time because several steps are necessary. First, of course, is application by the prospective payee to the Social Security office. Next, Social Security sends for confirmation of the patient's condition from the attending doctor or hospital administration. They also double-check by sending a letter to the designated recipient and waiting 3 weeks for a reply. Once a payee is appointed, the Social Security checks are issued to the payee until further notice.

But thank you for caring enough to ask. With so much fraud being perpetrated on our elderly, it's reassuring to know that holistic nursing really means "whole-istic."

Incontinence pad

Should a thin rubber sheet or plastic bag be used between the pad and sheet?

Q I work in a nursing home. On some patient beds, we use a convoluted foam mattress covered with a bed sheet, then an incontinence pad. Some of the staff think we should also place a thin rubber sheet or plastic bag between the pad and sheet. What do you say?

A When using a convoluted foam mattress, logic suggests that the fewer and thinner the layers you use, the better.

Use the plastic sleeve that comes with the mattress (which should be enough to prevent absorption into it), then one bed sheet. If *absolutely* necessary, use one incontinence pad.

Indwelling urinary catheter

Can a patient safely take a bath with one?

Q Can a patient with an indwelling urinary catheter safely take a bath?

A If the patient must, for some medical reason, have an indwelling catheter, showering would probably be better for him than bathing.

If the patient *must* have an indwelling catheter, however, and *must* take a bath rather than a shower, advise him to take the following precautions:
• Avoid traction on the catheter.
• Pass as much urine as possible from the tubing into the drainage bag *before* getting into the tub.
• Try to keep the drainage bag and tubing lower than the bladder to prevent backflow of urine into the tubing. A reflux valve will usually prevent this, but if a small amount of urine flows back from the bag into the tubing, this isn't likely to be a problem.

Should a patient scheduled for pelvic ultrasonography have water instilled into the bladder?

Q When a patient on our obstetric unit is scheduled for pelvic ultrasonography, instead of waiting for her bladder to fill naturally, we nurses are expected to insert an indwelling urinary catheter before she goes to the X-ray department.

Then, at the appropriate time, an ultrasound technician fills the patient's bladder retrogradely through the catheter and performs the test.

Most of us never heard of doing this routinely, and we think it's an added embarrassment and expense for the patient. What do you think?

A Routinely inserting an indwelling catheter to fill the bladder retrogradely seems like an unnecessary invasive procedure for the convenience of the technician. This procedure is usually done only when the patient has poor bladder control or for some other medical reason. Otherwise, routine procedure is to have the patient drink three to four glasses of water 1 hour before the exam, then tell her not to void.

Voice your concerns to your immediate supervisor.

Should insertion be done in the patient's room or in the operating room before surgery?

Q I'm an operating room nurse, and wonder about indwelling catheter insertion for a patient undergoing total hip replacement.

Should this procedure be done in the patient's room or in the operating room before surgery? Our orthopedic surgeons are concerned that inserting the catheter in the operating room can increase the risk of postoperative hip infection.

Do you agree?

A No correlation exists between the insertion of an indwelling catheter and postoperative hip infections. The catheter should be inserted when the patient is in the operating room and under anesthesia so his legs can be spread apart without causing excruciating hip pain. This positioning will allow better exposure for inserting the catheter, and the absence of pain will keep his urinary sphincter and perineal muscles from tightening. The net result will be a decreased chance of urinary tract infection caused by contamination.

What are the guidelines for sterile technique?

Q After giving a lecture on catheterization, I took some of my students to a local hospital for clinical experience. In teaching, I'd emphasized the following:

• Indwelling urinary catheters are inserted *only* if patients cannot void normally.

• Since an indwelling catheter is connected to a closed drainage system, the catheter must remain sterile and so should never be disconnected from the drainage bag.

• The drainage bag should be emptied only through the small drainage tubing, which should be wiped with an alcohol sponge before being replaced.

> *"We found one patient whose catheter was disconnected from the bag with the loose end of the tubing dragging in a puddle of urine under the bag."*

What we saw in this hospital, though, was quite different. *All* chronically ill patients had indwelling urinary catheters inserted— even those who could have used a bedpan or walked to the bathroom with some assistance.

We found one patient whose catheter was disconnected from the bag with the loose end of the tubing dragging in a puddle of urine under the bag. To help the busy staff and give my students some practice, I got a new collecting set from central supply. The students measured the urine left in the drainage bag, re- moved the old collecting set, discarded it, and replaced it with the new set.

Meanwhile, a nursing assistant who'd walked in to attend to another patient saw what we were doing. He told me, with some irritation, that collecting sets were expensive, and that if everyone discarded a set each time it became disconnected, the hospital would be spending a fortune.

The usual procedure in this hospital, I found out later, is to clamp the catheter and disconnect the tubing (letting it dangle) whenever a patient has to be moved.

Now my students are asking why *they* should wipe the drainage bag tubing with alcohol, since the catheter tubing has already been exposed to contamination. When I stick to my standards, am I too fussy?

A You are *not* too fussy. You're absolutely correct. Maintaining sterility in a closed system is important in order to guard against nosocomial infection. You should continue to stress these points to your students.

Why don't you and your students try to improve the questionable practices in your hospital? (Incidentally, it's hard to understand *why* the hospital would use catheters for all patients, even those who could walk to the bathroom. Start by having your students get a copy of the guidelines and regulations on the use of indwelling catheters put out by the Centers for Disease Control. These guidelines are so useful they'll not only be helpful in your present situation, but should also be posted in every nursing unit where catheters are used. Then have your students compile statistics on nosocomial infections associated with unsterile catheter procedures, and present the figures to the nursing supervisor.

If you can't get the hospital staff to change its practice, consider taking your students elsewhere for clinical experience—especially if you find other poor practices and poor examples for the students. If you don't have an alternative, though, remember you can teach dramatically by *negative* example.

But don't compromise *your* standard or those of your students. You're right—and have a right to be fussy.

When should they be changed?

Q I'm a recent graduate working on a medical/surgical unit for the first time. I've already run into a conflict between what they taught in nursing school and what the nurses on the unit say.

> *"Experienced nurses say there's no reason to change the catheters every 10 to 14 days, but in nursing school I was taught differently."*

In nursing school, I learned that indwelling catheters should be changed every 10 to 14 days. But on the unit, the experienced nurses say there's no reason to change the catheters that frequently. They think a patient can have a catheter in place for months as long as we perform the proper daily care.

When *should* an indwelling catheter be changed?

A Indwelling catheters should *not* be changed at arbitrary, fixed intervals. Rather, the entire drainage system (catheter and bag) should be changed when the system no longer drains properly, when it leaks, or when some crusting can be felt inside the tubing.

You're right, though, to be fussy about catheter care. Indwelling catheters can entail serious risks, such as urinary tract infections,

urethral strictures, epididymitis, and potentially fatal gram-negative sepsis.

Inexperience

Should a nurse refuse to care for children in ICU if she lacks pediatric experience?

Q I'm an intensive care unit (ICU) nurse at a large teaching hospital. Until recently, our unit was an adult ICU staffed for this purpose.

But the hospital's decided to develop a pediatric ICU. And now children of all ages—from newborns to teenagers—are being admitted to our *adult* ICU. However, my coworkers and I have no experience in caring for critically ill children.

What steps should we take to protect these children and ourselves? Would we jeopardize our jobs by refusing to care for the young patients? And what would a court say about our pediatric "qualifications?"

A This situation could eventually cause problems for you *and* the hospital.

If a nurse isn't properly educated in pediatric ICU procedures and techniques, yet is caring for pediatric patients in an intensive care setting, she's probably functioning *below* the accepted standard of care for pediatric ICU nursing. So, she could possibly be accused of malpractice.

If the quality of a nurse's care is ever questioned, a court would try to determine how a nurse with the same education and experience would behave in similar situations.

The hospital, by *having* a pediatric ICU, is saying it does have a facility for providing pediatric care in an intensive care setting—with the staff and equipment to do the job. If the nursing staff is *not* qualified to work in this setting, the hos-

pital could be held liable for providing inadequate care.

You'd probably jeopardize your job by refusing to care for these pediatric ICU patients—unless you have a written agreement with the hospital stating you're to work *only* in the adult ICU.

So ask your administration for a crash course in pediatric ICU nursing. Completing that course would be a plus for you if your qualifications as a pediatric ICU nurse were questioned in court. But more important, you'd be taking the first step toward protecting the children and protecting yourselves.

Infection control

Can uniforms that infants have burped, wet, and messed on be washed with regular family wash?

Q About 5 months ago, management decided that we should stop wearing scrubs in our newborn nursery and go back to wearing and laundering our own uniforms. Now with acquired immunodeficiency syndrome in the picture, we're wondering if we can safely wash our uniforms—which the infants have burped, wet and messed on—in with our family's wash.

A To be on the safe side, wash soiled uniforms separately from the rest of the family's clothing, using hot tap water, detergent, and bleach. That will eliminate any possibility of spreading resistant bacteria or virus to family members, especially to any of them who may be immunocompromised.

Can you recommend a good book on infection control?

Q We're trying to compile a booklet on infection control procedures for our isolation unit. What we need most is information about cleaning that we could pass on to everyone working on the unit—but especially the cleaning staff. We can find very little written about this. Suggestions?

A There's a book that fills the bill: *Infection Control in Intensive Care Units by Selective Decontamination,* edited by H.K. Saene, et al, (New York: Springer-Kerlag, 1989). In the chapter on isolation techniques, the book deals with cleaning and disinfecting everything from large pieces of medical equipment to everyday paraphernalia such as dishes, linens, books, money, and even children's toys.

Does suite sharing risk cross-infection?

Q I'm a staff nurse in the urology clinic of a large health maintenance organization. A few months ago, we moved into a new suite of rooms that we must share with a pediatric clinic. We use the suite from 9 to 5 Monday through Friday The pediatric staff uses it after 5 on weekdays and all weekends and holidays. With hours almost overlapping, our two staffs have a hard time keeping out of each other's way.

To add to the friction, our nursing supervisor has just issued a directive on nosocomial infections—to the *pediatric* nurses. To minimize possible cross-infections from urology to pediatric patients, the pediatric nurses must do the following at the start of every clinic session:
• Wash all horizontal surfaces, including examining tables and work counters.
• Change examining table sheets.
• Request the housekeeping department to empty linen hampers and garbage containers.
• Change the examining table sheet and wash all horizontal surfaces after a child with a communicable disease has been examined.

Our nursing supervisor also prohibits filling drinking cups at the sinks in the examining rooms. The directive no doubt refers to our practice of pouring urine down the examining room sinks—something we do to save time. The entire suite has only one toilet, at the far end of the row of examining rooms.

When the pediatric nurses come on duty and have to start scrubbing, they glare at us. Sparks are beginning to fly.

Does a possibility for cross-infection really exist? Are the supervisor's measures justified? Frankly, we don't see the need for all these precautions. Do you?

A *Every* clinic session—yours or anyone else's—should begin with clean work areas. In your case, *both* departments have to be as careful as possible. Scrubbing the work areas and emptying the hampers and the trash containers should apply to the urology clinic nurses as well as to the pediatric staff. And certainly, after a visit by any patient with an infectious disease, the cleanup procedures should be stringent.

However, it's not necessary to avoid using the sink to fill drinking cups. Generally, urine specimens will not contaminate the sink because they're usually sterile. Certainly don't allow the urine to splash around when you're pouring it out. But you shouldn't splash water around the sink either. Contaminating organisms can reside in a wet sink—whether it's wet from water or from urine.

But even before you work out the necessary infection control procedures, you'd better stop the sparks—or you'll have a blazing conflict. Get together with the pediatric nurses and try role-playing each other's problems. Then maybe you'll be ready to draw up some sensible procedures for sharing your working quarters. Your supervisor might also consider a full-time aide schooled in proper cleaning techniques. The

nurses could then spend their time on nursing activities.

This all means practice proper infection controls: Your health maintenance organization is a valuable community health resource—much too valuable to be put at risk.

Isn't there a risk of cross-contamination if pediatric patients and isolation patients are mixed?

Q I'm a staff nurse on a primary nursing medical unit that also takes pediatric patients. Because our hospital's short of staff, we sometimes have isolation patients assigned to our unit when we already have pediatric patients—even infants. We realize that on occasion this can't be helped. But lately, we see this mixture more and more. And we've become concerned about cross-contamination.

The infection control nurse shares our concern. But when we broached the subject with the nursing supervisor, her response was: "There's no problem as long as correct techniques are used."

Of course, theoretically, there *shouldn't* be any problem if correct techniques are used. But we worry, nonetheless.

Do you agree that this is a poor, even dangerous, policy or do you think we're overreacting?

A There's *no* special threat of infection, as long as correct septic techniques are used with thorough care and understanding.

Good infection control will protect an all-adult unit, an all-child unit—or one that's mixed.

Of course, this addresses only the narrow question of the danger of infection. Obviously, a patient—young or old—would be better off on a unit where nurses were knowledgeable about the characteristic problems and needs of that patient.

But to come back to the infection control issue: you must keep practical considerations in mind even while you're observing the principles. With a nursing shortage or some other common emergency, you might well face a mix of ages on your unit. You'd then have the nursing obligation to do your best for the patients under the circumstances.

Shouldn't there be a sink in every patient's room?

Q I work on a medical/surgical unit in the oldest wing of a community hospital. Not all patient rooms have sinks, so to wash hands after each patient contact I must go to a sink in another area. If someone stops me on the way, I may forget to wash my hands and go right on to my next patient.

Nurses on our unit have told the hospital administrator about this situation and suggested that sinks be installed in all patient rooms. He won't listen to us.

Isn't this setup in conflict with infection-control standards? Can you help us?

A Ideally, hospital personnel should wash their hands after every patient contact. Having a sink in each room certainly promotes this concept, but when no sink is handy, try using an antiseptic foam that requires no water and can be kept in every room.

Why not ask your infection control nurse to help you convince the administrator of the importance of using antiseptic foam? And ask again for more sinks—if not in every room, maybe in three or four locations. (Remember, he's thinking of the cost.) Also, nursing supervisors and infection control nurses should be on the hospital's planning committee to make sure that sinks are installed where the *staff* needs them.

What are proper infection control precautions?

Q As the infection control nurse at a skilled nursing facility, I'm wondering whether our isolation precautions for wounds infected by *Staphylococcus aureus* are current. What's the latest from the Centers for Disease Control (CDC) in Atlanta? Does an occlusive dressing provide sufficient protection against the spread of this organism? What about gloving, gowning, and masking? When are they necessary? And should we be treating the patient's linens as contaminated?

A The severity of the wound is the key consideration in determining the extent of isolation precautions for *S. aureus*. If the wound is minor—that is, if the dressing covers the wound and adequately contains the pus—then handwashing and gloving provide sufficient protection. You don't have to gown when caring for minor wounds.

A major wound, on the other hand, calls for more stringent precautions. The CDC defines a major wound infected with *S. aureus* as one that is draining or that otherwise can't be adequately covered or contained by a dressing. When caring for major wounds, wear gloves *and* a gown (especially when soiling is likely) *and* double-bag all linens.

Masking's unnecessary as long as you don't shake contaminated linens too vigorously, which is about the only way the organism can become airborne.

What can change a staff that's lax about infection control?

Q I work nights in a nursing home where the staff takes a rather casual attitude toward staphylococcal infection. Here are some of the disturbing details:
• Many patients have pressure sores, so I regularly take cultures

and send them to the laboratory. If a lab report reveals a staphylococcal infection, and I tell this to the day nurses, they're reluctant to inform the doctor. One nurse told me not to be concerned, because "we all have staph on our bodies."
• The director of nursing doesn't want us to tell the nursing assistants that a patient has a staphylococcal infection because that's "being an alarmist."
• Most nurses don't bother to wash their hands after caring for a patient, because they'd have to go back to the nursing station. (Proper washing facilities aren't available in the patients' rooms. And gloves are hard to come by because they're expensive.)

I've been away from nursing for 5 years. Have the standards I learned for infection control been relaxed while I was gone?

A If anything, infection control has become even more rigorous during recent years. Sorry to hear that this increased concern hasn't caught on yet in the nursing home where you work, and that the care is less stringent than the care you learned and practiced some years ago.

As you're well aware, without proper control and isolation, an infection could spread to other patients, staff, and families. Since many nursing home residents are chronically ill and debilitated, their susceptibility to an infection calls for painstaking identification and control measures.

Here are some suggestions: One, keep insisting on good nursing practices: Culture any suspicious lesions; use proper handwashing techniques; wear gloves as well as a mask and gown when these are warranted; and encourage the isolation of patients with highly communicable infections. Suggest that a staff development program be conducted by a local infection control practitioner—and arrange for periodic consultations with her.

Despite a 5-year absence, your conscientious approach to infection control is more current than the blasé, noninterventionist attitude of the other staff members.

What is a nursing supervisor's responsibility?

Q A patient recovering from a colon resection for adenocarcinoma was admitted to the intermediate care facility where I'm the supervisor. Fifteen days after admission, the patient's incision opened, draining a profuse amount of odorous, pinkish gray, thick material.

When I asked her attending doctor to culture the drainage, he refused, saying angrily that it wasn't *my* responsibility to ask for a culture. Besides, he said, he could tell the infection was *E. coli* by its smell.

Still worried about the danger of infection from unknown organisms for the other patients and the staff, I initiated certain isolation precautions, as well as good handwashing techniques. Fortunately, no infections developed among patients or staff.

Now the patient's wound has stopped draining, and she's ready to go home. But I still feel uneasy about a culture not being done. As a nursing supervisor, just what *is* my responsibility for infection control?

A In the serious matter of infection control, no one should be led by the nose—no matter how sensitive his nose might be. Certain organisms do have distinctive odors, but smell alone isn't conclusive identification. Only a culture can determine what organism is present—and therefore, what antibiotic's called for and what precautions are necessary to prevent the spread of infection.

Infection control is everybody's responsibility. Taking cultures is where responsibility divides. In some facilities, culturing is up to the infection control nurse. In other places, the doctors are responsible.

Clearly, the facility where you work needs a written infection control policy stipulating that all drainage wounds should be cultured immediately, specifying who's to do it, and how the staff is to be informed of the results.

What should a visitor do if she sees a nurse doing an unsafe practice?

Q Recently, I went to my hometown to visit my father, who was in the hospital recovering from a transurethral resection of the prostate gland. While we were talking, I noticed his I.V. bottle was nearly empty, so I turned on his call light.

The charge nurse, a new graduate, and obviously inexperienced with I.V.s, had trouble inserting the tubing in the new bottle. She dropped the tubing. From where I was sitting, I couldn't see the tubing land, but I'm fairly certain it touched the floor.

Much to my amazement, the nursing picked up the tubing, wiped it with an alcohol sponge, and inserted it in the new bottle. My first impulse was to scream, "That tubing's *contaminated!*" But I didn't want to be a "bad visitor," so I did nothing. Now I wonder—what *should* I have done?

A You certainly were in a bind. If you'd confronted the charge nurse with her error, you'd have risked jeopardizing your father's relationship with his nurses—and possibly his care. But by not doing anything, you risked more serious possible consequences for your father: He could have been exposed to contaminated equipment.

You should have said something to the nurse immediately—in a nice

way, of course. ("Isn't that tubing unsanitary, and shouldn't you get a new one?") Once you called her on her mistake, the nurse would've probably gotten a new I.V. set and inserted it, without an argument. Your father might have had to endure another venipuncture—but that's a minor inconvenience compared to the risk of having a contaminated I.V.

Finally, before leaving the hospital, you should've reported the incident to the unit manager or supervisor. A nurse who can't handle I.V.s properly should be replaced by a more competent nurse and be given some training in I.V. techniques, *stat*.

It's not too late for you to send a letter about the incident to the staff development director. This is a quiet way to ensure that the nurse doesn't repeat her mistake and risk the well-being of another patient.

Informality

Can't a nurse address a patient by his first name?

Q I'm a bit bothered about the double standard on names in our medical/surgical unit. We encourage patients and visitors to call us by our first names as part of our effort to create an informal, even "homey" atmosphere on the unit. But this seems to be a one-way street. Patients expect *us* to address them as "Mrs. James" or "Mr. Johnson." Any day of the week I can hear the wife of a patient say to me: "Anne, Mr. Johnson would like to see you." The same wife would never dream of calling the doctor by *his* first name.

But what's so important about a first name? I know that what's *really* important is my nursing skill. Yet I can't help feeling I'm entitled to some recognition as an adult professional. Do you think I have a valid point? How would you handle it?

A You've got part of the right answer: Your professionalism lies in your skill, not your name. What your patient calls you does not alter your skill. But how your patient regards you—reflected in part by how he addresses you—can undermine or reinforce your nursing effectiveness.

Maybe you take the wrong first step by *encouraging* the use of your first name. You and your patient are in a therapeutic relationship. You're not "all friends." With a manipulative or sexually aggressive patient, you're certainly better off as "Ms. E." than as "Anne."

How do you turn things around? Well, remember all that talk about assertiveness? If you *want* to be called "Ms." you'll have to *ask* for it.

When you're introduced to your patient or his family, simply say: "I prefer to be called Ms. E." Later, if you *want* to move to a first-name basis, you'll find it easy enough to go from the formal to the informal.

Injections

How do you give an injection to a frightened child?

Q The doctors at our clinic recommend preparing the injection outside the examining room, then giving it quickly (and accurately). I agree.

But what do you do when the child screams and hides behind his mother, or kicks and fights back? What else can I do to make it easier on the child (and me)?

A You might want to take the mother aside and find out how she's "prepared" the child for this visit to the doctor. Has she somehow conveyed anxiety of her own to the child? Or—hard to believe, but possible nonetheless—has she used the shot as a threat ("If you're not good, the doctor will give you a shot.")? Once you trace the origin of the child's fear, you're on the right road to calming him.

Then use this method:
• Approach the child calmly and matter-of-factly.
• Explain that the injection is necessary and that you *are* going to give it.
• Ask for help in holding the child (and possibly ask the mother to leave).
• Give the injection, *then* talk to the child a little more.

This should reassure the child that he isn't being punished—and should also keep him from associating a nurse only with pain. After all, you can give love as well as injections.

Is it safe to give infants I.M. injections in the gluteal muscle?

Q I've been on "leave" from nursing since my son was born 6 months ago. Last week, when I took my baby to our local pediatric clinic for his 6-month checkup, the nurse gave the baby a diphtheria-pertussis-tetanus injection in the gluteal muscle. (At this clinic, run by a group of pediatricians in private practice, the RNs and LVNs give the injection.)

My nursing's not rusty yet. And although pediatrics is not my specialty, I did learn that an infant should *never* be given an I.M. injection in the gluteal muscle. Yet, this is a common practice among the nurses at this particular clinic.

Looking back, I wish I'd insisted that the nurse give my baby son the injection in his thigh. But I didn't. Now I'm wondering: *Is* it safe to give I.M. injections to infants in the gluteal site? Is another site preferable—and safer?

A There are nurses who do it and doctors who do it. But the chief danger is the possibility of hitting the sciatic nerve.

A better site would be the quadriceps muscle of the leg or the ventral site. The principle is to use the needle in the most active area, where blood circulation is best. As the baby moves and kicks his legs, the drug will be picked up and quickly absorbed.

You can change the clinic procedure to protect other babies as well as your own, and your spirit is admirable. Start in the nursing department of the clinic. But don't be bashful about next taking the matter up with the doctors who own and run the clinic. They're responsible.

Write a letter or go in person. But either way—don't attack, especially if you plan to continue using the clinic. Argue with reason and information.

If the clinic won't change, *you* should. Find a group of pediatricians who'll listen to reason.

Injured nurse

Can a nurse sue a patient who injured her?

Q My shift was over and I was about to leave when I heard another nurse shouting for help. She and three other nurses were trying to restrain a man who'd had a total hip replacement 2 days before. Since then, he'd become increasingly disoriented. Diagnostic tests hadn't uncovered a reason, so his doctor had ordered restraints and observation.

As I came over to help, one nurse asked me to pick up a restraint that had fallen onto the floor. When I bent over, the man got his leg free and kicked me in the face, knocking me unconscious and breaking a tooth.

Later, we learned that the patient was an alcoholic suffering from alcohol withdrawal syndrome. He and his family had concealed his alcohol abuse from the staff. Now I'm wondering: Can I sue a patient who withheld information about his history and who physically injured me?

A Given the facts you describe, you couldn't successfully sue this patient. Although your shift was over, you were injured at work while performing a job-related task (helping other nurses restrain a disoriented patient). The reason he was disoriented isn't legally significant. Your only recourse is to file for workmen's compensation.

Innovation

What if a supervisor resists teaching new techniques?

Q Having graduated from an urban medical center, I now work in a small, rural community hospital. Several nursing assistants have noticed that I use the more current technique for total patient care rather than the old, functional approach. In fact, during my senior year I did an independent study on work simplification and received departmental honors. These assistants, interested in improving their skills and bettering patient care, have asked me to teach them. The unit manager on our floor, however, will not permit me to help them in any way. I offered to give my own time. But she is set in her ways and won't listen to anything new—no matter how good it might be for the patients and hospital. Because of commuting problems, I don't want to change jobs. But the situation is so frustrating. How can I work this out?

A Your generous offer to teach on your own time indicates that your intentions are certainly good. Probably the innovative ideas on work simplification that you brought from the urban medical center are

very good, too. But, please, *slow down*. There's apparently something you didn't learn at your school and that's how to handle a threatened superior. That's what you're facing.

Hospitals are traditionally conservative and your hospital, being situated in a small rural community, is probably doubly so. Very likely, your unit manager is interpreting your desire for change as a criticism of the existing system—*including the unit manager*. She might also feel that you're undermining her authority by working through the nursing assistants. If she continues to see you in that light, it's going to be "no way, all the way" for you and you'll never get an opportunity to innovate. Let's face it, you *need* your unit manager as a friend and ally, so use a little practical psychology. Pick out some problems or tasks you face and ask her how you should handle them. Incorporate her ideas into your work and let her know it. After all, the hospital was getting along before you came so they must have been doing something right. Continue at this level until you sense that you're no longer considered a threat, then try to introduce some of your new ideas.

> *"The unit manager won't permit me to teach the other nurses more current techniques, no matter how good they might be."*

Human nature being what it is, possibly the unit manager won't unbend. If that happens, you might go to the staff development director and discuss your ideas. If she's interested, she could bypass the personality conflict by ordering the new ideas into her program. You won't be getting the immediate satisfaction of having done it yourself, but that probably isn't the underlying reason for your actions. The pa-

tients will surely profit and that should bring satisfaction, too.

If all else fails, keep your eyes open for another unit manager who seems more approachable, and then transfer to her unit.

Inquisitiveness

How should a patient's personal questions be handled?

Q Any suggestions on how to deal with the patient who comes on like the entire panel from "What's My Line?" You know: "I see you're wearing a wedding ring. What does your husband do for a living? Your hair looks nice; who does it? How much do they charge? Do you like the unit manager? What kind of money do you make here?" and so on.

A Patients are people who just happen to be sick, and nurses are people who just happen to be taking care of them. This doesn't mean, however, that you respond to a patient as you would to any other person.

If some Polly Pry came up with these "20 Questions" in a social setting, you could properly give her the story of your life. . .or the cold shoulder. It would all depend on how *you* felt.

When a barrage of personal questions comes to you from a patient, however, the picture changes. "The nurse-patient relationship is a one-way focus on the needs and concerns of the patient...not a situation in which the needs of the nurse are met," says Dr. Hildegarde Peplau. So how *you* feel is not the issue. It's how the patient feels.

Why is she pouring out this frantic spate of questions? Is she really interested in the minutiae of your life?

No, the patient is probably using the mindless questioning to ease the boredom and loneliness of unfamiliar surroundings. It also distracts her from the real and anxious questions—What's going to happen to me? Is it going to hurt? What if?

The next time a patient begins to sound like a cross-examiner, answer her first few questions in an open, friendly manner. This will ensure a graceful, unobtrusive transition into the next step of the nursing intervention which is to pull up a chair and start referring each question back to the patient. If she wants to know about your husband's work; you answer, then ask her about her husband. The same with the hairdresser, and so on. You're neither sparring nor socializing conversationally. By getting the patient to talk about herself, you are working toward the solution of a health problem. Once you've established rapport and reversed the questioner's role, you can move on to a more directly professional question, "Is there something bothering you that you'd like to talk about?" Sometimes this will be the release the patient was unconsciously waiting for. Other times it will move the patient to end the conversation right there.

In either case, you'll get a clearer overall picture of the patient. And she'll have benefitted from your sympathetic attention.

Insecurity

What's the best way to help a new nurse without intimidating her?

Q I'm unit manager in an intensive care unit (ICU) where the staff usually has a close working relationship. But we're not working so well together anymore because of Betty—our new co-worker.

Betty transferred from our medical/surgical unit 8 months ago. She tries *very* hard to do a good job—she's enthusiastic, willing, and good to the patients.

But under pressure, Betty falls apart. During emergencies, she becomes anxious and makes bad decisions. Once, during a code, she was so shaken we actually had to ask her to leave the unit. She also has trouble setting priorities—a broken nail seems just as important to her as a broken leg.

But what bothers me most is how Betty treats me—she puts me on a pedestal; she thinks I'm "supernurse." When I'm around, she's so nervous that she makes foolish mistakes. But nothing I say to her helps. After 8 months, Betty should be well adjusted to the ICU, but she's not. We've all tried to talk to her, but we can't even get her to admit she *has* a problem. She thinks we simply don't like her.

How can we help Betty without intimidating her? I really don't want to ask her to resign—we've invested so much time in training her. Also, I'm afraid she'd be devastated if I asked her to leave.

A Betty *should* know the ropes after 8 months, so it's easy to understand why you're giving her another chance. You've invested a lot of time in her. While her respect for you is certainly a compliment, Betty's carrying respect to the outer limits.

Here are some further suggestions:

Why not discuss the problem with Betty and a nursing supervisor Betty feels comfortable with? Ask Betty why she transferred to a high-pressure unit like the ICU rather than stay on the medical/surgical unit.

To help Betty improve her performance, why not hold weekly conferences, evaluate Betty's performance, and discuss any problems. Or try the "buddy system"—having another nurse work closely with Betty for a few weeks. Another idea's role-playing. One nurse could be the "patient," and Betty could

act out what she'd do during an "emergency." One last suggestion: If you have enough staff, assign only nonthreatening jobs to Betty during a code until she becomes more comfortable.

Of course, keep a written record of your meetings and record the problems you've discussed and Betty's answers to your questions. Also keep a record of her progress.

You'll need to set a time limit for Betty to improve—say, 6 weeks. If in this time Betty still hasn't adjusted to the ICU, recommend that she transfer to another, less stressful unit. She might not be as devastated as you think.

Instructor's liability

Is reading charts an invasion of the patients' privacy?

Q The community college where I teach takes students to a local hospital for their clinical experience.

To supervise my students properly, I make sure to read their patients' charts. Now one of the hospital's anesthesiologists is challenging this: He says my reading charts is an invasion of the patients' privacy.

What do you think?

A How can you determine how well the students are caring for the patients *unless* you read the charts? Of course you have the right to read them. In fact, you'd be negligent if you didn't.

Remember, you are responsible for the quality of care your students are giving. The patients' charts will give you one of the significant keys to what that care should be.

There's no problem with what you're doing; but the anesthesiologist obviously has a problem understanding what you're doing. Maybe this should be your next teaching assignment.

What if a staff nurse doesn't agree with an instructor's assessment of a deteriorating patient?

Q I'm an RN teaching in a private-school LVN program. Our student LVNs get clinical experience in several local hospitals through contractual arrangements. But I'm still confused about my responsibilities (and my legal status) as an instructor working in a hospital where I'm *not* a staff member.

One situation in particular worries me. If I notice that the condition of a patient we're studying seems to be deteriorating seriously, I immediately tell one of the staff nurses so she can either call the doctor or take emergency measures. But the staff nurse doesn't always agree with me that the patient's getting worse.

When this happens, do I have the right to take emergency measures or to call the doctor myself? If I don't take *any* action, could I be held legally responsible?

A Your concern for the patient who appears to be in jeopardy is understandable. But since you're *not* an employee of the hospital where you're educating students, you *don't* have the right to take matters into your own hands. Staff nurses have the ultimate responsibility for patients under their care—and your disregard for the chain of command would be questionable nursing practice and would certainly not make for good relations with the staff.

What *can* you do? In a life-or-death emergency—such as a cardiac or respiratory arrest—and if a staff nurse isn't immediately available, you do have the legal right and responsibility to act. In a lesser emergency, you'll have time to notify the proper authorities (unit manager, team leader, supervisor, and so on). Then document what you've observed about the patient

on the chart. You might call for a conference later, and invite all those involved with the patient to participate. When you've taken these steps, you've covered *your* responsibilities—and then some.

Who's liable if students make a mistake?

Q I'm a staff nurse in an immunization clinic, which is attended mostly by children. Recently our local AD nursing school began placing student nurses in the clinic to expand their pediatric experience. The director of the nursing program asked me to let the students give injections, after assuring me that they had had experience in giving injections to adults. My supervisor told me to cooperate.

The first three nursing students just completed their 2 hours with me, and I was distressed by their obvious ignorance of injection technique and safety.

My question is, who's liable if they make a mistake and hurt somebody? Me? Or my supervisor? Or their instructor? Or, as my supervisor says, the director of the nursing program? I am the only RN present in the clinic.

A If an error occurs, the nurse present and supervising is liable. That's you. Demand that the instructor supervise the students. She also pointed out that the students are also liable for their own mistakes. If they don't carry liability insurance, they should.

Insulin

Can beef and pork insulins be mixed in the same syringe?

Q Can beef and pork insulins be mixed in the same syringe for a patient who's not allergic to either? Our pharmacy ran out of beef regular and mixed in pork insulin.

A It's okay to mix the two. In fact, many insulins are a combination of beef and pork.

Does the combination of NPH and regular insulin have to be given promptly after mixing?

Q On the medical unit where I work, our census often includes several patients with diabetes mellitus.

My practice is to prepare all the 7 a.m. insulin injections at one time, usually with one or two orders calling for a mixture of NPH insulin and regular insulin. That means that a half hour or so can elapse between preparation of the syringes and administration.

Recently I heard that the combination of NPH and regular insulin must be given promptly after mixing. Is this so, and why? I'd appreciate your input.

A The excess protamine sulfate in NPH insulin binds regular insulin. If a mixture of NPH and regular insulin remains standing for more than a few minutes, the regular insulin's potency will greatly diminish; however, the NPH potency won't be affected. Lente insulin, which contains excess zinc, also binds regular insulin, and letting this combination stand before administration also diminishes the regular insulin's potency. Don't prepare any syringe containing either of these combinations of insulin until you're ready to administer it.

Now for the exception to this rule: One pharmaceutical company, Nordisk-USA, manufactures an NPH insulin without the excess protamine that causes the binding problem mentioned above. It also manufactures a premixed NPH and regular insulin combination product. Ask your hospital pharmacist about this.

Is it legal for a nurse to give another employee an insulin injection?

Q A housekeeping department employee at the hospital where I work has diabetes. She keeps her insulin at the hospital, draws it up every morning, and has one of the medical unit nurses inject it for her.

When I floated to the medical unit, she asked me to administer her insulin. I politely refused. I just don't feel comfortable giving an injection of a drug I haven't seen drawn up to someone I hardly know.

She acted so insulted that I'm wondering if I might have been too cautious. Do you think I should have given the injection?

A You did the smart thing. Certainly you aren't obligated to give any medication that you're not sure about. If this woman had had an adverse reaction or mistakenly had drawn up too much insulin, which you then injected into her, you could have been held liable.

If you really want to help her out, you might gently tell her that treating employees is the responsibility of the employee health department, or the emergency department in smaller hospitals, not the staff nurses. She could also inject her own insulin after the proper patient teaching. Your hospital's malpractice insurance covers only *patient* care, so you should be cautious about giving care to fellow workers.

Should it be given I.M. or S.C.?

Q Last week, we received an order for regular insulin to be administered I.M.

I've often given insulin S.C., but never I.M. Can you tell me why and when this method of administration is preferable and whatever else I should know about it?

A Insulin is injected I.M. for rapid, overlapping response in the treatment of severe hyperglycemia. Sometimes it's used to treat diabetic ketoacidosis (although I.V. administration is preferred). The dosage is usually based on 0.1 unit of insulin per kilogram of body weight per hour until the blood glucose level falls to 250 mg/dl or less. Duration of action is about 3 hours, with peak action occurring about 1½ hours after an injection.

Unless your patient is overweight, you can use an insulin syringe and needle. Hold the skin taut against the muscle and insert the needle at a 90-degree angle.

Should nonlicensed assistants be taught how to give insulin?

Q A nursing home administrator has asked me to teach two nonlicensed nursing assistants how to give residents their insulin injections. I refused, explaining that I was concerned about my liability. But he persisted, asking me why this would be any different from teaching a patient's family how to administer insulin. I replied that a family has to learn about only one or two types of insulin, but the nursing assistants would have to recognize many different kinds. He finally backed off, but I know he's asking other nurses to do the same thing.

Do you think I am wrong to worry about this?

A You were wise to refuse. And you're right—the administrator's analogy is way off base. If he insists on implementing this scheme, he's asking for trouble.

Most nurse practice acts say that only RNs or LPNs can give injections, so what the administrator is asking you to do is illegal. Any nurse who agrees to teach nonlicensed nursing assistants to perform this function will find herself on the wrong side of the law—along with the administrator.

What's the right way to evenly disperse the particles?

Q A nurse on our staff has been debating with me about the right way to evenly disperse the particles in NPH insulin. I'm in the habit of inverting the vial gently several times, but my co-worker rolls the vial between both palms.

Which of us is right?

A This is one of those happy situations where you're *both* right. You can safely invert the vial gently, as you're doing; or you can roll the vial between both palms until there's no sign of sediment.

What's *not* acceptable is shaking, because shaking introduces bubbles. As you know, bubbles are difficult to clear from the vial and syringe in the aspiration step of the injection procedure.

Which insulin should be drawn up in the syringe first—regular or NPH?

Q Recently, my supervisor and I disagreed about which insulin should be drawn up in the syringe first when the patient is getting both regular and NPH insulin. She said regular insulin.

What do you say—and why?

A Your supervisor's right. The regular insulin should be drawn up first so the NPH insulin won't contaminate it. The NPH insulin contains protamine, which can precipitate some of the soluble regular insulin and change the onset and duration of its action. Another practical reason: If you're distracted while you're drawing up the insulins, you'll know by looking at the syringe whether you've drawn up only regular (clear) insulin or both regular and NPH (cloudy) insulin.

Insurance

Does being married to a doctor require extra insurance?

Q I'm returning to nursing after being home 12 years taking care of my family. Recently, I was discussing malpractice insurance with a friend who's also an RN. She was shocked when I told her I'd just purchased a standard policy. My husband, a doctor, makes a good living, so my friend thinks that I need three times more insurance if I don't want to risk losing everything we own.

Is this true?

A No, it isn't true. Your husband's assets aren't at risk for your actions as a nurse—nor would your assets be at risk for his actions. In fact, in most jurisdictions, any jointly owned property or property in his individual name wouldn't be subject to liability either.

> *"My husband, a doctor, makes a good living, so my friends think I need three times more insurance if I don't want to risk losing everything we own."*

Check with your insurance carrier. Most standard policies provide adequate coverage, with a single liability limit of $1 million and an aggregate limit of $2 to $3 million. So if multiple incidents occur during a policy year, the carrier will pay up to the aggregate limit of liability.

Remember, the vast majority of "reasonably prudent" nurses work day in and day out, year after year,

without ever being sued. So stop worrying and enjoy your return. America needs nurses.

How should a nurse go about getting it?

Q I'm shopping around for nursing liability insurance, but I'm confused about what to look for. Can you give me some guidelines?

A You're wise to investigate. Insurance regulators are concerned that some group insurance companies may not have stable underwriters behind them.

The American Nurses' Association recommends consulting Best's Insurance Reports and looking for companies rated A+, A, or A−. Companies rated A+ are judged by Best's as being superior in performance compared with the norms of the insurance industry. Ratings of A and A− indicate companies with excellent records.

Don't just check Best's, though. Before signing up for insurance, make sure you call either your state nurses' association or your state insurance commission to verify the company's credibility.

Shouldn't it cover overseas duty at a base considered U.S. territory?

Q My husband is in the Air Force stationed in Japan, and I plan on joining him soon and working on the base. My malpractice insurance company (and others I checked with) won't cover me while I'm overseas. Yet, the base is considered U.S. territory, and it operates under U.S. laws and regulations.

Why can't I get coverage?

A The promise of legal defense is an integral part of every malpractice insurance policy. And no insurance company wants to send

a lawyer to defend a client overseas, whether you'd be working on U.S. territory or under the laws of a foreign country. When you think about the possible hassle and expense the insurance company could incur, it's easy to understand why they don't offer coverage overseas.

You shouldn't have any problems, though. When you get to the base, ask what coverage you'll be given by the U.S. government while you're employed in a government facility. Then, relax and enjoy your stay—and nursing—in Japan.

Insurance physicals

Can a nurse be held responsible if the person she's examining is an impersonator?

Q I'm an RN working for a company that does insurance physicals. The insurance company gives my company the names, addresses, and phone numbers of potential insureds, and then I go to their homes and examine them.

All of my clients are total strangers—I've never seen a single one beforehand, and neither has anybody in my company. And that's what worries me. Suppose the person I'm examining isn't a client at all but an *impersonator?* Can I be held liable for the mistake?

I don't have malpractice insurance, but I'll get it if you think it might help. Also, do you think it might be a good idea to take a picture of each client so we could verify whether he was the "right" person?

A Impersonating patients in insurance physicals occurs rather freuqently. But nurses who act in good faith *aren't* held responsible in the case of impersonation. Just to be sure, consult a lawyer.

Also follow these recommended precautions. For instance, always ask the client for an identification with his signature, and then make sure he signs all insurance forms in your presence. If you're at all suspicious, you can compare the two signatures.

Malpractice would probably not come into play here—although carrying malpractice insurance is a good idea for *all* nurses.

Your taking pictures might be a good idea. But it would be even wiser to have the insurance company *agent* take the pictures of potential insureds beforehand. You'd have the pictures when you went to do the physicals. That way, you'd have a positive check on an impersonator.

Interviews

Does a prospective employer have the right to ask personal questions?

Q I'm an experienced and caring nurse. The trouble is, I didn't get along with my former supervisor; that's why I left my job. Now I'm having a hard time landing another one.

Today I applied for a job with a traveling nurse agency, and the recruiter needs a reference from my former supervisor before I can be hired. She's to fill in a form rating my appearance, emotional stability, attitude, ability to get along with others, initiative, dependability, and so forth.

Does a prospective employer have the right to ask personal questions like those?

A Yes, he has the right to ask those questions. However, the person who answers them might be opening himself up to a defamation suit. That's why most employers will confirm only the dates of employment and job titles of former employees.

Realistically, though, employers can discuss their employees with others who have a common interest in them. And as a fundamental legal principle, true statements and statements of opinion aren't defamatory even if they're hurtful. Employers are liable for defamation only if they knowingly or recklessly spread false information.

If you're concerned about what your former supervisor is saying about you, make a note on your job applications: "Before you contact my former employer, I'd like to explain a few things." Then tell your side briefly and without hostility. Or, if you can keep your cool, telephone your former supervisor and ask if she'd mind filling in the form you need. Tell her you hope that your differences from the past won't cast a lingering shadow over your future.

What are some taboo topics?

Q I've just been promoted to nurse-manager at a 100-bed rural hospital, and I'm now responsible for interviewing staff nurses who apply for jobs here. I've never conducted job interviews before, and I don't want to get off on the wrong foot. What types of questions should I avoid asking?

A Legally, you can ask only for job-related information, including education, experience, licensure, and citizenship status. You *can't* ask about religion, denomination, or custom; place of birth or national origin; union membership; credit rating; prior arrests; or marital or family status.

Your secretary can record an applicant's race and sex on an Equal Employee Opportunity-1 (EEO-1) job applicant log and you may establish that the applicant is at least 18 years old before you hire her. But you can't ask to see her birth certificate until *after* she's been hired.

To protect yourself and the hospital, make sure the job application form advises potential employees that they could be dismissed for providing written or oral misinformation.

What should a nurse do when an interviewer asks inappropriate questions?

Q I recently interviewed for a job to work weekends in our local hospital's home health department. I know that my experience and academic qualifications made me a strong candidate. But I wasn't hired.

Here's what happened. The interviewer began by asking whether I was married (yes), had children (yes), their ages (under 6), and who would take care of them while I worked (my husband). After learning about my recent work experience, she seemed anxious to hire me. We left it that I'd send in my references, and I'd probably start working in a month.

The next morning, the interviewer called to say she'd discussed staffing with the administrator, and they'd decided they wouldn't need me. Now, I'm wondering if they're just shying away from hiring anyone with small children. Was it right for her to ask me about my family? If not, what steps should I take now?

A The interviewer shouldn't have asked you whether you were married or who was going to mind the kids. Neither question has any bearing on your qualifications for performing the job.

You could file a complaint with the Equal Employment Opportunity Commission. However, even if they decided your complaint had merit, proving that you were discriminated against would take time, and maybe even a court appearance.

Why not contact the interviewer and ask her what tipped the scales against you—perhaps her administrator nixed hiring anyone. And ask her to keep you in mind for the next job opening—assure her that you'd like to work for them and could do a good job.

From here on, remember this when you're job hunting: Although you can't stop interviewers from asking inappropriate questions, you don't have to answer them. You could reply with a question: "May I ask how that relates to my ability to do this job?" The interviewer should get the drift—and respect you for your assertiveness.

Intuition

What should a nurse do if she senses impending death?

Q Recently, I developed a close relationship with one of our patients, a woman dying of lung cancer. When I was about to leave on a 3-day weekend, I had a feeling that I'd never see her again. But I convinced myself that she'd live at least until I returned.

I was wrong. She died the day before I got back. Now I feel sad that I missed out on saying good-bye—and angry that I didn't listen to my inner voice. Did I do wrong?

A We're taught to convert our observations into nursing diagnoses, and after caring for enough terminally ill patients, we usually know when death is imminent. But it's easy to tune out both the clinical information and the subtle signals from a patient. That way, you didn't have to risk acting on what you know or feel. Instead, we tend to borrow Scarlett O'Hara's philosophy and wait to talk to the patient "tomorrow." But too many times, there is no tomorrow—only an empty bed.

In the future, when you see a patient who you think won't live through the night, try to discuss that openly with the individual.

Say something like, "Emily, you seem so much weaker than you did this morning. I'm off duty for the weekend, and just in case you're not here when I return on Monday, I want you to know that I care very much about you and appreciate all I've learned from you."

Patients value that honesty. They know death is knocking, loudly. If you return to work and the patient is still alive, you haven't lost anything—and you have more time to talk. But if the patient does die, you can feel content knowing you shared your feelings in time.

Isolation

Is delaying it common practice?

Q On our medical/surgical unit, we sometimes admit a patient whose symptoms could indicate a contagious disease such as tuberculosis, hepatitis, or acquired immunodeficiency syndrome. Yet, because his doctor doesn't mention any suspicions in his progress notes, no isolation procedures are started until *after* test results are back—sometimes several days later. If the tests come back positive, we know that many staff members were already exposed. Infection control then has to audit the chart to find out who's had contact with the patient. Is delaying isolation like this common practice?

A It shouldn't be. Somewhere in the patient's admitting papers, it should state that his doctor wants tests made to confirm or rule out the contagious disease he suspects. The patient should be placed on isolation procedures *immediately* and remain on isolation until his test results come back negative.

Fortunately for both patient and caregiver, isolation procedures these days aren't generally so intimidating. In times past, isolation meant that you'd put on a hat, mask, gown, and gloves for working with

any patient thought to have a contagious disease. Now we know much more about disease transmission and use only what's necessary to protect patients and ourselves.

With a little investigation and teamwork, you could easily solve this problem. Ask your infection control nurse to help. It's her job to set up proper guidelines and to see that they're written into policy. You shouldn't have to worry that you're open to contagion.

When a patient's on isolation, should we keep his room door closed?

Q When a patient's on isolation, should we keep his room door closed? Most isolation patients at our small county hospital have tuberculosis, hepatitis, or skin disorders.

A Patients on respiratory isolation should be in private rooms—behind closed doors. As a general rule, if a patient has an infectious airborne disease, keep his door shut.

For more detailed guidelines on isolation for specific disease, use the Center for Disease Control's excellent reference, *Isolation Techniques for Use in Hospitals* (Washington, D.C.: Department of Health, Education, and Welfare, 1975). If you can't find it in your hospital library, try contacting the center at 1600 Clifton Rd. NE, Atlanta, Ga. 30333 (telephone: 404-329-3311).

I.V. bag

Is it okay to mark doses and times directly on the bag with a felt-tip marker?

Q One of my co-workers marks doses and times directly on a patient's I.V. bag using a felt-tip marker. Is this okay?

A No, the ink could leak through the plastic into the solution. Labels, not felt-tip markers, should be used on bags.

Tell her.

I.V. infusion pumps

Do they damage blood cells?

Q At a hospital where I used to work, we frequently used I.V. infusion pumps when administering blood. But many of my present co-workers claim infusion pumps damage blood cells. Are they right?

A Your co-workers may be basing their opinion on experience with early-model infusion pumps. Those pumps could do a lot of damage to cells because of their high output pressures. According to the guidelines of the American Association of Blood Banks, blood shouldn't be infused at a pressure exceeding 300 mm Hg.

If you have up-to-date equipment where you're working now, the I.V. infusion pump shouldn't cause excessive damage. Of course, it's smart to check the manufacturer's manual for recommendations. And remember, call in the service representative for demonstrations; you're his customer.

I.V. lidocaine therapy

Is it safe practice to abruptly discontinue a lidocaine infusion or is weaning necessary?

Q On our telemetry unit, we use I.V. lidocaine (lignocaine, Xylocaine) therapy for treatment of premature ventricular contractions. Some of the doctors order the lidocaine weaned by decreasing the

drop rate per minute over a period of time. Others just write a discontinue order.

Is it safe practice to abruptly discontinue the lidocaine infusion, or is weaning necessary?

A Lidocaine's unique pharmacokinetics allow the drug to be slowly metabolized and excreted from the body on its own. For this reason, lidocaine is often referred to as "self-weaning." So for patients whose cardiac rhythm is stabilized or for those who show signs of toxicity, infusion may be stopped abruptly and safely, no tapering off necessary.

However in patients with congestive heart failure or liver disease, lidocaine's clearance from the body is inhibited, causing buildup. So after a prolonged infusion of 24 hours or thereabouts, the doctor may order the dose reduced by 30% to 50%. This is considered dose reduction, not weaning. If the doctor wants the dose reduced over a period of time, he should specify how and when he wants this accomplished.

I.V. therapy

Can potassium chloride ulcerate vein walls?

Q Our I.V. team nurses are all experienced, and we've had no changes in equipment over the past 18 months. Yet our rate of infiltrations at every site, with all size cannulas, has increased. Most infiltrates seem to occur during administration of potassium chloride (KCl) or antibiotics. Are these fluids ulcerating the vein walls, or are there other causes?

A High doses of KCl and antibiotics can irritate vein walls and cause infiltration. So when you're administering drugs such as vancomycin (Vancocin), nafcillin

(Nafcil), aqueous penicillin, tetracycline (Tetracap), or KCl, be sure to add sufficient diluent and to carefully monitor the infusion. Infuse at the rate of 100 ml over 1 hour and 250 ml over 2 hours and flush with normal saline. For some antibiotics, the doctor may order sodium bicarbonate added to the infusions to raise the solution's pH and reduce irritation.

Infiltration may also occur if you place the catheter tip too near a point of flexion, where it might lodge against a vein wall, or if you leave an I.V. in place too long and the catheter gets stiff. Also, if a patient's had a lot of previous I.V. therapy, his vein walls may be abnormally thickened by fibrin deposits or they may be sclerosed. They can then be easily damaged by I.V. infusions of anticoagulants, long-term steroid or antibiotic therapy, or irritating drugs. Elderly patients have thinner, mored fragile veins, so infiltrations are common 2 to 3 days after an I.V. has been infusing satisfactorily.

Keep track of infiltrations on your unit for 3 months, noting placement site, catheter gauge, drugs injected, and length of indwelling time, to find out if there are any consistent factors.

If you're caring for an increasing number of older, compromised patients who may have received a lot of I.V. therapy, infiltration is more likely and may not be the fault of your technique.

Does disconnecting the tubing increase the chance of airborne contamination?

Q When collecting I.V. credits at the end of their shifts, some nurses on my unit are adding air to the I.V. bags to get "accurate" readings. They disconnect the I.V. tubing momentarily, allow air to enter the bag neck, then reconnect it. Does this increase the chance of airborne organisms contaminating the I.V. solution?

A I.V. solutions don't hang long enough for airborne organisms to multiply into large colonies. Of course, anytime the spike is removed and replaced, there's some risk of contaminating the spike or the bag neck. Readings obtained by this method won't be accurate. Collapsible bags are marked to be read as fluid infuses and the bag collapses.

The correct way to read the fluid level is to grasp the edges of the bag just above the level of the fluid and gently pull it taut. Or simply read the fluid level without touching the bag—a slightly less accurate, but acceptable, method.

What's important is that all staff members use the *same* method, for consistency.

Doesn't disconnecting I.V. tubing to change a patient's gown create a risk for infection?

Q As a nursing student, I've watched the staff disconnect I.V. tubing to change a patient's gown, then reconnect the tubing. Surely this creates a possibility for contamination of an otherwise closed and supposedly sterile system. With breakaway gowns readily available, this practice seems inexcusable.

The staff and clinical instructors I've discussed this with agree with me, but not one expected any change in the situation. They just said, "Look, this is Reality Street." Is it?

A It may be Reality Street, but you're right not to want to settle there. As a student, you probably lack the clout to effect immediate change. But never forget that a conscientious student often serves as a

catalyst, reminding seasoned staffers of the need to review and update procedures.

You've probably already done this, and you get an A+ for your good work.

How long can a patient remain on the same I.V. without a problem?

Q As an I.V. therapy nurse working in home care, I sometimes come across a patient with veins that are impossible to cannulate—"veins from hell," as we call them. When that happens, I usually nurse the I.V. along for a few days until it infiltrates. Recently, though, I took care of my most challenging patient. He needed 4 weeks of therapy after hospitalization, and his doctor wouldn't approve a central line. Luckily, I found a vein in his upper forearm good enough for starting the I.V.

However, every 5 days after that, I tried to find another vein as an alternate site and couldn't. So I kept the initial I.V. for 4 weeks—without problems. I babied it like a central line, and I stopped by every day, including my days off, to check the I.V. site for redness, sclerosis, swelling, or drainage.

This isn't something I'd want to do again soon. But just so I know, how long can a patient remain on the same I.V. without problems?

A Adhering to recommended standards is best whenever possible, but there's no set rule on how long a cannula can remain in place without causing phlebitis. Some patients receiving nonirritating fluids or medications had cannulas in place 5 to 7 days in hand veins and up to 6 weeks in larger arm veins with no apparent signs of harm. Actually, when there's little chance for success, you might do more harm sticking the patient re-

peatedly and traumatizing veins that are too small or scarred for access.

When you know the patient has poor veins and the doctor won't insert a central line for long-term access, ask him to write an order allowing you to leave the cannula in place longer than usual if necessary. Then be vigilant in observing and documenting the status of the I.V. site.

If the amount of air in the entire length of tubing isn't harmful, what's the concern?

Q On a recent visit to a friend in the hospital, I noticed about 5 inches of air in her I.V. tubing. I told her nurse, but she claimed that the air didn't matter, that it wouldn't create any problems for the patient. She said that in an emergency, she connects the tubing to the I.V. catheter with air in the entire length of it.

How well I remember being drilled and grilled in nursing school on the principle of keeping air out of I.V. lines. If the amount of air contained in the entire length of tubing isn't harmful, what's the concern?

A As you know, the most serious concern is that an air embolism will form and cause neurologic or circulatory problems—even death.

True, a few bubbles of air injected I.V. probably wouldn't hurt an adult patient—how *rapidly* air is infused is the crucial factor. Obviously, in an emergency it would be rapidly infused, thereby placing the patient in grave danger.

Just as obviously, you can avoid the problem by sticking to the principle you learned in nursing school: Keep air out of I.V. lines. One way to do this is to use a 0.22-micron filter on the distal end of the tubing to vent any trapped air. And connect the I.V. catheter with a needle-locking mechanism to prevent air entering the vessel or accidental disconnection.

Is it advisable to send a known drug abuser home with an I.V. line?

Q Today a known drug abuser suffering from bacterial endocarditis was admitted to our medical unit. The usual treatment is a 6-week course of I.V. antibiotics. Our policy is to discharge the patient as soon as he's stable, then have him continue the antibiotic therapy at home under the supervision of a home health nurse.

When I asked my supervisor about the advisability of sending a known drug abuser home with an I.V. line, she said, "As long as the doctor orders it, it's okay."

As a new discharge planning nurse, I may be overly cautious, but I don't find her answer very reassuring. What do you think?

A You have every right to be concerned. A drug abuser could easily use an established I.V. line to administer illegal drugs. Of course, this could possibly lead to reinfection or an overdose.

But the facts are these: Any person who wants to abuse drugs will, and you can't do very much about it. You can, however, discuss your concerns with this patient's doctor and ask him whether the patient can use an alternate administration route after discharge. Document your concerns in the patient's chart, and include mention of your talk with the doctor.

If this patient isn't in a drug rehabilitation program, ask a psychiatric nurse for a consultation. And be sure to alert the home health nurse that the patient will need close monitoring.

We want to do the best for all our patients. But at some point, you have to let go and rely on the next professional in line to take over the responsibility.

Is it a good idea to make sure an I.V. bag hangs in readiness?

Q In the labor room where I work, our unit manager instituted a new policy that has me concerned. We nurses must make sure an I.V. bag, with tubing inserted and flushed, hangs in readiness for when the next patient arrives. Some days patients arrive like clockwork. At other times, the bag will hang unused for close to 24 hours, when it's wasted and another one is prepared.

Is my concern justified?

A According to the Centers for Disease Control guidelines, I.V. bags should be changed every 24 hours and the tubing every 72 hours, so the new policy falls within these boundaries. At the same time, following the guidelines to the letter could lead to less than optimal practice. For example, what if a bag is hanging for 23 hours and a patient arrives? Will the bag be changed 1 hour later, or will the infusion continue past the 24-hour time limit? Another big concern these days is cost-effectiveness: It doesn't take an accountant to figure out that throwing away *any* supplies is a waste of money.

The bottom line here is that I.V. equipment can be set up very rapidly. It would be a lot safer and more economical to have unopened equipment at the bedside.

What considerations determine which base solution pharmacists use?

Q Our pharmacy mixes medications for I.V. piggybacks in either normal saline or dextrose 5% in water (D_5W). What considera-tions determine which base solution they use? Cost? Stability? Type of patient—specifically, how about a diabetic patient? I'd appreciate an expert's opinion.

A Normal saline and D_5W cost about the same, so that's not a factor. Stability, however, is important. Some medications (such as ampicillin) are stable longer in normal saline than in D_5W. Others (such as phenytoin) crystallize if the pH of the base solution is too low, so they can't be mixed in a D_5W solution.

D_5W diluent is generally considered safe for diabetic patients. There are only 5 g of sugar in 100 ml of D_5W, an amount considered too insignificant to adversely affect these patients.

What can patients do to build up their veins?

Q I read somewhere about I.V. patients building up their veins through exercise.

So many of my patients needing frequent I.V. therapy have fragile or small veins, and I'd like to have them try it. Do you have information on this?

A Have the patient squeeze a small rubber ball in each hand as often as possible every day. In a few weeks, veins should protrude above the dorsal surface of the patient's hands, making the I.V. insertion much easier and less painful.

What should you do if tubing disconnects from the cannula?

Q If a patient's I.V. tubing disconnects from the cannula while he's in bed, should you reconnect the tubing, replace only the tubing, or discontinue the I.V. and start over at another site?

A The essential rule to remember is that manipulation and touch contamination are major causes of I.V. complications. If you're present when the tubing disconnects and you're sure the cannula hub hasn't been contaminated, replace the tubing. While you set up the new tubing, attach a syringe filled with normal saline to the hub of the cannula and administer the saline as needed to keep the cannula patent. Then connect the new tubing to the cannula.

If you come across a disconnected line in a patient's bed, no way can you assume that the tubing or cannula is uncontaminated. Discontinue the I.V., use new tubing and cannula, and restart the I.V. at another site.

Who's responsible when hanging a premixed I.V. admixture?

Q I'm wondering about the relevancy of one rule we had drilled into our heads in nursing school: The person who prepares the medications administers the medications.

In the hospital where I work, we've adopted the unit-dose system. The pharmacists and technicians premix all medications, including I.V. admixtures. The registered pharmacist is responsible for the pharmacy technicians, but what about the nurses? Who's responsible when we hang a premixed I.V. admixture?

A Don't push the erase button in your memory bank just yet. Not all hospitals use the unit-dose system, and the axiom you learned is still a good one. With a unit dose, however, the pharmacy department *does* assume responsibility for preparing and labeling the premixed medications accurately. This doesn't mean you can totally relax. You must still hang the correct I.V. admixture or administer the proper medications to the right patient.

You can't just put blind trust in the system either. You could share some liability for a gross error with the pharmacist. If you suspect a pharmacy error—perhaps you notice a wrong color or dose—by all means double-check with the pharmacist before administering the medication.

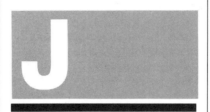

Jehovah's Witness

Can a blood transfusion be withheld?

Q An elderly patient of mine needed a blood transfusion because her hemoglobin count was dangerously low. She'd told me she was a member of Jehovah's Witnesses, and she didn't want the transfusion. I shared this information with her doctor and told him I couldn't ethically give her the blood. He went to my manager and told her I was endangering a patient's life by refusing to carry out an ordered treatment. She reviewed the chart, then told the doctor she agreed with me. Furious, he went to the unit's medical director—who also agreed with me.

> *"I couldn't ethically give a patient who was a Jehovah's witness a blood transfusion but felt torn when she died."*

Sadly, the patient died. Her daughter later thanked us for respecting her mother's religious convictions, but I feel torn. Another nurse on the unit told me she'd have given the blood. Maybe I should have. What do you think?

A Because this woman's religion was obviously a strong force in her life, you were right to voice your concerns on her behalf. By trying to force his values on this woman, the doctor nearly violated her right to choose her own course of treatment.

Another issue here is informed consent. Was your patient told fully and clearly about all treatment options—including blood transfusions? Did she specifically refuse transfusions on the consent form she signed?

If you're in a situation like this again, do just what you did this time—refuse to participate in the treatment, share the situation with your manager, and notify the medical director if necessary. One more thing: Make sure you chart any conversations you have with a patient about treatments she'd refuse on religious grounds. This documentation will back you up if a doctor tries to force the issue.

Job application

Should a hearing deficit be reported?

Q For several years, I worked as an instructor in a nursing school, then I left to get my MSN. I'll be filling out job applications soon, and I want to present myself in the best light possible. Some applications ask about any physical disabilities that would prevent the candidate from handling the position, and I'm worried about how to answer. I have some hearing loss in both ears, but with the help of aids, I can hear just fine. On the clinical unit, I wear only one aid in my worst ear so I can use a stethoscope.

Someone suggested I write "hearing corrected with aids" because the interviewer will see them. But people who wear glasses don't usually make a note like that on their application, and I say my problem is comparable.

Do you agree?

A Yes. When you're filling out a job application, your obligation is to answer questions honestly; you don't have to overexplain. So if your hearing deficit is corrected by aids, don't worry. If this question appears on the application, your hearing deficit isn't relevant.

Job benefits

Should an LPN lose them after becoming an RN?

Q As an LPN, I've worked full-time at the same private hospital for 15 years. Currently, I'm also enrolled in an associate degree program, with another year to go before I can take the state boards for RN licensing.

Recently, I've heard that when I become an RN, I'll be forced to resign my LPN position (with the hospitalization benefits and 5 weeks of vacation I've earned over 15 years). I'll have to go back to the bottom of the seniority list with a chance of being the first laid off. Worst of all, I may have to leave this hospital altogether if it can't offer me full-time work.

Is this any way to encourage LPNs to advance themselves?

A Fifteen years of dedicated service surely deserve some consideration.

Personnel policies vary all over the lot. Some hospitals would consider the LPN (now RN) a new hire for seniority status; but there would be some adjustment in the vacation schedule. Others would retain hospital benefits (including accrued vacation).

Don't listen to opinions. Ask the administration where you work if a 15-year employee might receive special consideration. And ask about the hiring picture for new RNs.

What's encouraging about becoming an RN? The *real* benefit you're earning is the opening up of your career possibilities. And that could prove to be its own reward in the shifting health care environment.

Job change

Is it realistic to switch from the ICU to psychiatric nursing?

Q I'm 45 years old, a diploma grad with 15 years' experience on the intensive care unit (ICU). Although I love my work, I'm finding the physical demands of ICU work too taxing. And if I'm ever going to make a career change, it better be now, considering my age.

I've thought a lot about what I'd like to do, and my first choice would be psychiatric nursing. Does this seem a realistic goal? If so, how should I go about reaching it?

A You have more to offer and less to fear seeking employment in the psychiatric setting than you may imagine. Your clinical expertise will be welcomed, and your life experience is a real plus. Don't ever forget that.

> *"Although I love my work, I'm finding the physical demands of ICU work too taxing. And if I'm ever going to make a career change, it better be now."*

Your best option would probably be applying for a job in a state facility. The educational criteria won't be as stringent there as in the private sector. Also, many state facilities are teaching facilities, and as such, they provide on-the-job learning opportunities. You'll get a good grounding and theory base, learn the jargon, familiarize yourself with psychopharmacology, and be able to use your clinical skills caring for patients. This temporary step could lead to a job in the private sector.

As with any career change, you must sell yourself. Answer ads; be persistent. Emphasize your strengths and assets, not the least of which are the emotional stability, compassion, and empathy that usually come with years of experience.

Is there a shortcut to finding out what hospitals are looking for?

Q I'm ready for greener fields this year. More than ready, since I've just been divorced. But even professionally, I've become restless after 3 years in the cardiac care unit of the university hospital in my city.

I've been wondering: Is there a shortcut to finding out what hospitals are looking for? And, in turn, what they're offering in salaries, benefits, and extras?

Any suggestions for me?

A You asked at the right time. The *Nursing Magazine Career Directory* is now available. The guide is free (while the supply lasts) and contains just the information you asked for about hospitals throughout the country.

Write to: *Nursing Magazine Career Directory,* 1111 Bethlehem Pike, Springhouse, PA 19477.

Job description

How can a nurse go about getting a new one?

Q I'm a nurse working in a large hospital's cardiac catheterization lab. We have a staff of five, all hired under the title and job description of cardiac catheterization lab technicians. However, three of us are RNs, and we perform nursing duties such as starting I.V.s and administering I.V. and I.M. medications. We must make nursing judgments and decisions in the course of our work. But because the present job description was written for technicians, it doesn't mention our nursing functions.

For safety and legal reasons, we nurses feel an updating and separating of job titles and descriptions is necessary. The director of the lab, a doctor, seemed to agree with us initially but now has changed his mind.

How can we get a new job description?

A Your campaign for a separate job description may rest on whether you were hired by the hospital's nursing administration or by the catheterization lab. If you accepted technician status when you were hired, you may have trouble getting your job description or title changed.

Collect your arguments supporting a change:
- Identify all the ways in which a nurse's responsibilities within the lab differ from a technician's (for example, administering I.V. and I.M. medications).
- Point out that most hospital departments need nurses for the special perspective they bring to patient care.
- Draft a suggested job description.
- Propose that the nurses in the catheterization lab report to a nursing supervisor, and the technicians report to a technician supervisor.

Present all your arguments to your hospital's nursing and medical departments in person.

If you get no results whatsoever, consider working in another department or even another hospital. However, your administration probably will fill your prescription for a new description so you won't have to move.

Job dissatisfaction

What should a nurse do when her heart's not in nursing anymore?

Q I've been active in nursing for 5 years. During that time, I completed my degree, and last year I was appointed assistant nurse-manager in our pulmonary-care unit. I regard myself as reasonably successful and, until recently, really enjoyed my work.

Lately, however, something's missing...the satisfactions seem fewer. I find myself going through the motions of being a nurse but my heart isn't in it. I don't know what's wrong. I'd welcome any suggestions.

A You know, people in television commercials aren't the only ones who come down with "the blahs." Real people get them, too. And you sound as though you've got a pretty good case going. Two things you should check out.

First, the physical. Have you been so concerned with others' health that you've neglected your own? How long has it been since you had a complete physical?

Second, you don't mention your home life. But is it possible that you're looking to nursing to fulfill some need—companionship, appreciation—that should really be fulfilled in your private life? Job satisfaction can be stretched only so far.

If you check out on those two points, then is the something that's missing in your life *challenge*? Anyone who gets her degree while working full-time and advancing herself to assistant manager has *got* to be a person who likes challenges. Is it time to set new goals for yourself?

Have you checked with your staff development office? Is there any program on pulmonary care you could develop—and teach—for

them? Or is there some way you could use your skills in another clinical area of the hospital?

Job evaluation

Any suggestions for writing them?

Q I was recently promoted to unit manager on a large medical/surgical unit. As part of my job, I'll have to write performance evaluations.

Although my own past evaluations were always good (reliable, cooperative, ambitious), I was often disappointed when an appraisal failed to mention what I considered to be my unique contributions to the department.

> *"I was often disappointed when my job evaluations failed to mention my good points. Now the shoe's on the other foot."*

Now the shoe's on the other foot, and I want to write the kind of evaluation for my staff that I'd like to receive. Any advice?

A Get yourself a copy of the book, *Effective Phrases for Performance Appraisals: A Guide to Successful Evaluations,* (4th ed. Perrysburg, OH: Neal Publications, 1988).

This guide lists over a thousand phrases that describe a variety of commonly rated performance standards. You can thumb through the phrases listed and plug in the one that says just what you want. Under the heading "Creativity," for instance, how about "seeks creative alternatives" or "originates unsought ideas"? Or instead of the hackneyed "reliable," try "works smarter, not harder" or "identifies and eliminates time wasters."

J
K

Writing an appraisal—good or critical—can be a tough job. Bravo to you for, as the book suggests, "giving maximum effort."

Can a supervisor continue to write statements that relate to past experiences?

Q In early April, my supervisor gave me a good overall appraisal for clinical practice. But she wrote that I am argumentative and abrasive with co-workers. This surprised me because my nurse-manager never mentioned this behavior in any interim conferences during this past year. So I asked the supervisor for specific instances. She said that her documentation referred to occurrences in early 1988 and that I had improved somewhat this year.

Can a supervisor continue to write statements in an evaluation that relate to past experiences? I'm confused and disappointed.

A And well you should be. Negative information from early 1988 shouldn't be mentioned in a 1989 evaluation unless the identified problem continued. Unfortunately, a busy supervisor might scan past evaluations and continue citing a criticism without fully investigating whether the problem behavior has changed.

Set up a second appointment with your supervisor. Before you meet, ask your co-workers for honest feedback about how you get along with them. And prepare a self-evaluation; if you've successfully resolved any problems you've faced, include them in your notes.

At the meeting, avoid "you" statements ("You didn't check"). Refer to the written evaluation only: "This statement doesn't give specific information," and so forth. You might offer, "For the record, I want to document some positive feedback I've received from my co-workers." Then ask the supervisor about problems you need to work on—and

also ask her to comment on any improvement she's seen in those areas.

Your efforts should be rewarded. The evaluation process, though far from perfect, can be a valuable learning tool—for the employee and for the evaluator as well.

Can someone objectively evaluate performance of a friend whose performance is below par?

Q Has anyone in the world ever written an objective evaluation of a friend who was not performing satisfactorily—and still have that person remain a friend? I'd like to know how it's done.

A Every day, some supervisory nurse in some part of the country sits down with a staff nurse (who also happens to be a friend) to review that nurse-friend's job performance. More often than not, some part of the evaluation will be less than positive. Yet, the two nurses remain friends. So, yes, it *is* possible. But you're wise to ask for particulars on how it's done, because it doesn't just happen "like zip." It takes planning.

Evaluation is *not* something that takes place for 30 minutes every 3 months. It's an ongoing process. If someone is not measuring up, and you let her go along for months thinking she is, you're asking for trouble. The element of surprise alone is likely to cause as much friction as the poor rating. Try this:
1. Keep anecdotal notes day by day. These notes will document behavior—both satisfactory and unsatisfactory.
2. If your official policy calls for trimonthly evaluations, give the nurse an evaluation report after 6 weeks. Ask her to judge her own performance for an unofficial review. A worker often has some question about her level of work performance and can take this chance to air her

uncertainty. If, however, there are discrepancies in your two views, this is the time to iron them out. Have your anecdotal notes on hand to give examples of what you're talking about. Give pertinent suggestions on how the worker can improve her performance.
3. Remember, you are evaluating the work performance—not the person. No matter how unsatisfactory the person's performance, there is always something commendable to say about the person herself. Make sure you get that across strongly. These positive views provide the balance in any judgment and are just as important as the not-so-positive comments.

How should a nurse handle her supervisor if she disagrees with her?

Q After working as an RN in the same nursing home for 10 years, I had to resign because my husband relocated to take a new job. The director of nursing gave me an excellent recommendation, so I had no problem finding a new position in another nursing home.

Everything seemed wonderful until today, when I received my 3-month evaluation. My supervisor gave me a poor rating, saying that I'm too involved with my patients and can't handle stress. Talk about stress: I feel like giving her a piece of my mind and then quitting.

How should I handle this?

A Keep calm. Storming into the supervisor's office and giving her a piece of your mind will only fuel her claim that you can't handle stress. Give yourself a day or two to gather your thoughts—and to do some self-evaluation. Make a list of your strong points and of the areas you know need improvement. And ask staff members for their honest opinions of your work. Then request a second meeting.

At this meeting, discuss what you've learned from your self-evaluation. And ask your supervisor for specific information—such as dates, times, and examples of getting "too involved" with your patients—to substantiate the poor rating she gave you. This discussion should suggest ways for you to improve your performance. Above all, don't be defensive or sarcastic.

What might you have done at that first meeting? When a supervisor takes you off guard like that, interrupt the session as soon as possible. Say something such as, "This comes as a surprise to me. Can we postpone discussing it until I've had time to think it over?" If your supervisor insists, sign the evaluation form. This doesn't mean you agree with it, only that you've seen it. You can add a comment such as, "I don't agree with this evaluation. Will discuss it at a later meeting." Before you leave, request a second meeting similar to the one suggested above, and proceed accordingly.

Your supervisor behaved in an unprofessional manner. Instead of waiting until your evaluation meeting, she should have been pointing out times when you were letting your feelings show or when you needed to handle stress better. And she should have offered suggestions for improvement.

If you decide not to accept the evaluation, you can present your side of the story, thoroughly documented, to the director of nursing—but only after first informing your supervisor. Since you worked in another nursing home for 10 years with a good performance record, chances are, that will weigh in your favor.

What can be done when it's late?

Q I work on the medical/surgical unit in our community hospital. My annual review and pay increase were due 3 months ago—but

so far, nothing. When I asked my supervisor about this, she said, "When I can get around to it, I will. Don't worry—your pay increase will be retroactive to the anniversary date."

My past evaluations were good, and I always work my assigned hours and holidays. Lately though, I've turned down extra hours and on-call duties because of family responsibilities. Now I'm wondering if this is why my review is late.

I don't want to go over my supervisor's head, but the delay is making me nervous. Do you think I'm being unreasonable?

A No way. Three months overdue is just too long. From what you say, it sounds as if your supervisor's probably up to her eyeballs in work, and she keeps putting your review on the bottom of the pile, hoping it will go away.

Grab a few quiet moments with her, and don't be afraid to speak honestly. Tell her, "Your feedback is important to me. I need to know what you like about my work—and what you don't. And I need my raise, too." Offer to do a self-appraisal to save her some time.

One thing about evaluations. Usually everyone up the line who gives one gets one. For this reason alone your supervisor should understand your feelings and get on the ball.

Job hunting

Any suggestions for a nurse planning to move?

Q As soon as I get my board scores, I'll be off to California to pursue my nursing career, a plan I've had in the back of my head for some time now. I consider myself independent and organized, but it still won't be easy. You see, at age 24, I've never been away from home before, and I'm naturally very scared about going alone—

particularly because California is 3,000 miles away, and I know very little about that state or its hospitals.

I've been too busy at school to plan the logistics. However, I want to move to a major city and work at a hospital that offers educational reimbursement. I'm thinking of taking a quick trip out for job interviews.

> *"You see, at age 24, I've never been away from home before, and I'm naturally very scared about going alone— particularly 3,000 miles away."*

Do you have any suggestions to help me plan my move?

A Our first suggestion is that you reread your letter and ask yourself if you really want to go now—alone. Or have you just become caught up in the *idea* of moving to California and disciplined yourself to fit the plan? True, the move could be great, but anyone with experience will probably tell you that making the leap from student to working nurse can be tough enough without going across the continent to do it. So, to avoid being miserable, you need to do a little soul-searching as well as logistical planning.

When you have a breather from your studies, sit down and put your thoughts on paper—weigh the advantages of moving now against the advantages of staying put and getting a year's nursing experience. Under reasons for going, you could list that you're psyched up to move. Or perhaps you have some personal reason for wanting to put distance between you and your present situation. Under the advantages of staying put for a year, you could list that you'll have more credibility when you're job hunting, you can save money toward your living expenses, and as an experienced nurse, you'll be eligible for a job with a traveling nurse agency—a good way to "try on" the California lifestyle and find out where you'd like to settle without spending your own money on travel and housing.

If you think it through and decide you still want to go now, get in touch with the California Board of Registered Nursing for licensing information (P.O. Box 944210, 1030 13th St., Suite 200, Sacramento, CA 94244-2100). Then go to a hospital library and check the *American Hospital Association Guide to the Health Care Field* (Chicago: AHA, 1990); you'll find the names, addresses, size, type of services offered, accreditation status, and so forth of every hospital in California. Contact the California Nurses' Association about joining, and ask for information on housing and nursing educational opportunities (1855 Folsom St., Suite 670, San Francisco, CA 94103). Once you're out there, you can attend their meetings and network with professionals who can become your friends. Best wishes.

How can a nurse convince potential employers that the economic situation was responsible for her job loss?

Q We hear a lot these days about the nursing shortage but very little about the scarcity of jobs for those of us who live in economically depressed areas. The hospital where I first worked my way up from staff nurse to management went bankrupt. Since then, I've lost three supervisory jobs in 2 years because of hospital cutbacks or bankruptcies. Now it's happening again: Yesterday, our administrator announced a cutback of supervisory staff—and as the most recently hired, I'll be the first to go. That

means job hunting again, and I'm dreading it.

How do I persuade potential employers that the economic situation and corporate strategies have done this to me? I'd hate to give up nursing after 10 years, but the uncertainty is overwhelming. Any comments?

A First of all, try not to feel defeated; the economy's picking up in your area. Start by asking for a staff job where you're working and already known. Or, get prepared for job hunting; ask former co-workers and managers (the more the better) to help you by writing references that you can take to interviews. On applications, explain your employment record with a statement such as, "I've held several jobs in the past few years because this area's economy...." List all of your previous employers; explain why each job was eliminated, and invite the recruiter to verify your story with the employers themselves. Ask the recruiter questions, too. Are any major organizational changes coming up? Stress that your hands-on and supervisory nursing experience will make you a doubly valuable employee.

> *"I've lost three supervisory jobs in 2 years because of hospital cutbacks or bankruptcies."*

Second, don't neglect networking. Your nursing friends may be able to tell you when jobs are opening up. Thanks to the grapevine, they often know who's planning to leave before administration does. Their inside information might help you get the next available job.

Finally, if you're willing to move, hospitals in other areas of the country would gladly snap you up and pay your transportation costs. You might have to be more flexible about

your job goals because most openings are for staff nurses, not managers, even where the nursing shortage is acute. Consider accepting a staff position and maneuvering for advancement later if you're satisfied with the salary, fringe benefits, and, most important of all, the promise of job stability.

If a nurse were to say that she was in a program for chemical dependency, who would hire her?

Q A few weeks ago, I was fired for absenteeism—and the experience was a real eye-opener. I'd been using recreational drugs off duty, foolishly thinking that I could handle them. I never stole any drugs or used them while working. Since then, I've entered an outpatient program, and I've really changed—I know I'm on the right road. But I have to make money, so I want to know how to apply for a nursing job. No one would know I had a minor drug problem. But if I say I'm in a program for chemical dependency, who would hire me? Do you think I'm out of luck for a nursing job?

A If you truly want to be on the right road and have come to terms with yourself, you ought to be honest about this problem with others. When you fudge answers on applications, you're jeopardizing your job and maybe your license.

Yes, job recruiters are leery when they hear about a former chemical-dependency problem of any kind. But attitudes are more positive these days, and many recruiters are willing to give a chance to someone who can prove she's straight.

It's great you're working your way through this, but your chances of getting a nursing job would be better if you were in recovery longer. In the meantime, why not take a stopgap job outside of nursing to make money? Then, when you apply for a nursing job, take along documentation from your recovery program and from your doctor attesting to your full rehabilitation.

> *"I'd been using recreational drugs off duty, foolishly thinking that I could handle them."*

For now, try calling your state nurses' association for the number of the peer-assistance program for nurses in your state. Remember, you're not the only one with this type of problem. Take advantage of all the help available.

What's the best way to handle an unfavorable reference caused by a personality difference?

Q My husband and I have just moved to a new city, where I'm having difficulty finding a new position. I think the problem's an unfavorable reference I received on my last job. This reference resulted from personality differences with the supervisor, *not* from the quality of my nursing care. I *know* my nursing care has always been above standard.

How should I handle this unfavorable reference in future interviews?

A Put the problem right up front when you're asked about your past experience. Tell your side of the story. Be brief, speak calmly—and don't show hostility. Some interviewers will accept your version. Even those who don't are more likely to take the unfavorable reference with a grain of salt.

Good luck in finding a position soon—and in reestablishing your record for fine nursing.

Job rejection

What's a wise approach after failing to get a new job?

Q I am 47 years old and have had considerable experience with recovery room nursing. When our hospital recently opened an 8-bed minor surgical unit, I applied for the position of unit manager. Quite truthfully, I was looking for an opportunity to give total care without the hassles of a larger unit and challenge of that position.

Although I had the most seniority of the applicants, I did not get the appointment. When I asked the director why, she said I was too valuable to waste in a unit like that! Can you explain the logic of that answer?

A Your director doesn't exactly have a gift for words, but if you weren't so disappointed at not getting the job you'd probably see her answer as the backhanded compliment she intended.

There are a couple of points at issue here, though. From what you say of your background, you seem to be an experienced and capable nurse. And you have seniority. None of these qualities, however good in themselves, would necessarily make you the best candidate for nurse-manager. Do you have leadership ability? *That's* what a director wants in a unit manager. If your answer to that question is yes, then look at it from the director's point of view.

Administrators are often loath to move good employees out of key positions—even when the move might very much benefit the employee—because the administrator is then faced with having to find a replacement.

If you think this is what happened in your case, then discuss it with your director. Sparing her an in-

convenience is no reason for depriving you a deserved promotion. Further, you should explain exactly why you want a job change. Don't be ashamed to admit you're looking for a new challenge. We all have different needs at different times in our careers, and your director will never know your needs unless you tell her.

Once you get these points straightened out, you ought to be first in line for the next suitable job opening.

Job responsibility

Can an RN floated to a unit be held liable for an LPN's actions?

Q Last week, I floated to a medical/surgical unit, where I was working under an LPN. My manager told me that because I'm an RN, I'd be responsible for the care of all patients on the unit, even though the LPN was in charge. I told her I didn't think that sounded reasonable—unless she made me charge nurse. But she wouldn't do that because my assignment was temporary. Where do I stand legally in a situation like this?

A Because you weren't in charge, you were responsible for the care of your patients only. Making assignments is a management duty, so ultimately your manager would have been liable for any problems that arose.

You would have been liable, though, if you'd seen the LPN do something that could have harmed a patient and you hadn't intervened. You have the same responsibility, of course, if you witness an RN or doctor endangering a patient.

You can't do much about what's already happened, but you can plan for the future. First, check your state's nurse practice act to see what it says about supervising LPNs. In

J
K

most cases, an RN must supervise the care and treatment given by an LPN. Then, document your concerns and put them in a memo that you send to your manager. Make sure you keep a copy of the letter for your files.

Can a nurse refuse to work a double shift?

Q I've been the only RN on the night shift at a small nursing home for over 2 years. The day-shift nurse calls in sick several times a month, and the owner, who is also an RN, expects me to stay until she finds another nurse. If she can't find anyone, she expects me to work the whole shift, until 3 p.m.

Since I have several children, two of them preschoolers, I have to be home when my husband leaves for work. If I'm not, one of the older children has to skip school to baby-sit for me. When I explained this to the administrator, she hinted that she'd fire me if I refused to stay.

What can I do? If she fired me and gave me a bad reference, I'd never get another job around here. But I can't keep on working double shifts.

A Since the owner is an RN and acts as director of nursing, she (not you) is solely responsible for nursing coverage on all shifts. Federal labor laws, do permit her to fire you for refusing to work overtime.

What should you do? First, be sure the administrator understands your feelings. Have you been open with her or have you just assumed she understood your problems?

Second, decide on the likely outcome. If you think the administrator is trying to solve the problem (maybe she's looking for a more reliable day-shift nurse), you might be willing to help out temporarily if you do so, you must be paid time and a half for over 40 hours in a week.

Can nurses delegate invasive procedures to nursing assistants?

Q I've just transferred to the intensive care unit. Some of the certified nursing assistants who work on the unit routinely do things like catheterizing patients, suctioning, and removing arterial lines. One nursing assistant told me she'd even helped a doctor intubate a patient and insert a pulmonary artery catheter. I'm concerned about their doing these types of invasive procedures—and about the legal ramifications for nurses who delegate the responsibilities. Are we headed for trouble?

A Unless forbidden by state law, hospitals may hire unlicensed personnel to perform the tasks you describe. And with the nursing shortage, more and more of them are doing just that, taking a cue from long-term care facilities that have been doing it for years. (Of course, if this type of delegation is prohibited by state law, you and your employer could be held liable—you for negligent delegation, and the hospital for illegally expanding the nursing assistant's role.)

> *"Some of the nursing assistants do things like catheterizing patients, suctioning, and removing arterial lines."*

The hospital should provide a course to prepare assistants for tasks allowed by state law and hospital policy. It should also set up a system to check the credentials of assistants certified at other hospitals and require them to pass a written examination.

After nursing assistants have been properly certified, you're free to delegate *appropriate* tasks. Just

make sure you know what they're allowed to do and how skillful they are. As you would when delegating to any other staff member, assign only tasks that fit the assistant's demonstrated abilities.

Does a nurse's responsibility end when the ambulance attendants take over?

Q I'm an occupational health nurse in a small manufacturing company. Recently, I had to order an ambulance for an employee, but I wasn't sure whether or not I should have accompanied him to the hospital.

Does my responsibility end when the ambulance attendants take over? Or when the hospital staff takes over? At what point am I no longer legally responsible for this employee?

A Once an emergency occurs, you'll have your hands full. You can't be expected to stop at this point and figure out "responsibility" and "policy." So work these questions out ahead of time with the ambulance people who serve your company, with the hospital the patient's likely to be taken to, and with the proper authorities in your company. Everyone involved should collaborate to write the definitive guidelines for emergencies.

Should you go in the ambulance with your patient? You must weigh all the circumstances each time. For example, your decision may depend on who's in the ambulance (how experienced, how skillful that person is, in your opinion), the need for your services back in your own department, and of course, the condition of your patient. If he's had a heart attack or a traumatic injury, you'd be more pressured to go with him in the ambulance, if at all possible. If he's going to the hospital for sutures, X-rays, or a consultation, you'd be less inclined to go with him.

And where does your responsibility end? At the hospital door. But here are some practical suggestions for protecting both an employee and yourself.

• Get to know the staff at the hospital that will receive your patient.

• Call ahead to the hospital with as much information as possible about the patient. Chances are their staff will then be in a better position to give "informed" care.

• Keep emergency telephone numbers posted where they'll be easy to find in a hurry. And be sure the numbers are written large enough so they can be read easily.

• Keep your next-of-kin file for each employee up to date, with the *latest* telephone numbers and addresses for the persons to be notified.

• Compose and distribute a leaflet to all employees about your company's medical care program, with a special section on emergency procedures. (Be sure that when a new employee is hired, he gets a copy.)

No matter how carefully you "plan" for an emergency, each situation will be unique and will call for an immediate nursing judgment. But with a well-defined written policy clearly established, you'll be free to handle an emergency—without having to figure out your "area" of responsibility.

How risky is giving injections when the doctor's away?

Q I'm a nurse in a small-town general practitioner's office. When he's out of town, he expects me to give injections—for instance, penicillin—to his "regular" patients who're complaining of sore throats or colds. He also expects me to give vitamin and allergy shots to patients who receive them regularly.

The last time the doctor left town, he even asked me to give flu and pneumococcal shots to patients after I'd examined them—but then have them sign a statement saying they wouldn't hold me responsible for any side effects.

I've never felt comfortable giving these injections, and I've told the doctor so. But he just shrugs off my remarks.

Please help me—I need to know *exactly* what I can and can't do while the doctor's gone. Will a statement signed by the patient really protect me? The doctor says "yes," but I think the answer's "no."

A The answer's "no"—the release statements can't relieve you of professional responsibility for your actions.

Aside from the issue of responsibility, what would you do if a patient *did* have an unexpected reaction to an injection? Is there another doctor on call to handle these emergencies?

And what if a patient does sign a statement releasing you from responsibility? Who'll accept responsibility? Your boss?

If you do it, administer certain injections during the doctor's absence—but only under specific conditions. Give injections only if the doctor left standing orders for those patients who need vitamin or allergy shots for preexisting conditions; and even then, only if another doctor were available to handle any emergencies.

Don't, under any circumstances, administer injections for *new* conditions. For example, don't give penicillin shots to patients complaining of sore throats or colds. If you did, you'd be diagnosing and prescribing for a medical problem, which could leave you open to charges of practicing medicine without a license.

Discuss this problem with your boss immediately—and don't let him shrug off your concern. Protect yourself now. If an emergency occurs, you'll need all the protection you can get.

If LPNs can perform the same duties as RNs, what's the need for more education?

Q After working as an LPN for 10 years, I thought going back to school to become an RN would be a wise move. Since graduation last May, I've been working as a staff RN at an extended care facility. Now I'm not sure I was so smart.

The director of nursing at the facility insists that LPNs have the same capabilities as RNs. I'm having a hard time swallowing this—I was always taught that RNs were responsible for LPNs.

And the director of nursing's philosophy has created some problems for me with one of the LPNs on my shift, who thinks seniority counts far more than education. She's never worked with an RN, and her defenses are up. I try to avoid conflict, but I think the nursing assistants sense this—and my authority's being undermined.

The last straw came when the director of nursing announced that LPNs can draw blood and start I.V.s after some instruction. When I questioned this, the one LPN who's been making my life difficult said, "Where have you been? I draw blood when I do insurance physicals."

Am I behind the times? If LPNs can perform the same duties as RNs, am I carrying a 5-year student loan for nothing?

A You're right to be concerned about this blurring of the lines separating the duties of RNs and LPNs. You're not alone in your concern—many nursing leaders are calling on RNs to defend their educational background and their right to perform specific duties that LPNs cannot.

Among the duties LPNs can't legally perform, according to a typical state board of nursing, are drawing blood and starting I.V.s. Make your director of nursing aware that her LPN-RN philosophy has led her into dangerous legal waters. Ask her for detailed job descriptions that you and your co-workers can refer to whenever a who-does-what question comes up.

Speaking up can be tough, especially when you're new on the job, but remember, defending professional standards *is* part of your professionalism.

If staff nurses are being exploited to act as unit managers, what can be done?

Q Our hospital does not employ assistant unit managers to replace the unit mangagers on their days off. Instead, administrative policy holds that the staff nurse with the most seniority will act as head on those days. For this, she receives no additional pay.

Our written job description does not state that a staff nurse must do this, yet nurses who refuse this additional responsibility seem to wind up with undesirable assignments or poor references when they leave.

We think we're being exploited and would like to know if a hospital can legally order a staff nurse to assume the responsibility of a nursing unit when she doesn't want to?

A Put simply, the nurse practice act directs that a nurse may perform only those duties for which she was prepared, tested, and found competent. If a staff nurse feels that she's unprepared or unable to assume responsibilities of a unit manager, then she has an obligation to her patients, herself, and her license to refuse such an assignment.

Further, if a hospital cajoles its staff into performing duties for which they are not prepared (thereby allowing them to practice

below-standard care), then the hospital will be held responsible for any malpractice that might occur.

If the obligation to fill in for unit manager is absent from the staff nurse's contract of employment, then the staff nurse does not breach her agreement by refusing to assume such responsibilities.

This endorsement, of course, will provide small satisfaction to the nurses you mention who did refuse and who were treated shabbily in return.

The problem of being expected to assume greater responsibility without commensurate payment is common to nurses everywhere. And it may never be solved until staff nurses organize into strong bodies to bring about enforcement of the criteria of the Joint Commission on Accreditation of Healthcare Organizations and the requirements of the hospital codes with regard to staffing. Nurses must also negotiate their employment contracts.

The written contracts of employment must spell out *in detail* the obligations of the employee and the obligations of the employer—especially with regard to financial compensation—so that such practices will be stamped out.

Is a private-duty nurse responsible for LPNs or graduate nurses even though they're hospital-employed?

Q I recently decided to try my hand at private-duty nursing in local hospitals. On my first night, a graduate nurse who was assigned to my patient told me I was permitted to give medications but she'd give the I.V. antibiotic. The next night, an LPN told me only staff nurses could give medications.

When I checked my patient's chart, I saw that his muscle relaxant was already an hour overdue, so I

alerted the LPN. She snapped that she was busy and that my patient would have to wait. Luckily, she was free in a few minutes, but it set me to wondering if, as an RN, I'm responsible for the LPN (or the graduate nurse) even though they're hospital-employed?

A As a private-duty RN working with a graduate nurse and an LPN, you're responsible for their actions only insofar as they affect your patient—and your patient only.

Hospitals usually maintain tight control over a private-duty nurse's practice and have written policies detailing how her duties and responsibilities relate to the hospital nurses'. Ask for a copy stat. Of course, if any limitation in the policy keeps you from giving quality care to your patient, contact nursing administration and—if nothing changes—the patient's doctor.

Knowing your responsibilities will allow you to do your job competently without pulling rank or feeling dependent on the staff nurses. Remember, you are, in effect, invading their "turf," so it's up to you to fit in, make the extra effort to be friendly, and communicate your needs. If you present yourself as a professional, the staff nurses will find out quickly enough that the more you can do for your patient, the more you'll help them.

Is it ever acceptable to refuse supervisory responsibilities?

Q I'm an RN in the laboratory of a public-health clinic that also has one LPN and three technicians on the staff. We all do venipunctures, handle the specimens, sort supplies, and that sort of thing. The LPN and I also train new technicians to do the venipunctures, help patients who get sick, and pass nasogastric tubes.

My problem is that a new laboratory chief has given us written job descriptions. (We've never had them before.) My job description says I'm *in charge* of the technicians who work with me.

When I complained, the chief said that was why I was hired—that an RN was expected to supervise.

The old chief, who hired me, never said anything about supervising, and I don't think it's fair for this chief to change my job now. What can I do about it?

A The first thing to do is to calm down. Then, analyze what has happened, how you've reacted, and why you've reacted that way.

What has happened? You've been told you're expected to supervise.

> *"The old chief, who hired me, never said anything about supervising, and I don't think it's fair for this chief to change my job now."*

How have you reacted? Your letter sounds threatened and angry. Is that how you'd describe your feelings?

If so, why do you feel threatened? Is supervising a new experience for you? Do the technicians' personalities or work habits make them particularly hard to supervise?

And why do you feel angry? Will supervising add significantly to the amount of work you have to do? Do you think someone else is ducking responsibility by telling you to supervise? Do you think supervising will adversely affect your job record or your relationships with the other employees?

Once you've analyzed the situation, you'll probably know what to do. If you feel unprepared for the job of supervisor, you might ask your chief for guidance, along with

a specific list of
you feel someor
doing the super
chief to explain w

Of course, onc
the situation, you
your initial resista
and welcome it.
seem overqualifie
described.

Is it legal for
an RN to perfc
duties?

Q I'm both an
cal techniciа
RN. I used to work
hospital in both ca
cently quit my nursing job to take a position elsewhere. But my community has a shortage of EMTs, so I agreed to continue working part-time at the hospital as an EMT.

Here's my problem: Because the hospital often has inadequate RN coverage in the emergency department, I'm asked to perform nursing duties. I'm concerned that although I *am* an RN, I'm no longer employed as a nurse at that hospital. Am I taking a legal risk?

A You bet. Here's why: If you committed a negligent act while performing nursing tasks, the hospital might not share liability with you in a subsequent lawsuit. That's because, as you say, you're not employed as an RN at that hospital. Legally, you'd be an independent contractor, solely responsible for your own negligence—and for paying any judgment against you.

But if you committed a negligent act as an EMT and a lawsuit resulted, you'd be partially protected by the hospital. Because the hospital has employed you as an EMT, it would share responsibility for your mistakes.

Remember, you're not responsible for providing nursing coverage; hospital administrators are. Don't take an unnecessary legal risk.

Yes, the hospital is liable. But so is the postanesthesia room staff, since they *know* about the dangerous practice of leaving the patie unattended—but have neither umented it nor remedied it.

Now for the more or les part: Ideally, an RN sh pany all patients fro esthesia room. In this is the routi anesthesia They feel and ab

If

me. If all the orderlies are busy, the patient may wait as long as half an hour at the door of the postanesthesia room. During this time, no one's checking his vital signs.

If one of these patients ran into trouble before he reached the medical/surgical unit, who'd be responsible?

Our unit manager claims the hospital would be responsible. I checked the hospital's policy book, and it's vague about transport and about the postanesthesia room nurse's role in discharging a patient.

Of course I'm worried about these patients. But I'm also worried about *my* responsibility as a postanesthesia room nurse. Is transporting a patient without a nurse standard policy in most hospitals?

A There's room for flexibility in the answer to your question—but not much. Here's the inflexible part:
• At no time should a postanesthesia room patient be left unattended.
• The responsibility for the postoperative patient remains with the recovery room staff—until that patient's been turned over to the staff of the medical/surgical unit and an appropriate report's been given.

J
K

flexible
...ould accom-
... the postan-
... hospitals where
...e practice, the post-
...room nurses love it.
...secure about the patients
...out their own responsibility.
...nurses can't go with *every* pa-
...ent, a nurse *should* at least accompany a high-risk patient—say, one with chest tubes. An orderly could accompany a patient less likely to develop difficulties.

In all cases, the recovery room nurse should call the medical/surgical unit and tell the staff the patient's on his way.

To remedy the situation in your hospital, try to get a sound policy in writing. Begin by finding out how the transfer of postoperative patients is handled in other hospitals in your area. Then document the risks of your hospital's current practice. Bring all this information to the attention of your immediate supervisor. If she doesn't take action, keep going up the chain of command. In calling attention to this risky nursing practice, you may get some flak.

Just tell yourself you're not *making* trouble—you're *preventing* it. If you need moral support, consult the Association of Operating Room Nurses, 10170 E. Mississippi Ave., Denver, CO 80231. They'll be able to help.

Should nurses carry out therapy ordered by respiratory therapists?

Q I work in the surgical intensive care unit of a Veterans Administration (VA) hospital that is about to make a disturbing change.

Until now, a doctor has been ordering all respiratory therapy for our patients, and we nurses have been *doing* the care, except for the setting up and checking of ventilators.

But now we're told a respiratory therapist (RT) will decide on treatment. That means we'll be participating in respiratory therapy ordered by an RT, but *not* cosigned by a doctor.

We don't consider this sound policy. Do you?

A No. In some hospitals, RTs operate with relative independence in setting up their equipment and administering treatments.

But in the situation you describe, an RT will be making the treatment decisions *and* prescribing the drugs, while depending on nurses to carry out the orders.

Where does that leave you?

In most states nurses give medication and treatment as prescribed or authorized by a person licensed to do so (an MD, DO, or DDS). Most VA hospitals will adhere to the nurse practice act of the state they're in. However, federal policy can vary.

Since your concerns seem to be well-grounded, why not take them up with your nursing and hospital administration? Involve someone in nursing education who has some clout—someone who would probably support your position.

Sure, an RT has an important part to play in patient care, but not if his part impinges on your nursing role and jeopardizes your license.

What can nurses do if they don't feel comfortable being unit managers?

Q For 11 years, I've been an instructor in the staff development department of a 600-bed hospital. Just recently, we've been told we're to rotate with the associate directors of nursing for administrative coverage on weekends and holidays.

Like most of the nurses in our department, I've never had nurse-manager or supervisory experience. Furthermore, because of the size of our hospital, we don't always know what's going on in other departments—or even if policies have been changed.

When I raised these objections with nursing administration, I was told "not to worry," an associate director would always be on call if any problems arose.

Any suggestions?

A If you're going to assume an administrative position, ask to attend all meetings that would be pertinent to these administrative duties. You must also make sure you're on the list to receive all memos and directives that might pertain to your administrative duties. And know where these memos are kept on file in the nursing office, too. You should have a list of all the key people who are on call that weekend—from the chief house officer on down.

Perhaps most important, you should make rounds on the Thursday and Friday before the weekend you are scheduled to work so you get your own "feeling of the house." Have the associate director who worked the previous weekend give you a rundown on what you can expect to meet on your tour of duty. Every system has its own quirks—maybe your hospital's turn up in the emergency department or the operating room on weekends. Just knowing that will help prepare you.

Despite all preparations, however, some questions are bound to arise and you'll be expected to come up with the answers. That's where you lean on your nursing education and experience. A large part of your professional life is making (and, in your case, teaching others how to make) good judgments. Here's where you'll be putting that background into practice.

As for the decisions you really aren't prepared to make—that's when you lean on your nursing administration's guarantee that there will be an associate director on call for just such situations.

What do you do when a supervisor assigns duties beyond a nurse's realm?

Q Our neonatal intensive care unit has a new supervisor determined to expand the role of nurses on the unit. While I'm comfortable with some of the changes she's implementing (nurses doing emergency endotracheal intubation, for instance), I'm concerned about some others. The supervisor sees no reason why nurses can't do bladder taps, umbilical arterial catheterizations, or needle aspiration of the chest. Are my reservations well-grounded, or am I making a mountain out of a molehill?

A You need to consult the nurse practice act in your own state. In your case, the Pennsylvania Board of Nursing *does* support nurses, like others, in intensive care units and emergency departments doing endotracheal intubation, *provided* they've been given the proper preparation, and *provided* they do the procedure under a competent supervisor. (The board does not, however, support nurses in other areas doing intubation as a routine procedure.)

But needle aspiration of the chest? Bladder taps? Umbilical arterial catheterizations? No way. The board views these as invasive procedures within the realm of medicine—not nursing.

Your best bet is to meet with other nurses and doctors on the unit and explain the board's views. You can then *all* agree that such procedures are best left to the doctors.

Job selection

Which would be the best position for a new graduate?

Q While in high school, I worked weekends and summers as a nursing assistant in a small hospital near home. I really enjoyed the people and the work, so I decided to become a nurse and take a BSN program in college.

> *"I have job offers from a large university hospital, a large county hospital, and my hometown hospital, but I'm not sure where to go."*

I graduate this summer and already have three job offers—one from a large university hospital, one from a large county hospital, and one from my hometown hospital. All things being equal, which would be the best move for a new graduate like me?

A Surely the welcome mat is out for you at all three hospitals. But all things are *not* going to be equal. You'll have to weigh each hospital's nurse-patient ratio, orientation and staff development programs, scheduling policy, salary offer, fringe benefits, and so on.

If none of these considerations tip your decision, maybe the small hospital where you had a happy work experience as a nursing assistant is your best bet. Being familiar with the physical setup and knowing how the hospital system works would help cushion the reality shock that so many new graduates experience. After you're "seasoned," you might consider moving to the university or county hospital if you decide that the larger scene has more to offer you professionally.

Job title

Does it affect the way others perceive authority?

Q A few weeks ago, I started working on a small specialty unit on a 3-month trial basis. Technically, I'm functioning as a unit manager; the job description I received was labeled unit manager, and my responsibilities are those of unit managers throughout the hospital. However, my title will be charge nurse because administration hasn't budgeted for a unit manager's salary. (My supervisor says she's willing to work with me in every other way. It took her a long time to fill the position, and she thinks I'm doing a great job.)

This may sound foolish, but I find I'm more disturbed about not having the proper job title than I am about the pay differential. It affects the way others perceive my authority and the way they respond to me. What do you think I should do?

A Stick to the arrangements you agreed to and wait until the trial period's over before you speak up. When your temporary status becomes permanent, and you've proven yourself on the job, you'll be in a better bargaining position for both the pay increase and the proper title.

In the meantime, use this settling-in period to hone your management skills. (Titles may grant authority, but your leadership skills earn your staff's respect and cooperation.) Get to know your coworkers; take time to meet ancillary personnel—respiratory therapists, X-ray and laboratory technicians; observe the movers and shakers at the hospital; and learn policies and procedures. Use one-on-one conversations and unit meetings with your staff to market yourself as the unit-manager-in-waiting. Discuss your goals for the department, your

J
K

ideas on delegating and problem solving. Let the staff know that you'll communicate their needs to administration and provide feedback on recommendations they've made. (It won't hurt to have them on your side.) Then, when the time is right, speak up.

Jurisdiction

Is it legal for nurses to accept orders from doctors who don't practice in the same state?

Q We are six RNs employed by a municipal health agency located practically on the border of where three states meet. We are expected to perform nursing procedures and administer medications that are ordered by doctors who do not personally practice in our state. We think this is illegal, but each of us has at some time approached our department head with this question only to have it brushed off with the unsatisfactory explanation, "Oh, everybody does it."

What are your thoughts on this?

A Ordinarily, the law does not allow a nurse to perform any nursing function based on an order signed by a physician who is not licensed in that jurisdiction. A few states, however, have so-called "border agreements" whereby an out-of-state doctor's orders or prescriptions can be fulfilled if he is licensed in a state that borders its own. If a state has no legislation to cover this situation, the attorney general is authorized to approve such a practice.

For definite information on the practice in your state, contact the state's attorney general or your local medical society.

If it turns out that you are *not* covered by the proper legalities, your health center should discon-

tinue the practice of taking orders from out-of-state doctors. Or it should have a local doctor countersign the orders.

Kerosene heaters

Can space heaters fueled by kerosene cause respiratory problems?

Q I recently read that air-pollutant particles released by wood-burning stoves can cause respiratory problems in small children. But what about space heaters fueled by kerosene?

A A kerosene heater can create an unhealthful level of air pollutants, particularly nitrogen and sulfur dioxides.

> *"I knew that wood-burning stoves could cause respiratory problems, but no one ever told me about space heaters."*

These pollutants probably won't cause a healthy adult any adverse reactions during short periods of exposure. But certain sensitive people should avoid even limited exposure: those with asthma, respiratory disease, allergies, angina, and very young children (because their lungs are sensitive and still developing).

Advise your patients that anyone using a kerosene heater should know the variables that affect pollution levels—room and heater size, ventilation, efficiency of room insulation, proper fuel grade. Emis-

sions can be minimized by following the manufacturer's operating specifications. One final caution: In some communities, portable kerosene heaters are illegal.

Kidnapping

Any suggestions for prevention?

Q Two months ago, a newborn was kidnapped from our nursery by a woman posing as a nurse. Luckily, the baby was found unharmed a few weeks later. We're still shaken by the incident—and reeling from the lawsuit filed by the baby's parents.

Our administrators are afraid this might happen again, so they want us to revise our nursing policies for the obstetrics unit. What advice can you give us that will help prevent kidnappings?

A Sadly, nursery kidnappings are an increasing threat. For the family and staff, the emotional fallout is devastating. And as you're finding out, security breaches can be costly for the hospital.

Several recent kidnappings have involved people dressed as nurses. One woman simply walked into a nursery and walked out with a baby. Another imposter entered a mother's room, identified herself as a nurse, and took the baby for "tests."

Vigilance is your best defense. Make sure you know the hospital's security policies and strictly adhere to them.

Here are some other ways to improve nursery security:
• *Identification.* Don't assume everyone in a white uniform or laboratory coat is a fellow employee. If you don't recognize someone, ask to see her identification badge. If she refuses to show it, call security immediately—don't try to take action yourself.

Of course, you should always wear *your* identification badge, too. Make a habit of introducing yourself to your patients and showing them your badge. Then ask them to call the nurses' station if anyone without a badge comes into their rooms.

• *Visitation.* An unwed mother can pose special problems. Because she probably has sole custody of her baby, the father doesn't have an automatic right to visit his child. So if a man shows up at the nursery and claims to be a baby's father, you must check with the mother first. She'll give the final word on who may see the baby.

• *Discharge.* You'd generally discharge a baby to his mother. But if she designates someone else to take the baby home, make sure you get written authorization witnessed by hospital personnel. Then carefully check the person's identification before releasing the baby.

Laboratory values

Is acting on them a nursing responsibility or a medical one?

Q A question about laboratory values came up at a recent nursing standards meeting. Some of our nurses think nurses should read a patient's lab values and act on them. Other nurses say that's a medical responsibility—and too much to ask of nurses. What do you say?

A Those *other nurses* must be older nurses, because reading laboratory values *used to be* strictly the doctor's responsibility. Today, though, most nurses consider lab values an essential part of the nursing assessment, particularly when the test results are obviously going to affect treatment. If a doctor orders hematocrit and hemoglobin tests for a GI bleeder, for example, the nurse caring for that patient should make sure the tests are done and notify the doctor if the results warrant it.

In some hospitals, the unit manager takes responsibility for tests, but, more often, staff nurses do. Because most labs list normal values next to the patient's actual values, nurses needn't memorize all the numbers.

Sounds as if your next staff meeting should define nursing assessment procedures and, perhaps, review the purpose of common laboratory tests. But tell the older nurses not to feel bad. Nursing's changing so fast, nobody's definition of nursing responsibility stays current for long.

Language barrier

When's an interpreter needed in obtaining consent?

Q I work in a hospital located near the waterfront, and some of our patients are sailors who don't speak English. Recently, when one of them needed surgery, a doctor and our surgical unit's nurse-manager persuaded him to sign a surgical consent form. They claimed he fully understood the proposed surgical procedure, and both of them signed the form as witnesses.

The more we nurses "talked" to the patient, the more we doubted he knew what lay ahead. We told the nurse-manager how we felt, but the patient had his surgery anyway without (in our opinion) ever fully knowing its reason or scope. Since then, we've wondered whether we should have insisted on getting an interpreter.

A The answer is yes. The informed consent doctrine requires that the patient be told about the care he's to get—unless he needs emergency care—so he can decide whether or not to accept it. And if you have to call in a translator to make sure the patient understands enough to give an informed consent, do it. There's a good chance this doctrine was violated in the case you describe. If the patient sues for malpractice, both the nurse-manager and the doctor could be charged with assault and battery.

So be prepared if this problem comes up again. Volunteer to research hospital records to find out how many non-English-speaking patients were admitted during the past year. What languages did they speak? Then enlist help from the hospital's auxiliary to sign up people in the community who'd be willing and able to volunteer as translators. Keep a list of their names and telephone numbers handy in your department.

Meanwhile, get yourself a copy of *Taber's Cyclopedic Medical Dictionary* edited by Clayton L. Thomas (16th ed. Philadelphia: F.A. Davis Co., 1988), which is available in plain and indexed versions. This book contains a section entitled "The Interpreter," which includes basic conversation needed for assessment, medical diagnosis, and treatment in French, German, Italian, and Spanish.

Lateness

What should be done about a nurse who's chronically late?

Q I supervise a nurse who's possibly the best nurse I'll ever get, but she is chronically late from 10 to 25 minutes every day. At each review, we discuss this; she promises to improve, is on time for 3 or 4 days, and then starts it all over again. Practically speaking, it's not a problem because she accomplishes more in her abbreviated day than any other member of my staff. But it is a problem for morale. Now, when others come in late, they resent being reprimanded. I hate to lose this good worker, but I don't know what to do.

A You can't close your eyes to the bad effect this woman's behavior is having on your staff...but wouldn't it be a crime to lose a paragon of nursing because of one aberration?

You've already talked to her about this at review time without altering her behavior. And *talking*—no matter how well intentioned on both sides—probably never will. Chronic lateness is too often related to a deep-seated psychological problem.

> *"She's possibly the best nurse I'll ever get, but she's 10 to 25 minutes late every day."*

So if you can't change *her,* how about changing her *schedule?* Possibly because of nursing's historical connection with the military and religious disciplines, we sometimes exhibit a certain rigidity of thought. Where is it written that we can nurse only from 7 to 3, 3 to 11, or 11 to 7? Why can't you have her contract with the hospital to come in a half hour later and stay a half hour later? A certain staggering of personnel could work to everyone's benefit. Be prepared, though. The original psychological problem could cause her to begin coming in late on her new hours, too. If so, hang loose. Make a definite understanding with her that for every minute—10 or 25—that she comes late, she stays that much later. The other personnel can't feel cheated so long as she's putting in the stan-

dard amount of time. And the patients won't be deprived of the care of "possibly the best nurse" you have working for you.

Law practice

Are many jobs available for nurse-attorneys?

Q For 11 years, nursing was my life—until a violent patient attacked me, injuring my back and ending my days as an active nurse. At first I was devastated, but time heals. Now, with renewed optimism, I've decided that I'd like to become a nurse-attorney. That way, my years of experience won't be wasted, and I can help patient-clients. But I'm not sure how to get started. Are many jobs available for nurse-attorneys? I'd appreciate some advice.

A You're a spunky lady. And it's great you were able to bounce back, rethink your goals, and move forward.

To start: Get a copy of the *Pre-Law Handbook Official Law School Guide,* published by Educational Testing Service. This paperback has the information you'll need. The Law School Admission Test (LSAT) is usually a requirement; you might find an LSAT study course worth the expense. Take the test before you apply to law school; apply to at least three schools. The field is wide open now for nurse-attorneys. They generally represent clients in nurse-licensing disputes and malpractice and product liability cases. They can also be risk managers, insurance claim specialists, legal auditors, or consultants for hospitals, health care corporations, related businesses, and so on.

Why not talk with a nurse-attorney in your area? Check the yellow pages of your phone book, or contact the American Association of Nurse-Attorneys, an active organization, for the name of a nurse-at-

torney near you. Their address: Dept. N89, 113 W. Franklin St., Baltimore, MD 21201.

Lawsuits

Are there warning signs to watch for?

Q One of my co-workers was just sued for negligence. We were taken completely by surprise, because the patient hadn't seemed unhappy with her care. So now we're wondering: Do patients who are likely to sue give warning signs we should watch for?

A Although not every unhappy patient sues, most who do give fair warning by:
• questioning everything
• complaining habitually
• requesting their charts just before being discharged
• asking for the names of their nurses
• taking notes of discussions with nurses and doctors
• continually behaving in an uncooperative, combative, or noncompliant manner.

When you're assigned to a patient like this, you may be tempted to run the other way. But don't. Instead, be especially polite and professional when you care for him. Going the extra mile now could head off a lawsuit down the road.

If a patient or a family member just can't be satisfied, contact the hospital's risk manager and ask administration to intervene. Patients are less likely to sue when their fears and complaints are acknowledged and dealt with promptly.

Can the doctor sue a nurse if she doesn't follow his demand?

Q I'm a charge nurse in a small community hospital where everyone knows everyone else. My problem involves a doctor who admits many patients to our unit and a nursing assistant who works on the unit.

The assistant's husband recently filed suit against the doctor on her behalf, and now the doctor is demanding that we assign the other two assistants to his patients. (The assistant gives excellent patient care and never discusses the case with co-workers or patients.)

The administration says the doctor has no right to demand this, but when I reported this to him, he told me I'd better check with a lawyer. Needless to say, all my nursing assistants are watching to see what I'll do.

Can the doctor sue me if I don't follow his demand?

A This is one of those situations where the facts only confuse the issue. A doctor prefers two of the nursing assistants over a third. This fact seems to suggest a simple response: When convenient, try to assign the third nursing assistant to other doctors' patients.

Because of the upcoming lawsuit, small-town gossip has no doubt divided people into two camps—pro-doctor or pro-assistant. And the hospital's pecking order has no doubt turned this into a David versus Goliath contest, with all the David supporters (your assistants) wondering if you'll stand up to Goliath.

Legally, of course, you don't have any problems if you follow your administration's policy in this matter. But in your daily life, you're going to have a hard time no matter what you do.

Call a meeting of all your assistants, including the one involved, and tell them all the facts. Discuss your options and ask their help in weighing the pros and cons of each one.

Such a meeting will help nip any rumors in the bud—you can be sure they're growing by the minute—and will help your assistants see all sides of the problem no matter what you decide.

Is the doctor taking chances?

Q In the small-town practice where I work, we test whole families for everything from bug bites to major psychological problems, so naturally, the doctor-patient relationship is quite personal. What worries me—make that *amazes* me—is the naivete of the young (and attractive) doctor associate.

When women come in for breast and internal examinations, he sometimes asks me to be present, but sometimes not—depending on how busy we are, how well he knows the woman, and so on. I took him aside and told him that in this age of lawsuits, one of the women could misconstrue his intentions, and without my being present he'd have only his word against hers. He just laughed and said, "Aw, c'mon, everybody knows I'm married and a good guy. You're just being old-fashioned." I don't think so, do you?

A Not really. Anyone who picks up a newspaper or watches TV knows that professionals are prime targets for lawsuits. Any charges of sexual impropriety (even if they're off the wall and later proven false) can ruin a doctor's reputation and his practice. Having a nurse present during breast and internal exams is professional and just makes good sense.

And who asks the *patient's* opinion? Even though the exams may be business as usual for the doctor, many women (who'd never have the nerve to speak up on their own) find them embarrassing and traumatic. Given the choice, they'd appreciate having another female present.

Unfortunately, you can't order the doctor to change the way he runs his practice—and he already knows how you feel. What you can change

is the scheduling of patients so that you won't seem too busy to be present in the examining room during the gynecologic exams.

Laxatives

How will the medication go down when a feeding tube's in place?

Q One doctor on our staff orders 1 teaspoon of psyllium hydrophilic mucilloid (Metamucil) for his patients who are recovering from a cardiovascular accident. However, because these patients usually are on fluid restriction to decrease their intracranial pressure, he insists that we use no more than 30 ml of water to dissolve the Metamucil. That isn't enough water to help the patient swallow. And if the patient has a nasogastric tube, using this small amount of water creates a real problem. Despite rapid mixing and trying to quickly force the mixture down with a syringe plunger, the small-diameter feeding tubes get plugged and must be replaced.

Our complaints to the doctor have gotten nowhere. What do you say?

A Go back to the doctor and ask him to order a different laxative. Psyllium isn't appropriate for patients on fluid restriction.

Here's why: The manufacturer recommends a daily dose of 1 teaspoon Metamucil in a full glass of water up to three times a day. As a bulk-forming laxative, psyllium absorbs water from the gastrointestinal tract and expands. This increases bulk and moisture content of the stool and encourages normal peristalsis and bowel motility.

So you can see that this laxative just isn't right for these patients. In fact, according to some reports, using a bulk-forming laxative without enough fluid can cause esophageal blockage and intestinal impaction.

L

Leadership

Is there any way to build confidence for team leadership?

Q I've resigned from two hospitals and one convalescent home because I lack the confidence for the team leadership that's expected of me. I have very good references as far as patient care is concerned, but as a team leader, I'm a flop.

Although I'm licensed as an RN in two states, I've thought about becoming an LPN so someone else will have to be the leader. Is this possible for an RN?

A Being in a position where you have to direct others obviously makes you uncomfortable. But after all your education, stepping down in the chain of command seems to be the simple, but wrong, solution.

Instead, first pinpoint what it is about leading a team that gets you so uptight. Is it the *leading* itself or having to criticize others?

If it's the leading, perhaps you're not sure enough of your own skills. You have to be pretty confident of your own ability before you can give orders with confidence. If it's the criticizing, ask yourself why this makes you so uncomfortable. Perhaps you may have trouble accepting criticism and think others will react the same way. Why don't you get someone you trust—perhaps one of your former teachers or supervisors—to honestly assess your skills? If you do need improvement, take a refresher course or ask your staff development office for help.

What's a good way to assert leadership and meet a challenge to authority?

Q I'm the newly appointed unit manager of a 68-bed medical/surgical unit in a suburban hospital, and I'm having a problem I'm sure

other unit managers have experienced. I'm talking about the problem of informal "leaders"—staff members who assume unofficial leadership positions.

I was brought in from the outside and now find that two old-timers are challenging my authority. One's an LPN who's worked on this unit for almost 10 years. The other's a seasoned staff nurse who, I hear, had hoped to become unit manager herself. These two women question my decisions and judgment, keep my policies from being carried out—and generally undermine my authority.

I know I *should* be in full control of the situation, but I feel threatened by these women. What would you suggest I do to assert my leadership and meet this challenge to my authority?

A You're obviously facing a difficult situation. You're new on the job, and you come from "the outside." You were bound to arouse some resentment.

You're also dealing with the threat of change. Management specialists have found that any staff will resist change when that change is major. Established workers equate change with some form of loss—whether the facts support that feeling or not. Unsettled, and threatened by the change, some staff members will attempt to support and strengthen the remnants of the old organization.

The emergence of your two "informal leaders" is a natural outgrowth of resistance to change.

What's the resolution?

It's never easy to satisfy "old staff," but try the following:
1. Look at your appointment through the eyes of your staff members. Their concern, anger, and hostility will be less threatening—once you've seen it *their* way.
2. Include the would-be leaders in the new changes. If you want to win them over, ask for *their* suggestions. And by all means praise any good ones. (And use the suggestions, if you can.)

3. Ask yourself if other stress factors in the situation may be provoking additional dissension.
4. Discuss the situation at length with all of those involved. Be direct and open. Talking it out is still the best way to let off steam—and to put the problem into a more sensible, less emotional perspective.

Once the problem's been aired, your informal leaders will no longer have their secret, tensive environment in which to operate. They'll back down or back away.

And if the staff sees your ability to handle conflict and tension with authority and common sense, they'll begin to have confidence in you and to acknowledge your role as unit manager. They'll react to you as boss because you're *being* the boss.

Liability

Can a nurse be held liable if a boxer she examines becomes ill during a match?

Q I'm a full-time hospital nurse, but to earn extra money, I do prematch physicals for a local boxing team. Before the last match, I discovered that two of the boxers had elevated blood pressures. Naturally, I recorded my findings and advised the men not to fight. But when I told the coach, he just asked the men to rest for a while before fighting.

After the men had rested, I took their blood pressures again, and the readings *were* lower. But I was a nervous wreck during the match, wondering what had caused the blood pressures to rise in the first place and worrying if the boxers would be okay. (Luckily, there were no problems.)

If this should happen again, I need your advice. Can I be held liable if a boxer becomes ill during a match? I have malpractice insurance *only* for hospital duty.

A If one of the boxers had become ill during the match he *might've* tried to sue you for malpractice. But unless you were actually *negligent* (which you weren't), he probably couldn't win the case. You really did do all you could.

Don't be lulled into a false sense of security, though. In a malpractice case, nobody's really secure. You already know that your insurance *won't* cover you unless you're working in the hospital. You'd better check with the state boxing commission: Maybe you're covered under their insurance plan. If you're not, you'll obviously need to get your own malpractice insurance.

But insurance aside, why would you want to continue working with this uncooperative coach? You and the coach seem to be in separate corners concerning what's best for the boxers, so try finding another moonlighting job—before *you* and the *coach* end up in a boxing match of your own.

Was it wrong to give a fellow nurse a shot of trimethobenzamide?

Q I can't believe what I did! An LPN on our unit came up to me the other night and told me she was nauseated and didn't think she could finish the shift. She asked me to give her a shot of trimethobenzamide (Tigan). She was already holding it in her hand. I took the trimethobenzamide from her and gave her the injection.

I don't know what I could have been thinking of at the time, but now I'm worried about what I did. I *know* I'll use better judgment in the future, but I'd like to hear what you think of this situation.

A You didn't mention any adverse reaction in your coworker, so you're probably in the clear. But from the wringing-hands tone of your letter, obviously you realize what you did was not desirable, to put it mildly.

You should certainly have asked her where the drug came from and when it was prescribed for her. The drug *could have* made the LPN dizzy or drowsy, and not in a condition to be working on the unit.

In the future, avoid such incidents by refusing to administer a drug without a doctor's order. If this nurse approaches you again to give her a drug, refuse and suggest that she go to the emergency department or employee health service or consult a doctor. It's the only way to give your professionalism the shot in the arm it clearly needs.

Who's liable if a nurse-orientee commits a negligent act?

Q Last week, we received a memo from administration asking nurses from our unit to volunteer as preceptors for the clinical orientation of new employees. Many of us would like to be preceptors—it seems like a great way to build team spirit. But we're wondering who's liable if a nurse-orientee commits a negligent act. Can you address this concern for us?

A The extent of your responsibility depends on how structured the orientation program is. If the nursing education department manages the program, your responsibility as a preceptor will be limited to answering the orientee's questions in the actual clinical setting and pointing out where equipment is located. The education department supervisors will be accountable for the orientee's actions. (Of course, the orientee is also responsible for her own actions, just as any nurse would be.) However, if there's no formal orientation program where you work and you agree to act as preceptor, you could share some legal responsibility for the orientee's errors.

You can certainly save yourself a lot of problems by finding out exactly what administration has in mind— before you volunteer.

Would a nurse be held liable if a former X-ray technician acted as a nurse?

Q I'm working in a doctor's office with a former X-ray technician who's acting as a nurse, even though she's not. Twenty years ago, the doctor took her under his wing and taught her to assist him in the office. She dresses like a nurse and performs the same duties I do: handing out drug samples, answering questions, making nursing judgments, and even administering allergy injections.

I'm concerned about my legal liability if she makes an error. What should I do?

A If you're willing to risk your job, you could report her to the local prosecutor or the state's nursing board. As long as she continues to perform functions limited to nursing or medicine, she could be fined or jailed. And because she's presenting herself as a nurse, she'd be held to the same nursing standards you would in a malpractice lawsuit.

Unfortunately, you and the doctor are at risk, too: Anyone who knowingly supervises or employs someone who's posing as a nurse could be fined or jailed. And your license is in jeopardy, because you're aiding and abetting unlicensed nursing practice.

But you can easily remedy this situation by redefining your coworker's role in the office. For instance, she could still take patient histories, but she should refer questions to you or the doctor. She could give out premeasured, premarked medications if ordered, but she shouldn't give injections. Of course, she could still do X-rays.

The point is to eliminate any tasks that only a nurse can legally perform. Then you can supervise her without getting into trouble.

Would a nurse be responsible for a monitor technician's negligence?

Q The 12 monitors on our 49-bed telemetry unit are supposed to be watched continuously by technicians who have been trained to detect arrhythmias. Recently, a doctor discovered—too late to call a code—that one of my patients had died. When I asked the technician why she hadn't noticed, she said, "He was off the monitor. One of his leads had fallen off."

Now I'm concerned about my liability if the family sues for wrongful death. Am I responsible for the technician's negligence? By the way, hospital administrators took no action against her and she's still on the job.

A Hospital administrators have put you in a difficult position professionally. As you know, you're responsible for all aspects of patient care, so you could share liability—even though administrators delegated one aspect of care to someone else. Still, they should bear primary responsibility.

To ease the nursing shortage or cut costs, many hospitals now use unlicensed personnel to perform traditional nursing duties. In the process, they may jeopardize patient safety. So if your patient's family sued, the lawyer would probably focus on the hospital's role, arguing that administrators were negligent for using technicians who were unqualified—and unlicensed—to perform a nursing duty.

What can you do to minimize your own risks in the future? Carefully assess each of your patients at regular intervals and document your findings. Make sure the technicians know they should notify you if a patient is "off the monitor." In other words, keep on top of the situation, even if the hospital has delegated certain nursing duties to someone else.

License

How can an LVN get licensed by endorsement?

Q Two of my married children want me to move away from California, where I've been working for over 25 years, and live with one of them—one is in Nevada, the other in Arizona. I'm tempted, but I don't want to give up working as an LVN. And I also don't want to take a board exam over again after all these years. So I guess my decision hinges on whether I can get licensing by endorsement in either of these states. What are my chances?

A If you took your licensing exam in California before March 1974, you can get licensing by endorsement in both Arizona and Nevada.

Why that date? Because California used its own state exam from March 1974 through October 1986 instead of the national licensing exam. So any LVN who took her board exam during that period must retake the national board exam for licensing in either Arizona or Nevada.

So what's a mother to do? Even Solomon might have to think twice before making the choice you're faced with. When you do decide, get the licensing paperwork done early.

Is it legal to give a relative narcotic injections without a license in the state?

Q I've just moved from Indiana to Florida. My mother-in-law, who's terminally ill with cancer, will be moving in with us soon. I'll be administering her pain medication, an injectable narcotic. I have a current nursing license from Indiana, but not from Florida because I don't plan to work in this state. Am I taking a legal risk?

A Relax. You'll be acting as a family member who's a caregiver, not as a nurse. What you'll be doing won't be considered the practice of nursing. These days, many patients have family members who administer premeasured, injectable drugs. Your mother-in-law needs narcotics to ease her pain, and her doctor would prescribe them regardless of her caregiver's professional status.

One more thing, though: You might want to apply for a Florida license if neighbors start asking for your advice about their medical problems—and you start giving it. Although you don't intend to actively practice nursing, you could get into trouble if you present yourself as a nurse and your advice later causes a mishap.

What happens if a nurse gives nursing care over the state line?

Q I sometimes accompany a patient being transferred to a hospital in Washington, D.C., across the Maryland state line. I don't have a D.C. license, so what happens if I give nursing care to this patient while we're in Washington? Am I violating the nurse practice act? And whose orders should I follow if emergency care's needed en route—the doctor at the hospital we left or the one we're going to?

A Don't worry. As long as you're just bringing a patient to Washington, D.C. and returning home, your Maryland license will cover you during transit. Such incidental professional service is recognized as a necessary part of your work and not as any personal intent to violate the practice act.

While en route, you should accept orders only from the doctor who dispatched the patient from Maryland. The patient remains his responsibility until the transfer's completed.

License reinstatement

How can a nurse get her license back if she forgot to renew it?

Q I've been so busy having babies and running my house that I forgot to renew my nursing license. While my problem's far less serious than the problem of having a license revoked, I have a problem, nonetheless.

How difficult will it be to get my license back and what steps do I need to take?

A Typically, to get a lapsed license renewed you must take the following three steps:
• Fill out a new application.
• Pay the required reinstatement fee (currently $45, but always subject to change). With the payment of this fee, you'll have the privilege of renewing your license for a second year *without charge*. At the end of the 2-year period, you'll then pay the usual renewal fee (currently $20) every 2 years.
• Meet the state board of nursing requirements at the time of your reapplication. These requirements are still being formulated, but there's talk of requiring the nurse with a lapsed license to take a refresher course or else retake the entire nursing exam.

If you move out of your state at any time, keep in mind that regulations vary from one state to another. Call the state nursing association in your new state for exact details.

You should be able to get your license renewed without a hitch. Better mark the next expiration deadline on your calendar. Or perhaps you should tie a string on your finger or a ribbon on one of the babies to remind yourself that E day (expiration day) is approaching.

Is there any advantage in maintaining a license in one state after moving to a new one?

Q I recently moved back to this state after working elsewhere as a nurse for more than 25 years. I thought I could get my license quickly and get a job immediately because I was originally licensed here 30 years ago. Wrong.

I've had to wait longer—and pay more—to reactivate my original license than I would have to get a new one. I waited 10 weeks for the wheels of bureaucracy to turn, and I lost out on several jobs.

I have a good job now, but this experience set me to wondering. Is there an advantage to maintaining a license in a state where you never plan on practicing again? And how long should it take to get a license? Any words on this?

A Your letter is a caution to all nurses: When you first start thinking about moving to another state, think first about applying for licensure—and mail early.

Getting a license by endorsement usually takes 4 to 6 weeks—about half the time it took to have your license renewed.

Before moving out of state again (whether or not you plan to return), have your name added to the inactive file, where it can remain for 5 years without charge. Anytime within that period, you can come back and activate your license without delay.

License revocation

Can a doctor revoke a nurse's license by making one phone call?

Q Twice within this past year, the medical director of our emergency department (ED) has threatened to have a certain staff nurse's license revoked.

He made the first threat when the nurse couldn't give an injection as scheduled because his written orders weren't clear; the second threat came when the nurse simply disagreed with him. On both occasions, the doctor claimed he could have the nurse's license revoked by making one telephone call to the state board of nursing.

Is he trying to intimidate our colleague, or can he really do what he says?

A The threats are empty. There's no way a doctor can have a nurse's license taken away "with one telephone call."

Look at it this way: If you had a legitimate complaint about a doctor, you'd take it through appropriate hospital channels first. If a doctor thinks he has grounds for a complaint against a nurse, he should also take *his* complaint through hospital channels. You do *not* take an inside problem to an outside agency without going through the hospital channels first.

Revocation of a nursing license is a serious step, used as a sanction only against those nurses who act unprofessionally or who disregard the state's nurse practice act.

If the doctor was hell-bent on acting against a nurse, he'd have to put his complaint in writing and have it notarized. The amount of paperwork involved could easily stop him early on—even if he had far better grounds for complaint than you've indicated in your letter.

However, if the doctor persisted and filed the claim, the state nursing board would investigate the nurse's side of the story fully. If the board concluded that the complaint was invalid or trivial, they'd dismiss the case. Afterward, there'd be absolutely no indication on the nurse's record that a complaint had ever been filed.

This information should set your mind at ease. The nurse in question, along with the rest of your nursing staff, would do well to reexamine the problem. Although the doctor

L

can't get a license revoked, as he contends, he can *still* make trouble for the nurse within the hospital. So tell her—or any nurse in a similar position—that for her own protection, she should document any run-ins she may have with him.

Can it be revoked for taking antidepressant drugs from a patient's medication drawer?

Q For the past year, I've worked double shifts when asked, come in on my days off, and skipped vacation time. My manager gave me glowing evaluations for my patient care and for pitching in when we were understaffed.

All that overtime has taken its toll. In 3 months, I've lost 45 pounds and look terrible; I'm so tired that all I do is sleep when I'm home. My teenage son doesn't need me anymore; I'm lonely and depressed. To make matters worse, I'm in trouble at work. Yesterday, I felt so down that, for the first time in my life, I took some antidepressant drugs from a patient's medication drawer. The director of nursing found out, and now I'm terrified I'll lose my license and my job. The sad truth is I have no real identity except as a nurse.

Any words of advice?

A Get back to the director of nursing right away (ask your manager to come along for backup and support) and tell her your story. She has your time sheets and evaluations at hand; one look at them—and you—should convince her that you need help more than discipline.

See your doctor for a complete physical to rule out medical causes for your depression and weight loss. Ask him to recommend a psychologist or psychiatrist. On your own, try some diversions: Take a short trip for a change of scene, start an exercise program, plan some activity (as simple as a card game) once

or twice a month with your son or someone you'd like to be friends with.

On the professional side, if you're called before the state nursing board, remember that the board members are human; they'll listen to you. Because substance addiction isn't involved, they may recommend psychiatric counseling with temporary suspension (not revocation) of your license until the counselor says you're able to return to work.

Back at work, know that you're only one person and there's a limit to what you can do. Know, too, that you're a worthwhile person for yourself, not just when others need you. Once you feel good about yourself, your relationships—on the job and at home—will become more satisfying.

Under what circumstances could a license be revoked?

Q Recently I've been hearing a lot about nurses losing their licenses. I consider myself a good nurse—I've been on the same medical/surgical unit for 5 years now—but tell me: Under what circumstances could my license be revoked?

A You'll probably never need this information for your own use—nevertheless, you're wise to ask. License revocations usually follow this scenario.

A complaint against you from a patient, an employer, a co-worker, the police, or the boards of medicine and pharmacy can cause your state board of nursing to begin license revocation procedures against you.

One study found the largest proportion of complaints against nurses involved drugs—drugs diverted from patients, stolen from hospital stores, or procured by forged prescriptions.

The next largest group of complaints involves patient neglect.

Less frequent complaints include verbal and physical abuse of patients, alcohol abuse, practicing with an expired license, criminal convictions, and so on.

Any complaint received by the board of nursing against you would be recorded and reviewed. The department of licensing and regulation and the attorney general's office would work with the board of nursing in investigating the complaint. If a probable violation is found, the attorney general's office would draft an official complaint for the board of nursing. The board would in turn send it to you via certified mail.

Because you must respond to the complaint within 20 days (with appropriate supporting documents), at this point you'd be wise to engage a skilled lawyer. (However, neither the state nor the nursing board *requires* you to retain counsel.) Also, you might present your case later at an informal conference and formal hearing.

Ideally, once you've told your story, the charges will be dismissed. However, because the board of nursing screens complaints thoroughly before filing its own complaint, dismissal of the charges is rare. Generally, the board of nursing or the hearing examiner will impose sanctions—possibly a reprimand, probation, suspension, or revocation of license.

Revocation of a license, which means losing the privilege to practice, is permanent—with no right to an automatic reinstatement. After a given length of time (and a hearing) you may apply for a new license, but you must then retake the state board examination.

Losing your license might not be the end of your troubles. You could face criminal action and perhaps even a malpractice suit—both separate and distinct from the license proceeding. A complaint against a nurse can open a series of possibilities: all undesirable, all to be avoided.

One final word to the wise: Become familiar with your state nurse practice act's definition of your proper nursing role. Your best protection against losing your license is well-informed "preventive nursing."

Lie-detector test

Could it find someone guilty when she's actually innocent?

Q Last week, while I held the narcotics keys, I made an honest mistake that's being blown all out of proportion. When I counted the narcotics, one vial of morphine was missing; I recorded that, but I should have reported it, too. Something distracted me and I just plain forgot.

Now the security people are bullying me. They want me to take a lie-detector test to "rule me out" as a suspect because, as they put it, "Your hand was in the box." It doesn't help me any that I'm a fairly new employee and not well-known.

Although my supervisor's on my side, she says any drug investigation is security's territory, and they're up in arms because there have been so many narcotics missing in other departments. That makes me nervous, plus I'm afraid that the lie-detector test could find me "guilty" even though I'm innocent. What do you say about this?

A You probably don't have to worry about the lie-detector test. Congress passed a law, effective December 27, 1988, that virtually bans lie-detector testing of private-sector employees. It is allowed in certain circumstances, but according to a *Lawyers Alert* report, there are so many restrictions that an employer probably won't have enough incentive to go ahead with it. The potential for lawsuits is too great. One restriction: a lie-detector test can't be used to rule out an employee who might have been involved in a theft when there's no further evidence available.

Another says an employee can't be disciplined for refusing to take a test—or for showing positive results—unless there's additional supporting evidence of his guilt (a potential jury issue).

You should let the nursing administration know how you've been treated by the security department. Ask them to stand with you—then see if the bullies back off.

Life support

Can't nurses be more compassionate?

Q Last week, a comatose patient's daughter decided to terminate his life-support system. Although she wanted to stay with him while we disconnected the ventilator, my manager said it would be too upsetting and asked her to leave. Then the doctor disconnected the machine and left the room with my nurse-manager. All he said was, "Call us when he stops breathing."

I was stunned. Why can't we treat dying patients and their families with more compassion?

A After making such a difficult decision, your patient's daughter needed to be supported and included, not ignored or dismissed. And she had every right to stay with her father if she wished.

Here's a similar case handled with more compassion:

A 78-year-old man had gone into cardiopulmonary arrest. He was intubated, stabilized, and brought to an intensive care unit. A week later, he was still unconscious. Eventually, after consulting with neurologists and cardiologists, his doctor diagnosed a persistent vegetative state.

The doctor told the patient's son that his father had only a remote chance of regaining consciousness. A few days later, the son decided to terminate life support.

After discussing his decision with him, the staff was convinced that

he was making the request with his father's best interests in mind. He felt his father would have made the same decision.

Before turning off the ventilator, the nurses told him his father might continue breathing on his own. He understood. They wrote a description of the conversation in the progress notes and had him sign it. They asked if he wanted to be in the room when the machine was disconnected. He didn't, so he returned home and waited for a call.

The nurses went into the patient's room with the attending doctor and resident. In case the patient could hear, they told him that they were going to take the tube out of his throat, then turn off the ventilator. During the half hour that he continued breathing, they stayed with him, talking in soft voices and holding his hands. They let him know that they were there and that he was loved by his son.

As his breathing faltered, they repeated over and over that he was loved. He took his last breath with those words filling the room.

After the doctor pronounced him dead, they called the son and described what they'd said and done. He seemed thankful to hear that his father died peacefully.

In a bereavement call several days later, they learned that the son was grieving but comfortable with his decision. He thanked the staff for supporting him and his father, and for allowing his father to die with dignity. He also said he was relieved that his father hadn't been left alone—and grateful that the last words his father heard were that he was loved.

Should a nurse comply with the patient's wishes?

Q As a critical care nurse, I recently admitted a 75-year-old man who'd had his fourth myocardial infarction. Both he and his wife told me they didn't want heroic

L

measures if complications developed. I wrote that on his chart.

Before I had a chance to talk with his doctor, the man stopped breathing. Immediately, a resident intubated him and asked me to get a ventilator ready. I refused, relating the conversation I'd had with the patient and his wife. The resident pushed me aside and got one of my co-workers to help him.

I'm wondering now if I did the right thing.

A By charting what the patient told you and informing the resident, you respected the patient's right to decide what treatment he wanted—and what he'd refuse. But you should have asked his doctor to write a do-not-resuscitate order.

You also could have asked this patient if he'd signed a living will or durable power of attorney. If he had, you could have made a copy of the document and attached it to his chart. This would have given weight to your assertion that the patient didn't want heroic measures.

Should a nurse talk over other options with the family?

Q Recently, I had a patient who experienced cardiogenic shock and cardiac arrest while recovering from coronary artery bypass surgery. She was resuscitated with difficulty and placed on a ventilator. In the following weeks, she experienced one complication after another and her prognosis worsened. Yet her doctor continued to treat her aggressively. Eventually, after many painful weeks, she died.

As I watched her steady decline, I saw her son become more depressed and withdrawn. I wanted to sit with him and discuss the option of withholding treatment. But I'd been working on the intensive care unit for only 6 months, and I was reluctant to say too much.

Although months have passed, I'm still troubled by my failure to act. What should I do if a similar situation arises in the future?

A Your sad experience illustrates the importance of early patient and family assessments. In the future, you can try to make sure family members (and the patient, if he's able) understand all treatment options early in his hospitalization and explore how they feel about prolonged life support. Ask questions like these:
• "What do you know about your loved one's illness and the plan for his care?
• "Do you have any questions about the course of the illness, including possible complications?
• "If your loved one takes a turn for the worse, what do you want us to do? For example, would you want us to initiate artificial life support? (Explain life support in terms they can understand.)
• "Who should be involved in deciding your loved one's treatment now and in the future?" (Their answer may tell you how involved they want to be in the decision-making process.)

Share what you learn in an interdisciplinary meeting. And throughout the patient's hospitalization, work to maintain good communication between his caregivers and his family. In situations like these, everyone needs support.

Lonely patient

How can a nurse help?

Q One of my patients is a nice, elderly widow. She has five grown children, all of whom live reasonably close. In the 2 weeks she's been here, she's had several short visits from one daughter. The other children don't even call her on the phone. My patient is depressed and becoming more so since her roommate has eight children who visit their mother daily

and call frequently just to chat. I'd welcome suggestions.

A You can't hope to improve relations that may have deteriorated over half a century. Nor can you discount the possibility that the children have legitimate commitments that keep them away. But you can try several tactics. First, tell the patient's doctor about the situation. If he doesn't know the family well enough to intervene, ask permission to call the daughter who visited. Urge her to tell the rest of the family that their mother's well-being depends on them.

> *"My patient is depressed and becoming more so since her roommate has eight children who visit their mother daily."*

If you sense that your patient gets depressed at seeing her roommate surrounded by eight doting children, why not move your patient? Try a roommate that might make her feel needed—possibly an older patient more alone than she is, or a younger one who could use some "mothering."

If that isn't practical, talk to her present roommate's family. Their concern for their own mother suggests they might be willing to share part of their visits and conversation with your patient.

Patients have all sorts of social problems, and obviously you can't solve them all. But you can try to help.

Where, for example, is it written that nurses must take their coffee break anywhere but in the patient's room? Ask different members of the staff to share morning or afternoon breaks with the patient.

If she is well enough, you might ask the patient to help you—making up new charts, delivering mail. Contact your volunteer or social services office. They're likely to have some activity—knitting, painting—to interest her.

Equally important, stay your own warm, concerned self. It doesn't take words to tell a patient you care.

LPN image

Why isn't it better?

Q Four years ago, after working very hard in my LPN program, I finished with a 3.9 grade point average and scored very high on the LPN state boards. Since then, while working in nursing homes, I've had patients tell me they wanted "a real nurse" to take care of them, which is very discouraging. Where did the attitude that LPNs aren't real nurses come from, and how can I combat it?

A The image problem you're experiencing isn't universal. In fact, in many areas of the country, LPNs are enhancing their image through expanded practice. (For example, the boards of nursing in both New York and Pennsylvania have allowed LPNs with the proper preparation and supervision to administer I.V. therapy.) As the president of the National Federation of Licensed Practical Nurses (NFLPN) said in a recent editorial, "The nursing profession is changing, and its members are all working out new identities to go with new responsibilities." And as we predict for the nineties, LPNs and RNs will become increasingly sophisticated in their practice, better compensated, and more appreciated.

You and your co-workers should work on positive public relations at the nursing home and in your community. Why not suggest having an LPN Appreciation Day? You might distribute printed sheets to the residents with information about the LPNs on staff, highlighting their experience, education, and the work they do. Then get some of this information to the general public by submitting items to your local newspaper.

To help enhance your practice, ask the administrator to arrange more staff development programs, including some sessions at an area hospital covering new procedures you're now allowed to perform. And don't forget that networking is a great source of support. Keep in touch with what LPNs are doing in other states by joining NFLPN (which recently celebrated its 40th year), P.O. Box 18088, Dept. N90, Raleigh, NC 27619.

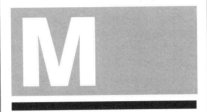

Male student

How can a male student nurse find a role model?

Q Although I share in the camaraderie typical of students, I'm the only male in my nursing class. I haven't any role models to identify with—not even another man to compare notes with in this female-dominated profession.

Any suggestions?

A Try this. When you're sent on clinical assignments as part of your program, look for a male on staff who can empathize. Then keep in touch with him, even if your assignment changes to a new hospital.

Meanwhile, don't become too preoccupied with finding a male role model. What you can look for are *qualities* to admire and emulate that are neither sex- nor role-specific. Qualities such as courage of conviction, initiative, curiosity, assertiveness, modesty, stick-to-itiveness, compassion, efficiency, and so forth.

Come to think of it, someone with enough grit to hang in there as a singular presence already has stick-to-itiveness and courage to boot.

Management

How can a recent graduate nurse prove she's management material?

Q I recently finished a BSN program at night and plan to continue working full-time in the same pediatric unit where I've worked part-time over the past 5 years. My goal is to move into a nurse-manager position as soon as one opens. I actively participate in our staff meetings, have good clinical skills, and have always received good evaluations. How else can I prove that I'm management material?

A You'll need better-than-average organizational ability and interpersonal skills, which you can demonstrate every day in the way you go about your work, do your charting, and get along with patients and others in your department.

Your chances for promotion will be better if you can also answer yes to the following: Do you take on new tasks without griping? Do you function with minimum supervision once you're comfortable with an assignment? Do you delegate fairly? Are you willing to help or teach newcomers on the unit? Can you handle supervising your friends? Can you accept and follow constructive criticism without rancor?

Are you still in the game? Then think of joining your state nursing and specialty associations, and start networking. Also consider attending some management classes at your community college.

Remember, the more you can exhibit the skills a nurse-manager needs, the better your chances.

Is hiring a nonnurse director wise?

Q Our hospital administrator's toying with the idea of hiring a nonnurse director of nursing. He's

M

had a constant problem with turnover and feels that a nonnurse director would be apt to stay in the position longer than the recent succession of nurse-directors.

The nurses at our hospital don't think he's be making a good move. What do *you* think?

A It's no more appropriate to hire a director of nursing who's not a nurse than to hire a director of surgery who's not a surgeon.

The director of nursing must provide personal leadership and direction to her staff—as well as perform managerial functions. A nonnurse as director of nursing could all too easily become one more bureaucrat in the hospital hierarchy. By default, the associate or assistant director of nursing would then become the one to make the real nursing decisions.

It's certainly not easy to find a good director of nursing. But looking for one outside of nursing should be the very last resort. *Before* the last resort, the administrator should analyze the reasons for the high turnover and resolve that problem. Bringing a nonnurse nursing director may only make matters worse.

Manipulative patient

How can this type of patient be dealt with?

Q I have a terminally ill patient who makes me so mad I'm at my wit's end! She won't do a thing for herself, and when I try to assert myself, she threatens to faint or vomit. Then I feel so guilty I end up doing whatever she wants. I know she's manipulating me, but what can I do about it?

A Sounds as if this lady is trying to see how far she can push you. You're understandably reluctant to show your anger or hurt her

feelings because she's already suffering enough. So you end up playing along with her.

Nurses get satisfaction from being needed, and this patient is certainly happy to be needy. What can you do? Instead of trying to control her behavior, you can help her get in touch with what she truly needs.

Simply ask her what she wants. She'll probably say, "to get out of this hospital."

That would give you a starting point. Then, you could help her identify what *she* can do to make that happen. Maybe it means helping with her own bath, feeding herself, or walking from the bed to the chair. Make suggestions. And get her family and other staff members involved. The secret is continuity—everyone working toward the *patient's* goal.

Sure, she'll have little setbacks. You need to be tolerant and kind but firm. Encourage her efforts, and don't forget to pat her—and yourself—on the back.

Remember, for a long time she got what she wanted by being dependent. So be prepared to accept whatever she can accomplish, even if she never reaches the level of independence you'd like.

Marijuana

What should be done about a group of young paraplegics who are smoking?

Q I'm a nurse-manager on a 48-bed rehabilitation unit. A group of young paraplegics who are long-term residents of the unit have been smoking marijuana and burning incense to disguise the smell. Although most of the unit staff aren't offended, a few have objected. Also, some of our other patients have complained about the smoke.

We discussed the problem and possible solutions in a meeting of

patients and staff—but none of our proposed solutions seem to work.

As nurse-manager, I have to think about the patients who complain about the smoke, the nurses who object to marijuana smoking, and the legal issues that are involved.

How should I handle this?

A Start by getting your priorities in order. Although you may be sympathetic to the young paraplegics, your primary concerns as nurse-manager are the health, safety, and comfort of *all* your patients. If the actions of one group impinge on the rights of another, you're acting reasonably and responsibly when you take steps to change the situation. And of course, keep in mind that using marijuana is illegal.

Then try finding out *why* the paraplegics are smoking marijuana. Are they using it to pass the time, to assert their independence, or to help them cope with their situation? (If it's the last reason, perhaps your staff psychiatrist or psychiatric nurse consultant should be called in.)

Call a conference of the paraplegics and the staff. When you speak, you'll have to choose your words carefully. You could say something like this:

"We hear that several of you are smoking marijuana. But in this hospital and this state, smoking marijuana is illegal. Also, we've had objections from patients and staff nurses.

"As nurse-manager, I'm accountable to my patients, the staff, the hospital administration and the state—so I *must* inform you that you're not permitted to smoke marijuana on this unit.

"There are certain hospital areas away from this unit where smoking *is* permitted—that is, the smoking of cigarettes, pipes, even cigars. What *you* smoke will be up to you. Of course, if you choose marijuana, you could still be held responsible for your actions and have to face any consequences.

"I'm not saying I approve or disapprove of smoking marijuana. I'm a nurse, not a police officer. I'm simply describing the situation in *this* hospital."

You'd be wise not to inject your personal views on marijuana; they're irrelevant and likely to involve you in controversy. Document your statements to the paraplegics and staff; keep a copy for yourself and send one to your supervisor.

If the paraplegics continue to smoke after you've made your position clear, you'll have to check with your administration about other legal steps.

Yes, this whole business is a nuisance as well as a challenge. You have to balance your legal and professional responsibility with your sympathy and concern for *all* your patients.

Married couples

Does any nurse practice act deal with a husband and wife working together or one supervising the other?

Q Where I work, there's an unwritten rule against spouses working together. That's why I was surprised last week when my wife, who's in the float pool, was assigned to the unit where I'm charge nurse. I didn't object; in fact, I joked with one of my co-workers that I would finally be "in charge" of my wife. We then went about our business, finished an uneventful shift, and went home.

My next surprise came the following day when the unit coordinator told me I should have reported this "dangerous situation" to the clinical supervisor. She said I could have lost my license if anything went wrong on the unit and my wife were involved. Is that true? Is there anything in the nurse practice act that even remotely deals with a husband and wife working together or one supervising the other?

A The practice act doesn't address the issue of married couples or relatives working together. So, you're in no danger of losing your nursing license over your wedding band. The ruling is probably a matter of hospital policy, but it should be a written policy that applies to everyone in the hospital.

Hospitals aren't the only employers with regulations like this. Many employers, both inside and outside health care, frown on couples or relatives working together, especially when one is a supervisor. Some employers won't even hire relatives—not because they're against marriage, home, and apple pie or because they don't trust the applicant's professionalism. They just want to avoid the appearance of nepotism or favoritism that might affect other employees' morale or performance. And they want every supervisor free to make an objective appraisal of an employee's work.

You'll agree that an unsatisfactory appraisal could put a real damper on many relationships and probably put the *marriage* license in jeopardy.

Medical assistants

Can they perform the same functions as nurses?

Q I am an RN employed by a group practice to work in their medical office. During recent months, after two more doctors joined the practice, we nurses began noticing subtle changes in our working atmosphere. Still, we weren't prepared for a memo stating that from here on in, medical assistants will be hired to fill vacated nursing positions. As the memo put it, RNs and LPNs will be hired only if they'll accept the lesser salary and the title of medical assistant. The reason: cost-effectiveness.

At first I couldn't believe that any RN or LPN would accept this condition. But just last week an LPN was hired, and a memo was sent around introducing and identifying her as a medical assistant.

As I understand it, medical assistants aren't licensed. Can they perform the same functions as nurses? And what about any RNs and LPNs who accept this condition to work as medical assistants? Are they responsible for their actions under their nursing licenses, or will they be responsible only as medical assistants?

Can you shed some light on this for us?

A With apologies to William Shakespeare: A nurse by any other name is still a nurse. Changing her title doesn't change her license or accountability.

Medical assistants aren't licensed. But in some states, the nurse practice act says that unlicensed personnel employed *in a doctor's office* may perform nursing or technical functions under the supervision of a doctor. These individuals are exempt from the educational and licensing requirements that apply to those performing nursing duties in hospitals, nursing homes, and other health care institutions.

Therefore, under this law, the doctor can train a medical assistant to give injections, apply casts, and so on. Here's the rub: The doctor is supposed to train, assign, and supervise these medical assistants. In practice, though, the training chore is frequently turned over to one of the nurses. So if you're asked to help out with the training program, be sure to have the doctor sign documentation that he's satisfied with the medical assistant's competence, and as the employer, he will be fully responsible for delegating tasks and

M

supervising performance. On the other hand, if *you're* not satisfied with the medical assistant's competence, document this both for the doctor and for your records.

Now, back to the cost-effective aspects of the situation. This may just be the perfect time to ask yourself what the new money-saving policy at the clinic is costing you—and your fellow nurses—in terms of your professional image and future employment possibilities. Think about it.

In the long run, if you don't protect nursing's professional image, who will?

Medical student's orders

Doesn't following them spell legal trouble?

Q At the teaching hospital where I work, hospital policy says that residents must cosign medical students' orders. When the residents are rushed, they don't always get around to it. But we carry out the orders anyway—cosigned or not.

I know we're supposed to take orders only from licensed doctors, not unlicensed medical students. Doesn't this practice spell legal trouble?

A Sure does. Not only is it dangerous, it's prohibited by the nurse practice act.

This sounds like a recurrent problem on your unit. To solve it, first take a close look at your hospital's policy and procedure manuals—chances are, they prohibit the practice you describe. Remember, medical students can't even function as physician's assistants, who at least are registered by the state medical board.

Then, talk with your manager. She should schedule a meeting with the directors of the residency program and medical education to discuss the issue and clarify their expectations.

If this doesn't solve the problem immediately, you and your co-workers should document your concerns in a memo and send it up through channels.

Meanwhile, refuse to carry out orders that aren't signed by a doctor. If necessary, remind medical students that residents must cosign their order sheets, but don't get involved in obtaining the signatures. That's the students' responsibility, not yours.

Medicare

Should a doctor's quick visits be documented?

Q Last week, one of the doctors stormed up to our nurse's station and blamed *me* because Medicare wants him to payback funds he received for inpatient visits. It seems that I'm at fault because I hadn't documented all the visits he made to patients.

The simple fact is that I did document all visits in which he examined patients or changed orders—but not every little "Hello. How are you?" visit. I'm not the doctor's "keeper" for Medicare. And in my opinion, any doctor who charges Medicare for such quick visits owes them a payback.

I don't know all the new regulations chapter and verse, so I couldn't defend myself satisfactorily. What do you have to say about this situation?

A Yelling and finger pointing solve nothing. What the doctor's telling you (and everyone else within earshot) is that he doesn't know much about current Medicare regulations either.

As things stand now, an attending doctor is reimbursed separately for inpatient visits only when he gives

the patient *medical* care. And the peer review organization (PRO) that monitors Medicare administration wants verification of exactly what care was given. Because the doctor's primarily responsible for documenting his care, the PRO will look for this information in his progress notes first. Then if his notes are missing or inconclusive, they'll look at your charting. If they can't find any proof of medical care in either place, Medicare can deny payment retroactively and ask for a payback.

Obviously, then, if quick visits don't warrant payment, the doctor shouldn't be charging for them, nor should you be documenting them.

Medication

Does contact with other pills or being out of the airtight container adversely affect the medications?

Q In the home health agency where I work, we set up a full week's medications at one time for many of our elderly patients.

We put each day's pills in a small envelope. For certain patients, this means putting four or more pills in one day's envelope.

I have some questions about this procedure. First, does being out of the airtight container adversely affect the medications? Second, does one pill's being in contact with others cause a chemical change?

A You're wise to raise these questions, but actually, the answer in both cases is no—with only minor qualification.

Unless you live in an intensely humid climate, there's only one drug that must be kept in its airtight container: nitroglycerin.

The biggest danger of the system you're now using is that an elderly patient may confuse pills that look alike. For example, haloperidol (Haldol) and diazepam (Valium) would be hard to distinguish from each other. So always make sure your patient recognizes and understands the different tablet markings. (If he can't consistently do this, you'll have to devise another system.)

Medication change

How long is too long to get signed orders back?

Q I left hospital nursing for a new home health agency in our area. I'm enjoying my work so far, but the paperwork takes some getting used to.

> *"The doctor told me to send him the medication order but the mail usually takes more than a day."*

For instance, when a doctor phones in a medication change for one of his patients, I'm supposed to note it in the medical record and send the order to him to countersign. But the mail usually takes more than a day, so I'm worried about my liability. How long is too long to get these signed orders back?

A If your home health agency participates in the Medicare program, you must conform to federal guidelines for documenting doctors' verbal orders. These guidelines are broad, but they do require a doctor's countersignature on any changes within "a reasonable amount of time." To most agencies, this means 7 days; this is probably addressed in your policy manual.

Keep a copy of the order change in the patient's record as a reminder until the signed original comes back and get used to some procrastinators. You'll have to follow up if a doctor takes a week or more getting

back to you. If this becomes a chronic problem, though, ask the agency to send a memo to the guilty parties so you don't have to police them yourself.

Medication confusion

Shouldn't the tablets be bottled separately to eliminate confusion?

Q The pharmacist at the hospital where I work will sometimes put two brands of the same medication (in tablet form) into one bottle. The tablets contain the same dose, but because they're manufactured by different drug companies, they *look* different. Don't you think such tablets should be bottled separately to eliminate confusion?

A You have good reason (and good sense) to question this practice. While putting two brands of the same medication into one bottle isn't illegal, it can create unnecessary confusion. A nurse spotting the different tablets in the same bottle might think the pharmacist has mistakenly bottled two different medications. She'd then probably delay giving the patient his medication until she could find out what was going on. But what if the patient should have his medication exactly when ordered? The nurse and the patient would have an upsetting situation to deal with—until the issue was resolved.

And that's not all. Did you know that variations in the manufacturing processes could cause tablets that are ostensibly the same to be absorbed at different rates? This could mean serious complications with medications such as lithium and digoxin, which are administered in therapeutic dosages extremely close to the toxic level.

Voice your concern over this questionable practice. If you take this issue up with your supervisor,

you should have no trouble getting other nurses to stand behind you. They don't want to cope with this problem, either.

Your hospital administrators should respond promptly—and they should recognize that they have an alert nurse at work.

Medication errors

Could a nurse be held liable when serving as a middleman?

Q Several weeks ago, an elderly man who'd cut his right index finger came to our emergency department for treatment. As the doctor was preparing to suture the wound, he asked me for procaine hydrochloride (Novocain). The charge nurse was standing next to the medication cabinet, so she handed me the vial and I gave it to the doctor. Ten minutes after the injection, the patient had a severe reaction. The vial contained *epinephrine* hydrochloride (Adrenalin), not procaine.

Now, the charge nurse tells me that if the patient files a lawsuit, I'll be liable, along with her. I don't understand why. After all, I was just the middleman. Is the charge nurse right or am I?

A Your charge nurse is right. No matter where you were in the chain, you're still liable for the mistake. When you handed the drug to the doctor, you were vouching that it was the *right* drug. Of course, the doctor was at fault, too—he shouldn't have given the drug without checking the vial's label himself.

Does one ever warrant suspension from work?

Q Several months ago, after a short orientation, I started working on the intensive care unit of our community hospital. Last

M

week, I made a medication error, my first ever in 10 years of nursing.

Here's how the error occurred: I misread our laboratory form (which has no lines separating test results) and reported my patient's potassium level, 4.8, as her serum calcium result, which was actually 15. I discovered my error after administering the I.V. calcium chloride her doctor ordered. I immediately told my charge nurse and unit manager, then left a message for the doctor to call me as soon as possible. Meanwhile, I monitored the patient carefully and held the calcium gluconate that was also ordered.

The doctor called back, furious. I explained how I made the error, that the patient was stable, and apologized profusely. He checked back several times for stat lab results and with new orders. I filled out an incident report and gave it to the unit manager with my apologies. As the day wore on, I felt too upset to stay, and my charge nurse said I could leave. Before leaving, I assessed the patient one more time to make sure her condition hadn't changed—then cried all the way home.

That evening the director of nursing phoned and told me I was suspended—and that she was considering notifying the state board of my actions. She didn't say how long I'd be suspended or let me tell my side of the story.

Now that I've calmed down, I don't feel I've been treated fairly. I'm thinking of getting a lawyer to go with me to see the director of nursing. What do you make of this situation?

A You picked up the error, then acted appropriately in notifying the doctor and making sure your patient didn't suffer any ill effects. So what went wrong? Unfortunately, you didn't help yourself. By losing your professional cool and overreacting, you focused more attention on the error than was warranted.

(And the director of nursing overreacted in kind.) By leaving early in an emotional state, you lost the chance to calmly defend yourself before the situation escalated.

You sound ready to assert yourself now. By all means, write up your side of the story for your personnel file and make an appointment with the director of nursing. She should know that you had at least expected some discussion of the circumstances—your flawless record on medication errors for 10 years in other hospitals, the short orientation you received on a stressful unit and, most important, a closer look at why the error occurred. The director of nursing should begin checking all of the forms used at the hospital for clarity and drop her plan to notify the state board about your error. If she doesn't, make another appointment with her—and take your lawyer.

Should the nurse have been truthful with the patient?

Q During a recent shift, I noticed redness around a patient's I.V. site; she was also complaining of itching and burning there. When I checked the label on her I.V. antibiotic, I realized I should have mixed it with normal saline solution, not dextrose 5% in water. I quickly discontinued the infusion, mixed a new bag, and restarted the I.V. in another vein. Within seconds, the patient said her arm felt better, and she asked if I'd changed her medication. Hedging, I said, "I thought this would be easier on your arm." She seemed satisfied with my explanation, but now I wonder—should I have told her the truth?

A Although telling the truth has its disadvantages, the ethical bottom line is yes, you should have been truthful.

On the plus side, telling the patient about your error would have informed her that the pain and itching weren't symptoms of her illness.

And you could have alerted her to symptoms of other problems your error might have caused.

But you would have had to be careful about what you said to avoid alarming her unnecessarily. Perhaps the best approach would have been something like this: "Mrs. Jones, I mixed your last medication with the wrong solution. I'm glad you spoke up so I could correct it quickly. The drug itself wasn't changed by the incorrect mixture, so you shouldn't have any other problems. But I'll continue to watch for redness and swelling, and please call me if you notice more itching or burning." Then you should have asked her if she had any questions.

Finally, you should have shared the situation with your manager and filled out an incident report.

Admitting a mistake isn't easy, but it *is* the best policy. A staff development program could help to make you and other nurses more comfortable answering questions in awkward situations like this.

Who's liable for a student's error?

Q A senior nursing student made a serious medication error when she was assigned to one of my patients. Luckily, he wasn't harmed. I was concerned about my liability, so I talked to the instructor. Because he often assigns his students to three different patient care areas, he can't supervise every student all the time. He told me not to worry because nursing students carry liability insurance and are accountable for their own errors. I find that hard to believe. Is he right?

A Only partly. A student nurse *is* liable for her own mistakes, so she should have insurance. But the nurse who's present and supervising her is also responsible for the error. If that patient had been harmed and had decided to sue, he probably would have named both you and the student nurse in his lawsuit.

The best remedy is to have the instructor supervise his students. Meet with him, other nursing school representatives, and the hospital's director of nursing to see if you can iron out your differences.

Would a mandatory corrective action program reduce errors?

Q Our nurse pharmacy committee reviews medication error incident reports twice a month. Occasionally, we find patterns of errors and identify employees who make an unacceptable number.

As newly-elected chairperson, I'd like a more complete review system that categorizes errors according to number and seriousness, and sets up a mandatory corrective action program. Would this kind of plan reduce medication errors?

A Any system attaching punitive action to incident reporting is likely to reduce the number of incidents reported rather than the number of incidents committed. In effect, staff members who *don't* report mistakes are the ones who will be rewarded.

Further, medication errors are hard to fit into neat categories. For instance, a "missed dose" can range anywhere from omitting a dose of multivitamins to omitting an antidote for a poisoned patient. How would you compare wrongly giving one patient a dose of penicillin with giving the same dose to a patient with a history of anaphylaxis?

To find and reduce the *cause* of medication errors, look to your nursing and pharmacy supervisors. An astute supervisor knows when problems exist and how to deal with them. Provide them with an atmosphere of encouragement and support—or, as the old song says, "Accentuate the positive."

Medication orders

Are nurses allowed to write prescriptions and sign the doctor's name?

Q One of the surgeons wants nurses on the outpatient surgical unit to write prescriptions for his patients who are ready for discharge. He says his office nurses do this all the time, but it doesn't sound right to me. Are nurses allowed to write prescriptions and sign the doctor's name?

A No. If permitted by hospital policy, you could take a verbal or telephone order from the surgeon, who'd have to countersign it later according to protocol. But this isn't what he's asking you to do. He wants you to assume a *medical practice*—prescribing drugs—which you obviously can't do. (Many states do allow nurse practitioners to write prescriptions, though.)

You might suggest instead that he have standing orders typed up for his signature. Then you could distribute the orders to his patients at discharge. This has been standard practice on some units for years (for example, in obstetrics/gynecology after dilatation and curettage). Not only is this system efficient, but it could also save you from charges of practicing beyond the scope of your license.

Can an LPN give ampicillin while the doctor's away?

Q I'm an LPN working for a general practitioner. He's asked me to cover the office when he's on vacation. One of his orders is that when patients come in with cold symptoms, I'm to give them ampicillin provided they've taken it before. I'd like to know if his permission gives me the legal right to give this drug.

A As you know, your license does not permit you to diagnose or prescribe. Under the circumstances you describe, your giving ampicillin to a suspected cold patient would be both diagnosing and prescribing.

Explain the scope of your license to your employer before he goes on vacation. This'll make his trip away from the office safe for you—and your patients.

Can nurses write them?

Q I've been a nurse for 20 years and am currently working as a float nurse on the night shift of a nearby community hospital. One night a patient asked, "How come I haven't had my Inderal and Tagamet for 2 days now? I always take these at home."

I checked his chart and found this notation: "Allow patient to take same meds as taken at home." But when I checked further, I learned that whatever medications a patient says he's taking are written by the nursing staff on the doctor's order sheet for that patient.

This is treated as a verbal order. Eventually, the doctor cosigns the order, the pharmacy sends up the drug or drugs, and the patient continues with the medications he *says* he takes at home.

Once I learned that nurses, not doctors, were routinely writing these medication orders, I refused to give the patient the propranolol hydrochloride (Inderal) and the cimetidine (Tagamet). But the other nurses gave him the medications anyhow because they said this doctor would get nasty if provoked.

I wanted to call the house doctor, but the other nurses *and* the supervisor said "let it be."

How would you have handled this?

A Pretty much the way you did. Orders for patient medications should be written by the doctor—not by the nursing staff on the

M

patient's say-so. The medications a patient routinely takes at home should be reviewed by his doctor on admission to the hospital. The orders for the patient's medications should then be written on the chart by the doctor. The doctor will decide whether or not to include the medications the patient's accustomed to taking.

> *"Once I learned the nurses were writing the medication orders, I refused to give the patient his medication."*

Before taking any steps, however, we think you should check your hospital's policy. Then express your concern in a memo sent through nursing channels. Let administration resolve this touchy situation legally and procedurally with the medical staff of the hospital.

You have your priorities in good order when you observe sound nursing and hospital policy rather than follow the arbitrary directions of a doctor who's cutting corners, perhaps for his convenience.

Do generic drugs meet the high standards of trade name drugs?

Q I'm a private-duty nurse to a 76-year-old cerebrovascular-accident patient. After watching a TV report on generic versus trade name drugs, my patient asked her doctor to prescribe her medicines by their generic names. The doctor refused, saying that generic drugs do not meet the high standards of trade-name drugs. What information do you have on this?

A Most states have enacted laws in the 1980s that allow pharmacists to substitute generics for trade name products (especially if the patient is on Medicare or Med-

icaid). Unless "medically necessary," the pharmacist *can* substitute a generic equivalent.

Another reassuring point is that generic manufacturers must submit data to the Food and Drug Administration that shows that their components are equivalent.

How much saline should be used when suctioning?

Q One of the interns on the pediatric coronary care unit where I work wrote a peculiar order for a patient with a tracheostomy. It read: "suction patient p.r.n., ventilate before and after, and use 30 ml normal saline with each suction."

I'm accustomed to using from 3 to 5 ml of saline, depending upon how dry or thick the patient's secretions are. Was the intern wrong in writing such an order?

A If the intern's order reads exactly the way you described, yes, he was wrong. However, could you have missed a decimal point? Or did the intern forget to include it? The 3.0 ml sounds about right. Did the intern mean for you to obtain the saline from a 30 ml bottle over the course of an 8-hour shift?

You didn't say if you followed the order as it was written. This is clearly a case where you're better safe than sorry.

The best way to moisturize the bronchial tree locally is to use a heated aerosol or nebulizer. Then, keep the area moist by systemically hydrating the patient.

Is following medical students' orders legally risky?

Q I suspect we've got the potential for trouble in the intensive care unit (ICU) where I work. Because we're in a university teaching hospital, we have senior medical

students writing orders for the ICU patients. According to the hospital's policy, a resident must cosign the students' orders within 24 hours. But if the residents are particularly rushed, they may not get around to cosigning the orders. Yet we're expected to carry out the students' orders—cosigned or not.

I've been taught that nurses take their orders only from licensed doctors. At our hospital, we're taking orders from unlicensed medical students.

I went directly to nursing administration with the problem, and was told not to worry. The director of nursing said whenever I had a question about an order, I could call the resident. I can't see this as a satisfactory answer; it still leaves me taking *some* orders from the medical students. It also wastes time and makes for sticky relationships with the medical students.

Before I take my concerns higher up the administrative ladder, I'd like your opinion.

A You're not worrying for nothing. You do run legal risks in the situation you've described. No nurse should carry out an order written by a medical student. She'd be violating the nurse practice act and jeopardizing her license.

Your hospital administration should take a second look at what they're permitting medical students to do. As for checking out a questionable order from a medical student: The residents and medical staff, not the nurses, have responsibility for supervising the medical students. The hospital's not paying you to do this, and the insurance company's probably not covering you in this role.

You and the other concerned nurses in the ICU should prepare a memo with the facts, and send it up through the regular channels. Probably your state's current nurse practice act specifies that nurses may take orders only from licensed doctors or dentists.

M

In states with there's no ruling on this matter, the hospitals themselves usually establish the policy. For example, they may require a senior resident or attending doctor to cosign a medical student's orders before the nurse implements these orders.

Is giving fluid challenges based on urine output considered practicing medicine?

Q On the intensive care unit where I work nights, we're expected to give fluid challenges or furosemide (Lasix) therapy as a patient's condition—based on urine output or pulmonary artery catheter readings—warrants it. We then write the order, and the doctor cosigns it in the morning.

Could this procedure be considered practicing medicine? We're worried that one of these days a doctor may not back up our judgment and we'll be involved in a malpractice suit.

A What you're doing is unwise. In the doctor's absence, nurses can use clinical parameters to administer the drugs or therapies he ordered—but they need specific, clear guidelines to follow. (That's what you do when you give p.r.n. medications.)

Use a printed standing order sheet for urine output (UO) and pulmonary capillary wedge pressure (PCWP). Have the doctor fill in the desired maintenance level of UO or PCWP. He should specify how much fluid and medication should be given if the patient's UO or PCWP either rises above or falls below this level. These order sheets should be signed by the doctor and evaluated daily. If a problem arises during the night—say the patient's condition deteriorates or the therapies don't work—contact a doctor according to your administration's policies.

Is it right to delay medication because of an incompatible order?

Q As charge nurse on a busy medical/surgical unit, I often have to skip lunch, but last Thursday, the unit manager sat in while I took a quick break. When I got back, she reported that one of the doctors came in for rounds and left a "now" order. Scanning the order, I noticed it called for digoxin I.V., but it didn't include an order for inserting a p.r.n. adapter. I told my manager that I wasn't comfortable giving this I.V. medication without one. She said, "You're the charge nurse, phone the doctor." I called him several times and left a message, but he never called me back. When my shift was over, I asked the oncoming charge nurse to call him and get the order.

On Friday, the director of nursing summoned me to her office. She had heard about the delayed order (the patient finally received the medication at 10 p.m.), and she blamed me. I was reprimanded and relieved of my charge nurse duties for 6 months. I don't feel that I'm the only one at fault. My manager could have checked with the doctor while he was on the unit, or he could at least have called me back. What do you think?

A Sorry, but the buck stopped with you. It was your job to make enough noise—through channels if necessary—and find a way to get that "now" order filled—pronto.

To avoid a recurrence, ask that your unit be given a standing order calling for inserting a p.r.n. adapter whenever I.V. medications are administered. That way, you won't need a doctor's order each time. And when you're reinstated to the charge position, remember this: Taking charge doesn't automatically mean you have to know all the answers; you just have to follow through and find someone who does.

Isn't informing the patient of medication risks a nurse's right?

Q A doctor prescribed meperidine (Demerol) for one of my patients to ease her pain after exploratory surgery. But this patient was 9 months pregnant, and I was concerned about giving her a narcotic. I know that meperidine is not advised during pregnancy. In addition, recent research has found that when meperidine is given to the mother during labor, the infant's earliest responses are adversely affected. (Although my patient wasn't in labor, she did have uterine contractions soon after her operation.)

After surgery, the patient frequently requested and received meperidine for her pain. On the fourth postoperative day, when she continued to request pain medication, I told her about the suspected ill effects of meperidine, during pregancy and labor—and offered her alternatives for her pain.

The patient became alarmed. She told her doctor if she'd realized the dangers of meperidine, she'd never have requested it so often.

The doctor and my charge nurse contended that I'd frightened the patient unnecessarily—and that for me to warn the patient was "outside the limits of nursing."

I disagree: The doctor did not inform his patient—although it was his responsibility. But none of this alters *my* responsibility—because I must administer the drug.

I could easily have administered the meperidine and kept my concerns to myself. But I believe that informing my patient of the risks certainly comes within the limits of nursing. Then why have I been reprimanded?

A A warning flag should go up in any nurse's mind when she sees a narcotic ordered for a pregnant patient. So you *were* certainly right on that score.

But about how you raised the question: You probably shouldn't have gone directly to the patient—bypassing the doctor. You should have discussed your concern about the order with the doctor, and together you could have planned an alternative approach for this patient. *Then* you would have been free to speak to the patient.

Of course the use of drugs during pregnancy is a touchy subject. Ordinarily, you'd advise a pregnant woman to stay away from *all* drugs (including over-the-counter drugs), particularly during her first and third trimesters. The exception is the woman who needs a certain medication to ensure her health.

Perhaps in this case, the doctor decided the benefits of meperidine outweighed the dangers to your patient. How do you know? You were absolutely right to question a narcotics order for a pregnant patient. But the next time be sure to take your doubts and fears to the doctor. Work closely with him—because this is also his province and his dilemma.

Was it wrong to withhold medication until the pharmacy opened?

Q One night soon after midnight a cancer patient in the intensive care unit (ICU) where I work developed a temperature of 104° F (40° C) and went into septic shock. The ICU resident came quickly and assessed the patient. The resident said he was ordering two antibiotics, and left to write the medication orders on the patient's chart.

I stayed with the patient to apply ice packs and set up the hypothermia blanket. I didn't have time to read the patient's chart until after 4 a.m.

The resident had written orders for cefoxitin (Mefoxin) and amikacin (Amikin). The cefoxitin was in stock on the floor, so I administered that at once. But we didn't have the amikacin.

Ordinarily, if a medication that's been ordered is not on hand, the night supervisor will get it out of the pharmacy (even though it officially closes at 9 p.m.). But I was under the impression that the night supervisor wouldn't get medication out of the pharmacy at 4 a.m. So I didn't say anything, figuring the amikacin had to wait until the pharmacy reopened at 8 a.m.

The next day, the nurse-manager reprimanded me for not giving the second medication immediately. She said the patient could've died because of my negligence. Was I wrong to do what I did?

A You were wrong, sorry to tell you. You'll probably want to know better for the next time.

Under certain circumstances, orders for an antibiotic *can* wait until the pharmacy opens in the morning. Your patient was in shock because of sepsis. Therefore, he *needed* those medications stat.

> *"I came into work and found the cancer patient I'd been caring for had a fever of 104° F and had gone into septic shock."*

You should have requested the medication immediately. The night supervisor would have procured it, even after 4 a.m. You can't put off administering a critical medication (amikacin is specifically indicated for septic shock, by the way) because the pharmacy is closed.

Fortunately your patient pulled through. But in the next life-and-death situation, don't rely on your "impression." Make sure you know

your nursing priorities and the hospital's policy. If you don't know, make it your business to find out.

What should a nurse do if the doctor's orders contradict the orders on the preprinted forms?

Q Our doctors use preprinted medication orders provided free of charge by drug companies. I'm afraid they're becoming too dependent on these orders, and on us.

One doctor, for instance, scribbles in his own orders, which often contradict those on the form. He also crosses out the ones we shouldn't follow. Worse yet, he doesn't tell us what to do when his written-in medication orders contradict the printed ones. He says we should decide which medications to give.

That sounds like practicing medicine without a license to me. What do you think?

A That's exactly what it sounds like. And if you're doing it, your license may be at risk. You're accountable for all orders you carry out, so you've got to make sure they're right. Next time you're faced with the situation you describe, ask the doctor to clarify his order. Tell him you don't want to second-guess him, so you'll need to know exactly what he wants before you'll administer any medication.

One more thing: Those preprinted orders are legal, as long as the doctor knows and agrees with what they say.

Who's liable if orders aren't countersigned by the doctor within the 24-hour period?

Q I work for a privately operated, nonprofit referral service for registered nurses.

Our policy is to keep nurses' notes on all home care cases, and when the patient's doctor changes a medication or procedure order by telephone, we note these changes in the patient's medical record as you would a hospital order.

We're worried about our liability, because these orders aren't countersigned by the doctor within the 24-hour period that's required in the hospitals in our area.

What's your opinion on this?

A Home health care agencies follow federal guidelines for documenting doctors' verbal orders. These guidelines are broad, but they do require a doctor's countersignature on any change in the patient's plan of treatment within "a reasonable amount of time."

What most agencies consider reasonable is documenting the verbal order immediately and sending the original to the doctor to be countersigned and returned within 7 days. A copy of the change order is kept in the patient's medical record until the original is returned with the doctor's signature. (Human nature being what it is, you should protect yourself by following up to make sure the doctor signs the order and returns it promptly.)

Any home health agency participating in the Medicare program must conform to federal guidelines.

Will dispensing medications jeopardize a nurse's license?

Q I work as an occupational health nurse for a large manufacturing company. The company doctor has signed standing orders allowing me to dispense medications to the employees in his absence. I can give methocarbamol (Robaxin) for lower back pain, an antispasmodic containing phenobarbital for stomachaches, and prophylactic tetanus injections for wounds. I can also give aspirin or acetaminophen (Tylenol) for head-

aches and over-the-counter products for colds and allergies.

That's not all. The doctor has also drawn up a list of ailments and the medications usually prescribed to treat them. If neither I nor the doctor is around and an employee complains of an ailment, the personnel manager, as well as the evening and night supervisors, is free to consult the list and give out the recommended medication.

This system for dispensing medications seems to require me to practice medicine without a license. Could I jeopardize my nursing license by doing this? Then there's the business of lay personnel dispensing medications so freely. Should *I* worry, or is this the company's problem?

A Your first concern is certainly justified. True, you're acting under a doctor's standing orders, but that's no guarantee that this couldn't jeopardize *your* license. The conditions you're being asked to assess may seem routine, but they can mask serious problems. For example, you're permitted to give methocarbamol for lower back pain. That's fine if the pain is musculoskeletal in origin, but lower back pain can result from kidney problems, too—or an aortic aneurysm about to rupture.

At the very least, a doctor should be available for consultation on these assessments. If that's impossible, document your concerns in a memo to management. Focus your criticism on the system, not on the doctor. Emphasize that, for professional reasons, you're uncomfortable with the present system.

About your second concern: It's one thing for a manager or supervisor to grab a few aspirins to give to an employee complaining of a headache. But when it comes to more powerful medications (the antispasmodic you mentioned contains phenobarbital, which is a controlled substance)—*no way.* Lay personnel shouldn't have access to

these kinds of medications, let alone be able to dispense them.

The company is ultimately responsible for the actions of its employees. But if you remain silent on this matter, it could be interpreted as condoning it—not good in the event of legal action. So we'd advise you to document the second concern, too, in your memo. Naturally, you'll keep a copy of the memo for yourself.

If, after receiving your memo, management refuses to change the system, you might tactfully point out the potential legal danger for the company. Maybe that'll make management sit up and take notice.

Unfortunately, this system of dispensing medications is not unusual in the occupational health field. If more nurses speak up, maybe some of the doctors would think twice about such laissez-faire attitudes.

Medications

Could forcing medications be considered assault and battery?

M

Q I've just started working on the hospital's psychiatric unit. In the past couple of weeks, I've seen three nurses force medications on paranoid or psychotic patients who'd refused to take them. Could this be considered assault and battery?

A In the last few years, many psychiatric experts, legislators, and lawyers have debated this very issue. As a result, some state laws now address the patient's right to refuse "excessive or unnecessary" medications. However, they don't define "excessive" or "unnecessary."

You may administer medication against a patient's will if he's in danger of harming himself or others. But if he isn't, you're in a gray area.

In those situations, forcing medications probably violates a patient's rights. Most likely he'd be successful if he filed assault and battery charges.

One more issue bears examining—that of patient advocacy. The type of patients you describe may be so severely impaired that they can't seek counsel to protect their rights. If that's the case, you and other nurses on the unit need to be their advocates. When you believe a patient is being excessively or unnecessarily medicated, you might discuss the situation with other members of the health care team.

Is it acceptable to drop off narcotics for home hospice patients?

Q We nurses sign for and pick up medications at a local hospital pharmacy for delivery to our home hospice patients. Many times, we just drop the drugs off without making a nursing visit.

We told our manager that we're uneasy with this go-between policy when Schedule II narcotics are involved. She said we shouldn't worry, that it's part of our job. What do you say?

A You can stop worrying because both your nursing and pharmacy boards have no problem with this policy. As far as the pharmacy board's concerned, you're acting as an agent for the patient, not the pharmacy.

Once the drugs are handed over to you for delivery, you assume responsibility for them. So both boards recommend that you have someone from the patient's family sign for the drugs as proof that you delivered them.

For comparison, a hospice nurse in the northeast says she tries to have a patient's relative pick up his drugs. But if she has to do it herself, she has someone—preferably the patient—

sign for the drugs. She doesn't run into this situation often, she says, because most of her patients receiving Schedule I or II narcotics use patient-controlled analgesia pumps, so the pharmacy delivers the drugs.

Nurses need to follow policy carefully in these touchy situations.

Is it ethical to send medications home with a patient or reuse them for other patients?

Q Our hospital policy says I can't give a discharged patient any of his unopened or partially used medications to take home. Yet, when the unopened items are returned to the pharmacy, his bill isn't credited for them. Those same medications will be returned to stock and eventually dispensed to another patient and charged to him. Isn't that double billing? What do you have to say about that and the whole question of sending medications home?

A There are no easy answers because your question involves complicated issues. Put simply, in your state, diagnosis-related groups (DRGs) determine how much your hospital will be paid for a particular patient's care, and payment is based solely on his diagnosis. Whether the medications are used or returned to the pharmacy won't change the DRG patient's bill one way or the other. But some patients' bills will be affected—for example, psychiatric patients, who aren't covered by DRGs in your state. So these patients should be credited for any returned medications.

As to the whole question of sending medications home, there are good reasons why your hospital has the policy it does (so don't be tempted to look the other way when a patient packs his bag). By law, patients must have a doctor's written prescription for any medica-

tions taken without hospital supervision. And the medications must be properly labeled—including instructions for use.

Fair trade is another reason for this policy. The pharmacy department, bound by pricing contracts with pharmaceutical suppliers, can't undermine private pharmacies' business by dispensing medications for home use. The only exceptions are those your pharmacy department policy classifies as an extension of hospital stay. In some hospitals, for instance, a patient may take home vials of insulin to use until he can obtain the same type of insulin from his local pharmacy.

Discuss any concerns you have with the pharmacy department. Where medications are concerned, nursing and the pharmacy departments should have an open-door policy.

Is there anything wrong with passing out medications someone else prepared?

Q Last week, a co-worker was called away on an emergency right after she'd prepared medications for several patients. As she hurried away, she asked me to pass them. I didn't have time to tell her that I felt uneasy about passing medications I hadn't prepared. Later, I mentioned my concerns to my nurse-manager. She said there was nothing legally wrong with the situation. Is she right?

A Technically, she is—the law permits you to administer a medication that another nurse or doctor has prepared. But the practice is risky at best—that's why most hospitals prohibit it. If you made a medication error, you, the nurse who prepared the medication, and the hospital would be liable for any injuries that resulted. In court, a lawyer could question whether you'd acted according to generally accepted nursing standards: A reasonably prudent nurse probably wouldn't give medications she hadn't prepared.

You were in a pinch this time, so you did what you had to do. Just make sure it's the exception, not the rule.

Is there a risk in administering epinephrine past its expiration date?

Q I work in a clinic where I'm required to give large doses of penicillin for treatment of gonorrhea and syphilis. In a routine check of the expiration dates of our drugs, I noticed by the date on the epinephrine that it had expired. (We keep epinephrine on hand for cases of anaphylactic shock.)

I reported this to my nurse-manager, who reported it to her supervisor. They agreed the date didn't mean anything because a drug could be potent long after its expiration date. Besides, they said, no new drugs were available.

I'm not satisfied with this response. On nursing units where I've worked before, drugs were replaced promptly once the expiration date passed. Should we or shouldn't we attach importance to the expiration date on a drug? Were they too cautious in the other places where I worked?

Would I be held responsible if I were to administer this epinephrine and the patient ran into a problem—*because* the drug had lost potency?

A Expiration dates are intended as a conservative deadline for the potency and shelf life of a drug. Of course, a drug with a July 31 expiration date wouldn't automatically become "ineffective" on August 1. But the date does mean that the manufacturer will guarantee full potency on the drug *only* through the July 31 date. With each week that passes after the expiration date, the drug presumably becomes less potent.

Whenever epinephrine turns pink or brown, do *not* use it, whatever the date. This discoloration, resulting from oxidation, tends to be linked with overaging.

The supervisor's statement that no new medication was available seems puzzling, since drug companies are usually willing to credit and replace drugs with an expired date.

Now, about your possible legal liability. You should refuse to administer the epinephrine with an expired date. Everybody—you, your nurse-manager, and the supervisor—could be held responsible for any problems.

In your situation, write a memo expressing your concerns (include *only* the facts, well documented), and send this to your supervisor and the nursing administration. When they recognize that using a drug with an expired date *could* lead to a lawsuit, you'll probably get a fresh batch of epinephrine.

Is there a safe way to transport them to patients' homes?

Q As a home health nurse, I often drive 40 miles to see patients, and I carry a few drugs (furosemide [Lasix], nifedipine [Procardia], and nitroglycerin [Nitrostat]) in my glove compartment just in case they're needed. I live in Arizona, and I'm concerned about whether the heat inside my car might affect these drugs. Is there a safe way to carry them? Or am I worrying about a problem that doesn't exist?

A The problem exists and, according to a recent study, may be more serious than you suspect. Temperatures in glove compartments can exceed outdoor temperatures by more than 50° F (25° C). This means that during hot months, drugs stored in glove compartments can be subjected to temperatures as high as 150° F (66° C).

The manufacturer's recommendations for storage temperatures of the specific drugs you mention are as follows:
• furosemide, 59° to 86° F (15° to 30° C)
• nifedipine, 59° to 77° F (15° to 25° C)
• nitroglycerin, 59° to 86° F (15° to 30° C).

As you can see, the temperature of your glove compartment can far exceed the ideal. As a minimal precaution, store the drugs in insulated containers on the floor of the car, protected from direct sunlight. Try to limit the supplies that you keep in the car, and rotate the stock often. A further precaution: Take the drugs inside when you're off duty.

Mercury

If a patient swallows some, will it hurt him?

Q I work at a large family practice clinic. Every now and then, a pediatric patient bites down on a thermometer, breaking it. If he swallows some mercury, will it hurt him? And how should I clean up any mercury that spills? I hope these questions aren't foolish, but this happens quite often.

A Your questions aren't foolish. In fact, broken thermometers and sphygmomanometers are the major sources of airborne mercury contamination in hospitals.

Fortunately for your patient, a glass thermometer contains only 0.1 ml of mercury, so he probably won't be hurt if he accidentally swallows some. It will oxidize too slowly in his gastrointestinal tract to be absorbed. However, mercury that's exposed to the air emits a harmful vapor that can be inhaled and absorbed into the body, so it should be cleaned up quickly.

Start by ventilating the area to disperse the mercury vapor. Then gather the visible mercury droplets into a pool with a stiff card. Use this card or a disposable dropper to put the mercury into an unbreakable container that you've set aside for this use. Cap it tightly, and when you've accumulated mercury from several spills, take it to your area hospital for recycling.

Why not consider using an electronic thermometer for your pediatric patients? The plastic sheath is unbreakable, and the temperature registers in seconds.

Mood swings

How do other nurses handle the physical and emotional challenges of the job?

Q I'm an LPN in a small hospital, and I frequently float to different units during a single shift. My problem is that I can't seem to switch my mood to fit different patients. I may start my day by lending an ear to a dying patient, then pass meds to an overjoyed new mother, then face a crisis in the emergency department.

I come to work cheerful, but I go home physically and emotionally exhausted. How do other nurses handle this?

A Everyone goes home exhausted some of the time, but no one should feel that way every day. If you do, you may be trying to give every hospital stay a happy ending, then blaming yourself when some don't work out that way. For your own mental health, you've got to accept the fact that, whatever the outcome, you've tried to help.

For some-of-the-time blues, many nurses value "rap" sessions

led by psychologists, psychiatric nurses, or others trained in counseling. In these sessions, nurses can let off steam and develop skill in handling the emotional conflicts patient care can cause. You might ask permission to hold such sessions at your hospital.

Finally, you must learn not to eat, sleep, and drink nursing. Taking your problems home with you won't help you or your patients. Try to develop outside activities with happy, healthy people to take your mind off work.

Morale

Is starting a "Nurse of the Month" contest a good idea?

Q I'm nurse-manager on a busy medical unit staffed by a great group of nurses. Although I'm not stingy with praise, I'd like to go further: to recognize certain nurses' special efforts in a special way. I'm hoping, as a by-product, to encourage other nurses to do more for their patients.

Do you think starting a "Nurse of the Month" contest is a good idea? Any suggestions on how to set up such a contest?

A Just be sure you're on the right track before you put your idea into motion. Personnel managers say that an employee recognition program is a surprisingly complicated undertaking.

First of all, what do you want the "Nurse of the Month" contest to accomplish? Most of your staff sounds well-motivated already. But do you really think the contest will supply the missing motivation for those who are lazy and apathetic? Could the contest possibly split your staff into two camps: the "superachievers" and the "underachievers"?

And who'll select the "Nurse of the Month"?

What qualities should the "Nurse of the Month" have? Determining the criteria for excellence in a service-oriented profession like nursing will be difficult.

What will the award entail? A prize at a hospital-sponsored luncheon? Or simply posting the employee's photo and a commendation on the bulletin board?

If you do get the program started, announce your winners regularly and on schedule so the contest doesn't become just a good idea that never came off.

Obviously the award idea raises some touchy questions. If you don't have the right answers ready, you may decide this isn't an idea whose time has come—but an idea you might better let slip off quietly into the night.

What should an overwhelmed nurse do?

Q When Hurricane Hugo devastated our island, it did more than wreck buildings—it destroyed our morale. At the geriatric facility where I work, we don't have enough nurses or equipment. Nursing assistants do most of the work. Unfortunately, they have little preparation and no way to learn. I've repeatedly asked the administrator for staff development sessions, but he doesn't respond. Sometimes I feel like quitting, but I won't because I know my patients would be worse off. What can I do?

A Hang in there as best you can—and don't expect too much of yourself. When you're faced with a situation this overwhelming, any action you take counts—and every action will help lift your morale.

Of course, the administrator should help you. He may be paralyzed by the enormity of the situation and focusing his attention elsewhere, but keep after him. Give him a list of your priorities along with a reasonable schedule for achieving these goals. Offer to contact another nursing home in your area and compare notes. Find out how they're rebuilding, recruiting, and preparing staff, and ask if someone could come over and make suggestions.

Meanwhile, until you can get formal staff development sessions for the nursing assistants, you'll have to teach them yourself. Nothing formal—just spend a few minutes every day on the care they should be giving. When you come across a particular problem, such as a pressure sore, call the nursing assistants together and show them what to do. Make signs and charts outlining certain procedures and display them prominently.

You may want to order a standard nursing assistant's manual, such as *Being a Long-Term-Care Nursing Assistant* (Connie A. Will and Judith B. Eighmy. Englewood Cliffs, NJ: Brady Communications, 1983). And ask your peers for support. Contact: Virgin Islands Nurses' Association, P.O. Box 286, Veterans Dr. Station, St. Thomas, VI 00803. They know better than most what you're up against and how to make the best of an ill wind.

Multidose vial

Will introducing air into a sterile vial contaminate it?

Q When we were revising our medication manual recently, we ran into a problem with our technique for withdrawing medication from a multidose vial.

Actually, our pharmacist raised the issue: He suspected that by injecting air into the vial to displace the solution (thereby making it easier to withdraw), we were inadvertently introducing contaminated air into the otherwise sterile vial.

We're worried. Is there any evidence to support our pharmacist's suspicion?

A According to recent studies, sterility is more securely maintained if all injections are drawn up under a laminar airflow hood. Preparing injections this way can be done only in the pharmacy and would be inconvenient for you.

On the unit, you really can't do anything about the air around you. But if your technique's efficient and careful, there's no need to change your procedure.

Mycostatin oral

Can the oral suspension be safely instilled in a patient's bladder?

Q Recently, when one of the patients on our coronary care unit developed a fungal infection in his urinary tract, his doctor ordered nystatin (Mycostatin) *oral* suspension instilled into the bladder at specific intervals. This solution is nonsterile and contains a form of glucose, so we checked with our pharmacist. He could find no literature supporting the drug's use as anything but an oral suspension.

> *"The doctor was so angry he threatened to go to administration if the procedure wasn't followed as written."*

We explained our concern to the doctor and suggested amphotericin B (Fungizone) as an alternative sterile solution. He was so angry he threatened to go to administration if the procedure wasn't followed as written. We still refused to carry out the order, but we're also worried about our jobs.

What do you think about this?

A Congratulations on sticking to your guns. *You're* responsible for your actions, not the prescribing doctor. The law protects you only when you follow orders that a "reasonably prudent" nurse would follow. Your rationale and your recommendation of amphotericin B are good.

Now for your worries about the doctor. Document your side of the controversy in a memo to your nursing supervisor, describing in detail the written order, your questions and what prompted them, the doctor's answers, and your response to him. Get the pharmacist to put his objections in writing, too. Keep a copy of this material for yourselves. If the doctor complains to administration about the incident, you'll have your documentation.

Chances are, when the doctor has time to think things over, he'll realize he should be sending you a thank-you note.

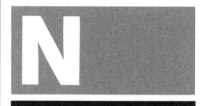

Names

How do other nurses feel about being called by their first names?

Q I'd like to know how other nurses feel about being called by their first names. The resident on our service, a former schoolmate of mine, thinks nothing of shouting down the hall, "Hey, Sheila, bring me this or that." Or, when I'm assisting him with a procedure, "Sheila, honey, adjust that light." How can I let him know I find this conduct unacceptable in a professional setting without sounding mid-Victorian?

A Using first names in a work setting is not necessarily unprofessional. We all know of units (especially when the staff have worked together for many years) where everyone is on a first-name basis.

What other nurses do, however, is not germane to your situation. You say *you* are made uncomfortable by this form of address. *That's* the issue here. Since mind reading is not yet part of the medical school curriculum, however, how can you expect this doctor to know what you're feeling if you don't *tell him?*

Take him aside tomorrow and tell him privately and kindly that you are uncomfortable being called by your first name in front of patients. You need no other explanation.

Once this doctor starts calling you Ms., Miss, or Mrs. it will also discourage him from adding "honey" or calling down the hall after you. These are unprofessional forms of address.

Narcotics counts

What are the legal implications for not keeping them?

Q Some of my friends contract directly with patients' families for private round-the-clock nursing care in the home. They recently asked me to join them for two or three shifts a week, which appeals to me because it pays more than agency work.

One thing bothers me: They don't keep narcotics counts, saying this is time-consuming and not necessary on private cases. But I'm not so sure this is legal, and I don't want to jeopardize my license. What can you tell me about this?

A There's no law in some states that says you must count the narcotics while you're doing private duty nursing in a patient's home. The drugs—once they're ordered by the patient's doctor and purchased by him or his family—belong to the patient.

However, whether or not the other nurses follow suit, count and note how many pills are there at the start and end of your shift. This practice just makes good sense these days. Then, if any questions do come up, you'll be glad you took time out for the count.

Who's legally responsible for reporting missing narcotics?

Q During a change-of-shift narcotics count, I discovered 16 prefilled cartridges of morphine sulfate with their plastic caps broken off. I immediately notified my supervisor, returned all the doses to the pharmacy, and completed an incident report. The 16 cartridges were tested and found to contain saline instead of morphine sulfate.

"I found 16 prefilled cartridges of morphine sulfate with their plastic caps broken off—they were found to contain saline."

Now I'm wondering—was *I* legally responsible for reporting the missing narcotics or was the hospital?

A You *weren't* responsible; the hospital pharmacy was. You did just what you were supposed to do—notified your supervisor, returned the doses to the pharmacy, and filled out an incident report. After that, the narcotics problem was out of your hands.

The pharmacy reports all narcotics incidents to the Federal Drug Enforcement Administration and notifies the hospital security department—which, in turn, notifies the local police. Your pharmacy keeps records of all narcotics incidents. If more than one such incident occurs on your unit, the

pharmacy will probably work with your supervisor to tighten up narcotics policies on your floor—and, perhaps, in your entire hospital.

Narcotics record

Is it legal to continue the record on the back of the form?

Q Our official narcotics-barbiturates record forms are produced on the hospital duplication machine. This machine can accommodate only 29 lines on one side of the paper. Because the pharmacy makes delivery in lots of 30, the last pill (or pills, if extra lines have been used to record mistakes) must be signed out on the back of the sheet.

We told the office manager that we think it is illegal to continue the record on the back of the form. His answer is that they can't change the machine. What are your thoughts?

A There's nothing illegal about writing on the back of the narcotics-barbiturates sheet. If, however, you'd prefer to see the record completed on a single side of the sheet, why not ask the pharmacy to send supplies in lots of 25 rather than 30? That way, even with a few mistakes, you still have room to accommodate all entries.

Nasogastric feeding

Should it be turned off before airway suctioning?

Q In the nursing home where I work, many of the patients receive continuous nasogastric feeding. If one of them needs airway suctioning, should I turn off the feeding during the procedure—and, if so, why?

A Yes, turn off the feeding before suctioning. Your primary concern is that your patient will aspirate his feeding, and by turning it off, you'll at least prevent his aspirating new feeding solution. However, because gastric emptying is sometimes delayed, he could still aspirate feeding accumulated in his stomach. So when you perform suctioning, make sure the patient is in an upright position and have a tonsillar suction device available. You can also decrease his chance of aspiration by using as small a feeding tube as possible and by keeping him in a semiupright or upright position during feeding.

If you can anticipate that your patient will need suctioning in 15 or 20 minutes, turn off his feeding at that point. And if you have a patient who will need frequent suctioning, it will be safer for him and easier for you if you can get an order for intermittent feedings.

Nasogastric tubes

How often should they be replaced?

Q Our unit disagrees on how often nasogastric tubes should be replaced. What do you suggest?

A Nasogastric tubes made of silicone and used for decompression can be left in place for as long as they function properly.

Those made of polyvinylchloride (PVC) become hard and brittle in the presence of gastric juices. They should be changed frequently (ranging from every three days to possibly every 1 to 2 weeks—according to the patient's needs.

Polyethylene tubes do not become hard and brittle and may stay in as long as the tubes are functioning, patent, and freely movable. This may be as long as a month or two.

Your best bet is to use your individual and professional judgment. Also, your unit should have a written nursing policy on this.

How should charcoal be administered?

Q Last week I tried to give a bottle of activated charcoal via a nasogastric (NG) tube to a minimally responsive alcoholic patient.

I shook the contents and squeezed out as much as I could into the NG tube. The bottle still felt heavy and full so I unscrewed the top and saw large lumps of charcoal. I added some tap water and started over. The bottle still felt full. In utter desperation, I used scissors to cut off the top and, much to my dismay, there was still a large amount of thick black goop in the bottle. Am I supposed to somehow mix the charcoal? If so, how?

By the way, the bottle was well within the stamped expiration date. More important, the patient is fine.

A The patient's fine, the nurse... exasperated. From your desperate tone, it sounds like you couldn't easily get another bottle of activated charcoal. That would be plan A. Barring this, adding more water to the unmixed charcoal is perfectly okay, says a manufacturer's representative. However, you should insert a tongue blade down into the bottle and *stir* the water and remaining charcoal, put the top back on the bottle, then shake vigorously.

The problem you had sounds excessive. Ask central supply whether the activated charcoal is stored properly—preferably upside down—at room temperature and not in a cold area (especially in the refrigerator, which is a common mistake). Before using any bottle, check whether the top jarred loose during shipment and allowed leakage. Although you could use this product in a real emergency by adding water as above, first choice would be to return the defective bottle to the manufacturer for replacement.

Should the cuff be deflated or inflated?

Q The nurses on our unit disagree about the proper procedure for placing nasogastric (NG) tubes in intubated patients, and we have no official policy to follow.

Who's correct? Those who say to deflate the endotracheal cuff or those who maintain (as I do) that the cuff should remain inflated. We'd appreciate your opinion.

A When inserting an NG tube in an intubated patient, the endotracheal cuff should remain *inflated*. In fact, deflating the cuff can cause tracheal trauma as well as misplacement of the NG tube in the trachea. Additionally, when the patient gags, a deflated cuff could result in aspiration of stomach contents or secretions.

Enough said. Why not write a policy and submit it to nursing administration for inclusion in the procedure manual?

Nasopharyngeal airway

Is it safe to use one for patients with liquid stool?

Q The other nurses on our intensive care unit use a nasopharyngeal airway (#34 French) attached to a urinary drainage set as a device for patients who have bowel incontinence. They insert the end that's normally exposed when it's used as an airway, and they keep it in place as long as the patient has liquid stool.

Is this method safe?

A Inserting and leaving this stiff tube in the patient's rectum for any length of time will irritate the bowel and may even perforate it.

N

A better alternative: Use a balloon-tipped catheter (#28 French with a 30-cc balloon). Insert the tip into the patient's rectum 2 to 3 inches (5.1 to 7.6 cm) to avoid pushing it into the sigmoid colon. Inflate the balloon with 20 to 30 cc saline or air, making sure the balloon rests on the internal sphincter to prevent stool from oozing; then, attach a drainage bag to the catheter. To relieve pressure and avoid trauma to the mucosa or sphincter, deflate the balloon for a few minutes every hour. Change the catheter and the drainage bag every day.

Another alternative, of course, is to use a rectal tube designed for this purpose.

Negligence

Could a hospital sue a nurse to recover part of the settlement?

Q My hospital was sued for my alleged negligence and settled the claim out of court. A friend of mine, who's also a nurse, told me that the hospital might now sue *me* to recover all or part of the settlement. That doesn't make sense. Am I at risk?

A In this case, no. Because the hospital settled the lawsuit out of court, it can't sue you.

> *"A friend told me that the hospital could sue me to recover all or part of the settlement."*

Theoretically, hospitals can seek reimbursement from negligent nurses for damages awarded by a court, but that rarely happens. For one thing, most nurses are covered only by their employer's malpractice insurance. So, as a practical matter, hospitals usually can't collect much from them. Perhaps more important, though, hospitals don't want to risk losing their nurses by adopting such an antagonistic policy.

Should a nurse speak up if she suspects substandard neonatal care?

Q I work at a large neonatal intensive care unit that accepts infants transported from many local hospitals. Their conditions range from asphyxia to septic shock, and some arrive with irreversible neurologic damage on full life support.

In many cases, I'm convinced by looking at an infant's records that his early treatment was substandard—even negligent. But how should I answer the parents when they question why the condition occurred and whether they should get a lawyer?

A However much your heart goes out to these parents, be cautious. There's no questioning your expertise or what your unit might have accomplished for any of these infants, given your specialized knowledge, experience, and equipment. But hinting at negligence or criticizing earlier care in another, less sophisticated setting may be unfounded and unjust. In such an emotionally charged situation, any criticism from you might be the only impetus the family needs to begin a long and arduous malpractice suit.

Of course, no one of principle can condone even unintentional negligence by doctors or nurses—or deny that it sometimes occurs. But you can help your patients and yourself better by recommending to the parents that they review their infant's condition with his doctor.

If they ask you point-blank about getting a lawyer, you can certainly tell them they have the right to do so, if they're dissatisfied.

What if a doctor ignores a urinary tract infection?

Q I'm an RN in a long-term care facility. One evening when I came on duty, I noticed that 86-year-old Mrs. Smith's catheter was draining thick, grayish yellow urine. When I took her temperature, it was slightly elevated. So I sent a urine specimen to the lab. The urinalysis showed a moderate amount of blood and packed white cells—in fact, the technician said the white cells were so packed he couldn't even *count* the bacteria.

Naturally, I called the doctor immediately. "Don't call me again unless it's an emergency," he snapped, and hung up.

The next morning I put a copy of the lab report in the doctor's mailbox. But it's been more than a week now, and he hasn't ordered any medication for Mrs. Smith.

Mrs. Smith's son, who visits every week, keeps asking me why his mother doesn't eat and why she's so listless. I make lame excuses.

I've discussed the problem with my supervisor, who advises me to *keep* making excuses. If I tell the son the truth, she says, I'll just cause trouble.

I approached the doctor and reminded him about Mrs. Smith's lab report. But he told me to tell Mrs. Smith's son that his mother is "doing fine."

This isn't the first time this doctor has ignored a possible urinary tract infection, and I know it won't be the last. I'm sick of all this deception, and I'm appalled at the doctor's outright *neglect*. What can I do?

A The situation you describe is a sad one and, unfortunately, also a common one. Here are some suggestions.

First of all, did you file an incident report right after your phone conversation with the doctor? You should have, and also should have reported that he hung up on you.

Putting a copy of the lab report in the doctor's mailbox was fine as a polite reminder—as long as you put the original report in the patient's chart. Trying to talk to the doctor in person was fine, too, but by this time he needed more than a reminder—he needed to be asked straight out why he hadn't ordered an antibiotic.

The next logical step was to go to your supervisor, and you did this. Unfortunately it didn't work. At this point you should've taken the problem to the director of nursing or higher, if necessary.

The "higher-ups" probably don't know that this doctor has a reputation for ignoring possible urinary tract infections—and if you don't tell them, who will?

This kind of problem should also be brought to the quality control committee or to the infection control nurse at your facility.

Some of your caring should rub off on the less caring members of your staff.

What if an accident victim dies because he was seen too late?

Q About a year ago, I became director of nursing at a small hospital and nursing home. Our long-term patients get a lot of TLC—but I'm concerned about the care of acute cases we handle. Last week something happened that both saddened and angered me.

Around 5 a.m., a young motorcycle accident victim was brought in. His vital signs were temperature 94° F (34.4° C), blood pressure 60/0 mm Hg, pulse rate 120, and respiration rate 32. He was restless and uncooperative.

The charge nurse called one of the doctors, who gave orders over the telephone. As the patient's con-

dition grew worse and the doctor still hadn't arrived, the nurse kept trying to call the doctor back. His line was always busy. At 6:25 a.m., she finally reached him. At 7:30 a.m., he arrived at the hospital.

At this point, the patient was in X-ray. At 8:20 a.m., as the patient was being taken back to his bed, he died.

I reported to our hospital administrator that this patient had been in the hospital for 3 hours without being examined by a doctor. But the administrator seemed reluctant to criticize the doctor.

I took the matter up with the board of directors. Again, nothing was done. The doctor (who's a board member) contended that he didn't hurry to the hospital because he didn't think the patient was in danger.

What can I do next? I'm afraid the problem is built in. The doctors get so angry at being "disturbed" that many nurses are afraid to call them at home.

I'm looking for another job, but I worry about the patients I'll leave behind. Am I running away or being wise to leave?

A The facts you've presented suggest that the key to the problem seems to be your hospital's identity crisis. The hospital-home should recognize the differences between acute and long-term care and set up clear-cut policies to meet the sharply differing demands of each. Nurses and doctors working in acute care should have the appropriate skills.

You've certainly acted responsibly, but perhaps you should have gone to the doctor involved and told him: "I have serious concerns about how we functioned in this case, and I'd like to talk to you about them."

What should you do now? Put your complaints in writing if further questionable incidents occur. Give copies to both the hospital administration

and the board of directors. Even though some nurses are timid about "annoying" the doctors with calls, try to enlist the nurses' support.

If the authorities remain unresponsive, you may have to take the rather drastic step of seeking help from outside the hospital—from your state medical association, for example.

No, you're not running away by looking for another job. But try to convince the administration to examine its policies and practices in acute care before they lose another patient—*and* a caring director of nursing.

Negligent doctors

What if doctors consistently fail to renew drug orders?

Q The doctors at my hospital have a laissez-faire attitude toward reordering medications—especially antibiotics. Our prescriptions for antibiotics cover 5 days only. But many patients need these drugs longer than that. Unfortunately, the doctors repeatedly forget to renew the antibiotics orders even though we do everything we can to remind them. We write drug expiration dates in red on the charts; we leave notes and signs on the charts; and we remind the doctors in person.

The doctors seem to pass the buck to each other—leaving the patient in the middle. The staff doctors tell us: "We have more important things to do." The attending doctors claim that reordering drugs is the staff doctors' responsibility.

The problem had become so sticky that our nursing administrators finally met with the chiefs of staff. But the doctors contended it "wasn't a nurse's job to be a reminder service." We're now at such an impasse that nursing administration last issued a directive automatically discontinuing all medications when they expire.

This could be a way to punish the doctors. However, what about the patients who must wait for their medications to be renewed—while their infections go untreated?

We hate to nag. But we'd like the doctors to do their job.

A Your problem is, unfortunately, all too common. But even though your intentions are admirable, you seem to be suffering from a common nursing condition: disproportionate guilt.

Nurses can't be responsible for *everything* and especially not for doctors. Sure, you want your patients to get the best care. But chasing after doctors and reminding them to do *their* job isn't *your* job.

So much for the guilt; now the real problem.

Your letting medications expire seems too drastic—particularly since it's the patient who'll suffer. If an order hasn't been renewed on time, call the doctor for his renewal rather than arbitrarily choosing not to give the patient medication. If you simply can't reach the doctor in question, try a staff doctor. He could help out with an order, even if reluctantly, and put pressure on the attending doctor to do his own work.

An internal problem with hospital staff communications should *not* become the problem of the patient, who has enough to cope with. But you do have to keep working toward a resolution. So:
• Talk with your staff doctors about your "bind," and explain the nursing position.
• Report the doctors who will not comply—using proper channels, of course.
• Make extra efforts to have the doctor adhere to the ruling.
• Use your hospital audit system, and your infection control nurse. You'll then be working *with* the administration—a far more effective method than nagging a doctor personally.

There aren't any foolproof solutions. But as we see it, you'll be applying your efforts and energies to the proper pressure points—and making progress toward the one real goal: the patient's well-being.

Neonatal ICU

Aren't there specific standards set for the staffing?

Q One year ago, I accepted the position of neonatal intensive care unit (ICU) unit manager with the understanding that in 6 months, when the new budget went through, we'd have assistant unit managers for every shift. In the meantime, three well-qualified nurses acted as "unofficial" assistant unit managers because of their loyalty to the unit.

It's a year now and other units have gotten their assistant unit managers but not the neonatal ICU. We've gone through channels right up to the director of nursing about this (and the director in charge of the unit has supported us all the way). I get a sympathetic hearing but it seems that because of hospital politics, we're still on the waiting list.

My "unofficial" assistant unit managers no longer feel they should continue with the added responsibilities because the administration hasn't kept its word, and I agree with them. Currently we're rotating the charge position among all the RNs, which means that the unqualified nurses are sometimes in charge.

I don't know what else to do. Aren't there specific standards set for the staffing in a neonatal ICU? I'll welcome any suggestions.

A Before the suggestions, first the compliments. You're some unit manager. You intelligently anticipated the staffing your department would need and made the assistant unit manager jobs one of

your conditions for accepting the position.

Since then, you've taken all the right steps, too, in trying to get administration to live up to its side of the commitment. There are no official figures on regulatory staffing for neonatal ICUs so you can't add them to the weight of your argument. Most statements on staffing, however, just seem to lean heavily on the catchall phrase that the hospital must "supply adequate coverage."

The only thing you can do at this point is keep your cool—and your consistency. Yes, keep going back to nursing service—it is indeed the squeaking wheel that gets the grease.

Trying to look on the bright side of it, now, you may find that by rotating all your RNs you'll be building a stronger staff for the future— one you can be completely confident about whenever you're off duty.

In the meantime, though, please don't give up. Keep fighting the good fight.

Nipple pinching

Is it acceptable for checking reaction to pain?

Q I'm appalled by something the staff is doing at the hospital where I've just started to work. They're squeezing or twisting a patient's nipples to check his reaction to painful stimuli. The rationale is that pinching the arms or legs would cause bruises, but pinching nipples would not.

I think the technique is cruel, but unfortunately it seems to be gaining popularity at the hospital. What's more, it's not being used just on comatose patients (which is bad enough); it's also being used on stuporous patients and those unresponsive to verbal commands.

I know we have more humane ways of eliciting response from patients. For instance, *I* always pinch the earlobe. Can you suggest any other techniques?

More to the point, though, is squeezing or twisting nipples acceptable practice?

A Squeezing or twisting nipples is *not* acceptable practice, and the practice is appalling. It isn't mentioned in any medical or nursing textbooks (unless the Marquis de Sade authorized a text). No *caring* nurse would use this technique.

> *"They're squeezing or twisting a patient's nipples to check his reaction to painful stimuli."*

Your question was put to 15 male and female health professionals, which included 5 staff nurses and a neurologic nursing instructor, 3 physician's assistants, 2 anesthetists, 2 anesthesiologists, and 2 neurosurgeons. Some of these professionals came from a city teaching hospital; others, from a small, local hospital. Here's a sample of their comments: "obviously unnecessary," "disrespectful," "aesthetically unsound," "sexist," and "downright barbaric."

But here's the real clincher: A neurosurgeon said that overzealous twisting of a nipple *can* cause bruises. It can even cause skin sloughing and the eventual *loss of a nipple.*

Here are two alternative techniques for eliciting response: pinching the trapezius muscle and applying submandibular pressure. Of course, these could cause bruising, too, but the potential complications are far less serious than the complications of injuring a nipple.

To stop the practice in your hospital, send a documented memo recording your observations up through the proper nursing channels. Why not solicit the support of your colleagues and supervisors by asking them to sign the memo?

"No code" orders

Couldn't a lidocaine drip be considered an extreme measure to prolong the patient's life?

Q On the intensive care unit where I work, our standing orders call for administering a bolus of lidocaine (lignocaine) and starting a lidocaine drip for any patient who has a 5-second run of ventricular tachycardia. But what about a patient who is designated "no code"? Couldn't the lidocaine drip be considered an extreme measure to prolong the patient's life?

What's your opinion on this, and how do you suggest we handle this situation?

A Follow the standing orders. Lidocaine is not an *extreme* measure and can be given appropriately to a "no-code" patient unless otherwise specified. Whether or not the lidocaine will prolong any patient's life is a judgment call. If the doctor doesn't want the standing orders followed, he should specify what he wants done for that patient. He may order something as simple as oxygen or potassium to control the patient's arrhythmia.

Does a nurse have authority to stop a code?

Q A doctor recently gave one of my co-workers a written do-not-resuscitate (DNR) order for a terminally ill patient. A short time later, that nurse left for lunch without telling anyone about the order. While she was away, the patient went into cardiac arrest.

Unaware of the newly written DNR order, a unit secretary trained in cardiopulmonary resuscitation (CPR) called a code and began CPR. Then the CPR team arrived and took over. When my friend returned from lunch, she tried to stop the code,

but team members told her that they couldn't stop without another order from the doctor.

She got the order, but not before the patient was revived and put on a ventilator. Should the team have responded to a call from a secretary? And should the team have stopped CPR when the nurse told them to?

A If your secretary was authorized to call the code, then the CPR team responded correctly. But even if she wasn't authorized, the team still may have acted properly if hospital policy requires the team to respond to any call.

So, whether your team's actions were authorized or not, they were legal *if the team followed hospital policy in responding to the code.*

As for stopping CPR, you again have to look at hospital policy. Some hospitals allow team members to stop when they know or believe the doctor has given a "no" code order; others require that the doctor give another order in person. If your hospital doesn't have a policy on stopping CPR once it's started, the team was probably right to continue CPR.

Hospital administrators should clarify who's authorized to call a code. And in case communication breaks down again, they should establish a policy for instances when the code team starts CPR on a no-code patient.

In this case, your co-worker caused unnecessary confusion by neglecting to tell anyone about the order. And that literally had life-or-death consequences for her patient.

How can a nurse be sure this is what the patient wanted?

Q When the doctor wrote a do-not-resuscitate (DNR) order for my patient with esophageal cancer, he told us to page him stat if the man's blood pressure dropped,

N

then administer dopamine. I'm not sure this is what the patient wanted when he asked for a DNR order. What should we do now?

A First, find out what a DNR order means to your patient. Perhaps he's willing to accept medication but draws the line at cardiopulmonary resuscitation.

As you talk with him, explore his feelings about types of resuscitative measures, including the use of dopamine to stabilize blood pressure. Also, make sure he understands his diagnosis and prognosis, or his decision won't be informed.

Document your conversation, including direct quotes from the patient ("I've had enough" or "I'm not ready to die"). Then discuss your findings with his doctor, who should clarify the DNR order with the patient if necessary.

Finally, make sure the doctor writes and signs a clear order—for example, "no code" or "limited code (dopamine only)." The order should include any special directions, too. Paging the doctor and administering dopamine shouldn't seem like an afterthought. These instructions should be explicitly written as an order on the patient's chart.

How can a patient's daughter be helped to accept his wishes?

Q One of my patients, a comatose, terminally ill man, was transferred out of the intensive care unit with a do-not-resuscitate order. His daughter objected to the order, but I'm pretty sure it's what the patient wanted—he'd briefly discussed his wishes with the doctor while he was still lucid. How can I help her accept this?

A Your patient's daughter may be denying the severity of her father's illness, or she may be having trouble letting go. If she equates "no code" with "no care," she might also fear that her father has been abandoned. Explain to her that this isn't so, that her father will be cared for and kept comfortable until he dies.

Gently ask her why she objects to the order. Let her know that doubts and confusion are normal at a time like this, and encourage her to talk with the doctor so he can answer her questions. If she can trust the doctor's judgment, she'll cope with her grief better.

You might also explore the ethical issues with her. When she's ready, talk about what "death with dignity" means to her. Ask her how she feels about honoring a patient's right to refuse treatment—and what she'd want others to do for her if she were terminally ill. You could even talk with her about living wills as a way to help her clarify her own wishes.

How can nurses keep other departments informed?

Q Recently, two terminally ill patients with do-not-resuscitate (DNR) orders were coded after they arrested in physical therapy or radiology—because personnel in those departments didn't know about the orders. What can we do to prevent this from happening in the future?

A You need to spread the word about DNR orders to all employees—many of whom may not know what a DNR order means or where to look for it. The hospital's code committee or team should find a way to educate them.

To help the code team identify patients covered by DNR orders, many hospitals are using colored bracelets or a small sticker on the patient's chart. Your hospital's code committee might want to adopt a similar practice.

How could nurses get a hospital to write a policy?

Q I work at a small hospital that doesn't have a written policy about do-not-resuscitate (DNR) orders. Naturally, we're concerned. Could you recommend guidelines that we could present to hospital administration?

A According to the U.S. Army's comprehensive policy and the Hastings Center's *Guidelines on the Termination of Life-Sustaining Treatment and the Care of the Dying,* the doctor should:

• write the DNR order, date it, and sign the order sheet
• note the medical rationale for the order
• document the patient's consent (if he's competent to give consent), or note that the patient is incompetent
• summarize discussions with the patient or family about the order
• record consultations with nurses, other doctors, or clergy
• determine the level of treatment to be continued
• reassess the patient periodically and change the order if appropriate.

The doctor should document all of this information in the patient's progress notes.

How ethical and legal is a "drug code only" policy?

Q Not long ago, our hospital amended its "no code" policy to include something called "drug code only." In essence, this policy means routine drugs included in emergency procedures (such as atropine for bradycardia, or lidocaine [lignocaine] for malignant ventricular arrhythmias) may be given, but chest compressions, respiratory assistance, and defibrillation are not to be done.

My co-workers and I aren't comfortable with this policy. For one thing, we feel that resuscitation should either be done at maximal effort or not at all. Otherwise, how could we justify raising the family's hopes that the patient could be revived—not to mention the major expense incurred by this limited treatment? We also wonder how a court would view such halfway measures.

We need another opinion.

A You're really asking two questions—one ethical and the other legal. Take the legal question first.

To date, no doctors or nurses have been successfully prosecuted in connection with a legal "no code" order. But the doctor must have thoroughly explained the situation to the patient or family and have procured patient or family acceptance of a "no code" order. This must be fully documented on the record. And the doctor's order to the nursing staff must be *written*—not given verbally. Then everyone involved would be legally protected.

Now, whether resuscitation should be all out or nothing at all is a sensitive *ethical* issue. In ethical matters there's usually room for more than one answer. But if a patient has a chance for survival, he should be given *total* resuscitation effort during a code. If the patient is dying—and there seems to be no hope for recovery—*using drugs to help him die comfortably* is ethically appropriate. But using drugs *to prolong the dying process* is ethically inappropriate.

Because you're the one who must administer these "drug code only" drugs, and because you're not comfortable doing so, you should report your concerns to the medical and nursing staff.

Request a meeting to explore the ethics of the situation you're dealing with, and work out a policy that will make you comfortable with your course of action.

Is it illegal to comply with a relative's wishes when there are no doctor's orders?

Q I work as a home health care nurse. Recently, one of my terminally ill patients arrested while I was visiting him. His son, who lived with him, asked me not to perform cardiopulmonary resuscitation. The doctor hadn't written a do-not-resuscitate (DNR) order, but I complied with the son's wishes and let the patient die.

Did I violate the nurse practice act? What should I do if this happens with another patient?

A From a legal viewpoint, you should try to resuscitate any patient who goes into cardiac arrest unless you have a doctor's order to the contrary. By not doing so, you make a medical decision—and that's clearly not allowed by any state's nurse practice act.

But as a practical matter, you needn't worry. If the patient had chosen to be cared for at home, he was making an implied decision not to be resuscitated. In situations like this, no one is likely to sue you for failing to resuscitate the patient.

Your agency needs to develop a policy about DNR orders. Then you should discuss the policy with terminally ill patients, their doctors, and their families when you start home care. That way, you'll know what to do *before* you're under the gun.

Isn't it unusual for an order to read "full code" when the ABCs of resuscitation can't be followed?

Q Last week, we admitted an elderly patient who was critically ill with pneumonia. When we asked for her code status, her doctor told us full code. And, although he

wouldn't put it in writing, he also told us not to perform cardiac compressions because this patient's sternum and ribs had been removed during a previous surgery.

We never had to act on the order, though; the patient's status was changed to "do not resuscitate" in a matter of days. But isn't it unusual for an order to read "full code" when the ABCs of resuscitation can't be followed?

A Technically, there's no such designation as full code—only code or do not resuscitate, and most hospitals' policies specify that these orders be written. In practice, some doctors want only one or two specific aspects of the code procedure used for certain patients (for instance, "no compressions"), and the term full code has made its way into the language to mean that all aspects of advanced cardiac life support should be used—airway management and breathing, I.V. therapy, drug administration, defibrillation, and cardiac compressions. Obviously, when you can't perform cardiac compressions, as in the case you cite, that information should be in writing.

Why not suggest a staff development session on code policies at your hospital? If there's no policy prohibiting verbal (or telephone) code orders, then one's needed.

Should a patient be allowed to choke to death?

Q I'm a new graduate who was assigned to help care for a terminally ill cancer patient with "no-code" orders. One night last week, the nursing assistant came running to the desk to report that she found him in distress. When my charge nurse and I got to him, we could see that although he was still alert, he was choking on vomitus. He looked at me with panic in his eyes—a look I'll never ever forget.

N

I wanted to do *something,* but the charge nurse said he was a no-code so we couldn't. I reached for his hands and held them. Several minutes went by before his respirations stopped.

I'm really torn up over this incident. Code or no-code, it doesn't seem right to watch someone die like that. What do you say?

A Code or no-code, every patient deserves to die as comfortably as possible—and choking to death is a terrible way to go. This patient should have been suctioned, which is a *comfort,* not a *resuscitative,* measure—whether or not clearing his airway might delay his death. What you cite is an unfortunate example of how the complex and murky legal and ethical issues surrounding do-not-resuscitate (DNR) orders can make a nurse—who's on her own to make a quick decision—hesitate to follow her nursing instincts. We suggest that you ask your hospital administrator to arrange an interdisciplinary meeting—doctors, nurses, social workers, your hospital lawyer, and a member of the ethics committee—to review the laws in your state and your hospital's DNR policy.

The bad news is that you probably *won't* ever forget this incident. But that can also be the good news—if you stop heaping guilt on yourself and simply learn from the experience. This time you were inexperienced and followed someone else's lead. But if there's a next time, you'll know for sure what needs to be done and be assertive enough to do it.

Shouldn't the patient's wishes be respected?

Q I'm caring for a 54-year-old man who has pancreatic cancer. Although weak and cachectic, he's alert, oriented, and competent. He isn't expected to live more than a few months, yet he insists on full-

code status. His daughter thinks this is irrational. I agree, but I know he's capable of making his own decisions, and I respect that.

Now his daughter is pressuring the doctor to sign a no-code order. What should I do?

A As his advocate, make sure his wishes are clearly documented. Using his own words, chart any conversations you have with him about code status. Also, assure him that *he* has the right to choose what treatments he does or doesn't want.

You might want to call a family conference to deal with the difference of opinion over code status. Ask the hospital's chaplain or medical ethicist to sit in on the meeting and help you focus the discussion. Include the doctor for an update on his treatment goals so you can devise an effective and appropriate care plan.

Your patient seems to be denying the seriousness of his condition. That may be beneficial for him, though. Consult with a psychiatric clinical nurse specialist, psychiatrist, or psychologist to learn more about this patient's need for control, assurance, and self-esteem.

Finally, try to sort out your ambivalent feelings about coding this patient. Do you feel obligated to carry out his wishes, no matter what the consequences? Again, a psychiatric clinical nurse specialist could help you balance conflicting feelings.

Should the family be told what it means?

Q One of my patients, an elderly woman, was hospitalized after her second cerebrovascular accident. She'd requested a do-not-resuscitate (DNR) order, and her relatives agreed. The doctor wrote the order. On my day off, the woman

developed ventricular fibrillation and was successfully defibrillated. Now her family is upset—and confused about what a DNR order means. They're looking to me for answers. What should I tell them?

A Before you say anything, double-check your hospital's policy on DNR orders. It may distinguish between "no code" (absolutely no intervention) and "limited code" (some interventions permitted). Then look at the patient's medical record. Did the doctor specify that defibrillation was (or wasn't) to be done if she coded?

Next, ask the doctor to clarify the patient's code status—no code or limited code, specific resuscitative measures permitted (if any), and duration of the order. The progress notes should indicate that he spoke with the patient about her options and that the order reflects the wishes she expressed.

These steps should tell you whether the patient's right to refuse treatment was compromised. Then you can speak to the patient and her family with confidence, clarifying any remaining questions and assuring them that her choices will be respected.

Should the nurse have called a code?

Q Last week, I was caring for a 4-year-old boy who was dying of leukemia. His parents told me they didn't want him resuscitated if his heart stopped. A little later, as I was checking his vital signs, he suddenly had trouble breathing. I picked him up and rocked him. He seemed to relax. A few minutes later, he died peacefully in my arms and I put him back in bed.

His parents returned to the room at about the same time as a resident, who asked me why I hadn't called a code. I explained that the patient was terminal and that his parents didn't want him resuscitated. But the resident pushed me aside and started cardiopulmonary resuscitation anyway. In the end, the father had to pull the resident off his son and repeat what I'd said.

The next day, my manager called me into her office and asked why I hadn't called a code. I explained the situation, but she reminded me of the hospital policy requiring that we call a code in the absence of a do-not-resuscitate (DNR) order, which hadn't been written.

Thanks to support from the hospital's chaplain, who knew the family and agreed with my decision, I was given only a reprimand. I still feel I did the right thing—and I'd probably do it again in the same situation. What do you think?

A This is one of those times when your role as a patient advocate conflicts with your obligations as a hospital employee. In your heart, you may feel you did the right thing for this patient and his family. But, as your manager pointed out, you also have a responsibility to follow hospital policy. By not doing so, you could have jeopardized your job.

To minimize similar conflicts in the future, you should press administrators to revise the hospital's DNR policy. Staff members need a way to identify potential no-code patients quickly—during the initial nursing assessment, for instance—and to document no-code requests.

A simple checklist added to the patient's chart would accomplish this. After getting a DNR request from a patient (or his parents or guardian, if he's a minor), you'd alert the doctor. Then you'd scan your checklist for evidence of appropriate documentation. Do you have a copy of the patient's living will or durable power of attorney, if those documents are legally binding in your state? Has the request been charted? Have you received permission for a DNR order from a legal guardian or the courts?

If you can answer yes to any of these questions, you'd call the doctor again and ask him for a DNR order. Of course, the hospital's policy must specify how to receive and document DNR orders given over the phone.

Finally, the policy should spell out what to do if conflicts arise. For example, what should you do if a doctor refuses to write a DNR order for a patient who requests one? A well-written policy would clearly define the steps you should take to protect your patient's rights.

What can a nurse do if she's uncomfortable with the hospital's policy?

Q Not long ago, our hospital amended its "no code" policy to include something called "drug code only." In essence, this policy means routine drugs included in emergency procedures (such as atropine for bradycardia and lidocaine ([lignocaine, Xylocaine] for malignant ventricular arrhythmias) may be given, but chest compressions, respiratory assistance, and defibrillation are not to be done.

My co-workers and I aren't comfortable with this policy. For one thing, we feel that resuscitation should either be done at maximal effort or not at all. Otherwise, how could we justify raising the family's hopes that the patient could be revived—not to mention the major expense incurred by this limited treatment? We also wonder how a court would view such halfway measures.

We need another opinion.

A You're really asking two questions—one's ethical and the other's legal. Here's the answer to your legal question.

To date, no doctors or nurses have been successfully prosecuted in connection with a legal "no code" order. But the doctor must have thoroughly explained the situation

to the patient or family and have procured patient or family acceptance of a "no code" order. This must be fully documented on the record. And the doctor's order to the nursing staff must be *written*—not given verbally. Then everyone involved would be legally protected.

> *"We feel that resuscitation should be done at maximal effort or not at all."*

Now, whether resuscitation should be all out or nothing at all is a sensitive *ethical* issue. In ethical matters there's usually room for more than one answer. But shouldn't a patient who has a chance for survival be given *total* resuscitation effort during a code? If the patient is dying—and there seems to be no hope for recovery—*using drugs to help him die comfortably* is ethically appropriate. But using drugs *to prolong the dying process* is ethically inappropriate.

Because you're the one who must administer these "drug code only" drugs, and because you're not comfortable doing do, report your concerns to the medical and nursing staff.

Request a meeting to explore the ethics of the situation you're dealing with, and work out a policy that will make you comfortable with your course of action.

What can be done to prevent a mix-up over code status?

Q I was taking care of an acquired immunodeficiency syndrome patient with end-stage *Pneumocystis carinii* pneumonia. When he went into respiratory arrest, the doctor immediately intubated him. I was shocked because I didn't think the patient would want to be resuscitated. What can be done to prevent this sort of mix-up in the future?

A As you'd probably agree, guessing what someone "would have wanted" is useless. That's why one of your main goals when caring for a patient like this should be to clarify his code status up front, before it's too late.

Many hospitals have policies for doing this when a patient is admitted with a serious condition or for complicated surgery. For example, a patient might be asked, "Do you have a living will?" If he says yes, a copy is put in the medical record and flagged so the doctor can write a do-not-resuscitate (DNR) order if appropriate. If the answer is no, the patient could be asked whether he's familiar with living wills and if he'd like more information. This would also be a good time to teach him about DNR orders.

If your hospital doesn't have a policy like this, share your concerns with your manager and ask her to talk with nursing administration about bringing the matter before the policy and procedure committees. You could even volunteer to help the committees.

What if a hospital's policy violates state law?

Q We have a new law in our state that worries me because it contradicts the policy of the hospital where I work. The new law says that a do-not-resuscitate (DNR) order must be accompanied by two doctors' signatures and one family member's consent. Hospital policy simply calls for the patient's attending doctor to issue and sign the DNR order.

I asked administration about this discrepancy, and they just told me to follow hospital policy until they investigated things further. But what happens in the meantime?

What if a DNR order following current hospital policy is written for one of my patients and that patient goes into cardiac arrest? Since I know the DNR order doesn't jibe with the state's new law, should I try to resuscitate the patient or what?

A The new law you're talking about—which does call for DNR orders to be accompanied by the signatures of two doctors and the consent of a family member—*is* on the books in your particular state. However, the law is classified as a *nonbinding statutory law.* As such, health care professionals and institutions are *not* absolutely required to obey it. Rather, the new law is an option that they may or may not choose to take. If your hospital does not choose to adhere to it, you must follow hospital policy on the subject.

For the sake of argument, however, say the law *is* binding. The responsibility to see that it's obeyed *still* wouldn't be yours. It would be the hospital's. You see, a new law sometimes takes a while to make it into hospital policy books. This delay is neither malicious nor neglectful. It's just that the hospital must familiarize its staff with the new law and policy. So before the new law becomes *official* hospital policy, you're to follow *existing* hospital policy—even if it contradicts the law.

You'd be wise, though, to remind administration about the new law (as you did), then document the situation to cover yourself. For instance, your documentation could read, "I'm following hospital policy regarding consents and signatures on DNR orders. I'm aware, though, of new legislation on this and I've contacted administration about it by memo (or phone)."

Who makes the final decision on "no code"?

Q Recently, we had an 82-year-old patient with terminal cancer. She'd been in and out of our unit many times, and we all felt that this would be her last admission. But for some reason, the doctor felt he could pull her through one more time, and so refused to write a "no code" order.

While she hovered between semiconsciousness and confusion, we worried that she'd have a cardiac arrest and we'd have to resuscitate her.

One night, when her blood pressure was fluctuating wildly, the charge nurse decided to talk to her daughters. The nurse told them how grave their mother's condition was and asked whether they'd ever considered requesting "no heroic measures" if their mother arrested again.

After discussing this with the rest of their family, the daughters decided they *didn't* want their mother resuscitated.

When the doctor found out, he was furious and let the charge nurse have it with both barrels. He told her she'd stepped out of line, had ruined his treatment plan, and that even though the patient was old, she was "still salvageable." Then he filed an incident report.

To our great relief, a few days later, the doctor's *partner* wrote a "no code" order for the patient.

This isn't the first time this has happened, and it won't be the last. Who makes the final decision on resuscitation? And was the charge nurse really out of line?

A Coding or not coding a patient should be a *team* decision—the doctor, the nurses, and the family should discuss the situation. Ideally, the patient himself should be involved in the decision, but of course this wasn't possible in the case you cited.

Ultimately, writing the order is the doctor's responsibility and his privilege. He's the one who must defend the order. However, many factors besides medical prognosis will have to be taken into account. For instance, is the family ready to "let go"? Is the patient himself ready to let go? Has the patient made a will? Since the nurse may be closer to the family than the doctor, she might know the answers to these questions. If she does, she certainly should inform the doctor.

About your second question— "Was the charge nurse out of line?" The nurse *was* out of line to approach the family *without discussing the problem with the doctor first.* (This would have been professional courtesy.) Maybe the nurse could've changed the doctor's mind, maybe not. But if the doctor *did* decide to write the order, he might've asked the nurse to discuss resuscitative measures with the family. He might've asked the nurse to be present when *he* talked to the family—or he might even have asked her to do the talking. (All of this, by the way, should've been done *before* the patient's "blood pressure was fluctuating wildly").

Keep in mind that the doctor has an emotional as well as professional investment in his patients. He may find it difficult to admit to himself that his patient will never recover.

So when it comes to coding, *everyone* involved in the decision needs support in order to prepare the patient for the most peaceful death possible.

Noises

What can be done about mysterious noises?

Q Three months ago on our medical/surgical unit, we became aware that every morning between 2 and 3, a loud knocking was oc-

curring on either of the two doors of adjoining private rooms.

In the beginning, we thought patients in these rooms were banging for attention. When we'd check, however, we'd find them sound asleep or complaining that we'd awakened them with our loud knocking. This became enough of a concern that I reported it to the director of nursing.

Since our floor has no lounge, we take our breaks in any room that's vacant. The night one of the private rooms was vacant, our director sat with us. She was closest to the door when the knock came; it was so forceful her chair vibrated. She and the head of maintenance have checked out every possible explanation with no results.

> *"Every morning between 2 and 3 we heard a loud knocking, but we never found the cause."*

So far, the staff has been very sensible about this but it definitely affects us. For example, we've had four dying patients in those rooms and each time "just by chance" there are always at least two of us in the room between 2 and 3 a.m. to see if that's when the patient will expire. So far, none of them has.

With one exception, we've kept all talk of the knocking from the patients. The exception was a middle-aged woman who wasn't very ill. She watched TV until the early hours of the morning and, when she first heard the knocking, wanted to know who was playing games. So we told her. After that when she heard the knocking, she'd call out, "Your friend just checked in."

I'd like to know how you'd handle this. Believe me, this is no joke.

A At one large city hospital, succeeding occupants of one room complained of loud organ music. From time to time, the staff

heard it, too, and they agreed that it was definitely loud, gloomy organ music. They searched for the origin but never did track it down.

In the course of remodeling, that block of rooms was torn down and "The Music Room" is now part of a hall. From time to time, though, reliable people say they still hear organ music in that part of the hall. There's still no explanation!

Perhaps in your case, the mystery will eventually be traced to some mechanical or electrical phenomenon that just happens to cause a knocking sound in that part of the building at that time of morning.

Or perhaps it will never be explained. Or it may stop as suddenly as it started.

No matter what the outcome, we'd like to commend you for handling an unusual situation in the best possible way. You've alerted your staff without alarming the patients. You've reported it to your director who checked it out as far as she could. And you're keeping your cool—and your sense of humor—about "your friend."

Nuclear accident

Should a supply of potassium iodide be kept handy?

Q The nuclear accident at Chernobyl made us all stop and think—what if? As a college health nurse in a school less than 20 miles (32 km) from a nuclear power plant, I want to be ready.

I read somewhere that after Chernobyl, the State Department sent potassium iodide to U.S. embassy personnel in the Soviet Union. What's the rationale for using potassium iodide? Would it be a good idea for me to keep a supply in the infirmary, just in case?

A To answer your first question: One of the hazards of a reactor accident is the release of a radioactive form of iodine (iodine 131) that causes thyroid cancer. Because the thyroid normally absorbs iodine, the goal is to have people who might be exposed to iodine 131 take potassium iodide to saturate the gland before the radioactive iodine reaches it. The radioactive iodine will then pass through the body rather than be absorbed by the thyroid.

> *"The nuclear accident at Chernobyl made us all stop and think...I work near a nuclear plant and I want to be ready."*

The answer to your second question is still up for discussion. Medical experts and health care organizations are actively debating the merits of stocking potassium iodide for full-scale distribution. The Food and Drug Administration (FDA) and the American Thyroid Association (ATA) recommend potassium iodide for people exposed to sufficiently high levels of iodine 131 (according to the FDA, enough to deliver 25 rems to their thyroids; according to the ATA, 100 rems). Opponents of stocking it say:

1. The construction of American nuclear power plants makes release of large amounts of iodine 131 unlikely;
2. Each treatment is effective for only 12 hours, and the drug must be taken *before* exposure;
3. Potassium iodide could have adverse effects on those with thyroid disorders and the 2% to 3% of the population who may have an allergic reaction; and
4. The evidence proving iodine 131 causes cancer is still inconclusive.

As things stand now, the single most persuasive reason for stocking potassium iodide could be that most of us want something, anything, available to shield us from even the threat of nuclear radiation. Look closely at your own situation (your proximity to the power plant, the student census, your facility's capabilities for organizing and carrying out an emergency program), weigh all the factors, then decide.

Nurse-doctor conflict

How can a nurse dispute the doctor?

Q I started working in this hospital right after passing my state boards, so I'm not too confident to begin with. Then last week, the director of nursing called me into her office and handed me a written reprimand for "willful conduct detrimental to patient care." She put me on probation and suspended me for 5 days without pay.

It all started when one of the doctors wrote on his order sheet that he wanted me taken off his patient's case. He stated that although his patient knew he had a poor prognosis, I had dashed all his hopes. He quoted me as saying, "You can take all of the treatments you want, but there's no cure for your type of cancer." Now he thinks he'll die no matter what's done.

I tried to tell the director of nursing that all I said was they've done studies and made a lot of progress and that I praised the patient for his positive attitude. She didn't comment.

I don't know what to do about it, but I surely don't think I'm being treated fairly. Do you?

A Not by any means. Perhaps this patient was anxious and depressed and just lashed out against you to the doctor.

These thoughts may help give you some perspective:
• Patients can misinterpret anyone's statements. Before taking any action, the doctor should have talked with you first and then discussed what you actually said with you and your unit manager. That way you could have gone in as a *team* to reassure the patient.
• Whenever a patient has a poor prognosis, his doctor should explain his treatment goals to the nursing staff. And because you were inexperienced, someone on the unit should have helped you prepare for the assignment.
• The patient's chart is a legal document for recording *patient* treatments, not staff problems. Even if you made the alleged statement, a reference like this sends up a red flag for any attorney looking for trouble and invites liability for the hospital. (The *doctor* should be counseled about inappropriate charting.)

Try to arrange a meeting with the director of nursing and the doctor, and ask your unit manager if she'll go with you for moral support. You'll probably be nervous, so take some written notes along to help you explain your side of the story again. Request that your suspension be rescinded and your pay restored. And ask the director of nursing to consider substituting a positive learning assignment—such as a staff development session. Of course, it takes courage to speak up. But this time, when your director of nursing hears your message for herself, she should give you support.

Nurse practitioners

Are they held to the same standard of care as doctors?

Q I've just become a nurse practitioner. One of my colleagues at the clinic says we're held to the same standard of care as the doctors we work with. Is she right?

A She could be. You're certainly held to a higher standard of care than an RN, even if the nursing board hasn't established separate regulations for nurse practitioners.

The court of appeals in one state recently ruled that a nurse practitioner is a specialist who should meet a standard of care appropriate to her level of knowledge and skill, even if she's working under a doctor's standing orders. In fact, the court said the standard could be the same as that applied to a doctor, depending on what the nurse practitioner does.

Nursery

Isn't it dangerous to hand-carry newborns to another floor?

Q Our hospital's labor and delivery room is located on the first floor, and our nursery is on the second. At present, newborn babies are hand-carried to the nursery. But we think this can be dangerous. What if the nurse trips or falls—and injures the new baby?

Then there's another kind of threat: As the babies are carried through the halls, the relatives converge (all adoring, of course). Some want to touch or kiss the new baby. While we don't want to be rude, shouldn't we be concerned about exposing the infant to infection?

Can you suggest a policy for our hospital that will be fair to both adoring relatives and the adorable infants?

A You may want to recommend the following policy for transporting babies:
• Babies should be transported between the postpartum unit and nursery by infant cribs only.
• When an infant has to be transported to X-ray or to some other area of the hospital, the baby must be transported in an incubator.
• Hand-carrying an infant will be permitted only in an emergency.

Because your delivery room and nursery are geographically separate, under these new regulations the baby would have to be transported in an incubator.

And now, about visitors being permitted near an infant immediately after delivery. Restrict visits to the immediate family—the father, grandparents, or siblings. Neighbors and friends should wait until the baby comes home to offer their warm welcome.

Nurses' pledge

Isn't there some official, universal nurses' pledge?

Q Recently I attended two graduation ceremonies for nieces who completed BSN programs. Much to my surprise, neither class recited a nurses' pledge. Later I learned that a nurses' pledge *is* usually recited during a separate pinning ceremony, but the pledge isn't a standard one. It could even be one composed by a class member. "In fact," both graduates were quick to point out, "there's no law saying nursing graduates must recite a pledge at all. Nowadays we're more concerned about what's in our heads and hearts, not what we recite."

All well and good, but isn't there some official, universal nurses' pledge?

A The International Council of Nurses' pledge is as official and universal as could be. Here's how it goes: "In the full knowledge of the obligation I am undertaking, I promise to care for the sick with all the skill and understanding I possess, without regard to race, creed, color, politics, or social status, sparing no effort to conserve life, to alleviate suffering, and to promote health.

"I will respect at all times the dignity and religious beliefs of the patients under my care, holding in confidence all personal information entrusted to me and refraining from any action which might endanger life or health.

"I will endeavour to keep my professional knowledge and skill at the highest level and to give loyal support and cooperation to all members of the health care team. I will do my utmost to honor the international code of ethics applied to nursing and to uphold the integrity of the nurse."

Nurses' titles

Why do they keep changing?

Q I left active nursing about 5 years ago, but I continue to read nursing journals. What surprises me sometimes is how terms have changed. Tell me, what happened to the head nurse? Now she's a unit manager. Singers, sports teams, and supermarkets have managers. And why did patients become clients? Lawyers have clients. Are we trying to dehumanize our care?

A To borrow from writer Gertrude Stein, a patient is a patient is a patient. However, the trend is to use the term client for someone who contracts for nursing service outside the hospital setting. It reflects the increased emphasis on professionalism.

This same trend affects hospital nurses. One good example is scrapping the ambiguous title head nurse for unit manager, which identifies a distinct role and rung on the management ladder. And in a subtle but significant way, it also changes the style of the unit's working relationship from that of a head nurse directing subordinates to a manager working with her team of professionals.

Nursing

When is it too late to start?

Q After 20 years of caring for a developmentally disabled son, I considered myself a natural for nursing. So I attended nursing school. As a new graduate, I got my nursing license in the mail with some birthday cards—for my 50th birthday.

Then I started working, and instead of the rewarding experience I expected, I've ended up feeling like a klutz. I've even heard the young unit secretary and nurses laughing behind my back. My unit manager says that I do my work well enough but that I lack confidence in my own decisions.

Was I wrong to think I could start something new at this late date?

A No, you weren't wrong. You're a gutsy lady who may be too uptight to give herself a fair chance.

Small wonder you feel insecure. After all, you've just come off 20 years of being both provider and decision maker at home. Now you're in an entirely new situation, receiving assignments and criticism from "old pros" maybe half your age. That's scary, all right, for anyone. It might help you to realize that self-confidence is just another skill, and you can learn it as well as anyone.

Start by confiding in a staff member you trust. Ask her if you can observe how she works with patients and families. Then imitate her coping behaviors, and eventually some of her confidence is bound to rub off on you.

To expand your clinical skills, attend staff development and continuing education classes. Try to identify a specific skill that's frequently needed on your unit (for example, teaching new diabetic patients how to perform insulin injections). Become expert in this skill, and before you know it, you'll be the designated resource person (and you might be sought after by other departments as well).

Relish your successes, even little ones, and replay them in your mind over and over. As your confidence grows, your attitude will become more positive.

And smile. As the old saying should have said, "She who laughs, lasts."

Nursing home

Does the JCAHO require 90% of patients to eat in a dining room?

Q At the long-term care facility where I work, we expect a visit soon from the Joint Commission on Accreditation of Healthcare Organizations (JCAHO). Our administrator told us that JCAHO requires 90% of the patients on each unit to eat their meals in a community dining room, so we're to enforce this more rigorously as the big visit approaches. Included in this 90% are many very ill patients, and some who get a lot of vigorous rehabilitation therapy. Some days, I've seen tired, frail women cry as they're pushed to dinner in wheelchairs.

I've told my director of nursing that I'll try to persuade patients to go to the dining room, but that I won't force anyone. At a time when there's so much focus on patient rights, I wonder whether there really is such a requirement. Do you know?

A There's no JCAHO requirement specifying a number or percentage of patients who must eat in the dining room.

According to JCAHO guidelines, patients who are able should be encouraged, not forced, to eat in the dining room so they'll benefit from socializing and retain some vestige of a normal routine.

When the surveyors visit, they'll be checking whether patients' nutritional, therapeutic, and special dietary needs are being met; they'll look at menus, food service, and the dining area itself. And to meet their standards, the dining room must be attractive, well-lighted, ventilated, readily accessible, and large enough to accommodate all of the patients—including those in wheelchairs—who are able to eat outside their rooms.

So get the word back to your administrator right away so he can modify this "requirement" before another patient's tears are shed.

What will convince the administrator that nurses should be able to make independent judgments?

Q At the nursing home where I'm day-care coordinator, nurses aren't allowed to telephone doctors to ask them to see patients—not even in emergencies. Only the director of nursing, his assistant, or one of the administrators is permitted to call a doctor. Theoretically, the doctors instigated this policy.

As a result of this unusual ruling, patients with possible fractures aren't X-rayed until at least 48 hours after an accident or injury.

Our present administrator just resigned, and we've been hoping his replacement would be more up-to-date in his thinking about nurses. The new man does seem caring and competent, but we're disappointed. He agrees with the old boss that nurses shouldn't make independent judgments, or even make suggestions to doctors. What's more, he labels nurses who *do* make suggestions as troublemakers.

We've tried talking to the new administrator, without success. Can you help us get through to him? We're discouraged, and our patients aren't getting the care they deserve.

A No wonder you're discouraged. Nurses certainly *do* have the right to call a doctor and the right to an opinion about when the patient needs immediate nursing care or medical care. A work situation that discourages calling for competent help in an emergency situation is questionable. And you do seem to be describing genuine emergencies.

What can you do? You tried talking to your administrator, and got nowhere. Ask for help from the department of accreditation and standards of your state association of nursing homes. Then you'll probably get somewhere.

Write a letter documenting each incident that worked to the patient's disadvantage because the nurse was not allowed to call the doctor. You need not sign your name to the letter; in fact, if you *do* sign your name, you will probably be putting your job on the line.

Don't worry about your unsigned letter being ignored. When state inspectors make their surprise visits, they have an uncanny way of zeroing in on a problem. If you've documented an instance in which a doctor wasn't called immediately after a patient fell out of bed, the inspector will probably comb the nursing home's records for evidence of other such incidents. If he finds any evidence, he'll require the nursing home to remedy the problem before approving the inspection and renewing the license.

In the meantime, as new incidents occur, don't hesitate to write on the patient's chart that the administrator has been notified of the patient's condition. Give the date, time, and all pertinent facts.

If your new administrator is as caring and competent as you think he is, don't write him off. Perhaps he *will* set things right—by revising the policy, so nurses can make the nursing judgments they're being paid for.

Nursing responsibility

Isn't checking pupil responses within the scope of an RN's responsibility?

Q Help! I work in an emergency department (ED) and feel very confident of my nursing abilities. Last weekend, we received a car ac-

cident victim who wasn't in acute distress but whose face was covered with blood—indicating he *might* have had a head injury. I noted that the patient's vital signs were good and that he was oriented to self, but not to day or time.

I'd been using a flashlight to check his pupil response and was just about to chart the response when the ED doctor approached and asked, "Hey, what are you doing with that flashlight?"

When I said I was checking pupil reaction, he hit the roof. He said that wasn't my job. I was so taken aback I couldn't say a word in my defense.

Later my unit manager told me that this doctor apparently feels *no* nurse should be responsible for checking pupil reactions. He wasn't singling *me* out. The unit manager had already taken the matter of this doctor's attitude through channels, she told me, but hadn't received any satisfaction from hospital administrators.

I *know* that checking pupil response is well within my scope as an RN. In fact, if I *didn't* carry out this basic procedure, I wouldn't be fulfilling my professional obligations—I'd be jeopardizing my patient's life, not to mention setting myself up for possible legal liability.

What should I do? If I quit, I won't be solving the problem. By the way, this doctor is *head* of the ED.

A According to just about every nursing and neurologic textbook in the field, you demonstrated sound nursing assessment by checking pupil reactions. You'd have been remiss if you *hadn't* done so.

You've discussed the matter with your unit manager but you haven't talked with the doctor himself. Why don't you? Discuss *his* perceptions of a nurse's responsibilities.

Try showing him the sections on assessment in a nursing curriculum and the chapters on nursing assessment in your neurology textbooks. You could also write or call the Emergency Nurses Association

(230 E. Ohio, Suite 600, Chicago, IL 60611, 312/649-0297) for material on nursing assessment in the ED.

He has to be made aware that you're not usurping *his* role by checking pupil response—your responsibility is a *nursing* assessment. His is a *medical* assessment. Obviously, this doctor isn't up-to-date about the nurse's expanding role. If you *hadn't* checked the pupils, you wouldn't have been meeting the standards established for a *student* nurse, much less for an RN.

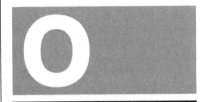

Observation

How can nurses keep from feeling "spied upon"?

Q Last week a staff nurse from another unit came to observe each shift in our unit. When she visited, she'd sit silently, observing the staff and taking notes. When any of us asked what she was doing, she'd say: "I'm not allowed to discuss it."

Now, I can understand that if the subjects of a research project knew all the details, the results might be influenced—and the validity of the research questionable. But this nurse was upsetting our staff. Several of our nurses felt uncomfortable and "spied upon."

We'd like your opinion. Do we have a valid complaint?

A Yes, you do have a valid complaint. Whoever's conducting this research is behaving in an unethical and unprofessional manner. Observation's certainly a proper way to collect data. But the subjects of the research are entitled to some explanation of the project—an explanation detailed enough to satisfy their natural curiosity and concerns but not so detailed that the project would be jeopardized. Besides, when the subjects of research are made uncomfortable, the researcher is hardly seeing "normal circumstances"—and the results would be questionable on this score.

Why not arrange a meeting with your supervisor or your director of nursing? You have to clear the air, and the nurse-researcher has to learn one of the basic rules of good research: An observer should "melt" into the background—not disrupt the subjects and the scene she's observing.

Obstetric nursing

Can a nurse perform an episiotomy in an emergency?

Q As an obstetric nurse, I've worked for 10 years in labor and delivery at the same small hospital. One night last week, when I realized a doctor wouldn't arrive in time for his patient's delivery, I scoured the hospital looking for another doctor to take over. The few doctors in the hospital were all busy, so I had no choice but to deliver the baby myself.

As the delivery progressed, I knew that an episiotomy would be necessary. So I asked both my patient and her husband (who was present for the delivery) for permission, and they agreed. Both mother and baby were fine, and the couple was pleased with the delivery. In fact, the obstetric unit staff and the patient's doctor complimented me for performance under fire.

The compliments ended there. When administration found out about the episiotomy, I was suspended, without any discussion, for 6 weeks. When I return to work, I'll be assigned to the medical/surgical unit; I was told never to set foot in the obstetric unit again.

This doesn't seem fair. Should I have delivered the baby and let the mother's perineum tear without doing anything to prevent it? What's your opinion?

A Some people would agree that there are times (especially in a small hospital) when a doctor just isn't available or can't get to the delivery room in time. And that by taking action, you were thinking of the patient and did your best in a difficult situation.

Others would say that your heart was in the right place, but you should have been ruled by your head. And that if you'd described the urgency of the situation, you could have persuaded one of the doctors to help.

Arrange a meeting with the hospital administrator before you're slated to return to work, and ask that both the patient's doctor and the director of nursing attend. Explain your story in detail. After 10 years' hard work, you deserve support, not suspension.

Can a physician's assistant legally deliver babies?

Q The private hospital where I work has just gotten its first obstetrics/gynecology doctor-physician's assistant (PA) team. So far, the PA has been handling most of the deliveries by himself. The doctor's usually present—but not always. During late-night or early-morning deliveries, he'll often sleep in the doctors' lounge. However, he'll respond quickly—if he's needed and called.

Many of us on the unit feel uncomfortable with the PA's perinatal practices. If we call the doctor in because *we* think there's a problem, the PA gets furious. He's convinced he's handling everything satisfactorily.

Actually, can the PA legally deliver babies? We need some facts. Can you help us?

A Can PAs deliver babies—legally? Most likely, yes. Most states' medical practice acts on physician's assistants say that the PA's ultimate role can't be rigidly defined because of variations in practice requirements caused by differing geographic, economic, and sociologic factors in the state. Delivering babies isn't specifically listed among the acts' permissible activities, but deliveries could very well be "indicated" under the broad *general* duties delineated for PAs.

> *"Many of us on the unit feel uncomfortable with the PA's perinatal practices, but if we call the doctor in, the PA gets furious."*

What about the PA's making deliveries while the doctor sleeps in the lounge? Again, this is *probably* legal. The PA practice acts don't demand the personal presence of the doctor—although the doctor retains the ultimate responsibility for supervision of the patient's care. The doctor's presence in the nearby lounge would *seem* to meet this criterion. (Of course, all this applies only if the PA has already met your state's requirements for practice: if he's a graduate of an approved PA program and if he's passed the Physician's Assistant's Certification exam.)

Even after you have the legal provisos clear, *your* responsibilities are still not discharged. With the serious doubts you have about the PA's perinatal practices, you must speak up. Document the behaviors you find questionable and make them known to the doctor-PA team in a nonhostile, let's-solve-this-one-together manner. And ask for a conference of everyone involved.

And then? How about going back to the delivery room? Your patients need you.

Should a father be allowed in the OR to witness a cesarean-section birth?

Q I'm a charge nurse in labor and delivery. Our hospital policy states that fathers can be present for vaginal deliveries if the couple has had childbirth preparation classes. But the policy also states: cesarean sections are surgical procedures, and fathers are *not* allowed to be present for such births.

On three different occasions, one of the obstetricians allowed husbands to be present for their wives' cesarean sections. I assisted at these deliveries and know for a fact that the women enjoyed having their husbands at the births.

Although paternal presence at cesarean-section births proved satisfying for the fathers and mothers, it still violates hospital policy. Should I play it by the book and refuse to let a father in the operating room (OR) to witness a cesarean-section birth?

A You can play it by the book or you can try to rewrite one of the chapters—that is, revise the policy.

A study conducted by the University of Michigan Medical school indicates that mothers who give birth by cesarean section benefit by the father's presence in the OR

Of the 26 women surveyed, all described the birth as joyful and said that they'd want the fathers present should they again deliver by cesarean section. The fathers, too, said they'd want to be there for another cesarean-section birth. Some of the couples added that the experience brought them closer together.

With such positive response to paternal presence at a cesarean-section birth, perhaps you should set your sights on revising the hospital policy rather than refusing to allow the fathers in the OR. This way, you're bound to make the birth process happier for a lot of couples.

What does gravida 2, para 3 mean?

Q I'm the proud mother of three—a 5-year-old boy and twin 3-year-old girls.

Recently, while being admitted to a hospital for tests, the nurse noted in my patient history that I'm gravida 2, para 3. I asked her, "are you sure?" I remember learning in nursing school that "para" refers to the number of viable pregnancies and twins are considered as one pregnancy and delivery. Am I right?

A You're right. If you'd delivered quadruplets instead of twins, you'd still be rated gravida 2, para 2 (1 for your son and 1 for the multiple birth). Gravida tells how many times a woman has been *pregnant,* whatever the pregnancy outcome. Para refers to the number of pregnancies that reached the stage of *viability,* not the number of fetuses delivered. Some practitioners, to be perfectly clear, record 4 numbers: gravida, para, number of children, and number of live births.

What's the legal risk for a nurse who's asked to take responsibility for the sponge count but took no part in the procedure?

Q In the labor and delivery unit where I'm nurse-manager, we have as many as 2,000 deliveries a year. In our unit, the medical students usually scrub and assist at vaginal deliveries; the nurses do not. Yet the perinatal department recently asked nurses to conduct the sponge counts for the vaginal deliveries. (This action came after one of the doctors on our staff was sued for leaving a sponge in a patient.)

I was asked to collaborate with the perinatal nursing director in writing the policy for taking the count. But she and I see the matter differently. I think that since the RN doesn't scrub and has no control over the use or disposition of the sponges, she should only *assist* with the count, not take ultimate responsibility for it. I see the nurse as having the job of checking the doctor's count.

The perinatal nursing director thinks otherwise. She contends the circulating nurse should collect and count the sponges, then document the count, as RNs do for cesarean deliveries. But I don't see that the two procedures are comparable. The nurse involved with a cesarean delivery scrubs and takes an active part; the nurse involved in a vaginal delivery does not.

I'm concerned about the possible legal liability of the nurse in the labor and delivery unit who's being asked to take responsibility for the sponge count when she takes no part in the procedure.

Can you straighten me out on this score?

A If the nurse doesn't have a direct role in the delivery, she shouldn't be held totally responsible for the sponge count. Those actually *doing* the delivery have to take their share of the responsibility. Drawing a parallel between the vaginal and cesarean delivery isn't valid because the nurse takes a different role in each procedure.

• Because a vaginal delivery employs so many $4'' \times 4''$ sponges, they're hard to count accurately. As a result, in some labor and delivery rooms, no one even *tries* to count the sponges.

• The legal climate has changed dramatically. In the past, if a woman discovered that a sponge had been left in the vaginal area after delivery, she might not express overt concern (especially because a sponge remaining in the vaginal area is not normally considered life threatening). But today the same "lost" sponge could precipitate a

O

lawsuit, with the hospital, doctor, and nurse getting sued.

• In case of litigation, who could be held legally liable for overlooking the sponge? The doctor would probably become the chief target of the suit, especially if the lawyer could establish that the doctor was theoretically "the captain of the ship" in the labor and delivery room. If the nurse's responsibility is written into hospital policy, then the lawyer will also try to hold *her* legally liable. The lawyer might argue that while the nurse didn't participate in the delivery, she was present in the labor and delivery room, recorded the sponge count, and probably did the routine charting.

Even though written policy assigned responsibility to her, the nurse expects the doctor to share the responsibility with her under the captain-of-the-ship doctrine mentioned above.

For more information on national practice standards, you might want to contact the Nurses Association of the American College of Obstetrics and Gynecology (NAACOG). Write NAACOG at 409 12th St., SW, Washington, DC 20024 or call (202) 638-0026.

To protect yourself, the nurse in the labor and delivery room should count the sponges, just as an operating room nurse would do, *and* carry adequate liability insurance.

Who should examine the patient?

Q At the small, rural hospital where I work, an obstetric nurse examines pregnant women who come to the emergency department (ED) in labor. She reports the stage of labor and the amount of dilation to the ED doctor, who then decides how to proceed.

As obstetric nurses, my colleagues and I don't think this should be our responsibility. We believe the doctor should examine the patient

as part of his assessment. Legally, is this policy putting us at risk?

A In the event of a mishap, the doctor *and* nurse could be held liable. As your employer, the hospital would probably share your liability.

However, that doesn't mean you should stop doing these assessments. Keep in mind that doctors routinely base medical decisions on nurses' findings. An experienced obstetric nurse is certainly qualified to examine a patient in labor and give her opinion. Of course, the doctor should also examine the patient. As always, make sure you both record your data and report these findings to each other. You should welcome such collaboration.

Occupational health nursing

Should nurses be expected to do "busywork"?

Q I'm an occupational health nurse (OHN) in the medical department of a large manufacturing company. Sometimes we're very busy; other times we're not.

Last week the personnel manager came into our health suite twice while I was chatting on the phone with a friend. This week he began dumping clerical work (alphabetizing personnel forms, filing, and other busywork) on me and my colleague to fill our downtime.

The other nurse doesn't mind; she feels we should accept whatever tasks we're assigned. I say we're *nurses,* not secretaries; the busywork is demeaning and bad for our professional image. Do you agree?

A Your professional skills are vital to the employees where you work. But no company these days can afford employees with down-

time. Instead of filling time with busywork, get busy finding ways to expand your *nursing* role and establish a high profile for the medical department.

As an OHN, you have a fantastic opportunity to plug into the fitness fervor sweeping the country. By helping employees stay healthy, you'll decrease absenteeism and save the company enough money to make your managers sit up and take notice.

Some ideas: Coordinate and promote a fitness program that includes blood pressure screening, supervised lunchtime exercise, and education sessions on stress reduction, weight control, alcohol and tobacco use, and drug abuse. Campaign for smoke-free work areas and reduction of environmental stresses such as excessive noise levels. Arrange sessions where working mothers can share coping ideas—for example, how to find baby-sitters who specialize in taking care of sick children. Schedule video programming in the cafeteria on self-help topics (time management, safety precautions, choosing a doctor, sensible eating habits). At one large corporation, the health and fitness program influences the food choices served in the cafeteria: The caloric content is prominently displayed, and nutritionally sound selections are subsidized by management.

One final suggestion: Join and become active in the American Association of Occupational Health Nurses, 50 Lenox Pointe, Atlanta, GA 30324. Members can recommend a nurse consultant who could help you set up such a program.

Go for it.

What's a nurse's liability when she treats employees?

Q I've been working as an occupational health nurse for a small manufacturer for about 3 years. I have two questions. First, I'm concerned about my liability when I treat employees. What protection does the fellow-servant doctrine offer?

Second, my job description says I can diagnose employees' illnesses and prescribe treatments. A new co-worker questions this policy. She says we could be accused of practicing medicine without a license. Is that true?

A In the past, the fellow-servant doctrine prevented co-workers from suing each other for injuries suffered on the job. Today's workers' compensation laws, which supersede this doctrine, contain similar provisions. So, if you're caring for co-workers who come to the employee health office or if you're responding to in-house emergencies, you needn't worry about lawsuits. Unless flagrantly negligent nursing care contributed to his injury, an employee could seek remuneration from your employer only.

To answer your second question, your colleague is right to be concerned. Your employer can't legally expand the scope of nursing practice to suit his needs. If he's asking you to diagnose illnesses and prescribe medication without a doctor's standing orders, you're overstepping the boundaries of your state's nurse practice act.

In this situation, you'd be wise to obtain standing orders to treat common ailments and injuries. But if any problem comes up that you feel unsure about, refer that employee to his doctor. Or, if he needs emergency care, take him to the emergency department.

Off-duty nursing

Is it risky to give injections off duty?

Q A neighbor of mine has two sons with hemophilia. She's asked me if I'd inject them with synthetic Factor VIII if they'd need it. Would I be taking a legal risk if I agreed?

A You could be. Because you'd be establishing a professional nurse-patient relationship, you'd be held to the same standards as any other nurse giving that type of care. If you failed to meet those standards, your neighbor could sue you for negligence.

Legally, that could leave you out on a limb—your hospital's malpractice insurance probably doesn't cover you for off-duty care. Before agreeing to help, read your own policy to make sure it extends to this type of situation.

Would a nurse be liable for giving wrong advice?

Q I have a common, annoying problem: When people find out I'm a nurse, they ask me for advice about their ailments. I try to be careful, but suppose I give the wrong advice? Could I be held liable?

A Theoretically, yes. But the risk of someone suing—and actually collecting—is very small. Even so, take the following steps to protect yourself:
• Find out if your professional liability insurance covers you off the job.
• Make sure your advice is up-to-date and reflects accepted professional nursing standards.
• Give only *nursing* advice. If you give *medical* advice, you're practicing medicine without a license.
• Don't speculate about the person's illness.
• Don't suggest that he change or ignore his doctor's orders.
• Don't offer any advice that, if wrong, could result in a serious or permanent injury.
• Don't accept money.

Of course, you can decide not to dispense free advice—the law doesn't require you to do so. But if you *do* give advice, ask yourself, "If I were at work and one of my pa-

tients asked the same question, what would I tell him?" Then use the same standards.

On-call policy

Is this type of policy legal?

Q Administrators at the hospital where I work have come up with a new policy: We have to be on call 4 days out of every 6 weeks to cover the second and third shifts if too many nurses call in sick. We don't get paid for being on call (of course, we are paid if we have to work). Is this policy legal? Also, can we be reprimanded, fired, or sued for abandonment if we refuse to come in?

A To answer your first question, yes, this policy is legal. Unless you're covered by a collective-bargaining agreement that limits it, you have to comply.

If you don't show up, you might be reprimanded or fired for insubordination. But you couldn't be charged with abandonment, because you wouldn't have established a duty to care for the patient. Hospital administrators would be liable though, because a hospital owes that duty to any patient who's been admitted.

You might want to talk with nurses at other hospitals and see how administrators there handle on-call situations. If your policy seems out of line, consider presenting your research—objectively, of course—to administrators where you work.

OR

Who's responsible for missing narcotics?

Q In the recovery room where I work, we have a double-locked narcotics box, and we nurses are responsible for ordering and counting the contents.

The operating room (OR) has no narcotics box. So when patients need I.V. sedation, one of the OR nurses comes into the recovery room to get the drugs. She's supposed to sign them out and return any that are unused to the narcotics box. However, we frequently are faced with an incorrect count at the end of the shift; we're not sure who's the culprit, and the OR nurses aren't around to help us investigate.

We're tired of this hassle, and we don't see how we can be held accountable. Don't you agree?

A Absolutely. Every OR should have its own narcotics box, period.

Would walking out be abandonment?

Q I work in a large operating room (OR) as a scrub nurse. Whenever a procedure isn't going well—for any reason—the surgeons tend to take it out on one of us nurses, yelling and belittling us in front of our peers. Lately, I've been the scapegoat.

Several times I've wanted to walk out—in fact, one surgeon recently told me I should *get* out. If I did walk out, would that be abandonment? Or am I supposed to stand there and take it? Are other ORs like this?

A The OR is notorious for these prima donna routines; some surgeons seem to enjoy their reputations as the hospital's "temperamental stars." But the fact is they really are under extreme tension, especially if a case isn't going well. They're stuck at that table—and can't leave or give up. So, they may unload their pent-up frustration on nurses.

You, on the other hand, are putting up with this as a professional because of your commitment to the patient. If you've agreed to the case assignment, you're committed to

remain until the case is over. Outside the OR, however, you can work to change this situation.

Get together with the other nurses, and ask to meet with the chief nurse of the OR and the chief of surgery to report what's going on and to enlist their help. What will it take? Some hospitals have an offending doctor hire his own scrub nurse and assign a select few circulating people to work with him. Others will suspend the surgeon's OR privileges for a short time (the wallet being mightier than words). No matter what efforts are taken where you work, noticeable changes might take a long time.

An interesting side note: Women surgeons are still a rarity, but their numbers are increasing, says an article in *The New York Times*. That could be good news for OR nurses. As the article suggests, these women surgeons are bringing more sensitivity, calmness, and a collegial atmosphere to the operating suite.

Organ donation

How can a nurse ask relatives about a patient's high-risk behaviors?

Q When I ask a deceased patient's family members if they want to donate their loved one's organs, I must also get permission to test the patient for human immunodeficiency virus (HIV). And I have to ask about high-risk behaviors. I'm uncomfortable asking a grieving family this type of question. How should I handle it?

A Try role-playing with other nurses so you can work through the questions and find ways of asking that are clear but not accusative. Make sure you explain your reasons for asking; that is, you want to minimize the risk of anyone

receiving an HIV-infected organ. Keep the questions and explanations matter-of-fact. For instance, you could say, "Your decision to donate your son's organs for transplantation is a valuable gift. I need to ask you some personal questions about John and get your consent for special testing. This will help us make the transplant a safe one. May I ask the questions now?"

Isn't it unethical to disregard a patient's wishes?

Q At the hospital where I work, we have to get permission from a patient's next of kin before removing that patient's organs for transplantation—even if the patient signed an organ donor card before he died. If the next of kin says no, we abide by that decision.

By following this policy, we're ignoring a federal law that allows us to take organs if that's what the patient wanted. And I think we're acting unethically by disregarding a patient's wishes. What do you think?

A What's legally permissible isn't always prudent, as your hospital's administrators have apparently decided.

In this situation, they're not alone. Many hospital administrators believe it's unwise to harvest organs if the patient's family objects—even though the federal Uniform Anatomical Gift Act permits them to do so. After all, the family members are already struggling to cope with a loved one's death. Forcing them to agree with his wish to donate organs may only intensify their grief.

Community education could help you avoid such painful situations. Suggest that the hospital sponsor a program to inform people about the value of organ donation. You can prominently display literature in the hospital to make patients and visitors more aware of the need for donors.

Finally, examine the language you use when you're asking families about organ donation. You might say something like this: "We understand that Joe carried a card saying he wanted to donate his organs for transplantation. When anyone takes the time to sign a donor card, it's because giving the gift of life is so important to him. The hospital would like to honor Joe's wishes." The family members will be more likely to agree—and to feel good that their loved one wanted to make such a generous gift.

OR nurse

Why is it so difficult to become one?

Q For the past 3 years, I've worked on a medical/surgical unit, but I want to be an operating room (OR) nurse.

The problem is that no hospital will hire me because I don't have any OR experience, and I can't get the experience without working in an OR.

I have friends who went to other specialized units without experience and got on-the-job preparation. Why is it so difficult to be an OR nurse?

A The Association of Operating Room Nurses (AORN) says the problem began when undergraduate programs removed OR experience from the nursing curriculum. To fill this void, many postgraduate courses for inexperienced nurses and those seeking a refresher course in perioperative nursing are either in the works or already available in various locations around the country. The AORN has compiled a directory of known postgraduate courses, so you can request a copy from the Continuing Education Division, AORN, Dept. N86, 10170 E. Mississippi Ave., Denver, CO 80231.

But what if you live in an area where no courses are offered? Contact your local AORN chapter (there are 358 chapters nationally); someone there will know about area job openings and orientation programs. Right now, the local chapters are working together on Project Alpha, "an organized effort to inform nursing educators about the advantages of including perioperative nursing in the curriculum."

Amen. And thanks for bringing this problem to light.

Ostomy

Any recommendations for reading material on ostomy care for nurses?

Q At work, I'm an emergency department (ED) nurse in a small community hospital; at home, I'm the daughter of a 60-year-old woman who recently underwent colostomy surgery.

> *"My mother wants me to help her, but, to tell the truth, I've never had to do ostomy care."*

My mother received TLC in the hospital, plus lots of instruction and reading material. And she's talked twice with an ostomy visitor from the United Ostomy Association since returning home. However, she still counts on me to help her because I'm a nurse. I don't want to shake her confidence, but the truth is that since I've worked in the ED, I've never had to put on or change an ostomy appliance.

Can you recommend any reading material on ostomy care for nurses?

A Kerry Anne McGinn, RN, and her mother, in a situation very similar to yours, produced *The Ostomy Book* (1980) written for patients *and* their families. Ms.

McGinn also wrote *The Ostomy Book For Nurses* (Palo Alto, Calif.: Bull Publishing Co., 1985), in which she shares what she has learned through her deepening commitment and involvement in ostomy care. As caregiver, resource nurse, and teacher of health professionals, Ms. McGinn has this to say about her experience: "Victories are sweet. Leading the new ostomate from despair to full participation in life is both a challenge and a thrill. Giving the longtime ostomate a new piece of information is very satisfying."

You might also be interested in a new journal, *Ostomy/Wound Management, The Journal for Extended Patient Care Management.* Published quarterly, the journal focuses on ostomy, wound, and incontinence care. For further information, contact Health Management Publications, Inc., 550 American Avenue, King of Prussia, PA 19406.

Otoscopes

Can they spread infection?

Q As a student nurse, I observe pediatricians in the emergency department. After examining a child with otitis media, one doctor placed the same earpiece into another child's ear—even though disposable attachments were at his fingertips. When I asked whether an otoscope can spread infections, he said not to worry.

Is there a rule for this situation?

A There's a risk for contamination whenever *any* device is transferred from one patient to another without some infection-control precautions.

The outer ear isn't a sterile area but a combination of skin and mucous membrane. So using a disposable attachment is optional. If these aren't used, the doctor should at least wipe off the earpiece with soap and water between patients and use some disinfectant.

Here's three rules of thumb from the Centers for Disease Control:
1. Devices entering sterile areas should be sterile.
2. Devices entering intact mucous membranes should be disinfected (with alcohol or the disinfectant hospital policy requires).
3. Devices in direct contact with intact skin should be cleaned with soap and water.

If you can remember these rules, making decisions should be as simple as 1-2-3.

Overbearing nurse

How can she be dealt with?

Q My problem is an older nurse who's worked in our urgent care center since the doors opened many years ago. She literally runs the place, and the owners don't want any complaints about her, period.

This woman is an overbearing nitpicker. She talks about me behind my back; she leaves me notes on every little thing; she shouts at me in front of patients—all of which makes me feel inadequate and nervous.

My husband is tired of having me come home depressed and wants me to quit. But I know I'm a good nurse, and I hate to admit defeat at her hands. Any suggestions?

A You've got to stop thinking of your relationship with this woman as a contest—with your self-esteem at stake. Decide truly whether the grief you're enduring is worth the money; if it isn't, give yourself permission to quit and find another job. Or, if you choose to view this as one of life's experiences, go at it wholeheartedly. You can learn a lot about yourself and how to grow.

When you can't control a person's problem behavior, try to control the

way it affects you. Look at how this nurse makes you feel now—tense, defensive, unsure of yourself, angry. These negative reactions are hurting you, so you must get rid of them.

Start by replacing them with positive thoughts about yourself. Make a list of your good qualities; remind yourself every day on the job that you're a good nurse and why. But admit to yourself that you're afraid of this bossy lady because she has power—from the owners, yes, but also from you because you've allowed her to intimidate you. Only action can cure fear.

> *"One of my co-workers is making my life miserable and my husband's tired of me coming home depressed."*

Next time, and every time that you're the victim of her put-downs, confront her directly. Let her know that her remarks hurt your feelings and distract you from your work, that you'd appreciate a more open working relationship, and that you want to deal with disagreements before they get out of hand. Even if she doesn't improve a whit, you'll be changing your feelings about yourself.

When your shift ends, try to leave your problems at the care center. Use your time at home to rest, relax—even laugh, if possible, at the absurdities of life so you can come back stronger the next day to deal with them.

Overdose

How should the transfer be charted?

Q On the medical/surgical unit where I work, we recently admitted an elderly patient who had taken an intentional overdose. Two

days later—after his medical crisis had passed—he was transferred downstairs to the psychiatric unit.

According to administration, diagnosis-related group (DRG) rulings prevent Medicare from paying for both the medical/surgical and psychiatric unit stays under one hospitalization. Administration's solution to this dilemma was to discharge the patient from the medical/surgical unit *on paper* but actually readmit him to the psychiatric unit. The unit manager told me to chart that the patient was discharged by wheelchair in stable condition at the time I received the order, even though he remained in my care for 3 unaccounted hours until the psychiatric unit was ready for him.

The ethics of this procedure seem so borderline that I'm worried I'm participating in a fraud. I'm also concerned about my responsibility and liability while the patient's in limbo—discharged but still in my care.

Can you shed some light on this for me?

A Here's the drill. Medicare patients on a medical/surgical unit, including the intensive care unit, are paid on a DRG system payment rate (that is, a predetermined fixed payment based on the diagnosis). It doesn't matter how much the hospital charges; the payment is what the government has already determined.

Psychiatric units, however, can be exempt from DRGs. Services provided on these units are paid on a cost-based retrospective payment system, which basically means that the bill is paid according to the individual charges—the payment is *not* predetermined by the government.

The government will not pay an acute care stay (DRG rate) and a psychiatric stay (cost-based rate) from the same bill.

For the hospital to be appropriately paid, then, the patient must be discharged from the medical/surgical unit, readmitted to the psychiatric unit, and two separate bills prepared bearing different account numbers. The government calls such arrangements "transfers to an exempt unit." To prevent unnecessary transfers requiring two payments (double-dipping), the peer review organization must approve and review a sample of transfers to exempt units.

All discharges should carry specific codes such as home, skilled nursing facility, and so on. Many hospitals use the code "discharged-transferred to DRG-exempt unit," which is perfectly okay, and the written discharge summary noted "to be readmitted to psychiatric unit."

So far, so good. But here's where your system is off base. Hours of care aren't considered part of the DRG system—days are. So it's both pointless and a lot of risk to have any patient without authorized care between stays. Chart discharge at the correct time you turn the patient over to the other unit— you're responsible (and liable) until then, and so is the attending doctor and the hospital itself.

If a nurse is on duty and believes a patient's life's in danger, couldn't she be liable for not administering naloxone?

Q I just started working in a drug-treatment clinic, and I'm concerned because the clinic doesn't permit standing orders for any drugs.

If a patient comes into the clinic showing signs of overdose, and the nurse can't reach a doctor, what should she do? The nearest ambulance service is a 30-minute ride from here. We do have naloxone (Narcan), a narcotic antagonist, in our emergency box, and an injection could save a patient's life.

If I'm on duty and I believe a patient's life is in danger from an overdose, wouldn't I be liable for *not* administering naloxone?

A You wouldn't be liable for *not* administering naloxone if such a patient died. However, your employer might be held liable for insufficient medical coverage.

Would you be liable if you *did* administer naloxone to a patient dying from a drug overdose? Again, it's unlikely, provided your action was reasonable for a nurse of your experience and education in that situation. You wouldn't be expected to ignore your training and expertise and helplessly watch someone die.

For more specific advice, why not ask your employer the same question you asked us? Certainly, you should have a protocol to follow in such a situation; a doctor to call in an emergency, supportive measures to take, and so on. Who knows, you may even end up with a standing order for naloxone.

Over-the-counter products

Is slipping over-the-counter preparations to patients both illegal and dangerous?

Q I'm a recent graduate of nursing school now coping with the "reality shock" of hospital nursing. I confess: I'm having more than a little difficulty dealing with the "slipping" of antacids, pain relievers, laxatives, and other over-the-counter (OTC) preparations to patients without a written order.

I was taught that slipping OTC preparations to patients is both illegal and dangerous. An OTC medication, which has been neither ordered nor recorded in the patient's chart, could alter the clinical data and skew the medical assessment of the patient's problems.

There are reasons why we shouldn't give these preparations to patients, but there are also understandable reasons why it's done. I've seen patients experience prolonged headache, indigestion, constipation—even fever—while a nurse struggles to get a doctor's order for a remedy. One nurse told me that to avoid this common hospital hassle, she's been slipping these preparations for 30 years. She claims she's never run into a problem.

> *"I have problems giving antacids, pain relievers, laxatives, and other over-the-counter preparations without a written order."*

But I refuse to do this, even though other staff nurses look upon me as a stickler for regulations. Their reaction makes me feel inexperienced and inadequate. How do you suggest I handle this?

A What you were taught is absolutely correct. You cannot give your patient an unordered, unrecorded preparation. One danger of doing so, as you pointed out, is that the OTC ingredients could alter the clinical data; it's also possible that the OTC preparation could interact adversely with your patient's other medications or mask significant signs and symptoms.

But what's the answer if the patient has a need and you can't get a doctor to fill the need (and write the order)? In many hospitals, nurses are now authorized to write an order for OTC preparations— which, after all, are nonprescription products. If your hospital doesn't permit this (but does permit the frustration and waiting you've described), why not work to change the policy?

There are good reasons not to give OTC preparations unless you have an order. You're showing good sense by adhering to the policy—at least until you can change it.

Overtime

Can nurses protest by refusing to adhere to the "self-coverage" policy?

Q The hospital where I work has a "self-coverage" policy. When a nurse calls in sick, another nurse is required to fill in for her. This usually adds up to a double shift for the nurse filling in.

Although we've all done our share of filling in, the consensus is that the practice is unfair to us *and* to our patients. We're not exactly giving optimum care by the end of two 8-hour shifts, are we? We think that the hospital should use nurses from a temporary agency to fill in—or better yet, hire more staff.

The nurses on my unit want to protest by refusing to adhere to the "self-coverage" policy. Can we do this legally, or can we be held liable if we leave the unit? We don't want to get into trouble, but we've talked it over, and we think the "direct approach" would work best.

A Walking off the unit sounds more like avoiding the problem than confronting it. *Don't* leave the unit. If you do and a patient suffers because of your inattention, you could be charged with abandonment.

When you accepted your job, the self-coverage policy was in effect and you were duly informed. In accepting the job, you implicitly agreed to fill in for co-workers when necessary. (That doesn't mean this situation has to remain unchanged.)

Your hospital's self-coverage policy is unfair to nurses and patients. You can't give the best care if you're exhausted (as well as angry and resentful) after working a double shift.

The only responsible approach is to write a formal complaint and send it through channels. Get as many nurses' signatures as possible; present your case in a reasonable, logical, unemotional way; offer some solutions.

You might also try this: Next time you fill in for a nurse who's ill, make every effort, as you always do, to give good patient care. Then, when the shift is over, prepare a written report showing why you can't, in good conscience and with good professional judgment, accept such duty again.

This will take courage and persistence. But since hospital administrators are usually conservative types, an unemotional approach will probably work better than walking off the unit in a huff.

Does malpractice insurance cover nursing care while officially off duty?

Q At the hospital where I work, administration won't pay overtime for any reason. A recent policy says that when we can't get our work finished, we must clock out on time, then come back to the unit and continue working.

I have my own malpractice insurance, but am I covered when I'm officially off duty but still working?

A You probably are. Most malpractice insurance policies cover you around the clock for nursing actions on and off the job. (Check with your carrier to be sure, though.)

Now that you're reassured on this count, there are some additional concerns. For instance, you might have a hard time qualifying for workers' compensation if you're injured after clocking out. You'd have a *chance* only if you could prove you were ordered back to work.

Moreover, clocking in and out at the correct time is a matter of honesty not to be taken lightly. The Fair

Labor Standards Act says that an hourly employee *must* be paid for all the hours worked—and you can't waive this right. As exceptions to the usual rule, hospitals and residential care facilities may use a 14-day, 80-hour work base and arrange schedules to limit the amount of overtime due.

Rather than making waves where you work, you can contact the nearest office of the U.S. Labor Department, Wage and Hour Division. They'll investigate your situation and keep your report confidential.

Is it fair that the hospital forces nurses to work double shifts?

Q I'm a staff nurse at a large teaching hospital, working the evening shift of a busy emergency department. Our contract negotiating committee has backed a mandatory overtime policy—meaning we can be forced to work a double shift if one of the night nurses calls in sick.

The double shift falls to the staff nurse who's worked the least recent overtime. No excuses—she's suspended if she refuses to work the extra shift. I've seen a nurse dissolve in tears because she had a final exam that night. And I've heard the director say to a nurse with a child waiting at home, "That's not my problem."

The other nurses and I never know until after we report in if we'll have to work the double shift. The committee's told us that we can do nothing, since mandatory overtime has been upheld.

Before I'm forced to resign, I want to know: Is this policy legal?

A Yes. A hearing's officer at the National Labor Relations Board stated that if a contract provision prohibited mandatory overtime, you'd have a basis for disputing such a policy. Such a provision would allow you to use the grievance procedure in your contract to resolve the problem. And without this provision, the policy is legal.

A spokesperson at the Department of Labor's Division of Labor Standards (Department of Wages and Hours) agrees. If the policy doesn't violate labor law it's legal. You can only modify work arrangements through contract negotiations.

So your employer *is* within his rights when he asks you to work a double shift. However, it's surprising your committee supports implementing and backing a policy that favors management more than the nurses it represents. If this is actually the case, you'll have to wait until contract renegotiations come up to get that policy changed.

Although you can't resolve this problem through your contract, you can confront your employer (preferably through the hospital's nursing practice committee) with a request for policy changes.

When you prepare your arguments, remember: health care's an industry, and as in any industry, the worker must take a professional rather than personal stance when making her argument for change.

For example, a nurse's personal problems (a final exam or child care arrangements) just won't wash. But slant your argument toward your employer's point of view, get him to see the connection between an ill-advised policy and a breakdown in quality patient care, and you've got a better chance of getting a policy changed.

Oxytocin drips

What do you think of this new policy?

Q Several of us nurses in the obstetrics unit are concerned about a new policy on induction and augmentation of labor using oxytocin (Pitocin) drips.

We were all taught that oxytocin drips should be increased at a rate of 1 to 2 microunits/minute every 15 minutes. Our new policy calls for "increase by 2 to 5 microunits/minute every 15 minutes × 3, then: increase by 5 to 10 microunits/minute every 15 minutes until maximum dose of 40 microunits/minute or until a normal labor pattern occurs."

Are we wrong to be concerned over such an aggressive approach?

A This practice falls somewhere between conservative and aggressive approaches currently used in oxytocin administration. The conservative approach calls for starting with 1 microunit/minute, increasing 2 to 2.5 microunits/minute every 20 minutes because plasma levels peak at 20 minutes. Dosage shouldn't exceed 30 to 40 microunits/minute. (Most patients require only 20 microunits/minute to establish adequate contractions.) The aggressive approach calls for starting at 1 to 2 microunits/minute and increasing by doubling the amount: 1-2-4-8-16 microunits/minute every 15 minutes until reaching a maximum.

> *"We're concerned about a new, more aggressive policy on induction and augmentation of labor using oxytocin drips."*

A word of caution: Oxytocin drips must always be accompanied by fetal monitoring. Adverse reactions can happen suddenly, and with two patients involved—mother and infant—the consequences can be doubly disastrous. Also keep in mind that the decision to use oxytocin and the medical management of the patient are the responsibility of the doctor who, under these circumstances, should never be more than 5 minutes away from the labor and delivery suite.

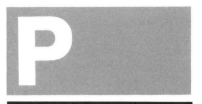

Pacemaker

Could a nurse with a pacemaker lose her nursing license if she experiences blackouts?

Q A medical/surgical staff nurse at my hospital has had a permanent pacemaker for over a year. Do you think she should give up nursing? We've heard that she's had at least three blackouts—all happening at home. Could she lose her nursing license if there was evidence of these blackouts?

A Pacemakers are more common than you might think—and many people with pacemakers lead very active lives. This nurse should be able to continue working on the medical/surgical unit unless her condition clearly deteriorates. Certainly her employer has a legal duty to protect patients against a nurse in questionable health. But before the hospital could fire this nurse for a physical ailment, the administration would have to prove she's physically unable to work.

About the reported blackouts: If this nurse *is* experiencing blackouts, her pacemaker could be malfunctioning. She should have it checked out.

And her license? Legally, the nurse's license is probably not threatened. To remove her license to practice is to remove her source of livelihood—this would require due process of law, meaning a hearing must be called, and the nurse must be *proven* dangerous to her patients.

Let's not be quick to discard a good nurse on the basis of "hearing" about her blackouts. Instead of worrying *about* her, why not be a good co-worker and worry *with* her? If you give her the opportunity to share her problems with someone sympathetic, she'll probably be grateful for the support.

And the next time your unit is frantically busy, you'll be grateful for an experienced nurse you helped keep on your staff.

Pain medication

Should the nurse refuse the patient's last request?

Q When a patient's preparing to go home after a stay on our orthopedics unit, he'll sometimes ask me for one last "pain shot" to make his trip home easier. The patient's already been discharged and usually has a take-home medication such as acetaminophen with codeine (Tylenol with codeine no. 3).

> *"Some nurses will give a patient one last pain shot before he goes home, but I feel it's wrong."*

I've been refusing this "last request," but some nurses on the floor *will* give the shot if their patient insists. Am I wrong in refusing a patient's request? When I refuse, am I causing him needless pain on the trip home?

A You're correct in refusing the patient's request. One of your responsibilities in medication administration is watching for side effects. Because many I.M. analgesics can cause potentially dangerous side effects, such as decreased blood pressure, you should be watching the patient for a good hour after you administer the drug. Obviously, you can't observe a patient who's left for home.

If the doctor decided the patient was ready for discharge, do you think he should need I.M. pain medication for the trip home? No.

Remember: As a professional nurse, you have the right to refuse to perform an action you're uncomfortable with because, as in this situation, it could be dangerous to the patient. You should, however, document the patient's request and your refusal.

To give you your own security blanket, ask for the hospital administration to establish a written policy for this special situation.

Paramedics

How can a paramedic tell a doctor he's in charge?

Q At the family practice office where I work, the doctor sometimes wants a seriously ill patient sent directly to the hospital. We call the emergency medical transport, and we state the diagnosis; but when the paramedics arrive with all their equipment, they forget the patient has already been evaluated by his own doctor.

One night last week, they were at our office for 30 minutes before a patient with cardiac insufficiency was even wheeled to the ambulance. The paramedic began communication with the hospital, then took an in-depth history, ran an electrocardiogram, administered oxygen, and began I.V. therapy. Finally, the doctor stepped in and told him that the other patients in the office are getting jittery; the hospital is waiting; please just take the patient out, now. The paramedic ignored him, saying he was in charge. How can this be?

A Once you contact the emergency medical transport, the paramedic who arrives must follow instructions from the doctors in medical command; he can't take orders from anyone on the scene—not

even the patient's private doctor. In effect, by your call, *you* put the patient in his charge. The paramedic's role is legislated by the Emergency Medical Service Act. And if he doesn't respond appropriately and perform the procedures called for, then he's legally liable. So you see, 30 minutes for a cardiac call is not unreasonable.

If you're routinely going to call the emergency medical transport, then make sure the doctor you work for sets up a dialogue with its medical command so both of you will know what to expect. Then if your employer decides that all he wants for his patients is transportation to the hospital, your office should simply contract with a private ambulance company.

Parenting

How can a nurse do her job and be a working mother?

Q I love hospital nursing and am good at it. But working rotating shifts and weekends makes it hard to get good, consistent care for my 9-month-old daughter. How do other working mothers handle the problem?

A The overall issue of good child care is filled with controversy, pitfalls, and guilt. But the crux of your immediate problems seems to be your work schedule. Talk to the director of nursing and see if she'll assign you to a permanent shift. This should help some.

If she can't or won't reassign you, look for a job with regular hours at another local hospital. Some area hospitals may even offer child-care services as a benefit. Also explore other options, such as working in a doctor's office or working as a school or industrial nurse. These usually offer better hours and will allow you more time to be with your baby daughter.

P

You're facing two big demands: nursing *and* parenting. Doing both will take some juggling. Lots of women *are* trying to do both, but the matter remains private and personal. What's important is not what *they* are doing but what works for *you.*

Parking

What can be done about poor parking facilities?

Q For my first few months in a new job, I rode to work with a co-worker and shared gas expenses. Now she's working nights, and I'm stuck with driving my own car. This wouldn't be bad except that the hospital issues parking permits for its lot on a first-come, first-served basis, and I'm last in a long line of those waiting. With no parking available on the streets near the hospital, I have to use a public lot two blocks away that costs plenty.

How do other hospitals handle this? And shouldn't the hospital reimburse me for the parking fees?

A Reimbursing you would be a nice gesture, but unless promise of a parking space was part of your hiring contract, you may be out of luck.

But don't give up yet. Try brainstorming with other employees who have the same problem. Together, you might think of solutions the administration could live with, too. A van pool, for instance, with the hospital paying the van rental and the riders sharing operating expenses. (Many businesses discovered that van pools increased employee morale and decreased lateness and absenteeism.)

Or consider this: Some hospitals charge all staff members a monthly parking fee for reserved spaces and then ask these employees to "rent" their spaces on their days off to those who need parking. Names and extension numbers of potential "renters" are posted on the bulletin board. Another idea: Ask the public lot management about contracting for a set number of spaces at group rates, and so on.

As with most problems, you can usually find a solution when driven to it (if you'll pardon the pun).

Patient abuse

What can make the nursing assistants realize patients should be treated humanely?

Q I'm a nursing assistant on the evening shift at "the best nursing home in the area," and I'm sickened by the way the patients are treated.

Our shift consists of one LPN, who does medications, treatments, and charting, and four nursing assistants, who feed the 35 patients and get them ready for the night.

The feeding is bad enough: most of the assistants mix all the food together and shove it in as quickly as they can. But what really upsets me is in the assistants' behavior when we make rounds at 10:30, to see whether the patients have been incontinent. (Most of them *are,* because the assistants won't take them to the bathroom.)

The patients go to bed about 8, so by 10:30, they're usually asleep. Yet I've seen assistants go into a room, throw the covers back, abruptly turn the patient on his side and rip the incontinence pad out from under him, then roll him abruptly on to his other side and rip out the other incontinence pad. If the linen is wet, the assistant yells at the patient for wetting so much and causing her so much work.

This is supposed to be my summer job (I'm starting nursing school this fall), but I don't think I can stomach it all summer. Is there anything I can do to make these assistants realize these are nice people and not sacks of potatoes?

A Patient neglect—or abuse—is deliberate in most cases. It usually occurs because the staff doesn't recognize the patients' needs or understand their problems.

At one nursing home, the supervisor put the staff on the *receiving end.* It was one of those try-it-you'll-like-it things, but nobody liked it. Every staff member had to take a turn at being a patient, but no one knew who was next or when it would happen—just like real illness.

Without warning, a nursing assistant or nurse was put into a wheelchair and restrained securely. If she was on her way to the bathroom at the time, too bad. If she had a cold and needed a tissue, too bad. If she needed an aspirin for a headache, too bad. *Because nobody listened to her!*

Cotton was put in her ears so sounds were slightly muffled, but she could still hear the nurses talking *over* her and *about* her.

A plastic band was loosely tied across her eyes, so her vision was clouded.

Then she was taken for a couple of quick spins up and down the halls, at a speed that was terrifying because she couldn't see where she was or where she was being steered. Even though every nurse had to take her turn, the experience was devastating.

You could imagine carrying this experiment even further: being fed a meal of pureed foods that are all stirred together, and spooned in, or—better yet—forced in with a bulb-fitted, blunt-tipped syringe... being rolled about in bed, stripped of privacy and modesty, and reduced to the potato stage, mentally and physically...maybe having your britches stripped down, be popped on the bedpan, with the doors open and everyone watching, and told to void. And being left on the pan until you did. Brutal treatment? Yes. Exactly.

But what can *you* do? You're in a frustrating position. Start by asking for a private meeting with the

P

charge nurse (who should have been making rounds anyway). If you're convinced she doesn't care, you could go to the administrator or the director of nursing.

Taking these steps might cost you your job, but having someone with your rare ability to recognize emotional needs and your willingness to speak out is particularly vital to elderly patients, who may not be able to speak up for themselves.

Patient advocacy

How can a nurse be a patient's advocate without getting into trouble?

Q Last week, when I disagreed with a doctor's diagnosis, I considered telling the patient that he should get another opinion. My unit manager warned me that I would undermine the patient's trust in his doctor. How can I be a patient's advocate without getting into trouble?

A You *are* the patient's advocate, but you may be confused about what that means. Yes, you should act in the patient's best medical, emotional, and legal interests, but it's not your duty to tell the patient that you disagree with his doctor. After all, you may not know all the facts or reasons behind the doctor's decision.

So what should you do? Share your doubts with your manager, and ask her to take the matter to the medical director for his opinion. That way, you can protect your patient while preserving his relationships with both you and his doctor.

How should a family's questions about a doctor's competence be handled?

Q I'm the unit manager on an intensive care unit. Recently, an anesthesiologist had difficulty intubating a young man on the unit.

After four attempts, he finally placed the endotracheal tube. The experience was traumatic not only for the patient but also for his family members, who were on the other side of the curtain. Later, his father asked me if doctors commonly have so much trouble with this procedure. I sidestepped the question that time. But what should I say the next time someone asks me if a doctor has performed a procedure competently?

A As the patient's advocate, you have an ethical duty to answer honestly. But in this case, you needn't have assumed that the doctor was incompetent. As you know, intubation can be difficult. So, rather than discussing the doctor's skill at performing the procedure, you could have educated the family about intubation and explained why it's sometimes hard to perform.

In the future, ask family members to step outside during potentially troublesome procedures. Take them to a comfortable waiting area and explain what's being done. That way, they'll be prepared for what they'll see when they return to the patient.

Should a nurse call a doctor even if her supervisor refuses her request?

Q Hospital policy where I work forbids nurses to call a patient's doctor after 11 p.m. unless the call is okayed by the night supervisor. We all know of times she refused because, as she said, the doctor needs to sleep.

I maintain that my responsibility is to the patient; if the supervisor refuses my request and the patient's doing badly, I'm going to call the doctor anyway. Do you agree with me?

A You're right on target about your responsibility and liability for your patient. You can certainly judge when he needs

immediate nursing or medical care. And you can call the doctor even over the director of nursing's head if necessary.

But such drastic measures *shouldn't* be necessary. What you need is a closer look at why this policy was written in the first place and then how to get rid of it. Was the problem too many needless calls? Or doctors on staff exerting too much pressure on nursing service? Logic dictates that only the direct caregiver—you—can relate the patient's problem and answer questions; therefore, *you* should be the one to make the call. Applying logic again, when you're not sure whether the call can wait, consult first with another staff nurse or the supervisor.

Don't make this issue a power struggle. Get staff and supervisory people together; use a little teamwork; and get this policy off the books.

What can a nurse do if her patient's suffering needlessly?

Q One of my terminally ill patients suffers constantly because her doctor won't prescribe morphine. He says that if he prescribes a narcotic, she'll know her bowel cancer has spread and she's dying.

I'm shocked that he would allow a patient to suffer needlessly simply to conceal her prognosis from her. I'd like to speak up, but I'm afraid I might get into trouble. Any advice?

A When in doubt, risk it! This patient needs an advocate. So, speak up, loud and clear. If the doctor won't listen, talk to your manager. Insist that she relay your concerns to the chief of staff if necessary.

Next, talk with your patient. She knows she isn't getting better, whether the doctor has told her or not. Explain that her pain *can* be controlled and that she can change doctors if she's unhappy with the level of pain relief she's getting. Then, give her the names of three competent, compassionate doctors who could help her.

What if two doctors give the patient conflicting prognoses?

Q Last week, two doctors on the same case gave the patient different interpretations of his prognosis—one optimistic and one pessimistic. Understandably, that put the patient on an emotional roller coaster. What can I do to help him?

A As your patient's advocate, you should mediate. Talk to him and find out what he thinks—and how he feels—about the information he's gotten. You might say something like this: "What did each doctor tell you? How do you feel about this information?" Questions like these will help him link his thoughts to his feelings—and help you decide whether he's missing the connection. Also ask him if he has any questions.

> *"The patient's on an emotional roller coaster because one doctor says he'll be fine, and the other predicts doom."*

Carefully and nonjudgmentally chart your patient's answers and your observations about his response. But don't interject your values or try to interpret his feelings.

The doctors must be involved in the solution, too. Talk with each one—preferably together—about what the patient has told you. Show them your documentation and ask them how *they* want to address the

patient's concerns. You might say: "I need your help with my patient's questions. He's wondering when he'll go home and if he'll be able to return to work. He wants to make important decisions about his future. I need to give him answers that we all agree on so he won't be confused about what to expect."

As part of your teaching, provide the patient with information about community resources and give him a copy of the American Hospital Association's Patient's Bill of Rights.

What should a nurse do if a doctor insists on a procedure?

Q A few weeks ago, a resident made several unsuccessful attempts to do a lumbar puncture on one of my patients. Finally, the patient begged him to stop and let his own doctor do the procedure. When I called the patient's doctor and explained the situation, he said to tell the patient to cooperate with the resident or go home.

I did as the doctor told me, but I felt I'd let the patient down. He shouldn't have had to suffer from the resident's inexperience. What should I do if something like this happens again?

A Stick up for your patient—he has a right to refuse treatment in most circumstances. If he asks to stop a procedure but the doctor ignores him, you have an obligation to support him. You might say, "Doctor, I believe Mr. Smith has decided to discontinue the procedure now. Is that your choice, Mr. Smith?"

To prevent a repeat of the situation you experienced, suggest that the director of the hospital's residency program convene a committee to draft a policy on such practices and volunteer to serve on it yourself. In many hospitals, a resident defers to a more experienced doctor (but not necessarily the patient's doctor) if he can't complete

a procedure in one or two attempts. Whatever policy you adopt, it should assure residents that other doctors will support them if they run into problems.

Patient-centered nursing

How can the administrative and nursing personnel be converted back to patient-centered thinking?

Q I've been working in a hospital for 9 months, and with each passing day I see a further turning away from the "patient-centered" nursing care approach toward a more "staff-centered" approach.

How can a sincerely dedicated RN try to convert the administrative and nursing personnel back to patient-centered thinking?

A Unless you are emotionally constituted to enjoy the role of "a voice in the wilderness," a single person really can't change the policies of any large institution. Ah, but what if you had a large number of like-minded co-workers? Numbers could make your goal not only more realistic, but a reality.

Continue a patient-centered approach in *your* dealings with *your* patients. Take time to explain what you're doing to your co-workers. Talk up your theory. Your patient-centered approach will probably prove demonstrably more successful than any other approach. And since success *does* breed success, isn't it possible—even likely—you'll convert some of your co-workers to your way of thinking? Then, once there are enough of you, you'd have a good chance of making your voices heard and getting the administration to listen to your views.

The biggest obstacle in situations like this is discouragement. The bigger the institution, the slower the

P

changes. So try to adjust your sights to a long-range goal. Don't get discouraged. If only for the patients' sakes, hang in there.

Patient injury

Could a nurse be liable for a nursing assistant's mistake?

Q Recently, I transported a patient to a surgical holding area to wait for the results of an intestinal biopsy. I had to leave, so I asked a nursing assistant to stay with her until I returned. When I got back, the nursing assistant was gone and my patient was on the floor with a fractured arm.

> *"When I returned, the nursing assistant was gone and my patient was sprawled on the floor."*

The patient later told me that just after I'd left, another nurse had asked the assistant for help in another room. When the patient was alone, she tried to sit up. The side rail collapsed, and she lost her balance and fell. Am I liable for her injuries?

A Because the incident involves a custodial rather than a professional action, the hospital's administrators have more reason for concern than you do.

You delegated a patient's safekeeping to a nursing assistant who's trained to handle this task. You expected her to stay with the patient, and you didn't know that she'd left. Under those circumstances, you probably wouldn't be held liable for the patient's injury. But a court could hold the hospital liable for failing to provide a safe environment for the patient.

Patient privacy

Is it an invasion to write patients' names and room numbers on a board by the nurses' station?

Q At the acute care hospital where I work, we've recently started using a wipe-off communication board at the nurses' station. The patients' names, room numbers, and scheduled treatments are written in large letters and can be seen by our staff, patients, and visitors. This seems like an invasion of patient privacy to me. Do you agree?

A Sure do. Some patients don't want anyone to know they're in the hospital, much less know about their treatments. Sure, jotting down reminders is a good way to make sure no patient or treatment is forgotten. But find a place out of public view (the report room, for instance) for this checklist.

These days, when it comes to a question of patient privacy over staff convenience, there's no contest.

Is it an invasion of privacy to allow students to observe procedures?

Q Recently, I was irrigating a patient's colostomy when my manager brought in three student nurses to observe the procedure. Later, the patient complained that I'd let the students invade his privacy. I explained that students routinely observe procedures in teaching hospitals as part of their education, but that didn't satisfy him. He says he'll speak to his lawyer.

What do you think? Did we invade his privacy?

A Yes, you did, because you disclosed private facts about your patient to those not directly involved in his care. And your ra-

tionale is incorrect. A patient doesn't automatically waive his right to privacy—or imply consent to have students observe his care—just because he's receiving care in a teaching hospital.

You could have easily avoided this problem. After telling the students to wait outside, you should have asked your patient if he'd allow students who'd studied the procedure to observe you performing it. That would have given him control. Chances are, he'd have said yes if he'd only been asked.

Under the right conditions, many patients enjoy talking about their conditions with student nurses. So next time, ask first. You probably won't be turned down.

Is it legal for a nurse to show a coroner a patient's record?

Q Recently, a 3-year-old boy was brought to the hospital where I work. He was dead on arrival, an apparent victim of child abuse. When the coroner arrived, he looked at the child, then asked me for a copy of our emergency department admissions record. Without thinking, I gave it to him. Now I'm wondering if he had a legal right to this kind of information.

A He did, but you shouldn't have been the one to give it to him. Hospital records belong to the hospital—and only to the hospital. Rules vary by state, but certain legal steps must be followed to obtain all or part of a medical record. These procedures protect a patient's right to privacy—and protect you and the hospital from liability for invasion of privacy.

Before a situation like this occurs again, review the hospital's policies and procedures manual to find out what action would be appropriate. You'll probably discover that you should refer such requests to nursing or hospital administrators and let them handle it.

Is it legal to search a patient's belongings if a police officer requests it?

Q Recently, two police officers brought a gunshot victim to the emergency department where I work. After they finished questioning the victim, one officer took me aside and told me that he'd recognized another patient as a suspected drug dealer. He wanted me to search the patient's belongings for evidence. I did so but didn't find anything. Now I'm afraid I violated this patient's privacy. What should I do if this happens in the future?

A That depends. If the patient is under arrest, you could legally search his belongings. But in the situation you describe, the patient wasn't under arrest and you shouldn't have agreed to help. (If drugs or weapons had been in plain view, though, you could have confiscated them.)

In this case, you violated your patient's right to privacy and his right to protection from illegal search and seizure. The officer acted improperly, too. He had neither a warrant nor probable cause to search your patient.

In the future, ask to see a search warrant before you agree to help. When in doubt, refer police officers to a hospital administrator or the hospital's lawyer.

Isn't it cruel to deprive patients of sexual intimacy?

Q I work in a veterans' home where most of my patients are middle-aged or elderly men. One patient, a 50-year-old paraplegic, is visited regularly by a woman about his age. I know the couple would like to be alone, but the patient is on a 20-bed unit, making privacy impossible. I'm sure that many of the other patients would like some privacy, too, when they are visited by women friends.

Many of the men are long-term patients, and depriving them of any chance for sexual intimacy seems unfair and cruel. Do you agree?

A Certainly. Patients, especially long-term ones, need sexual intimacy like everyone else. And with the trend toward treating the *total* patient, we're putting more emphasis on meeting a patient's emotional needs—this includes his sexual needs as well

In some states, the department of health has regulations saying that "A patient shall be afforded an opportunity to meet in private with visitors. When a husband and wife are patients in the same facility, they shall be permitted to share a room, if they desire to do so, unless it is medically contraindicated." This supports your point of view. Unless a patient is too ill, he should have the opportunity to meet privately with his wife or friend.

Giving every patient privacy during visiting hours simply isn't possible. However, your hospital should be able to set aside a room or two where patients and visitors can be alone. If the administrators balk at the idea of "privacy" rooms, you have to be the patients' advocate.

Should a nurse have documented something heard while eavesdropping?

Q A 14-year-old girl was recently admitted to our pediatric unit with head trauma from a fall at school. She offered several explanations for her fall, but I suspected she was hiding something. So when several of her friends visited, I listened through the intercom. They spoke freely about using drugs, and the patient said she'd been smoking marijuana before her accident.

I charted what I'd heard (including the fact that they didn't know I was listening). Although I feel guilty about eavesdropping, I think I should tell the parents about their daughter's drug use. What do you think?

A Your intentions were good, but listening through the intercom violated your patient's privacy, and that's hard to justify. Telling her parents what you overheard could damage her relationship with them—and with you.

Remember, you have no proof that your patient uses drugs. If you confront her parents with suspicions based on dishonestly obtained information, they may question your credibility and professionalism.

Rather than acting alone, tell your unit manager what you've done and enlist her support. She'll probably want to discuss the situation with the patient's doctor, who may decide to handle the matter privately with the patient and her parents.

For the future, work with your unit manager to draw up a policy to follow when you suspect a minor is abusing drugs. Include specific guidelines for obtaining and documenting information and a protocol for informing parents.

P

Would discussion of a patient's disease in front of the patient's roommate be considered an invasion of privacy?

Q We're finishing our first month of delivering change-of-shift reports in the form of "walking patient rounds."

So far, we're pleased with the results. The reports are more meaningful when the oncoming staff actually see and talk to the patients.

Because all of our rooms are semiprivate, however, the discussion of a patient's disease or condition often takes place in front of another patient. Could this ever be considered an invasion of privacy? Are there legal implications?

A Reports on other "walking patient rounds," are good, so it would be a shame to see this promising innovation compromised by poor judgment. Because that's what's at work here.

If you're truly professional, you'd never discuss in the presence of one patient anything that could legally be considered damaging to another patient. But there's more than immunity from legal actions at issue. There's common sense and sensitivity.

Common sense tells you that no one likes being talked *about*. Our sense of self suffers when we are the object of discussion—even by a group of professionals. But *what* is said about us is an even touchier matter.

As a nurse, discussing such an ordinary thing as constipation might not be an embarrassment for you, even if it's *your* constipation being discussed. But for someone else who has kept this problem her dark secret for 50 years, such a discussion—especially in front of another person—could be very distressing. Because patients come to the hospital to be *relieved* of their distress, you should be supersensitive to their feelings.

So here's a suggestion. Continue making the rounds. If a patient is unconscious, examine him and discuss only the most superficial aspect of his care while in the room. If the patient is conscious, include him in your conversation as you check him out. Once again, stick to the superficial aspects.

Save all detailed accounting of the patient's disease or condition until you're in the hall, or at the nursing station, or somewhere you're sure you can talk privately and professionally.

Patients' rights

Should a nurse fight for them?

Q In our surgical unit, I was recently called in to help with an emergency cesarean section. The patient was a frightened 18-year-old girl. When the anesthesiologist told her she was to receive spinal anesthesia, she balked. She wanted to be "knocked out" for the birth. The anesthesiologist kept insisting on a spinal. The patient was just as adamant about having general anesthesia.

When the doctor tried to override the patient's wishes, I showed him the young woman's surgical consent form—which stated her preference for general anesthesia. Grudgingly, the doctor gave in.

After the patient had safely delivered a baby boy under general anesthesia, I told the doctor I thought the patient's choice should have been respected from the beginning. His overpowering manner, I said, was out of line and clearly added to the young woman's fear and tension.

Although no action's been taken against me, I've heard that the doctor reported my "rudeness." I think I was justified in confronting the doctor with my feelings—but being human, I'd like a backup. Can you give me one?

A This anesthesiologist *was* a bit out of line, but perhaps only a bit. We all know that spinal anesthesia is preferred over general anesthesia for delivery, but his approach did not take account of the patient's near panic. He should have *persuaded* her of the advantages of spinal anesthesia rather than trying to ride roughshod over her objections and anxiety.

A patient has the right to be informed of her condition and to make up her own mind about treatment on the basis of the information. Apparently, this doctor did *not* extend this right to his young patient. You

may have been a bit heavy-handed with the doctor, but you were acting as the patient's advocate—and that's applaudable.

However, if you find yourself in a similar situation with this anesthesiologist at some future time, take your complaints through hospital channels. Start with the chief anesthesiologist, and go all the way up to the medical director, if necessary. You'll still be working for a good cause: your patient's rights.

Patient teaching

How can a nurse comfort the patient?

Q A 54-year-old patient with chronic obstructive pulmonary disease was recovering from a serious episode of respiratory distress. She heard one resident tell another that he'd almost had to "tube and ventilate" her. Frightened, she began asking questions: What did he mean by "tube and ventilate"? Would he do it if she had trouble breathing again?

I've asked the doctor to discuss this treatment option with her, but he's refused. What's more, he told me not to talk with her about it myself. What recourse do I have?

A First, you should find out why he doesn't want her to have the information. Perhaps he believes that she won't understand intubation and mechanical ventilation. Or maybe he's worried that when she knows, she'll choose an alternative that he doesn't believe is right for her.

When you talk with the doctor, point out that not knowing what to expect is making your patient unnecessarily afraid and compromising her nursing care. Remind him that she has a right to answers to her questions and that she'll be more likely to comply if she understands what's going on.

If that doesn't help, schedule a patient care conference with the doctor and your manager. Then check hospital policy for guidelines on a patient's right to refuse treatment. Take that information with you to the conference, along with documentation of your patient's questions and your responses. Tell the doctor that the patient needs more information so she can exercise her right to decide what treatment she will—and won't—accept.

As a last resort, you may have to ask the unit's medical director to intervene.

Patient transfer

Could a nurse be held liable if the patient's harmed by a delay?

Q Recently, an emergency department (ED) doctor ordered us to transfer a patient to another hospital. Before I could do that, two accident victims came in and I didn't get to the transfer for almost an hour. The doctor was furious when he found out, and he told me I'd have been liable if the patient had been harmed by the delay. Was he right?

A Yes. Once he signs the transfer order, you're responsible for seeing that it's carried out. In this case, you knew you were going to be delayed. You should have informed him immediately so he could have taken steps to see that the transfer was accomplished.

Another nurse from Texas discovered this a few years ago. A doctor in the ED had asked her to transfer a toddler who'd fallen and fractured her skull. He suspected that she also had a cerebral hemorrhage, so he wanted her to have a computed tomography scan at another hospital. For some reason, the transfer was delayed by about 2 hours. Despite surgery, the child later died of a massive cerebral hemorrhage. Her parents sued the hospital, as the nurse's employer, for negligence—and won.

What if a doctor seems to procrastinate over the transfer of a severely ill patient?

Q I work on the intensive care unit (ICU) in a small hospital. We have a 50-year-old patient diagnosed as having multiple brain abscesses. The neurosurgeon consultant isn't due in until the end of the week, and the patient's doctor wants to wait for the consult rather than transfer the patient immediately to a nearby city hospital.

> *"We're watching our 50-year-old patient's condition deteriorate and his wife becoming increasingly frightened."*

All of us nurses on the ICU (including the supervisor and unit manager) feel that with our staffing and equipment, we can't give this patient the extensive care he needs now or later. We're watching his condition deteriorate and his wife become increasingly frightened. Yet no one has spoken to his doctor about transferring the patient.

What do you suggest?

A Ask to speak to the doctor in private. Then, in a calm manner, simply tell him, "We're not prepared to handle this patient, and we need to consider a transfer." (You're probably not telling him anything he doesn't already know.) If he asks, "What do you mean?" be ready with some nonthreatening reasoning. "We do the best we can, but we're limited. This complex case needs sophisticated services available on a 24-hour basis. You might remember what a difficult time we had handling such-and-such case..." Then be sure that you let your unit manager and supervisor know you've made the observation to the doctor. He apparently has trouble deciding when to pass. Help him.

Pay

Should an increase be expected with a promotion?

Q Sixteen months ago, I was the first to accept one of several newly created charge nurse positions in this hospital. I was told I'd receive no pay raise then, but one assistant director of nursing seemed confident that it would come in time—probably after the other charge nurse openings were filled. Since then, my responsibilities have grown; I'm now doing the work of a nursing care coordinator—the next step up from charge nurse. But I'm still being paid staff nurse wages with no raise in sight. In fact, management now says the hospital can't afford to pay charge nurses extra money. The attitude seems to be that "nice nurses don't ask for money."

Yesterday, I told my supervisor that unless the raises come through, I plan to return to staff nurse status and I'll encourage the other new charge nurses to do the same. She asked me to reconsider, saying that she's already recommended me for nursing care coordinator. Now, I'm torn. Should I stick with my fellow charge nurses to fight the pay issue? Or take this new promotion? And do you think management is just trying to shut me up?

A Going back to staff nurse status will net you nothing and brand you as a troublemaker. Go for the nursing care coordinator position if it's offered to you; instead of muzzling you, it'll put you in a better position to influence those who can help. And you'll be gaining even more management experience.

In the interim, while you're still officially a charge nurse, call the others together and prepare a statement of what raise you expect (and deserve), when, and why; have everyone sign the statement; and send it through channels. Wait 2 weeks, then arrange for all the charge

P

nurses to meet and discuss your concerns with the nursing supervisor, the director of nursing, and the hospital administrator. Management will probably react more generously to this positive action. And you'll come away looking like a strong leader, not a sore loser.

Should nurses get paid for on-call time?

Q In the gastroenterology unit of our hospital, I'm expected to be on call every other week and to carry a beeper. If I'm called in, I'm paid double time. That's fine. But if I'm not called in, I'm not paid for being on call. How come the surgical nurses in this hospital *are* paid for being on call? What's the standard practice?

A You *should* get paid for on-call time—whether the compensation is in time off or in additional money. But why *shouldn't* you be compensated? Do you know any businessman, lawyer, or doctor who'd do this for nothing?

If you want to work toward changing the on-call payment policy in your hospital, start by surveying what other hospitals in the area do about this. Then review the on-call situation in your own hospital. Do base salaries reflect the added on-call responsibility? If not, assemble all the pertinent facts, take them to the nursing administration, and ask for a review of on-call payment policy—with an eye toward making change.

The review and the revision are certainly called for.

Payroll deduction

Can a nurse be forced to donate?

Q Our hospital administrators have been planning a building campaign and are soliciting donations from *all* employees. Each em-

ployee is expected to sign a pledge card authorizing a regular payroll deduction over the next 5 years. Even if we don't want to donate, we still have to sign the card.

Can the administrators do this? If I refuse to donate, can they note the refusal in my employee file and use it against me in salary and job evaluations?

A No, you're not *required* to accept this. If you want to donate, fine. But no one can force you to. In any event, you—and any others who also feel the administration is "pressing"—should seek a meeting with the administrators. Ask for a clarification of their policy on employee donations. Suggest they issue a statement that such donations are viewed as purely voluntary.

Suppose you refuse to donate: Can they use this against you? They shouldn't, but they might. Fortunately, most states have an Open Records Act that gives you access to your file. After the solicitation's completed, arrange to see your employment file. If it contains a record of your refusal to authorize a donation, don't be bashful. Ask why this information's in your file. If you suspect it'll jeopardize your chances for a promotion or raise, consider seeking legal help.

Pediatric oncology unit

Is there a good book to help prepare parents for the care of a child with cancer?

Q I'm new on the staff of a pediatric oncology unit and need some help preparing parents for the physical and emotional care of a child with cancer. Can you suggest an inexpensive book or pamphlet I could hand out to parents?

A A 93-page paperback publication called *Young People With*

Cancer: A Handbook for Parents, may just fit your bill.

The handbook explains the disease in simple, but graphic terms, and provides information about the child's hospitalization and treatment, and about possible adverse reactions. In addition, the handbook offers supportive suggestions for coping with the emotional impact of the disease on both the child and his family.

The handbook is free: Write to the National Cancer Institute, Building 31, Room 10A18, Bethesda, MD 20892. You can also call 1-800-422-6237 to get a copy.

Peer evaluations

Are they a good idea?

Q At the hospital where I work, our geriatric unit was chosen to initiate a new form of performance evaluation that administration terms "peer review." We received no written guidelines. We're just supposed to get together at reviewing sessions to assess each other's work. Eventually even our merit raises will depend on our reviews.

In the last 2 months, certain unit changes have taken place, all of them bad. Review meetings are nothing more than gripe sessions; one or two of the most vocal (not necessarily most sensitive) nurses have assumed self-appointed leadership roles; the RNs resent criticism by the LPNs; we've lost our sense of unity.

In my opinion, we're building resentment and tearing down morale. How does this "new age" review experiment sound to you?

A Like something out of George Orwell—all staff members are considered equal, but some are more equal than others. What you're involved in is someone's half-baked notion of what peer review entails.

As the name suggests, peer review means professional evaluation by those on a similar level in education and experience (for example, clinical specialists reviewed by clinical specialists, unit managers by unit managers, and the same for nurse educators, intensive care unit nurses, community health nurses, and so on). A mixed group reviewing one another's performance is not peer review. Even among closely matched peers, review by one's colleagues can be threatening and embarrassing unless you can guarantee willing participation, strong administrative support, clear guidelines, and some demonstrable *benefit* to be gained by turning to this management method. The policy your unit is struggling with strikes out on all counts.

For most of us, achievements on the job and recognition by our colleagues intimately affect our feelings of self-esteem and confidence. No one who's constantly worried about survival can function well. Quickly, before any irreparable harm's done, get word to the administrators so they can start a little reviewing of their own on this questionable policy.

Personal disability

Is there any place for a nurse with chronic fibrositis in nursing?

Q I am a 27-year-old diploma graduate, and for 6 years I was one of the happiest—and in honesty, I think one of the best—staff nurses you could find. I really worked well with patients. At the end of the day, I went home with a sense of satisfaction and accomplishment. Now, because of chronic fibrositis, which prevents me from lifting even the lightest load, I can no longer do general nursing. But I don't want to do any other kind of nursing—like office, occupational health, or school nursing. I want to work at the bedside. Can you think of any place for me?

A The first place to think of is school—if you can afford it, and you need not work right away. Because you're no longer capable of general duty, you'll need a specialty, and this almost always calls for a degree.

You say you relate well to patients. Have you ever considered becoming a thanatologist so you could work with the dying and their families? It's a most challenging but rewarding kind of work. Or how about patient teaching in orthopedics or obstetrics—or almost any other field you can name? Furthermore, a number of hospitals have instituted a position called patient advocate (or patient representative) in which one specially-trained person—often a nurse—is the designated representative of any patient with hospital-associated problems.

Any of these (and many other nursing specialties) will keep you working at the bedside and in good patient contact.

Personal journal

Should a nurse keep one in case she's sued for malpractice?

Q I've been keeping a journal of incidents I'm involved in at the hospital. (I'm worried about lawsuits.) My journal came up in a conversation I was having with a nurse who's new to the hospital, and she told me I shouldn't be doing this. She said that if I were ever sued for malpractice, I'd have to share my journal with lawyers from both sides. Is she right?

A Yes, your journal could be read by both sides in a lawsuit. Also, you could be questioned about any conversations you may have had about an incident.

In fact, virtually anything you write or say is subject to scrutiny, with the exception of communication protected by lawyer-client privilege. In other words, you wouldn't have to disclose any letters or conversations between you and your lawyer. Similarly, a lawyer wouldn't have to reveal thoughts and impressions he developed as he gathered information about the case.

Should you stop writing in your journal? No—you never know when you'll need to refresh your memory of an incident. Just be aware that someday, eyes other than yours could be reading your private thoughts.

Photographs

Can the emergency department legally take photographs when they suspect child abuse?

Q Recently, a social worker brought an 11-year-old girl to our emergency department (ED). The social worker suspected child abuse and asked us to photograph the girl's black eye and other injuries to document them.

We could all see the need for photographs, but we didn't know whether we could legally take them. Can the ED staff take such photographs? What sort of release would we need? It would be absurd to expect the parents to provide it.

As it was, no one would go out on a limb. Please tell us what to do before the poor kid comes in with new injuries.

A Every state has a law requiring doctors and social workers (among others) to report suspected child abuse in children under age 16 or 18, depending on the state. These laws also offer some immunity from liability, as long as the professional acts in good faith.

Some states have designated state reporting agencies. These agencies have 24-hour-a-day coverage and will send a caseworker to investigate. Either the caseworker or the local police can photograph injuries without parental consent.

In states that don't specifically mention the right to photograph, the examining doctor has the responsibility to authorize photographs if he agrees that there is a duty to report possible child abuse, because the duty to report implies a responsibility to preserve any evidence. If the parents are present and object to photographs, the doctor should contact law enforcement officials to secure a court order.

Child abuse reporting laws are far from standardized, so ED personnel should request a specific procedure from the hospital administration. Obviously, the administration should design a procedure that meets all state reporting laws.

Picketing

Can a hospital make a picketing staff nurse's life miserable?

Q On the medical/surgical unit where I work, we admit quite a few gynecologic surgical cases that lately include an increasing number of induced abortions. The pro-life organization I belong to plans to picket the offices of three of the doctors I work with. Because these offices are located in an adjoining wing of the hospital, we'll actually be demonstrating on hospital property.

My union attorney said the hospital can't do anything to me as long as I demonstrate on my own time and I'm not in uniform. I feel very strongly about abortion and I want to picket, but I'm nervous about maintaining my professional relationship with these doctors. They'll probably recognize me because I'm a charge nurse, and I'm afraid they may try to make my life miserable at the hospital.

What's your opinion?

A Your union attorney has already filled you in on your rights; certainly you're entitled to fair and equitable treatment on the job even if you demonstrate. Unfortunately, though, no court in the land can order the doctors to *like* you after you picket them or mandate that they include you in any of the social activities at the hospital.

Making even hard decisions will be easier if you follow a few steps. Define the problem (how concerned are you about pleasant association with these doctors?); weigh the risks (you'll be part of a group reaction and can't control other demonstrators' behavior); look at alternative solutions (are there other effective ways you can support the pro-life movement?); compare the alternatives; and last, but not least, remember that decisions are almost always choices between less-than-perfect alternatives.

The only way to be sure a decision's right for you is to make it yourself.

Piggybacking

Does it make any difference which tubing is attached directly to the patient's I.V. site?

Q We need an outside opinion to settle an argument that keeps surfacing on our unit. When piggybacking antibiotics or other medications, does it make any difference which tubing—the primary I.V. tubing or the piggyback tubing—is attached directly to the patient's I.V. site?

A You'll decrease the risk of contamination if you avoid manipulating the primary tubing any more than absolutely necessary for tubing changes. So, using the primary tubing for the I.V. solution and attaching it directly to the patient's I.V. site is best. Use the piggyback line for infusing the antibiotics and other medications that usually run for a short period of time.

Pilfering

How do other hospitals combat it?

Q Our hospital loses huge quantities of money each year on pilfered objects. I see employees leaving with shopping bags suspiciously full. The administration keeps busy sending out memos on this problem—but not doing anything about it. How do other hospitals try to combat pilfering?

A Hospital costs are everybody's business and you're right to be concerned about pilfering. You're also right that a virtual blizzard of memos isn't going to change the situation. For reasons unfathomable, some people act as though the commandment, "Thou shalt not steal," has a little-quoted rider that says, "...except from the government, corporations, or large institutions."

Certain large metropolitan hospitals now post guards at every exit to examine every package, shopping bag—even large handbag—of every person leaving the building. If an employee shops on her lunch hour, the bags are sealed as she returns. If the seal is broken, the package must be reexamined before she is allowed to leave. There are no exceptions—visitors, supervisory personnel, kitchen help—*everyone* gets the same treatment. It's been said that the decrease in thefts makes up for the extra guards' salaries. But at what cost to the morale of employees who have to work in such a prisonlike atmosphere? How much better for everyone if the stealing could be stopped at the grassroots level—on the units—before it starts.

Some hospitals have reported partial success by placing tighter control on supplies. Before any item leaves central supply or pharmacy, a requisition slip stating what it is, who it's for, and when it's taken must be filed. With this method, stock supplies on the floor are kept to a minimum, reducing the chance for pilferage. Critics of this system, however, point to an increased expenditure of time and paperwork.

Any system of theft prevention will depend on a number of variables, including the size of the hospital and its physical layout. The one constant is that honesty, like most virtues, is best introduced at home. So why don't you talk this over with the unit manager in *your* department? If she feels the same as you, she could announce her concern at the next staff meeting and call for ideas on how to "police" your own area.

Should a nurse blow the whistle if she doesn't have proof?

Q Several months ago, I saw one of my co-workers pilfering drugs from the medication cabinet on our floor. I thought about it, so later in the afternoon, I confronted her and told her that next time, I'd report her to our supervisor. Naturally, she was very embarrassed. She swore she'd never stolen before and it wouldn't happen again. I thought that was the end of it.

Yesterday, another co-worker mentioned to me that several drugs were missing from the cabinet. Since I don't know that the first nurse took them, I'm in a real quandary about what to do. Should I assume that she kept her promise? Should I ignore the situation or confront her again? Should I "squeal" to my supervisor?

A There are drugs and there are drugs. You don't say *what* the nurse was originally pilfering. But surely it wasn't a controlled drug—a narcotic, amphetamine, barbiturate—or you would have confronted her immediately and gone right to your supervisor. Public interest re-

quires that a profession regulate itself. Nursing must do so as well, to maintain public trust in its activities.

A co-worker who pilfers drugs is a thief, is in violation of the American Nurses' Association's Code of Ethics, and should be disciplined by her peers—the one who observed the infraction, then the peer group that reviews violations of the profession's code of ethics, the Board of Nurse Examiners. How far the matter should go would, of course, depends on the frequency and nature of drugs taken. Most nurses look the other way when a co-worker takes a single aspirin for personal use. Few would hesitate to report a nurse who takes a narcotic for personal use. In between is a gray area, and each situation must be considered separately.

Now that the incident you described has passed, report the latest incident of missing drugs to the supervisor. Request that she keep a closer check on the medicine cabinet, watching for a pattern. Do drugs continue to disappear? Is it always the same drug? Is it from the same shift? If her answers to these questions point to your suspected co-worker, then you should tell the supervisor about that worker's role in the original pilfering. If the surveillance does not point to the original pilferer, the surveillance should be continued until the guilty one is found. Remember, so long as no one is guilty, all are suspect.

Placebos

What should patients be told?

Q At the hospital where I work, one doctor often prescribes placebos for a patient who requests something for pain or anxiety. If the patient asks what drug he's receiving, the doctor's told us to reply "Oblacep," which spells placebo when unscrambled. I feel this is dis-

honest, although I know that in some cases placebos do relieve pain.

What's your opinion?

A A nurse shouldn't lie to a patient, nor should she be asked to do so by someone else. First of all, she has her own self-image to maintain. Second, when the patient discovers it's a placebo (most do), he'll lose his trust and respect for the doctor and the staff.

Instead of answering directly, simply refer him to the doctor.

Postop hemorrhage

If a patient keeps hemorrhaging and dies, who would be liable?

Q I'm an emergency department (ED) nurse in a rural clinic where tonsillectomies and adenoidectomies (T & As) are performed as ambulatory surgery cases. ED nurses don't assist with the surgery, but if a patient should hemorrhage after discharge, the ED nurse on call *is* responsible for caring for that patient. We notify the doctor immediately, but we have a standing order to pack the patient's mouth and give a coagulant. The doctor doesn't usually appear until the next day. Our total "preparation" for this procedure consisted of watching *one* T & A, and packing *one* patient who was under anesthesia.

Suppose some night one of us can't stop a hemorrhage? We worry. If a patient were to suffer from loss of blood, or God forbid, to bleed to death, would we be liable?

A Yes, you *are* liable for any patient you're caring for, so you must protect yourself as well as your patient.

Before you're faced with an emergency, do some checking. Ask your

P

state board of nursing if the packing and coagulant procedure *is* within the realm of nursing practice in your state. If nurses *aren't* allowed to do this procedure, then the doctor *must* come to the clinic immediately. However, if nurses *are* allowed to do this procedure, we suggest you brush up on your techniques.

From your description, your preparation for this procedure sounds dismally inadequate. The clinic is responsible for teaching you how to do it well. So ask your manager to schedule staff development classes on packing techniques, possible complications of hemorrhaging, and danger signals of excessive bleeding.

Incidentally, if you really couldn't stop a patient's bleeding, surely a doctor would come immediately. You can probably ease your mind on this score.

Postpolio syndrome

How many people suffer from it?

Q My best friend is a teacher with postpolio syndrome. For years, she had no problem standing all day teaching or with the hiking she did for exercise and recreation. Lately, though, she's noticed her leg muscles and joints becoming progressively weaker and more painful. She takes ibuprofen (Motrin) for pain but won't change her habits.

She might listen to me because I'm a nurse, but I have little information on this. How many other people suffer from this syndrome? Do you have any helpful advice I can pass on to her?

A A recent study showed that about 50% of the 300,000 people who survived polio have some postpolio symptoms. And 20% of those experience significant symptoms, though they're still not as devastating as the original illness.

Many postpolio patients either don't recognize or deny encroaching weakness. They may keep pushing themselves to continue activities that once helped them—and instead experience muscle strain, joint inflammation, and weakness.

Try to convince your friend to go to a medical center for assessment. A physical therapist or rehabilitation specialist could suggest some changes, even small ones, in her everyday routine to spare her overworked muscles and minimize her symptoms. For instance, a sensible diet for keeping her weight down will help—so might sitting on a stool while she teaches, and doing mild stretching exercises or swimming instead of hiking.

Such a reappearance of symptoms must be terribly disheartening for her. But your support can make a big difference for her mental outlook. Encourage her to contact one of the 200 polio support groups throughout the country. There's also an excellent resource in the Gazette International Networking Institute (GINI); tell her to write to GINI, Dept. N89, 4502 Maryland Ave., St. Louis, MO 63108.

Preemployment exam

What if failing a math exam blocks employment?

Q I recently moved to California and interviewed for an LVN position at our community hospital. The nurse-manager gave me a surprise math exam that included I.V. medications, and I flunked. (Where I come from, LVNs aren't taught to administer I.V.s.) She said I could retake the test the following week, which I did. That time, I missed two questions. When I asked her to explain why my answers were wrong, she threw down her pencil and said she doesn't hire incompetent peo-

ple who can't pass the test. She told me to go take a medications and math course and not to come back until I do.

I left the interview angry and embarrassed. What's your opinion on this?

A Sorry you were treated badly. Next time, when you set up an appointment, ask what's expected of you during a job interview. Find out how practice for LVNs varies in California from that in your home state; then be prepared to explain to a potential employer just how you plan to make up any deficiencies.

> *"On an interview, the nurse-manager gave me a surprise math exam that included I.V. medications, and I flunked."*

For now, concentrate on sharpening your skills and establishing a good work record, perhaps in another facility. Meet with the nursing faculty advisor at your local community college and arrange to take a medication and math course, as suggested. You might even want to go back to the community hospital when you feel at home performing the required skills. And if you do, good luck taking the test.

Pregnant nurses

What should pregnant nurses avoid?

Q What patient assignments should pregnant nurses avoid? We're looking for a safe rule of thumb to go by because it seems that more staff members are becoming pregnant these days.

A The cardinal rules of safety when caring for any patient are good handwashing technique and strict observance of isolation precautions. But when you're pregnant, you must also use good judgment about accepting patient assignments.

According to guidelines from the Centers for Disease Control (CDC), cytomegalovirus and rubella pose serious risks to a developing fetus. Pregnant nurses who work in the nursery or pediatrics, or with patients who have acquired immunodeficiency syndrome, should take special precautions and might judiciously consider asking for reassignment.

Hepatitis B is another danger. The CDC suggests immunization for pregnant nurses if they work on units where they might be exposed. Barring this, they should at least avoid working in hemodialysis units and laboratories where blood and body fluids are handled extensively.

Radiation is a risk to the fetus, too. In the case of diagnostic X-rays, any pregnant nurse whose fetus could receive more than 0.5 rem should either reduce her exposure or request reassignment. Pregnant nurses should avoid caring for patients with radioactive implants or material injected into body cavities.

Finally, nurses who are trying to conceive or who are pregnant or breast-feeding should neither prepare nor administer parenteral antineoplastic drugs.

Pressure sore

How can it be brought under control?

Q A patient at the nursing home where I work is elderly, malnourished, and blind. She also has severe arthritis, a chronic chest condition, and a recurrent urinary tract infection. But right now we're concerned with another problem the patient has: a coccyx pressure sore she's had for more than a year.

Although the sore looks clean, it's more than 2″ (5 cm) in diameter and will sometimes have a copious green discharge.

We've tried everything to bring the ulcer under control: normal saline compresses, medicated packing, polyurethane dressings, surgical debridement, and peroxide as a cleaning agent. But with each treatment, the area only seems to become redder and larger.

We've run out of things to do. Can you give us a new suggestion?

A Perhaps you're not getting a result because you're switching treatments too quickly.

Although you'll find a long, long list of therapies for pressure sores—each therapy backed by a different authority—you'll note that they all have the same fundamental approach. Keep the area clean and dry. Position the patient so she's not sitting or lying on the sore. Use a consistent treatment.

The new polyurethane dressings come well-recommended. You say you've already tried this type of dressing, but maybe you simply haven't used it long enough.

To help solve the patient's problem, get together with a dietitian (inadequate nutrition can be a key factor in the failure of the sore to heal), an enterostomal therapist, and a dermatologist at your facility. Go over the problem as a team. When you come up with an agreed-upon approach, give that treatment time to work.

If you're persistent and consistent, you'll probably be surprised and pleased with the results.

Prison nursing

Could a nurse be asked to participate in an execution by assessing, monitoring, or even injecting the solution?

Q I'm really concerned that as a prison nurse, I could be asked to participate in an execution by lethal injection by assessing, mon-

itoring, or even injecting the solution. Any word on this?

A Yes. The American Nurses' Association's Committee on Ethics is strongly opposed to all forms of participation by nurses in capital punishment. In a statement on this issue, they conclude, "It is a breach of the nursing code of ethical conduct for nurses to participate either directly or indirectly in a legally authorized execution." State nurses' associations also affirm that a nurse administering such an injection would be in violation of the nurse practice act, which defines the practice of nursing as "diagnosing and treating human responses to actual or potential physical and emotional health problems through the provision of care supportive to or restorative of life and well-being."

Private-duty nursing

How can staff nurses be prevented from taking cases?

Q At the hospital where I do private duty, the staff nurses work 12-hour shifts. Recently, they've begun taking private cases on their days off, often on the very unit where they regularly work.

The staff nurse gets first crack at assignments by making arrangements directly with the private-duty secretary. Those of us who count on private-duty nursing for a living get the cases the staff nurses don't want, if any. Naturally, this causes a lot of animosity.

What can we do when we're on the outside looking in?

A Alone, not much. The staff nurses are in a power position. Early on, they learn what cases need private nurses, and they move on this information.

P

You and the other private duty nurses will have to band together to make your own case. Draft a memo to administration—market yourselves. What have you got going for you? You're reporting for duty refreshed (not after putting in 36 to 48 hours' work); you're not hemmed in by a regular work schedule; you're free to accept a case and remain on it as long as necessary. And even without the benefits accorded regular hospital employees, you fill a definite need by providing an immediate, dependable reserve of experienced, oriented nurses.

Once alerted to the problem, administration should react and reconcile this touchy situation. Avoid personal confrontation with the staff nurses. Remember, infighting won't lead to job satisfaction for anyone—no matter who wins.

How should a nurse handle a doctor who puts down private-duty nursing?

Q As head of the department of private-duty nursing in our hospital, I received a written complaint from one of our members.

She'd been engaged by a neurosurgical patient for 2 days after his operation. When the neurosurgeon (whom she'd never met) made rounds, he belligerently demanded to know why she was there. As the nurse started to explain, he turned to the family and roared that he didn't want private-duty nurses on any of his cases because they're all "old retirees who have come back to nursing and no longer have the skills." (Just for the record, the nurse is 47 years old—6 years younger than the doctor—and she's been steadily employed for the past 17 years!)

He said his patients do better on general care and because he hadn't ordered a private nurse, he wouldn't authorize insurance payments for her salary.

The family, embarrassed by the doctor's behavior, assured the nurse they would pay her out of their own pocket. Other hospital visitors were shocked, and the nurses on the floor were angered by the doctor's humiliating treatment of the nurse.

The doctor must have heard about these reactions because he sent me a letter "explaining his position on private nursing." The gist of it is that, over the years, he has trained the staff of the neurosurgical unit in the way he wants things done. And since private nurses don't have that training, he'd rather not have them. No apology for his treatment of the nurse or anything like that.

I'm not sure how I should handle this. Should I answer the doctor's letter? Should I report it to the hospital? Are there any legal steps I should take?

A First of all, you should send the doctor a simple acknowledgement of your receipt of his letter. No additional comments should be necessary. Then notify your membership of the doctor's attitude toward private nurses so they'll be well-prepared if they're ever asked to do duty for a patient of his. Also file copies of this correspondence with the hospital administration so they'll know exactly what's going on.

> *"The doctor turned to the family and roared that he didn't want private-duty nurses on any of his cases because 'they're all old retirees.'"*

As to the possibility of legal action, the situation doesn't seem to justify such fears. This appears to simply be a case of an ill-bred, ill-tempered person rudely venting his spleen on a co-worker. Interpersonal conflicts pop up every day in

all walks of life and, while not pleasant, they scarcely call for court action.

As a matter of fact, you could take an optimistic view and be grateful that now—with things spelled out—you won't have to be dealing with such a disagreeable man. Pity the poor nurses in the neuro unit who have no such silver lining to look to.

How should a private-duty nurse address the nursing staff's neglect?

Q I'm an RN in private practice. Recently, I was hired to feed and provide companionship for a woman in a nursing home. When I arrived, she was in deplorable condition: She had two recent pressure sores, her hair was filthy, she hadn't had a proper bath in days, and her sheets were dirty. So I cleaned her up and changed her sheets.

I know I should approach the nursing staff about this situation, but I'm afraid they'll resent my intrusion. What should I do?

A You're the patient's advocate, so you can't ignore the situation. With the proper documentation in hand, approach the nurse in charge. If that doesn't get results, speak with the director of nursing.

Your report on the situation should be as complete, accurate, and *specific* as possible. Don't write "the patient hasn't had a proper bath in days"; instead, say "her hair was matted with bits of dried food; gown and sheets were soiled with pus and urine." Remember to remain nonjudgmental, focusing on the facts, not on personal impressions or conclusions.

Also, get a copy of the nursing home's policy on private-duty nurses so you're clear about your responsibilities.

If the care doesn't improve, don't give up. You're morally and legally obligated to report abuse, neglect, or abandonment of a nursing home patient to the proper law enforcement agency or the department of health. And, of course, you'd want to advise the patient's doctor and family members of any treatment that's endangering her health, welfare, or safety.

Will a hospital let a nurse care for her own mother?

Q My mother has asked me to be her private-duty nurse when she has a cholecystectomy next month. Do you think the hospital will let me care for her?

A There are two schools of thought on this subject. One would advise: Before your mother has her surgery, make it your business to find out about policy in her hospital. If you *are* allowed to do the nursing care, you'll have the deep satisfaction of knowing that your mother's needs are being met by someone with a personal interest. But don't let your emotions interfere with professional objectivity. Are you sure you'll be able to assess your mother's condition with detachment—under any circumstances? Can you carry out a doctor's orders—even if they mean discomfort for your mother?

If you *can* handle it, the personal and professional rewards will be large.

Another school of thought would follow this reasoning: Why not let the hospital staff care for your mother? They know the hospital's policy for emergencies, procedures, and medications. You probably do not.

Instead, visit your mother in the hospital and do all the nice things you can for her. Save your strength for when she gets home so you can help then. In other words, don't confuse your role as daughter and as nurse. The result could be too draining for everyone.

Prolixin

What are the dangers of injecting this drug so often?

Q As the only nurse at the mental health center in our area, I'm responsible for administering the antipsychotic drug fluphenazine decanoate (Prolixin) to outpatients once a week or once every other week. The drug in these I.M. injections improves their mood and behavior. But I worry about injecting as much as 2 ml of fluphenazine decanoate per week into the same general area (even though I use the gluteal site because of its large muscle mass and rotate sites regularly).

What are the dangers of injecting this drug so often?

A None. In fact, both forms of long-acting Prolixin (fluphenazine decanoate and fluphenazine enanthate) are so benign to tissues they can even be given subcutaneously.

You're quite right to rotate sites, but you don't have to restrict your injections to the gluteal area. You can also use any of the other I.M. injection sites, including the deltoid area.

So don't worry about injecting your patients once a week or once every other week with fluphenazine decanoate or fluphenazine enanthate. And, whatever you do, don't lose the concern and caution you've shown for your patients.

Promotion

How can friendships be continued without losing authority?

Q For 7 years, I worked as a general duty nurse on an unusually congenial floor. We had exceptionally good relationships,

even outside the hospital, and when I was promoted to supervisor 6 months ago, everyone seemed genuinely pleased. In the past few months, however, our relationship has deteriorated to a point where my "friends" not only shun me socially but resent and resist any changes I make in our work—even though I try to consult them before making the change.

How can I let them know that I'm still the friend they once knew, without losing my authority as supervisor?

A You seem to have two problems here. One concerns your working day, the other, your social life. Let's start with the first.

Perhaps your friends have been unable to accept you in your new supervisory role because *you* haven't been able to accept it. You speak of yourself as "still the friend they once knew." But during the 7-to-3 shift, you're *not.* During those hours, your staff members think of themselves as "us" and of you as "them"—that catch-all term for all supervisory figures.

Keeping in mind the difference that now exists, consider your statement, ". . . even though I try to consult them before making a change." "Try" is not good enough. A good supervisor *always* consults with her staff before initiating change. Otherwise, she's justifiably considered high-handed and authoritarian. Could this be one of the reasons why your co-workers "resent and resist any changes"?

In what seems to have been a period of "separation anxiety," you've gotten off to a slow start. But it's not too late. Here are a few steps.
1. Call a conference to discuss with your staff members some plan you have for solving a practical nursing problem in your department. Perhaps the problem will be as simple—but frustrating—as late laundry delivery. Arrange a joint

P

meeting with the unit manager and the laundry supervisor. Explore how you and your staff can help get the laundry to your floor on time. Even simple exercises in problem solving will, if repeated often enough, define your role to your staff—and *you*.

2. Come to the conference prepared to listen. Ask your staff members for *their* ideas on work-simplification programs, new training programs, and staff development classes. Be positive about their suggestions and put the good ones right into action.

3. Remember that a good supervisor does not stay in her office all day. She's out on the floor and she makes a point of knowing everything that's going on in her department. That does not make her a "snoopervisor"—it makes her a good nurse *and* a leader. And she's *there* when her nurses need her.

4. Look around for some management development courses. You'll be relieved to learn how common some of your problems are and how many different ways they can be solved.

As to the second part of your question, on socializing with your staff, you'll find it works out on an individual basis. Some people will want to keep up the camaraderie that existed. Others, regardless of the supervisor's personality, are simply not comfortable with a supervisor in a social setting. But that works out, too. These people are apt to be replaced with new friends—usually other supervisors!

Pronouncing death

Can the RN on duty or the manager pronounce death?

Q When a patient dies in the nursing home where I work, my manager pronounces death if a doctor isn't available. She says the RN on duty or the manager can legally do this. I disagree. Who's right?

A You are, in this case. Some states, such as New Jersey, permit nurses to pronounce death. But most require a doctor. (Emergency medical personnel sometimes may pronounce death, but only under special circumstances.)

Your manager is placing her license in jeopardy because she's making a medical, not a nursing, diagnosis. She may report physical evidence of death to the doctor, but only he can legally pronounce the patient dead.

One more thing: If the doctor isn't present, he can pronounce death over the telephone after a nurse calls him with the necessary information. She should then clearly chart that the doctor made that decision based on her findings.

Psychiatric nursing

Should a strict lights-out policy be enforced?

Q I work the 11-to-7 shift on an adolescent psychiatric unit. My problem is a strict lights-out policy, which I'm expected to enforce.

Most of the kids are suffering from depression and loneliness, and many of them have insomnia. Not surprisingly, they dread lying alone in their rooms at night, and I often find them in one another's rooms talking quietly. I'm supposed to report them, but if I do, they lose their privileges. If I *don't*, I may lose my job.

What's your opinion?

A Doing what's best for the kids is important but not at the expense of breaking the rules to do so. Knowing that adolescents can be experts at manipulation, most hospitals find strict enforcement of a few rules the best policy in adolescent units.

With this warning, devise a new policy and submit it to your night supervisor or director of nursing for approval.

Define the problem, then suggest ways to solve it. For example, perhaps sleepless teenagers could meet in a conference room, with or without a therapist. Or perhaps they could come to the nursing station for a snack and a visit when they can't sleep. If these solutions aren't acceptable, you might at least get permission for the teenagers to read or work on crafts in their rooms.

You might also want to look at the other end of the problem— preventing insomnia. Possibly, the kids can't sleep at night because they nap during the day or simply don't get enough exercise. With all three nursing shifts cooperating, you might be able to plan workouts in the hospital gym and other stimulating activities early in the day, to ensure that the kids feel tired by evening.

Psychiatric patient

Should statements like "Maybe today I'll jump out the window" be documented?

Q One of the postoperative patients at the hospital where I work has had a history of paranoia and other psychiatric disturbances. He used to be depressed and ill tempered—but during this postoperative period, he's seemed quite cheerful and pleasant. We though the present medication was helping.

However, two nights ago he told a nurse on the 3-to-11 shift that he couldn't take the pain. If it didn't stop, he said, he'd kill himself. The charge nurse told me this when I reported for the 11-to-7 shift.

The next morning, the patient seemed in an even mood, so I asked him about his threat. "Maybe today I'll jump out the window," he said. I charted his exact remark.

The next day, my nursing supervisor, the patient's doctor, and the staff psychiatrist reevaluated the patient.

My co-workers say I *shouldn't* have charted the statement because the psychiatrist concluded that the patient wasn't really suicidal.

Now I'm having second thoughts. Should I have charted the statement or passed it along verbally? Was I wrong to notify my supervisor and the doctor? In other words, did I overreact? What should I do if I face this situation in another case?

A No, you didn't overreact. In fact, you were right in two ways. First, because patients have been known to attempt suicide when seeming to come out of depression, your alarm was justified. Second, notifying your supervisor and the doctor was good nursing judgment.

All statements made by a patient should be charted if they relate to his problem or progress— according to accepted nursing practice. Your patient's suicide threat certainly fits into that category. If any question about your handling of the problem were to come up later in court, your accurate charting would speak in your favor.

So if you're faced with a similar situation in the future, follow your own example. If your best nursing judgment is to chart, then chart. By protecting your patient and your legal interests, you'll be doubly safe, instead of doubly sorry.

Psychiatric problems

How can untrained nurses be expected to handle them?

Q I'm the unit manager on a medical/surgical unit at a large city hospital. After a nearby mental health institution announced plans to close its medical facility, our administrator agreed to accept any of

its patients with medical emergencies. And guess whose unit these patients would be transferred to?

Preparations for the potentially troublesome new admissions included immediate installation of safety windows in the three rooms set aside for them, requisitioning leather restraints, and so on. We nurses received *no* special preparation in the care of psychiatric patients.

> *"The patient broke two beds and a telephone, threw excrement all over the walls, spit at anyone who came near her, and kicked one nurse in the breast."*

Recently a 17-year-old girl from the institution was admitted to our unit after taking an overdose of diazepam (Valium). During her stay, she broke two beds and a telephone, threw excrement all over the walls and ceiling of her room, spit at and threatened anyone who came near her, and kicked one nurse in the breast. We used our new leather restraints.

All in all, these patients are putting our unit in an uproar, disturbing our other patients and demoralizing my staff.

I've complained to nursing service and the administration, who profess to be sympathetic. But the transfers keep coming. What do you suggest I do before I transfer myself?

A Remember that these patients, difficult as they may be, have a *right* to nursing care. Your administrator has signed a contract that obligates the hospital to provide this care. That means both the physical environment *and* the staff must be prepared for these patients.

For proper preparation, have a psychiatric consultant counsel your staff on the techniques and approaches commonly used to handle

the aberrant patient behavior you describe. If possible, the consultant should be on call, available to you whenever a situation becomes too hot to handle.

Also consider sending members of your staff, in rotation, to conferences on care of psychiatric patients. Each staff member could share what she learns at her particular conference with the rest of you.

You'll have to work closely with administration in making these plans. But in the meantime, for your protection, write a memo on how disturbing the new admissions policy is, and list your suggestions for remedying the situation. Send copies to both the nursing and the medical directors, and urge a meeting of everyone involved.

If you see help is on the way and decide *not* to walk away from the challenge, any success you have— no matter how small—will add inestimably to your self-esteem and your professional growth.

Pulmonary artery catheter

Should a nurse refuse to care for a patient who doesn't have his own monitor?

Q I work the 11-to-7 shift in a 10-bed intensive care unit/cardiac care unit. On several occasions we've had two patients with pulmonary artery catheters sharing our one and only monitor. Although our nursing supervisors don't approve of this practice, the doctors involved don't seem to think there's a problem.

But I do. I feel strongly that every patient with a pulmonary artery catheter should have his own monitor. I'm very uncomfortable with this sharing practice, and I'm wondering if I should refuse to care for a patient without a monitor next time the situation arises.

Are my fears unfounded? Would I be justified in refusing care under these circumstances?

A Your fears aren't unfounded. A patient with a pulmonary artery catheter *should* have continuous electrocardiogram (ECG) and waveform monitoring whenever possible. But if the equipment isn't available, you can still maintain both patients' safety by:
• having continuous ECG monitoring for both patients, and
• selecting the more critically ill patient for continuous pressure monitoring.

Then, when you want to take a reading on the less critically ill patient, remove one transducer and exchange it at the monitor outlet with the second transducer. Allow the equipment 10 minutes to warm up before taking your reading.

"We've had two patients with pulmonary artery catheters sharing our only monitor, but I'm very uncomfortable with this practice."

If you find that you must share monitors more and more often, then you and your nursing supervisors should consider documenting how often you're called upon to do this; also report the problems sharing entails. Such documentation may convince the doctors and hospital administration that you need more monitors.

In the meantime, continue to assess both patients—checking vital signs, listening to heart and lung sounds, and documenting your findings. Signs of trouble include frequent premature ventricular contractions, caused by the catheter irritating the right ventricle, and respiratory distress. (This can develop if the catheter becomes wedged in a pulmonary capillary.) Both findings require quick inter-

vention by the doctor, who'll either reposition or remove the catheter.

There may be some question about the need for one or two monitors, but there's no question about the patients' need for nursing care.

Should patients who have them get out of beds and into chairs?

Q I work on an intensive care unit, where we have many patients with pulmonary artery catheters.

Recently, the doctors have been telling us to get these patients out of bed and into chairs. But I'm afraid this activity will cause the catheter to slip out of the pulmonary artery and into the right ventricle, causing life-threatening arrhythmias.

I'd like an expert's opinion.

A Moving these patients is fine as long as you take the usual precautions:
• When moving the patient to a chair, avoid pulling or kinking the tubing.
• Use a lounge chair so he remains in a semireclining position. (That way, the patient's more comfortable and the lines are less likely to kink or pull.)
• Monitor the waveforms frequently and know your tracings.
• Keep antiarrhythmic drugs and defibrillation equipment on hand.
• Notify the doctor if you suspect the catheter has slipped into the right ventricle. While you wait, try inflating the balloon or positioning the patient on his left side. This may cause the catheter to flow back into the pulmonary artery.

Pulse dosing

What does this mean?

Q I hear the phrase "pulse dosing" used to cover a method of administering certain medica-

tions, but I'm not sure *exactly* what the phrase means. The other nurses on my unit would also appreciate hearing your definition.

A Actually, "pulse dosing" is jargon, so not all professionals use it. Pulse dosing means giving a large amount of drug in a relatively short period of time to ease a crisis. For example, transplant patients showing signs of rejection are admitted for a "pulse of methylprednisolone."

Pupil size

What's the correct practice for measuring it?

Q On the intensive care unit where I just started working, we can't agree about the correct practice for measuring pupil size and reaction. Some of us say to measure the patient's pupil before using a light; others say to measure what size the pupil contracts to after light is applied. We're all charting our findings, so we should all be using the same rule, but who's right?

A Generally speaking, you are. Examine pupils for size, shape, and equality *before* you apply light. (The average pupil size is 3.5 mm, and both pupils should be equal in size—unless the patient is among the 17% of the population who normally have unequally sized pupils.) Next, apply the light to test the pupils' reaction. Do they react briskly to both direct and consensual light, and do they contract equally? If they *don't,* note what reaction did occur (for instance, sluggish, unequal, ipsilateral, or contralateral dilation or contraction). Some experts recommend measuring the pupil size again after it contracts for better comparison as the patient's status is monitored.

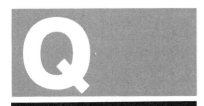

Quadriplegia

Can an administrator legally force a nurse to resign because she cares for a patient in her home?

Q After much consideration, I decided to allow a quadriplegic patient from the nursing home I work in to move into my home. My husband and I are buying a home, and it would allow this well-adjusted quadriplegic to have his own room.

He is 40 years old, and he wants very much to get out of the nursing home. Medicaid and Medicare would pay most of his expenses, and he could pay the rest out of his Social Security check.

Since I'm a part-time student working toward a BSN, this would be an ideal situation for me. I could do private duty in my home and work only part-time as a staff nurse at the nursing home.

When I talked with the administrator of the home, he said I would have to resign if I carried out my plan. Can he legally force me to resign for caring for a patient in my home? He also implied that I would be putting my license on the line by caring for this patient in my home. Is that true?

A There are four issues in your letter—two that you raise and two that you don't. The first is the question of your resignation. Obviously, the administrator feels that you are competing with the nursing home for this patient. Even if he can't legally ask you to resign for this reason, he can undoubtedly find some justifiable reason to dismiss you. You should expect him to try.

The second issue is your license. You wouldn't be "putting your license on the line," if you take the following precautions: Be sure the patient changes his legal address to yours. Be sure he has a doctor for necessary medical orders and that you are equipped to carry them out. Be sure you meet all state licensing and inspection regulations. And be sure you have your own malpractice insurance policy. Then, caring for the patient will be legal and safer.

The third issue is compensation. Neither Medicare nor Medicaid is apt to pay for long-term private home care, so you need to do some checking. Ask representatives of Social Security and state welfare for precise information about the benefits available to this man as a patient in your home.

Finally, the fourth issue: your plans to do private duty at home, work part-time at a nursing home, and work toward your degree, all at the same time. Whether you can manage all of that is a question that only you can answer. Give it some further thought.

How should BSA be calculated?

Q We recently admitted a 50-year-old quadriplegic with a left midthigh amputation and a disarticulated right hip. During surgery to repair a penile fistula, he developed severe hypotension. The operation was discontinued, and the patient returned to our unit with a pulmonary artery catheter.

Because he's an amputee, we're not sure how to calculate body-surface area (BSA) to help us determine cardiac output and systemic vascular resistance. Also, will limb loss and quadriplegia affect his hemodynamic status?

A You can calculate BSA for an amputee just as you would for any patient—by plotting his height and weight on a BSA nomogram.

(Remember that your amputee patient's weight will be considerably reduced because of limb loss.)

Quadriplegia and limb loss, either separately or in combination, won't affect normal pulmonary capillary wedge pressure and pulmonary artery pressure in a patient with normal cardiac and respiratory status. However, quadriplegia may cause some decrease in venous return because of the relaxation of smooth vascular muscle.

Quota system pay

Any suggestions for dealing with the treadmill of overtaxing assignments?

Q Nurses at our home health care agency are concerned about a new salary policy: Instead of hourly wages, we now have a quota system. Our pay gets docked if we don't make five visits a day (or three to four for more remote visits). Making the quota wouldn't be so difficult if daily paperwork, frequent meetings, public relations, and phone calls didn't eat up valuable time. To top it off, we don't get paid for assessing prospective patients who end up ineligible for home health care.

We like our work and our patients. We don't like the treadmill of overtaxing assignments. Any suggestions?

A Changing from hourly rates shouldn't be a problem as long as total pay still matches the hours you spend nursing. And although docking pay for incomplete quotas hardly seems fair, many agencies require six or more visits a day—regardless of time traveled. So your caseloads don't seem unreasonable.

Paperwork *is* time-consuming. But it needn't take hours for each patient. Why not use a dictaphone and have office personnel tran-

Q R

scribe your notes? Delegate other nonnursing tasks (that you weren't hired for in the first place). And let your fingers do the walking before you go out on visits. In most cases, good advance telephone questioning can weed out the ineligibles and spare you unrewarding trips.

What you're experiencing is the spillover effects of diagnosis-related groups. More and more, agencies are competing to minimize costs and maximize contact with patients. You'll need to budget your time judiciously so the agency can meet its budget.

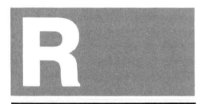

Radiation monitoring

What's the cutoff point for a safe reading?

Q In our busy cardiac catheterization laboratory, we do everything possible to protect ourselves from radiation exposure. Lately, we've had an unusually heavy caseload, and we've noticed increased readings in our radiation monitoring badges. Can you please tell us the cutoff point for a safe reading?

A To reduce the risks of radiation exposure for medical personnel, the National Council on Radiation Protection and Measurements has established a safe level of exposure called the maximum permissible dose.

Here are the guidelines: For nurses who usually don't work around radiation sources, 0.5 rem per year is the maximum dose; for nurses classified as radiation health

care workers who are routinely exposed to ionizing radiation in their work, 5 rems per year; for pregnant nurses—whether classified as radiation workers or not—0.5 rem over the 9-month gestation period.

Check your hospital policy manual as well. You may find that 0.5 rem per year is considered the maximum permissible dose for all personnel.

Remember, to protect yourselves, you must also protect your monitoring *badge*. To ensure accurate monitoring, don't expose the badge to heat, moisture, or intense light. They can inactivate the monitoring tape, causing inaccurate readings. And don't wear the badge outside or take it home.

Radium implants

Should nurses be responsible for them?

Q As an operating room (OR) nurse, I'm responsible for the radium implants we use to treat endometrial cancer. I don't think I should be responsible. Why can't the radiologist take responsibility?

As it is, I have to inspect the radium capsules when they're delivered, assist the radiologist in the OR during insertion and removal of the radium, and wash and disinfect the capsules after use.

Who takes responsibility in other hospitals?

A Responsibility for radium capsules varies with hospital policy, but you're probably in the minority: Radiotherapists usually take responsibility for the radium. Also, in many hospitals, radium is inserted and removed in the patient's room rather than in the OR, to expose fewer members of the hospital staff to radiation.

If your primary concern is legal liability, ask the radiotherapy department and nursing service for copies of hospital policy on re-

sponsibility for radium implants. If there is no policy, consult the radiation safety officer (either a staff member or a consultant) for advice. If you're still not satisfied, call your state health department for guidelines.

Send for these publications: Precautions in the Management of Patients Who Have Received Therapeutic Amounts of Radionuclides (Report #37); and Protection Against Radiation from Brachy Therapy Sources (Report #40). Both reports are available from: National Council on Radiation Protection and Measurements, 7910 Woodmont Ave., Bethesda, MD 20814.

Recreation program

Where can volunteers be found?

Q In the privately owned nursing home where I work, the head of our recreation program plans activities and outings for our residents. But there's a catch. She can't find volunteers to help with her programs. We've tried working with our local social service agencies—without much luck. Do you have any suggestions?

A Don't get discouraged. Volunteers *are* out there. The problem is getting the volunteers together with the organization that needs help. As a solution to the problem, some communities have set up a local clearinghouse for volunteer services.

Look in the telephone book for "volunteer" or "voluntary" groups in your community. You may locate a clearinghouse for volunteers close to home.

Get in touch with your local churches, the YMCA and YWCA, the Girl Scout and Boy Scout troops in the area, and the community's health department. Call the guidance counselor in your school district; perhaps he'll refer you to students willing to volunteer evenings or weekends. And students in your area nursing schools will often volunteer for summer jobs in health care facilities. Don't overlook the other end of the age spectrum: Try the retired senior citizens' volunteer group in your neighborhood.

While you're looking for help, remember that volunteering is *mutually* beneficial. The volunteers need you as much as you need them.

References

Any suggestions for getting reliable references and for choosing applicants?

Q As the staff development coordinator for a small home health agency, I'm responsible for interviewing and hiring applicants. Few nurses respond to our ads because we can't compete with the salary, bonuses, and broad benefits being offered by larger institutions. So, out of desperation, we're hiring some applicants who might not be the best-suited for home health nursing.

Do you have any suggestions for getting reliable references and for choosing among those who apply?

A Phone the applicant's references. Some people refuse to put anything negative in writing, fearing liability, but they'll speak openly on the phone. And finding out everything possible about a prospective employee is especially important for home care because the nurse will be working on her own with the patient.

Besides references, take the applicant into patients' homes to find out if she has good "people skills." Does she stand far from the bedside? How does she interact? Do the patients like her? What do your instincts tell you?

Clinical skills can be taught or brought up-to-date. New employees at some agencies attend I.V. and total parenteral nutrition courses. And both seasoned and new staff members regularly are sent to classes on new dressing techniques and complex care at an area hospital.

Yes, choosing the right applicant for home health nursing takes more than checking the paperwork. You also have to put your heart into it.

Do prospective employers have the right to ask personal questions?

Q I'm an experienced and caring nurse. The trouble is, I didn't get along with my former supervisor; that's why I left my job. Now I'm having a hard time landing another one.

Today I applied for a job with a traveling nurse agency, and the recruiter needs a reference from my former supervisor before I can be hired. She's to fill in a form rating my appearance, emotional stability, attitude, ability to get along with others, initiative, dependability, and so forth.

Does a prospective employer have the right to ask personal questions like those?

A Yes, he has the right to ask those questions. However, the person who answers them might be opening himself up to a defamation suit. That's why most employers will confirm only the dates of employment and job titles of former employees.

Realistically, though, employers can discuss their employees with others who have a common interest in them. And as a fundamental legal principle, true statements and statements of opinion aren't defamatory even if they're hurtful. Employers are liable for defamation only if they knowingly or recklessly spread false information.

If you're concerned about what your former supervisor is saying about you, make a note on your job applications: "Before you contact my former employer, I'd like to explain a few things." Then tell your side briefly and without hostility. Or, if you can keep your cool, telephone your former supervisor and ask if she'd mind filling in the form you need. Tell her you hope that your differences from the past won't cast a lingering shadow over your future.

What should go into an employment recommendation?

Q One of my co-workers surprised us by announcing that she's getting married soon and will be moving out of state. We're happy for her, but we'll miss her. She knows her stuff clinically and is good with her patients.

Because we've worked together the longest, she has asked me to write a letter of recommendation for her. The problem is I've never written one before, and I'm not sure how to go about it. Any suggestions?

A Before putting pen to paper, find out whether your co-worker will be applying for a specific position, to whom you should write, and whether she has some particular points she'd like you to make.

Begin your letter by mentioning that you're writing at your co-worker's request. (Recruiters won't consider letters of recommendation that the applicant hasn't solicited.) And be sure to tell the recruiter where, when, and in what nursing positions you and the applicant have worked together.

Of course, most recruiters expect to receive good recommendations, so your tone may be more persuasive than what you write. Mention some of your co-worker's nursing

Q
R

strengths, such as starting I.V.s or responding well in an emergency, and zero in on some personal qualities that make a difference to your unit—maybe she's quick to offer help when needed or willing to adjust her schedule in a pinch. Finish your letter with an invitation to the recruiter to call for more information.

Taking the time and effort to organize your thoughts and write a letter of recommendation is a big favor to your co-worker. But you can be doing yourself a favor at the same time. First of all, you'll realize that your opinion—offered as one professional to another beyond your immediate work setting—has weight and value. And secondly, by making you look objectively at which skills and qualities might impress a prospective employer, you'll get a better perspective on what you're already doing, or should be doing, yourself.

Refusing nutrition

How can a nurse get a patient to comply?

Q My patient, who knows he's terminally ill, has refused medical interventions, so we've been providing comfort measures only. Now, though, he refuses to eat. His doctor has ordered parenteral nutrition, but we're reluctant to give it. What can we do?

A The issue of withholding food and fluids is legally and ethically complicated. In this case, though, your patient is competent and clearly understands his prognosis. Restraining him and forcing him to accept parenteral nutrition would be difficult—and unpleasant—for you both. It would also be unethical and unprofessional: Besides violating his rights, you'd destroy his confidence in his nurses and doctors.

Negotiation is the key to resolving this dilemma. Go to your man-

ager with documentation of your patient's refusal, plus your own assessment of why this treatment would be inappropriate. Together, arrange a conference with the doctor and other members of the health care team so you can discuss your concerns about violating this patient's right to refuse treatment. Involve the hospital's ethicist or ethics committee if possible.

Meanwhile, continue to discuss parenteral nutrition with the patient, including why it might make him more comfortable (by preventing dehydration, skin breakdown, and so on). If he still refuses, document his choice, but don't argue with him. Continue to assess him for pain and other symptoms, and provide appropriate comfort measures as his nutritional status deteriorates.

Relatives

Could there be conflicts if a nurse's husband is an administrator at her hospital?

Q My fiancé is currently serving his residency in health care administration in a hospital 15 miles from the nearest major health care facility. In 2 weeks, I'll receive my nursing diploma and in 3 weeks, we'll be married. Because of the transportation problems, I'd like to work in the same hospital as my husband but I'm concerned because I'll be a staff nurse and he'll be an administrator. Could this cause any professional conflicts?

A The situation you describe *could* cause professional conflicts. Judging from the good sense and foresight you display in anticipating that possibility, however, conflicts probably will *not* happen. There are some things you might want to consider, though. It sounds

as if the hospital is a small facility. This lends itself to agreeable homogeneity, and general meeting and mixing among employees. At the same time, it could make the working situation between nursing service and administration more intense. Keeping this in mind, be most judicious in sharing with nursing service people anything your husband might tell you about administrative policies or procedures. Further, your husband must be most discreet about anything you tell him concerning *your* working day. Most of all, you must not be lured into playing the role of unofficial mediator between nursing service and administration. Not only will you wind up in the middle, you'll find yourself on the outs with both sides.

All these are cautionary considerations. On the positive side, your working together could be a real opportunity to improve understanding and rapport between nursing service and administration. That's an experience that could help you both in your careers. And it won't hurt your marriage, either.

Should a nurse do private-duty nursing for her ex-husband?

Q My ex-husband, a spoiled baby of 37 who once again lives with his parents, wants me for private duty in the hospital and at home following his minor operation. His parents are pushing this, and I know they'll pay handsomely. I hate getting involved with that family again, but I could use the money. Any thoughts on this?

A This is one time when "ex" doesn't mark the spot. You closed the chart on that case once; we suggest you keep it that way. But do have the family call the registry. There are sure to be many nurses on call who love pediatrics.

Should a nurse get involved in a relative's mismanaged case?

Q My sister-in-law's mother was hospitalized for a "simple" hysterectomy. This was the beginning of a horror story—trips in and out of the intensive care unit, all kinds of complications, and inexplicable setbacks.

Finally, after 3 months, the doctor transferred the patient to a large medical center where, within hours, a specialist properly diagnosed her problem as an abdominal cyst. The woman is now coming out of a long convalescence.

In discussing the case with my sister-in-law, I agreed with her that her mother's care certainly sounded as though it had been mismanaged. Now the family is thinking of starting a lawsuit against the original doctor and want me to put in writing my professional opinion that the doctor was negligent.

The last thing I want is to get involved in a lawsuit. But I don't want my in-laws mad at me, either.

A Be a good nurse—and a good relative—by advising your in-laws that the first professional opinion they need is that of a malpractice attorney. (Malpractice litigation is a legal specialty of its own and the family can get the name of a malpractice specialist from their local bar association.)

Such a lawyer will be able to preliminarily evaluate the case. After that, he may consult with a medical expert. He may even call in a nurse for her professional opinion. Most likely *that* nurse won't be you. The lawyer will want an expert who has demonstrated skills in analyzing medical records. Your letter suggests you have no such expertise.

For what it's worth, you might also explain to your relatives that although you (as you suggested in your letter) felt that your in-law's case was handled negligently, a de-

tailed evaluation of the records may show that it was an unfortunate medical event—but not malpractice. Poor medical results do not *necessarily* constitute malpractice.

Religion

Should a nurse secretly administer pain medication to a Christian Scientist?

Q I work in an extended care facility, and one of my patients has terminal cancer. But she's a Christian Scientist, and she's refusing all pain medication.

Since she's mentally alert and seems competent, I feel we have to abide by her decision. Of course I explained the consequences of not taking pain medication, but she still won't change her mind.

All of us are upset to see her in so much unnecessary pain (especially since the most we can do is help her feel as comfortable as possible). Since she *will* take vitamins, one staff nurse suggested we administer pain medication along with the vitamins—and just not tell her.

I think this is a violation of the patient's rights. Do you agree?

A Yes, and legal experts would agree too. Here's one: Mary W. Cazalas, RN, JD, says in her book *Nursing and The Law* (Rockville, Md.: Aspen Systems Corp., 1984) that "adult patients who are conscious and mentally competent have the right to refuse any medical or surgical procedure....failure to respect this right will result in liability for assault and battery."

You'd be in legal hot water if you gave the patient pain medication without her permission.

This is also an ethical question. By participating in this deceptive practice, you'd be violating this patient's autonomy. *She* is the only one who can decide what treatment she will or won't allow. You may regret

her decision, but you can't impose your wishes on her.

Document in the patient's chart and nurse's notes the patient's refusal and conversations on the subject. Then communicate this to your manager and the patient's doctor.

But you *don't* have to rely on drugs to help your patient in this situation. Why not be creative? Use your nursing skills. Get away from the medical model. You have resources other than drugs for relieving pain.

You could use imagery and relaxation, biofeedback, acupuncture or transcutaneous electrical nerve stimulation. A psychiatric clinical nurse specialist can help you with these techniques.

This doesn't have to be an either-or situation.

Relocation

What can be done about a backward administration?

Q All my previous working experience has been in big-city teaching hospitals. Because of my husband's tour of duty, we're now stationed in a rural area for the next 3 years. Three months ago, I got a job as staff nurse in the community's 50-bed hospital, but I'm not a bit happy with it.

The administration here is backward; the nursing office not much better. However, I guess I could learn to live with that. What I can't bear is the mismanagement on my unit. Things are totally disorganized and nothing goes right because of the unit manager. Personally, she's a nice woman but, after 2 years in the job, she still can't cope. Once or twice a week, she leaves the floor for an hour or more and returns with eyes red from crying.

Because of our location, this hospital is, so to speak, "the only game in town." I do need the money, but the ulcers I don't need. I don't know where to turn.

A Unfortunately, your problem is not unique. Too often the selection of a unit manager is thought of as a promotion for a loyal staff member rather than as the hiring of someone who's competent to be unit manager or who shows good leadership potential. This is what seems to be operating in your situation. And 2 years on the job or not, your unit manager doesn't seem to have unveiled any latent management skills.

So your course seems pretty well charted: If you're going to have to work under this unit manager for the next 3 years, then *you* are going to have to bring some order to the floor.

We suggest you analyze your working day. Determine the chief cause of the disorganization and study possible ways to correct it. Think back on the way similar situations were handled at other hospitals where you've worked. Perhaps you can adapt those methods to your present circumstances.

Once you've hit on a workable plan, approach the unit manager with your ideas. Be honest, but kind. Let her know that you're a team player—that you want to support her, not usurp her job. We suspect she'll welcome all the help she can get.

Report

What should be done if the existing policy isn't working?

Q I'm an LVN on the 3-to-11 shift in a post-coronary unit. A few weeks ago, the unit manager, who works the 7-to-3 shift, decided that the three LVNs on our shift should go directly to the unit and begin taking vital signs and assessments while the RN listens to the taped report from the previous shift. She said this would ensure that the 7-to-3 shift got off on time. Our RN

is to give each of us a brief report on our assigned patient—when there's time.

Here's how it's working out. Yesterday, I found Mr. R. in rotating tourniquets, Mr. S. very pale with increased shortness of breath, and Ms. C. with a barely palpable radial pulse. Then I found three new patients, whom I knew absolutely nothing about. How am I supposed to assess these patients without information?

Worst of all, when I found Mr. V. quiet and withdrawn instead of his usual chatty, jolly self, I tried to cheer him. My jokes fell flat, and no wonder. I later found out he was scheduled for open-heart surgery. How differently I would have approached him if I'd known!

> *"I found one patient to be in rotating tourniquets, another very pale, and a third with a barely palpable radial pulse."*

Another problem is that I never get report on patients I'm not assigned to even though I'll answer their call lights many times during the 8-hour shift. What are your thoughts on this situation?

A You need to hear report on all the patients. If the unit manager's purpose is to get her shift off on time, she'll probably accept any report system that accomplishes this. You and your charge nurse should document your objections to the new system (as you did in your letter), then suggest another system that will meet everyone's needs.

For example, could everyone on each shift come in 10 minutes early? Could you make walking rounds with the day shift? Could you cover for each other while you hear the tape?

Meet your unit manager halfway with a constructive alternative. Employees *should* get off at the time

they're contracted for, but not at the patients' expense.

Reporting

Does a nurse have a legal obligation to tell the patient she's committed a nursing error?

Q In a recent clinical conference, a nursing student asked if she had a legal obligation to let the patient know if she had committed a nursing error. I recognize the moral and ethical implications involved in reporting an error to a patient. But what's the legal angle?

A A nurse does *not* have a legal obligation to let a patient know about an error involving his care. The courts *imply* that a patient has a right to be told the truth, but the issue of who's responsible for telling this to the patient has never been resolved.

You're right to think about the moral and ethical aspects of this question, though. The honest thing would be to promptly tell both the patient and the doctor as soon as you commit an error in patient care—even if this isn't easy to do.

Reputation

How can a nurse get hired if she's considered a "troublemaker"?

Q A few months ago, I made some waves about poor working conditions in the hospital where I worked. Now, I'm paying the price.

Besides voicing my concerns to my manager, I put signed and unsigned complaints in the suggestion box. When I got no response, I circulated a petition requesting an investigation. The local newspaper printed the petition (signed by more than 200 nurses), along with a signed letter to the editor detailing my complaints.

Since then, I resigned my job to go back to school, but I'd like to continue working part-time. Although the assistant director of nursing said this wouldn't be a problem, the director of nursing later told me she couldn't hire someone who'd caused so much trouble and bad publicity. She also told me not to bother looking for work at the local nursing home—the director of nursing there has been advised that I'm a troublemaker.

How can I prevent them from getting away with this?

A The federal labor relations act allows you to engage in efforts to improve working conditions. If the director of nursing refuses to rehire you solely because of your past activities, she and the hospital have violated this act.

Contact the National Labor Relations Board (NLRB) to file a claim of unfair labor practices. The nearest office should be listed under Federal Government Agencies in your telephone book.

Here's what will happen. After you file a written charge (which you must do within 6 months of the alleged unfair labor practice), the local NLRB office will investigate. If the investigation supports your charge, the NLRB will issue a complaint against the hospital and set a date and time for a hearing. The hospital has a right to file an answer to this complaint.

During the hearing, you and your former employer will have a chance to testify. If the NLRB decides that your charge has been substantiated, it'll order the hospital to stop engaging in unfair labor practices. The order will include a remedy, such as reinstating you and possibly giving you back pay. If either side is unhappy with the outcome, this order can be reviewed in the United States Court of Appeals for the federal district where your hospital is located.

Resentful doctor

What can be done when a doctor resents ED patients?

Q I work in a rural hospital that offers 24-hour emergency department (ED) services. We use three family practice doctors on call, and our system works great—except for spring and summer. That's when vacationers flock to nearby campgrounds and begin using our ED.

One of our doctors resents the invasion by campers and their "emergencies," which range from insect bites to alcohol or drug problems. He ordered us to send one such patient "somewhere else. Maybe back home. I don't become involved in those things." He won't come out at all unless he judges the complaint a "true" emergency.

Our hospital policy says we're to report any problems to the administrator (a young business type). But he knows business, not health care, and he usually sides with the doctors.

Naturally we're concerned about our liability, so we document everything. But we also resent the uncomfortable position we're put in and the bad name the hospital's getting. How would you handle this?

A If your administrator is the business type you say he is, he should know that nursing care and ED service represent two excellent public relations investments. As a matter of fact, the care given in the ED can make or break a hospital's reputation. Contrary to what the doctor's attitude suggests, statistics say that "true" emergencies account for 10% or less of any ED business.

A resort area hospital should expect to accommodate vacationers—especially in the ED. For starters, a visitor won't know the local doctors, who themselves may be unwilling to take on a new patient for one office visit. Short of

posting a "No Campers Allowed" sign in the ED, your entire health care team must decide which emergency services will or will not be provided. The doctors at this hospital should examine the specific provisions in the hospital bylaws on what services the emergency department will provide so if litigation develops, there won't be one set of criteria for care in the bylaws and another being used in actual practice. The point is that each doctor should either agree to participate in your emergency department or withdraw.

Meanwhile, you must protect yourselves. Keep documenting. And if the covering doctor won't come out, telephone the supervisor and expect her to either get the recalcitrant doctor in or arrange for another doctor. Join together and send your documentation through channels. Be sure to include the other doctors on call. If the administrator's really on the ball, he'll make a review of ED services his first order of business. By acting now, in the winter of your discontent, you can ensure a tranquil summer ahead.

Responsibility

Can a doctor just dismiss a patient and refuse any further responsibility for her care?

Q Ever hear of a situation like this? Ten days ago, our unit admitted a middle-aged woman complaining of lower back pain. Two days ago, her doctor dismissed her and flatly refused to have anything more to do with her. The problem is, this lady won't leave the hospital; she says she has nowhere to go. The administrator told the nursing staff to stop all medications and treatments because we have no doctor's order for them. All we need to do, he said, is serve the patient's meals (and hope she leaves without causing too much trouble).

We feel caught in the middle. Can a doctor just dismiss a patient and refuse any further responsibility for her care? And is the administrator right about *our* responsibility for the patient?

A A nurse has a legal duty to care for a patient within the parameters of a reasonable standard of care. This standard does not change until the patient is discharged and leaves the premises. (The doctor, incidentally, may be leaving himself open to charges of abandonment should this patient initiate suit.)

Back to your concerns. No administrator worth his salt would put nurses in the middle like this. What ever happened to referring such cases to the social worker, whose job it is to know how and when to make suitable arrangements for patients who need them? With a little more caring all around, this entire scenario could've been avoided.

For now, continue routine care you can perform without doctor's orders. Send an SOS to the social worker. Document your concerns through hospital channels (mark the memo "For Your Immediate Attention"). And keep copies as proof that you acted as the patient's advocate.

This case may be an isolated one now. With diagnosis-related groups (DRGs), sicker patients are being discharged earlier—some to empty houses, others without the money for the care they need. If your hospital administrator has any smarts at all, he'll plan now.

Restraints

Is it okay to restrain someone without doctor's orders?

Q Yesterday, an 85-year-old patient on our unit got out of bed, walked onto the fifth-floor fire escape, and began waving to passersby. We didn't know this had

happened until someone saw him and alerted us. (I'd checked him only 15 minutes before, and he seemed fine.)

After much cajoling, we got him back into bed and put up the side rails. He suddenly became violent and started hitting us, giving one of the nurses a black eye. Feeling this was an emergency situation, we put him into restraints without getting his doctor's permission.

> *"Yesterday, a patient walked onto the fire escape, and began waving to passersby."*

Should we have waited for the doctor's orders? Can we be held liable for our actions?

A When and when not to restrain a patient can be a complicated issue, but your situation seems pretty clear cut—and your solution correct.

The key in deciding for or against restraints is the *danger* that the patient might injure himself, another patient, or a staff member. Certainly your patient fit all three requirements. He not only became so violent that he injured a nurse, but he could have also injured another patient or himself. If you hadn't restrained him, he might have tried to escape again—possibly falling to his death.

A doctor's order for restraints *is* necessary except in an emergency such as yours. In that case, you apply the restraints, then get orders from the doctor—verbal if necessary. Then get written orders as soon as possible (usually within 6 hours), making sure the orders are renewed every 24 hours.

For your protection, remember to document:
• the behavior that called for use of restraints
• the type of restraints used
• the exact times your patient was put into or taken out of restraints

• your notification of the doctor
• the care you gave while the patient was in restraints.

You know this, of course, but it bears repeating: No form of restraint can be used as a legitimate substitute for nursing care or as a convenience for you. Never keep a patient in restraints any longer than absolutely necessary. When he becomes more stable and cooperative, remove them as ordered.

Is it risky to restrain a suicidal patient?

Q Because of an incident last week, I'm concerned that some co-workers and I may be facing an assault-and-battery lawsuit. Police and emergency personnel brought in an intoxicated woman who'd threatened to kill herself with a diazepam (Valium) overdose. She refused to enter the emergency department (ED) until I called her personal doctor. As soon as I hung up the telephone, she bolted down the hall. I pursued her, with another ED nurse, the police, emergency personnel, an X-ray technologist, and a security guard close behind. We captured her, wrestled her into a room, and strapped her down with four leather restraints. I can still hear her screaming, "I'll sue every one of you!"

Were we wrong to restrain her?

A Your concern about using so much physical force to restrain this patient makes sense. Perhaps her lawyer *could* make a case for assault and battery. But he's not likely to try.

An intoxicated patient is legally incompetent. You had a duty to protect her from harm until she was sober enough to make her own decisions. Plus, she'd threatened suicide. You had to make sure she couldn't carry out her threat—even if that meant restraining her temporarily.

Retirement village

How do other retirement villages handle health care?

Q I'm an RN working the night shift at a health center that is part of a new retirement village. Only one other person—a nursing assistant—covers the shift with me. According to my job description, I must respond to all calls from the village residents. I'm often called away from my patients for such "emergencies" as headaches or upset stomachs. Sometimes all the person really needs is someone to talk to.

I sympathize with the residents, but I'm worried. What if a real emergency occurs at the health center while I'm on a nonemergency call at the village? The nursing assistant would have to handle everything alone until I returned.

A You're right to be worried. In a typical state, Pennsylvania, for example, licensure regulations require one licensed nurse (RN or LPN) on duty at a "skilled nursing center" with a census of 59 or fewer patients. And that nurse is not permitted to make visits; she must remain at the center.

In your case, you could make a quick assessment over the phone, but unless another licensed nurse is on duty with you, you shouldn't leave the infirmary.

Some retirement villages use a "buddy system" in which each resident is "buddy" to another resident, whom he calls every day. If the buddy isn't well, the caller alerts the health center. A nurse then calls the sick resident, assesses the situation, and acts accordingly. Additionally, a "home visitor" makes daily visits to the village. The visitor isn't necessarily a nurse but is someone who has some health care background and who's close in age to the residents. She checks on the residents and ed-ucates them to the uses of the health center, telling them not to wait until an emergency occurs before they contact the center.

Some villages have an "off-hook" system, installed by the telephone company. A resident in a medical emergency needs only to knock the phone off the hook to trigger a light at the main switchboard. If the switchboard has closed for the night, the light goes on at the nurses' station.

Meet with your supervisor or management to discuss your concerns about staffing and the possibility of using these systems. Since this is a new facility, management may not be aware of the problems stemming from your job description.

Alert them—immediately.

Return to nursing

Any suggestions for a nurse who's fearful?

Q After 7 years of critical care nursing, I left in 1979—vowing never to return. I resented the way the doctors treated nurses. I was sick of the emotional drain and the erratic scheduling that kept me from leading a normal life with my children. I felt exhausted yet unable to relax even on my days off.

With this latest nursing shortage, I'm tempted to come back. But as much as I enjoyed working with patients, I'm afraid I'll run into the same turnoffs again. What do you say?

A Don't stay away from nursing just because you were burned out in the past. But don't come back because of sentiment either. If anything, nursing is even more stressful now; the physical and emotional demands are still part of the territory.

However, you and your responsibilities at home have changed in 9 years. Life experience—and chil-dren—are great teachers. Chances are, you've learned how to stand up for yourself and to set more realistic goals. And your children have probably taught you that you can't always change people's behavior—but you can control your reaction to it.

Practically speaking, you'll need a refresher course before you start job hunting. Some other suggestions: Go to an area hospital and check the bulletin board for staff development sessions you can attend. Use their hospital library; bone up on current practices in the nursing journals, and ask the librarian for information on any upcoming clinical or legal seminars or nursing association meetings. Stay for lunch in the cafeteria and observe whether the atmosphere is friendly.

When you're interviewing for jobs, ask about the orientation and current nurse-patient ratio. And, as a final suggestion, don't request critical care nursing until you're really comfortable with your nursing skills; you may be surprised by the patient acuity level in all departments now. As someone coming back with lingering doubts anyway, you'd be best to ease yourself in.

How can a nurse keep her skills sharp while she's not working?

Q After more than a dozen successful and rewarding years in nursing, I married, resigned from my job, and started a family. I'm expecting my second child later this year. By the time the baby is born, I'll have been away from nursing 4 years; by the time my children are in school, 10 years. But I do plan to return to nursing.

I continue to read nursing journals and take CEU tests, but I'm concerned about keeping my skills sharp. Aside from taking refresher courses, do you have any suggestions?

A You're wise to be thinking ahead. With a little planning, keeping your hand in nursing during these interim years shouldn't be too difficult.

Here are some suggestions: Start graduate school, even if you're able to manage only one course per semester. Sign up with a temporary agency and work an occasional shift in a high-skill area if possible (the emergency department, recovery room, critical care unit). Continue your reading and keep an eye out for trends in health care. Last but definitely not least, keep your professional network operating. Some of the nurses you'll meet in graduate school may be in administrative positions by the time you're ready to return to full-time work. Perhaps they'll help you land the job you want when the time comes.

How should a nurse prepare for her return?

Q Although I've kept my license current, I haven't worked for several years. Now my husband is threatening to leave me and the kids, and I have no means of support if he does. I'd love to go into private-duty nursing, but most hospitals won't hire anyone who hasn't worked in the last 3 years. And in nursing homes where I worked previously, the responsibilities have expanded to include supervisory duties. I've never had management training, so I really don't know how I could measure up.

I've tried to keep current by reading journals, and I've taken a cardiopulmonary resuscitation course and attended several programs offered by our local hospital. (I don't have the money for a formal refresher course right now.) But if I can't get a nursing job, I don't know what I'll do.

Other women, I'm sure, have survived this sort of crisis, but as you can imagine, I need help. If you have any suggestions, I'd appreciate hearing them.

A By focusing on the practical issues at hand, you've already begun helping yourself. Here are some suggestions: Keep cool and continue your job search. Set small goals at first. Budget the minimum cash flow you'll need, and look for a job—inside or outside nursing—that will pay you enough to get by and give you some breathing time.

Don't despair if you have to take a job outside nursing. Remember, you can always come back to it at a later date; with the continuing shortage of nurses, more opportunities are available. Plus, it's always easier to get the job you want when you're already working.

Find out whether your community offers career counseling. And call your friends—some of the best jobs are found through networking. Speaking of friends, is there someone you admire who came through a similar situation? She's someone you can talk to.

Last, but not least, don't let this life crisis become all-consuming. Be kind to yourself; make sure that you get enough exercise and other diversions. You may be scared sometimes—that's understandable. But in the long run, you'll probably find out that you're a survivor.

Right of refusal

Can a nurse refuse to participate in diagnostic tests for an elderly patient?

Q I'm a new graduate with only 5 months' working experience. Nevertheless, on two occasions I have been seriously upset by the misery I had to cause elderly patients in preparing them for diag-

nostic tests that were seemingly unrelated to their illnesses.

This morning, for example, one of my patients was an 80-year-old woman who'd been admitted for pneumonia. Her doctor ordered a series of upper and lower GI X-rays. So, instead of letting the patient rest and recoup her strength, I had to administer a series of enemas that left her so weak she almost blacked out.

I know I have a legal right to refuse to participate in an abortion, but what are my rights in refusing to participate in a situation such as I've just described?

A Every nurse has the right to refuse to participate in any procedure contrary to her moral or religious beliefs. Is such an issue being questioned here, though? The problem here seems to be one of judgment. The doctor judges that a patient needs certain tests. You judge that the patient doesn't.

Why are you questioning these tests? You say they are "seemingly unrelated" to the patient's illness. But unless you have access to the doctor's detailed medical history of the patient, how can you have the full picture? Maybe the pneumonia with which your patient was admitted is minor compared to GI problems the doctor suspects. Unless you have proof that the doctor is stupid or ill-intentioned, you should follow his orders for his patient.

Talk to the doctor. Not to challenge his judgment. Talk to him in the spirit of one who is honestly seeking knowledge. Explain that you're a new nurse and you'd like to learn. Tell him of your concern. Ask his reasoning. Most doctors will accept your queries in the spirit that you deliver them. As a matter of fact, if he's one of the many doctors who have a strong professional bent, he'll actually welcome the chance to discuss what he's doing...and why.

RNLP

Aren't these initials misleading?

Q Recently, our unit supervisor hired a graduate nurse from Chicago who signs the charts with the initials RNLP after her name. She tells us LP stands for license pending.

Although it may sound like a really small point, we think these initials are misleading. Do you agree?

A Small points can often cause big hassles. Your question has come up so often that many nurse practice acts specify which initials graduate nurses should use.

In Idaho, for example, a new nurse must use the initials GN (or GPN for LPN candidates) after her name until she has her license in hand. But in Illinois—your new co-worker's home state—the rule calls for RN, Lic. Pend., and any variation violates the nurse practice act.

The question may seem minor to an RN-to-be, but the nursing boards consider it important enough to make a regulation.

Robots

What harm could a robot do in bringing a few laughs to the unit?

Q I work on a medical/surgical unit where many of the patients are on postoperative bed rest. Last Saturday, the husband of a patient brought a robot to visit. Omnibot talked to many of the patients, took them their mail, and was obviously the bright spot on our unit that day. Our unit manager thought this very unprofessional.

What harm did Omnibot do in bringing smiles and a few laughs to a sometimes cheerless unit?

A A little fun's no harm at all as long as Omnibot didn't interfere with patient care. Ironically enough, the unit manager is the one whose thinking is programmed. A little laughter helps promote healing. And a sunny atmosphere doesn't hurt the spirits of the staff either.

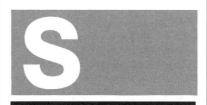

Safety straps

Is it a nurse's responsibility to check all the recovery room stretchers?

Q I'm an RN in a 15-bed recovery room. Last week, when we were admitting a restless postoperative patient, I was upset to discover that the safety straps on the stretcher didn't work. I tugged and tugged, but the straps couldn't be secured because they'd been improperly attached. I reattached them, secured the patient, then reported the incident to the unit manager. She told me to check *all* the recovery room stretchers.

I objected, since I consider it a nursing assistant's job, not mine, to maintain the equipment. I was reprimanded for my attitude. Was I right or wrong?

A Checking stretchers may not be a stated part of your job description, but *patient safety is.* Back up a little, and consider some ways of putting safety first:
1. Check the safety straps on other stretchers, as requested.
2. If you're too busy with other duties, delegate the checking to an assistant. But check on *her* checking.
3. If you find other stretcher safety straps out of order, obviously the assistants who do the work need

training—or retraining. Report *this* to the unit manager.

Once the assistants have been taught to do the job, *they* then become accountable for their own actions. But this does not eliminate *your* responsibility to protect your patients. When a patient could be in jeopardy, do you consider it *professional* to quibble over the letter of your job description?

School nursing

Should sixth graders be allowed to cover the nurse's room while the nurse is teaching health classes?

Q I'm a school nurse, and the principal recently informed me I'm to train sixth-grade students to cover the nurse's room while I'm teaching health classes. He says we can't spare the money for an aide, period.

Now I'm reluctantly teaching simple first aid (stopping nosebleeds, applying ice to bruises, taking temperatures) to some of the brighter students. Already the word is out, and some parents have complained.

I don't blame them. Don't you agree that we're gambling with safety in a situation like this?

A You can bet on it. When you've a gut feeling a situation's not safe, chances are you're right. Sure, children can be trained to apply an adhesive bandage or an ice bag. No one, heaven knows, can teach them the *mature* judgment that comes with time and experience.

Send out a call for parent volunteers, and arrange first-aid training for them at your local American Red Cross chapter. You might be surprised how many parents (a.k.a. taxpayers) welcome the chance to help out at school and keep the budget trimmed. Help yourself out, too, by

S

organizing your time: Keep track of your busiest office hours, then make sure you're not scheduled to teach at those times. Also, arrange for an intercom or telephone hookup between the nurse's room and classrooms so you can be summoned quickly for emergencies.

Remember, you have a lot to offer the kids—as nurse and teacher of health and early sex education. Don't settle on a no-win situation. Budgetary concerns shouldn't jeopardize the students or keep you out of the classroom.

School's medication policy

Should nurses insist that doctors renew medication orders on a more regular basis?

Q In my job as a public health nurse, I'm the "backup" nurse at a school for physically disabled children. In this school, nurses are allowed to dispense medications.

In my opinion, the school has a much too casual policy on dispensing medications. When a student needs a medication, the doctor writes a single order at the opening of school, which has to cover the whole year. If there's a change in a child's medication, his caregiver (either a parent or someone from the nursing home where the student lives) is supposed to inform the school nurse. Unfortunately, not everyone understands this policy. The other day I learned that we'd been giving 100 mg of phenytoin (Dilantin) daily to a girl whose medication order had been canceled 3 months before.

My supervisor tells me we weren't at fault because no one relayed the information to us. But I think we were at fault for not insisting that the doctor renew medication orders on a more regular basis. What do you think?

A A lot of people were at fault—the doctor, the nurses, the school administrators, and the nursing home staff. You could all be held liable if the student were to suffer any ill effects from the medication mix-up.

You have quite a few problems to iron out, but they all boil down to a communication gap. Obviously, you need to be in closer touch with the doctor. He shouldn't be issuing blanket medication orders for a whole year. And you have a built-in communication problem with the adults responsible for the children if no one is informing you of drug changes. (These adults may have their *own* communication problem with the doctor.)

To prevent similar occurrences in the future, sit down with all the students' caretakers and try to get *written* policies on drug orders. The nurses, doctors, and nursing home and school administrators should feel free to question each other about all aspects of student-patient care. So be sure you have the telephone numbers of everyone involved in each child's care.

School transcripts

Is it ethical for administration to ask for them?

Q I've been working in a community hospital for 5 years now. Recently, our director of nursing asked all staff nurses for copies of their school transcripts because, she said, she's concerned about the increase in fraud. I personally feel this is an infringement of my rights. What do you think?

A Since the state board of nursing is responsible for reviewing transcripts before they test and license nurses, a transcript review by your director of nursing is an unnecessary duplication of effort. A copy of your current, valid

license should certainly be sufficient to resolve any question of fraud.

Your director's real reason for reviewing transcripts is probably to pinpoint the staff's strengths and weaknesses. With the growing emphasis on continuing education, many directors want to learn where their education budget will be put to best use. For example: Will the majority of the nursing staff profit more from an I.V. refresher course, or a course in patient psychology?

One long and tiring way to determine this would be to pore over school transcripts—weighing the merits of various courses from various schools, along with the individual nurses' grades. An easier way is simply to issue a staff questionnaire. Surely the nurses themselves are the best judges of the kind of education that would help them the most.

Scrub gowns

Shouldn't nurses in ICU wear them?

Q I think the nurses in our intensive care unit (ICU) should wear scrub gowns. For 2 years, I've been asking our nursing administration to make a ruling on the matter, but until recently, they've ignored the request. Now they say I must document my reasons.

Unfortunately, I'm unable to find any authoritative literature to back me up. The fact that ICU nurses in many hospitals wear scrub gowns doesn't constitute "documentation" for our nursing administration, so my co-workers and I are reporting on the advantages of scrub gowns in the hope of supporting our argument.

What's your opinion? Do you think we're right?

A You're on the right track. Scrub gowns are good because they're loose and easy to move around in, and because they're usually made of cotton—which eliminates the static electricity you often get with polyesters. The scrub gown is much more practical—because some nurses' uniforms are too short, some are too tight, and some are not as clean as they should be.

As an extra protection, scrub gowns are laundered by the hospital and are traditionally worn only inside the unit. If you do go to the coffee shop in your scrub gown—or to any place in the hospital other than the pharmacy or the supply rooms, be sure to wear a lab coat over your scrub gown.

Your efforts to gather evidence on the advantages of scrub gowns sounds like exactly the right approach, and should help persuade your administration. Good luck!

Search

Can a nurse search a patient's belongings?

Q Recently, when one of our cancer patients began mentioning suicide, the doctor asked him whether he had brought any medication from home. The patient admitted having oxycodone with aspirin (Percodan) and pentazocine (Talwin) in his bedside table. The doctor told him he would have to give them to the nurse for safekeeping until discharge. Then, the doctor told me to get the medications.

> *"The suicidal patient denied having any medication, but I knew he had Percodan and Talwin in his bedside table."*

A few minutes later, I asked the patient for the medications, and he denied having any. I told the doctor, but nothing more was done. The patient was discharged a few days later.

What should I have done? Can I legally check a patient's belongings in a situation like this? If I find medication can I take it without the patient's permission?

A Legally, you're obligated to take the patient's medication, but it's obviously a sticky situation requiring tact as well as documentation.

You might get the doctor to take the medication, explaining that he could take it without a confrontation since the patient admitted to him that he had it. Or, you might ask a family member to take it, explaining the hospital policy against self-medication in the hospital.

If *you* have to search a patient's belongings and take the medication yourself, your best protection is a step-by-step hospital policy that tells you how to proceed when you think a patient has medications or some other possibly dangerous substance. If your hospital doesn't have a policy, ask nursing service to provide one.

In the meantime, if this happens again, document everything: the doctor's order to get the medication; your explanation to the patient and his reaction; your action; and the results. If you anticipate any problems, you might want to take another nurse with you as a witness.

Should a patient's belongings be searched if he doesn't seem suicidal?

Q One of our doctors suspected an elderly patient admitted with recurrent chest pain was taking more than the prescribed dose of his pain medication (from a supply he'd brought with him to the hospital). The patient denied this, so the doctor asked me to search his belongings. I felt this was an invasion of privacy, and my supervisor agreed. Naturally, the doctor was upset, saying that "patient safety overrides the right to privacy."

The hospital's present policy on searching a patient's belongings comes under suicide precautions. Even though we considered the patient to be somewhat depressed and unreliable, we didn't feel he was suicidal.

We need your advice.

A You have legitimate concerns. Under the Fourth Amendment, any *unreasonable* search of a person or his personal effects is prohibited. As a general rule, health care providers don't have the authority, right, or responsibility to search patients or their possessions. But remember the "reasonable nurse standard" that courts use to determine applicable standards of care in malpractice lawsuits.

A possible exception to a patient's right to protection under the Fourth Amendment can be explained this way: If a reasonable health care provider would conclude from the known facts that the patient may harm himself, then she has a duty to act to protect the patient. In your case, it could be argued that the patient is overmedicating himself and therefore endangering his well-being. As the health care provider, you must take action equal to the danger. If danger is not imminent but a potential exists for the patient to harm himself, then you should notify nursing and hospital administration.

If the doctor asks the patient for permission to search his things, you could avoid the constitutional issue altogether. But if the patient refuses and the doctor insists on the search, do the following:

• Get the doctor's written order to search.

• Notify the nursing supervisor, hospital administration, and possibly the hospital attorney.

• Fully document your explanation to the patient, his reactions, and the fact that you notified the proper authorities.

• Take along another nurse to serve as a witness.

S

Secrets

How does one know when to keep a patient's confidences confidential?

Q Many teenagers admitted to the adolescent unit where I work come back again and again with drug and psychological problems. After several admissions, these kids become friends as well as patients. That creates a problem because they tell me everything. How do I know when to treat a patient's confidences as confidential—and when to chart what I've learned?

A You shouldn't protect any patient's secret if doing so could harm him or anyone else. Tell that to your teen patients up front. Assure them that you won't go to their parents or gossip about their confidences. But if the information affects their treatment or safety, you have an ethical duty to share those confidences with doctors and other caregivers.

You could have another problem, though: becoming too involved with your patients. Sure, some involvement helps your adolescent patients feel comfortable talking with you. But you must remain objective or the friendship could turn ugly.

If you're starting to feel as if you have to "rescue" your patients, step back and examine the situation. Talking to your manager and colleagues about what's happening may help you get a better perspective on avoiding overinvolvement and handling confidential information.

Should a nurse break her friend's confidence?

Q Last week, a senior nursing student confided to me that she's pregnant. Because she isn't sure she's going to have the baby, she asked me to keep her condition a secret. School policy, though, says we must report to the dean a student's serious emotional or physical problem, including pregnancy. Pregnant students are required to take a leave of absence. I think this policy is unfair, so I've decided to keep quiet. Am I doing the right thing?

A Yes. This policy discriminates against students with certain medical and personal problems, and it may violate their right to privacy. As long as this potential exists, you shouldn't break your friend's confidence. How can a school teach students to respect a patient's confidentiality if it doesn't respect theirs?

> *"A senior nursing student told me she was pregnant and asked me to keep it a secret...but I'm not sure I should."*

Your friend needs more time to make some difficult choices. Continue to protect her and to be available when she needs to talk. Your willingness to stand by her during a very stressful time in her life may make a crucial difference in her future.

If you feel strongly enough, you could take this situation a step further. Without mentioning a name or giving specifics, ask for a copy of the school's policy on nondiscrimination. Does it conform to antidiscrimination laws that prohibit schools from penalizing students or treating them prejudicially on the basis of age, sex, race, and so on? You might also talk with instructors at other nursing schools to find out if they have a similar policy (or if they've revoked a policy like yours).

With documentation in hand, ask the dean to consider whether the school's policy fosters illegal discrimination or invasion of privacy. Suggest that she review the policy with a lawyer, paying particular attention to these issues.

Sedation

Should a sedated child be sent home without any staff supervision?

Q A child coming through our otolaryngology clinic and going on to our affiliated speech and hearing department for a hearing test is sedated beforehand. The resident doctor writes the order, and one of our nurses administers the sedative.

We know the drug is considered mild enough for pediatric use and it will calm a child going through unfamiliar testing techniques. But when the test's over, the child is sent home without seeing either the doctor or a nurse from our clinic. No one checks on the child's response to the drug.

We feel negligent in allowing a sedated child to be sent home without any staff supervision. What if he were to have an adverse reaction to the drug?

A Your protective feelings toward the child are understandable, but you can stop worrying. In a one-dose situation, the child is probably safe.

Of course, both the child's parents and the audiology technician should be alerted to possible adverse effects of the drug.

The biggest problem may be drowsiness, so the parents and the audiology technician must protect against injury, particularly if the child's left alone. The nurse administering the drug should certainly tell parents about possible adverse effects and caution them about the need for protection. But chances are, the sedative will help the child sleep off his clinic experience on the ride home.

Self-confidence

How can an out-of-practice nurse master venipuncture?

Q My problem is lack of self-confidence. I worked full-time for 3 years after graduation from nursing school—but that was 25 years ago.

Since then, I've worked part-time now and again. Now, with my children all grown, I've gone back to full-time work and, after 6 months, still find myself very anxious about starting I.V.s. I've completed the I.V. course and watched other nurses, but I just can't seem to master the skill of venipuncture. Can you advise me?

A Nursing's changed a lot in 25 years—and so have you. But if you're confident of your theoretical knowledge (equipment, location of veins, methods, complications), you *can* become proficient. The secret lies in three little words: practice, practice, practice.

Here are a few suggestions: Ask the hospital's staff development department to arrange venipuncture practice sessions for you in the intensive care unit or operating room when they have a patient with good veins. (Young to middle-aged men are most likely to have large, easy-to-locate veins.) Also, anesthesia personnel are experts in this skill and can give you some good tips.

Don't give up if you've made one or two unsuccessful attempts. Stick with it (excuse the pun) and you'll be sure to master the technique.

Self-discharge

What's a nurse's obligation when a patient signs out against medical advice?

Q I'm puzzled about the patient who signs out against medical advice (AMA). From what I've seen, such a patient's usually smarting about some neglect or slight (real or imagined). He wants to leave immediately—and signs himself out AMA, assuming responsibility for his own abrupt departure.

But I wonder what our responsibility is. Should we let him fend for himself at this point, since he no longer *wants* our nursing care? Or should we escort him to the door and to his car—as we do for any patient being discharged in the regular way? If you tell us we *should* escort him, would this be a matter of courtesy on our part, or a legal obligation?

We've been trying to get a policy statement on this point from our nursing administration, but so far we've had no response.

A You've raised a small but nettlesome question. Even though your hospital hasn't ruled on this, you'd be wise to assume that your responsibility doesn't end when the patient signs an AMA form.

The legal yardstick—to give a "reasonable standard of care"—is still in effect. If it's policy in your hospital to escort discharged patients to the door, this should also be done whenever possible with patients who are leaving AMA.

In many cases these patients will be angry and hostile and refuse to have you escort them to the door. In such cases, this must be documented in a patient's record.

Outside of the legal question, you should be leery of letting any patient—even an angry, hostile one—"fend for himself," even though he's declared he no longer wants your nursing care. While he's fussing and fuming, there's still the risk that your hands-off response could make him even angrier and more recalcitrant.

Stay on the side of courtesy and caution. See the patient leaving AMA to the hospital door, if you can, while maintaining your dignity and your professional demeanor till the last good-bye.

Self-esteem

How can it be improved?

Q I graduated from a diploma program 6 years ago, and made exceptionally good scores on my boards. Since then, I've worked in varied positions from charge nurse in a small hospital, to evening supervisor in a large nursing home, to office nurse. I'm conscientious, take all possible continuing education courses and really care about my patients as people. But regardless of what job I take, I just don't seem to have any confidence in myself. I'm always afraid that some situation or problem will arise that I won't know how to handle.

This constant fear keeps me from concentrating on my work and from functioning as well as I should. I'm a nervous wreck every minute I'm at work. Although most of the time my judgments prove correct, I'm always afraid to act on them until I've found someone to check with first. Many times, the other nurses I turn to don't know what to do either.

I truly love nursing and can't think of any other profession I'd rather be in, but what if I can't act wisely and quickly at some time when a patient's life might depend on it? These worries prevent me from finding any satisfaction in my work and make me feel like a real failure. Have you any helpful suggestions?

A You say you've been a nervous wreck in every job you've ever held. In your job as supervisor in a large institution, however, you must surely have met vastly different problems than you did as an office nurse. Yet you responded to them both with the same degree of anxiety.

So the problem probably doesn't lie with the pressures of the individual job...or with the profession itself. Your problem is probably one of self-confidence in general. And

S

this is a pity. Because as much as you doubt your capabilities as a nurse, you're probably not only a good nurse—you're probably an excellent one.

Seek psychological counseling to help you work out your problems of self-doubt. Until then, however, when you start feeling anxious about your capabilities at work, try repeating this to yourself: "When I passed my state boards, my peers judged me professionally competent. So what's my opinion against so many?"

That's partly in jest, of course, but mostly in earnest. You *have* been judged competent. What you have to do now is convince yourself.

Self-medication

Is it legally risky to let patients take their own medications?

Q I work in the retirement home of a religious order. A few of the nuns who are elderly and frail live in the infirmary. They're all alert and oriented, so we let them take their own medications, as instructed, from stock bottles kept in their rooms.

Lately, we've read so much about legal liabilities that we're wondering whether the nurses should dispense the medications. But we'd like to help these older nuns retain a little independence if we can.

What should we do?

A The current trend *is* toward self-medication for patients who can manage it safely. Hospitalized patients typically are given a 5- to 14-day supply of medications—not stock bottles—and checked regularly to make sure they're taking the medications correctly. (Of course, every facility should have its own self-medication policy.) But in your situation, with only a few infirmary patients and

with the close contact between them and your staff, we see no problem with using the system you describe.

Your sensitive approach to the older nuns in the infirmary and your concern that they retain their independence is quite admirable.

Shoplifting

Can one immature mistake ruin a nurse's chances of taking the exam?

Q Several years ago, my high-school senior class migrated to a popular resort for a week of sun and fun during spring break. On a dare, I very foolishly shoplifted a souvenir sweatshirt and was caught, jailed overnight, fined, and sent home—chastened, humiliated, and a lot wiser. I had never done anything like that before or since.

Now I'm ready to take the nursing board exams, and that old specter is back to haunt me. One question on the exam application asks whether the candidate has ever been convicted of any offense other than a minor traffic violation. Does this mean that after all my studying, one immature mistake can kill my chances of taking the exam and ruin my future? Suppose the board decides I can take the exam: Will information about this arrest be kept in my file and follow me to future employers?

I really feel discouraged. I know I'm a good person, and I could be a good nurse.

A Meeting life's challenges day to day can be hard enough without having mistakes dredged up from the past that are long since learned from, paid for, and (one would hope) laid to rest.

However, the question you mention appears on the exam application in your state, and you must

answer it honestly. You can explain the circumstances on a separate piece of paper. The *good* news is the board is looking for convictions that bear directly on the applicant's suitability to practice nursing: drug-related incidents, driving while intoxicated, assault, and so forth. They're not intent on locking out those who've made juvenile mistakes like yours and learned from them. But *they* want to be the ones to make this determination. The information you supply remains with your file, but no mention of it will appear on your license or be forwarded to any future employer.

Now stop worrying and start cracking the books. And good luck.

Sick leave

Are insurance forms sufficient?

Q In the industrial plant where I'm the occupational health nurse, I think we have a problem: Employees returning after a sick leave are supposed to drop by our office before reporting to work.

Company regulations require that the employee bring a doctor's note telling us what was wrong, and giving some indication of any remaining physical problems we should be aware of.

No one—absolutely no one—bothers to turn in a doctor's note. However, most employees will hand in their completed insurance forms.

My supervisor thinks that the insurance form is sufficient. But I disagree. I'd be more comfortable having the insurance form *and* the doctor's note so we'd be aware of any physical problems the employee might still have.

What's your opinion?

A Both are not essential. While *you* may feel more comfortable having the doctor's note, what about the employee? Won't he feel a bit like a child returning to school with an "excuse" note in hand?

The solution to your problem's easy enough, in our opinion. When the employee stops by your office with his insurance form, *ask* him how he's feeling and if he's coming back with any special problems. Chances are he'll be only too glad to give you the details you need, including the name and address of his doctor. You'll have the information you need—and one less piece of paper.

Should doctors' notes be required for sick time?

Q I'm a staff nurse in an acute-care hospital. We started working 10-hour days a few months ago, and the schedule seems to work well for us. But last week, our clinical supervisor announced that, starting next month, anyone who calls in sick must either bring a slip from a doctor or report to our emergency department. The supervisor justified it by saying sick time and overtime have markedly increased since we shifted to 10-hour days.

I don't think this is fair, and I wonder if it's legal.

A Management has the right to establish its own sick time policies, so there's no legal issue here.

Still, maybe this is a case of a solution being chosen before the problem's identified.

The solution was obviously chosen to discourage abuse of sick time, but is abuse occurring, or is just sick time being used? A study of individual attendance patterns could determine whether there's widespread abuse or whether increased sick time and overtime are occurring for other reasons, perhaps related to the 10-hour day.

Usually people who abuse sick time can be identified by illness patterns, such as calling in on weekends, on Mondays and Fridays, and on days before or after time off.

Even if there's widespread abuse, your hospital's solution is no solution. Abusers can easily get a doctor's certificate, yet nonabusers with self-limiting illnesses will be inconvenienced and embarrassed.

One hospital noted a sudden increase in sick time abuse after a code-a-phone system went into effect. This automated system made abuse very comfortable.

The hospital abolished the system and began requiring nurses to call their supervisors directly. Under this system, people who called in excessively had to discuss their need to stay out with their supervisor, but those who didn't abuse the system weren't inconvenienced. Sick calls decreased greatly.

Certainly, you should express your views about the new policy and help select another fair and effective policy. Of course, the only solution may be a return to the 8-hour day if longer days are causing this expensive problem.

What can be done about a nurse who's not being reprimanded for abusing sick time?

Q One of my responsibilities as unit leader is staff assignments. When our medical/surgical unit is busy and a nurse calls in sick, I must find someone to cover for her. Naturally, we all need a sick day now and then, but one nurse on our unit is absent 30 to 40 days a year—usually in conjunction with a weekend off. It has gotten to the point where the entire staff is talking about it. And I feel frustrated. You see, our unit manager and the chronic absentee are close friends. So instead of acknowledging my concerns, the manager feels sorry for her friend and says I should be more sympathetic.

What do you say?

A We say that whether your co-worker is legitimately sick or not, her chronic absenteeism shouldn't be your headache. Our advice: Start by talking with her directly. Let her know you feel genuine concern for her health, but that you'll need to plan accordingly if her absences are likely to continue. Ask her for feedback. Would part-time work be a better option for her?

Document your conversation, then make an appointment with the unit manager. Take examples of how scrambling around for staffing coverage interferes with your own performance, and discuss the overall effect of this one nurse's chronic absenteeism on staff morale. Remember to focus on personnel, not personal, issues.

Everyone's willing to pitch in now and then to help a sick co-worker, of course, but there's a limit to what's fair and reasonable, and perhaps you've reached it. If your unit manager is worth her salt, she should get your message—and share it with her friend.

Where do you draw the line?

Q The small hospital where I work has no set policy on when to stay home when we're sick. So, some nurses come to work with severe colds, and others stay home as soon as they sneeze.

When we asked the nursing administrator for guidelines, she said it was up to the individual. But we're still a little confused.

Can you tell us when to stay home?

A If you have a sore throat and fever, with a suspected flu or strep infection, you shouldn't have any trouble deciding to stay home—both for your own and the patients' sakes. But if you have a cough resulting from an allergy or

S

perhaps from a cold you had the week before, you don't have much reason to stay home. You should simply take extra precautions working around your patients.

You could ask the hospital administration for some general rules. (Some larger hospitals have an employee health nurse who has the say in this case.) But on the whole, administration's likely to sit on the fence. They *want* you on duty because they need you. However, if you're spreading infection, they don't "need" you.

In the long run, the decision comes right back to you. As a nurse, you make the judgment for others; now you have to make it for yourself. The nurse in you is going to have to monitor the human in you, who might wish to pamper herself a bit. But let your nursing conscience be your you-know-what.

Signature

Is it legal for a nurse to sign a doctor's name if he can't use his hands?

Q In our mental health clinic, we have a young doctor who, through an auto accident, has lost the use of his hands. In his own office, his secretary signs all his papers. Here, he wants us nurses to sign his name on records and prescriptions. Is this legal? How should we handle this?

A What the doctor is asking is acceptable under the circumstances, and there shouldn't be any legal problems. For your own peace of mind, however, and to forestall any problems that *might* arise, here are two things you should do.

First, have your director issue a statement authorizing the nurses to sign the doctor's name on the prescriptions at the doctor's request. Second, have the nurse who signs the doctor's name indicate it on the prescription (for example, John Doe, MD, by Mary Roe, RN), then have it initialed or countersigned by a second nurse.

These precautionary measures will protect you from any possible allegation that a prescription was not authorized by the doctor.

Silver nitrate

Can a woman who's free from gonorrhea refuse treatment for her infant?

Q I have reservations about the regulation that requires putting silver nitrate drops into an infant's eyes right after birth. I know this is designed as a prophylaxis against ophthalmia neonatorum—in case the mother has gonorrhea. However, I've observed that the silver nitrate often causes extreme irritation of the infant's eyes; the infant's resulting discomfort interferes with the vital bonding between mother and child.

Is there any way that a woman who knows she's free of gonorrhea can make a choice: refuse treatment for her infant and take responsibility herself for any consequences?

I'm expecting my first child in 6 weeks. But I'm *not* being purely subjective: I've heard other pediatric nurses, other expectant mothers, and other nurses who are expectant mothers question this seemingly inflexible regulation.

A You'll probably be pleased to hear you *can* refuse to have the nitrate solution put into your baby's eyes after birth. The hospital where you deliver will probably ask you to sign a consent form to release them from any liability that might ensue.

Remember, a mother can harbor the gonorrhea organism without realizing she has it. So the overall policy of prophylaxis remains fixed.

However, in some states, two important concessions have been made: Erythromycin (0.5%) or tetracycline 1% ophthalmic ointment (both less irritating than the nitrate drops) may be substituted as the agent for postnatal ophthalmologic prophylaxis. (These alternative treatments have the full approval of both the American Academy of Pediatrics and the Centers for Disease Control in Atlanta.)

An hour's delay can be permitted before application of the prophylactic agent. This should give mother and child uninterrupted time immediately after the birth for the first step in the bonding process.

But check with your state to see what it allows.

Sleep

Should nursing home patients be kept up until bedtime?

Q I was out of nursing for 22 years. Then, at age 60, I suffered financial reverses and had to go back to work.

I got a job as evening charge nurse in a nursing home. I like working with the elderly, and had good rapport with my staff. I left after 7 months because another nursing home offered me better money for the same job.

In this second nursing home, patients are gotten up at 6 a.m. and kept up until bedtime—between 8 and 9 p.m. Those who are not ambulatory are put in chairs and kept there for hours. By the time I come on duty, many of them are aching from sitting and begging to be put to bed. The nursing assistants make them wait until bedtime, however, because they believe that the patients will go to sleep faster and sleep longer if they're exhausted.

I told the assistants that since the institution is the patients' home, the patients should be allowed to go to bed when they want. I then typed a notice to this effect and put it on the bulletin board. Later on, I found that someone had torn up the notice.

Many of the assistants have been here for years. They are also members of a union, if that makes a difference. I'd like to know how to handle this.

A A union contract can provide for many things, but poor nursing care isn't one of them. And that's exactly what your patients are getting. You're right in insisting on change.

But you're not working in a vacuum. You're working with people, and, as a species, we're notoriously resistant to change. Propose something new, and in almost any circumstances the programmed response will be: "But it's always been done *this* way."

That natural reaction plus the fact that you yourself represent a change to the staff suggest that you'll need some help.

Go to your supervisor and tell her your problem. Explain that you understand the human dynamics of the situation and offer to hold staff development classes for the assistants.

Teach them that exhaustion does not necessarily ensure a deep, lengthy sleep. It can sometimes produce a troubled, interrupted rest. Teach them the problems of poor circulation. If they genuinely understand the patients' need for position changes and the dangers of pressure sores and contractures, they'll be more amenable to new directives. Then, with your supervisor's knowledge and support, reintroduce your order that patients be allowed to set their own bedtimes. And be there to make sure it's carried out.

Since you're likely to be working with nursing assistants for a long time, why not begin collecting suit-able material for teaching? Both the American Hospital Association, 840 N. Lake Shore Dr., Chicago, IL 60611, and the American Health Care Association, 1201 L St., NW, Washington, DC 20005, have good instruction books.

Should stable patients be awakened?

Q Recently I switched from day to night duty on a busy medical/surgical unit. One change in routine has me confused and uncomfortable.

> *"My co-workers tell me I shouldn't wake up certain patients when I'm on night shift because they become angry."*

On the day shift, I did a total assessment of all my patients as soon as I arrived on duty so I could note any changes that occurred during the shift. Now, on the night shift, my co-workers say I should wake up and assess only the unstable patients and those with orders for medications or treatments. The other patients need the rest and become angry when awakened "for nothing." Then they have trouble getting back to sleep.

What's the right way to handle this?

A There's no *one* right way. Whether or not to perform a total assessment on any patient is a judgment call, not a matter of routine. But every patient should be observed at least once every 2 hours during a shift.

You don't necessarily have to awaken every stable patient to assess him. You can check dressings, assess color, observe breathing, and touch the patient's skin for signs of diaphoresis or change in temperature. Check each patient's medical history: You may have a patient who appears stable but who still needs more thorough assessment (for instance, a patient who's a brittle diabetic).

Remember, too, that any time you observe a patient, you should turn the light on so you can see properly. Don't worry excessively about the patient's being angry if you wake him. After all, you're not an intruder in the night; you're a nurse working for that patient's welfare.

You need to protect yourself as well. Nowadays, nurses are being charged with abandonment if a plaintiff's attorney can prove that patient injury was caused by infrequent observation.

Enough said.

What's the proper way to document it?

Q I wonder if nurses on the night shift in the rural hospital where I work are charting properly when they write: "From 11 p.m. to 7:30 a.m., patient sleeping soundly."

I'm concerned on two scores: Shouldn't they write "patient appears to be sleeping soundly"? And how about charting in large blocks of time as they've done? Would this practice be legally defensible in case of a legal problem?

A You're raising excellent questions. Neither "seems" nor "appears" is acceptable; using them detracts from the validity of your charted observations. The sleeping patient is an exception here. It's both logical and acceptable to note that the patient "seems" or "appears" to be sleeping. However, if the patient *tells* you "I really had a good night's sleep," you can strengthen your charting by reporting his words.

About your question on block charting: Covering large chunks of time with a single notation could

S

have legal pitfalls. How can a nurse say for sure that the patient seemed to be sleeping soundly from 11 p.m. to 7:30 a.m. unless she was with him for most of that time? She's better off to chart more accurately and precisely. For example, "12 midnight, patient *appears* to be sleeping soundly. 3:30 a.m., patient still *appears* to be sleeping soundly. 7 a.m., patient reports he slept through the night."

Charting in this manner won't take the night-shift nurses much more time, but will afford them more protection.

Smoking

Shouldn't an 84-year-old resident be allowed to smoke if he wants to?

Q Our nursing home has an 84-year-old resident with no relatives or friends who visit. His main enjoyment in life is smoking cigarettes—if he had his way, he'd smoke two packs a day. (He doesn't inhale, so they burn up fast.) To curb his habit, a few staff members limited his supply; so he started stashing his butts in his pocket for later (a practice they found appalling) and wandering the halls looking for cigarettes or bumming them from everybody, including visitors.

After that, at a behavior modification program, we were told to put him in a geri chair every time we found him wandering looking for cigarettes. That didn't stop him, though—he'd forget the rules, start searching for cigarettes, and end up in the geri chair every day.

Some of us are very upset with this program. Sure, he can be pesky sometimes, but we feel he should have the same rights as the other residents—including the right to smoke.

We'd appreciate an unbiased opinion.

A No matter how strongly anyone objects to smoking itself, this resident has the right to smoke as many cigarettes as he wants as long as he follows your nursing home's policies. In fact, withholding cigarettes from him and not from others is a violation of rights and borders on emotional abuse.

Perhaps your co-workers were concerned about safety—for example, does this resident always remember to put his cigarettes out? Does someone supervise forgetful or confused patients while they smoke? Are there designated areas for smoking? Your policy should be clear, written, and strictly enforced for all.

For behavior modification, try positive reinforcement, not punishment. A little praise or extra attention might provide some of the comfort this gentleman finds now in his cigarettes and encourage him to cut down. Schedule a care conference and call in a geropsychiatric consultant. She can offer specific strategies for managing an older adult with poor recent memory and help you put the problem in perspective.

What can be done about nurses who smoke in front of patients?

Q Off in the corner of the large room that serves as our intensive care unit, we have a small supply area where we take breaks and give report. The door is seldom closed, so smokers are clearly visible to the patients and, at times, the smell of cigarette smoke invades the very air the patients are breathing. Some of them even comment, "Why do they tell me not to smoke when they sit in there doing it in plain sight?"

I'm a nonsmoker, and I agree with the patients. I've talked to both the unit manager and the smokers themselves, but all I've succeeded in making is enemies—not changes. Any ideas?

A If you try telling someone that her cigarette smoking is polluting your space and jeopardizing your health, chances are she'll consider you a pain and a crank.

If you keep after someone who's working in a stressful situation to quit smoking and be a role model for patients and the public, she'll probably resent your intrusion—even if she agrees with you in principle.

But if you speak up as the *patients'* advocate at a general staff meeting of medical, nursing, and support personnel, your chances of striking a responsive chord are better. Point out that smoke, wafting onto the unit, is unfair to the patients, especially those who may have been heavy smokers and now have to quit as part of rehabilitation.

Keep on talking—ask for stop-smoking programs, staff development sessions, and the removal of cigarette vending machines from hospital premises. At the very least, insist on an effective ban against smoking by *anyone* within whiffing distance of the patients.

Socializing

Could a nurse be fired if she refused to agree to never socialize with patients?

Q I work on a unit where we care mostly for drug- and alcohol-dependent patients. Recently, the administration drafted a new policy stating that an employee—whether a nurse, counselor, or secretary—cannot meet socially with a patient or with a former patient until a year after his discharge. The policy, I'm sure, is an indirect way of dealing with one particular nurse who does date patients, but handles the matter indiscreetly.

However, I interpret the policy as an attack on *my* professionalism. Is

S

such a policy legally binding? Could I be fired if I refused to sign a form saying I'd comply with the policy?

A The new policy *does* seem like an indirect way of handling a problem that calls for direct, one-to-one discussion. The policy probably wouldn't hold water *if* the case ever came to court.

Get together with your colleagues and ask the administration to draft a new policy dealing solely with off-duty behavior—perhaps prohibiting the staff's social interaction with patients *outside* the hospital.

Your question about being fired for refusing to comply with the current policy is a difficult one. Unless you have a contract with your employer, either individually or through a union, the employer can discharge you at any time. (But by the same token, you can *resign* at any time if no contract exists.)

You should be able to work with your employer to achieve a fair policy that doesn't insult your professionalism—but which would deal more effectively with the nurse who originated the problem.

Is having an off-duty drink with a patient unprofessional?

Q My nursing supervisor recently reprimanded me for having an alcoholic drink with a patient-friend in his room. Although I was still in uniform, I thought this was okay, since I wasn't on duty. The doctor had written an order for an occasional drink on the patient's chart.

But my supervisor told me I was "acting unprofessionally." I just don't see how having an off-duty drink with a patient is unprofessional. Do you?

A The answer will depend upon whom you ask. A relatively easygoing nurse might say she has no objection; a social drink might

be a pleasant interlude for a patient. But even then, she'd advise keeping visibility low.

But another nurse might say *she* wouldn't do it. She wouldn't risk her reputation. Visitors and other patients might misinterpret or misunderstand the situation. Besides, the important thing to the patient is your presence—*not* your having a drink with him.

Your question invites differences of opinion rather than a comforting agreement. Here's a case where you'll have to make a nursing judgment that concerns *you*.

Is it wrong for a nurse to have a sandwich with her patient's husband?

Q I work evenings. One of my patients is a neurotic who has been in and out of the hospital many times with nothing drastically wrong. Her husband, who's attractive and well-to-do, keeps asking me to go out with him for a sandwich after I finish work. He also told me that they are thinking of a divorce. So far, I've been able to put him off. But would it be unethical for me to just have a sandwich with this man?

A If you thought it was only going to be a sandwich, why are you giving it a second thought? Having a sandwich with *anyone*—even a patient's husband—is a neutral act that can hardly raise a question of ethics. In this particular case, however, what it will raise is a question of your good sense. Look at your query. It's packed with loaded phrases—she's neurotic; he's attractive and well-to-do; they're thinking of divorce; you work evenings; he keeps asking you to go out. Put them all together and they do not spell m-o-t-h-e-r.

No, you apparently don't see him as a patient's relative who needs

mothering and emotional support. But if all you *really* want is just to innocently share a sandwich with some *man* after work, then you've got a wide selection. There's you and Colonel Sanders...you and Mighty Mac...you and Gino...you and Roy Rogers...

What are the risks of romantic involvement with a staff doctor?

Q I work at a large rehabilitation center and have been seeing one of the doctors socially. Will this jeopardize my job?

A Here's a story you might benefit from—a true story from a nurse who did socialize—and then had to live with the consequences. The nurse, call her Mary, had never met the doctor but learned they'd summered at the same small resort all their lives, so they got off to a friendly start.

This doctor was a stickler about his work, and a lot of nurses didn't want to work with him. Since Mary got along with him well, the director of nursing assigned her to him almost exclusively.

Over the period of a year, one thing led to another, and although they were both happily married, they became entangled in an infatuation. It was nothing serious—a few kisses and embraces, a few telephone calls outside of work. When the grapevine got hold of it, though, the stories were vicious. Mostly, it was whisperings behind Mary's back, but some people actually asked her to her face about her "passionate affair." She denied such a thing.

The director of nursing called Mary to her office and told her—kindly—that she was assigning another nurse to work with the doctor. She further told Mary that if she was going to be romantically involved with the doctor, she'd better do it

S

on her own time because such things were disruptive for staff morale. She later told the doctor the same thing.

The doctor called Mary at home to discuss it, and they decided three things. First, Mary would not quit her job. Quitting would solve nothing and only make the two look guilty of something more serious than it was. Two, they'd never again give anyone anything else to talk about. And, three, they'd call the director of nurisng and tell her, without giving any further details, that the problem situation was solved.

> *"I was always told not to mix work with pleasure but then I met a very attractive doctor."*

Those next few months were hell, Mary says. She dreaded going on the floor and felt everyone was talking about her (sometimes they were). But she dreaded going to other parts of the hospital even more—knowing that near-strangers were talking about her, too. As a professional, she just held her head high and made sure she got her work done.

A year later, and with the constant turnover in staff, the present employees couldn't care less about old gossip. Mary occasionally works with the doctor, but it's a very natural exchange. The director of nursing and Mary get on well—and she still loves her work.

Mary states that this situation could happen to anyone. Not necessarily a romantic involvement—it could be a violent personality clash, it could be some error in treatment or professional judgment. It could be anything that makes you dread going to work, ashamed of facing your colleagues. If something like that should ever happen to you, Mary advises to remember that, no

matter what else, the professional gets the work done.

What can a nurse do if she falls in love with a comatose patient's husband?

Q I've gotten myself into a terrible predicament, and I don't know where to turn.

Eleven months ago, I started caring for a young woman who was comatose. The doctor told the patient's husband that his wife's brain was "dead," and her chances for recovery were nil.

Since the patient's husband visited every day, I got to know him and tried to give him emotional support. He confided in me that he'd cried for 5 months. But now, knowing his wife wouldn't recover, he'd decided to make a new life for himself and had started dating other women. Although his family and friends didn't approve, I understood his need for companionship and told him so.

One night when he came out of his wife's room, he seemed more depressed than usual, so I suggested we go for coffee after my shift. Well, one thing led to another and we fell in love.

I know I could be jeopardizing my job, and I know, too, that many people would think what I'm doing is unethical. That's why I've told only three close friends at work—and they support me. I probably should let my head rule, not my heart, but I don't want to give him up. What can I do?

A You're in a predicament. Although you say you should probably let your *head* rule, you sound like you've already made the decision to let your *heart* rule by continuing to see your patient's husband. *Don't* tell anyone else at the hospital about your romantic involvement. You've already told three too many people.

If your supervisor learns your secret, she could have you fired. And, if you do get fired, the reason for your dismissal will be on your record forever. And you'll have a hard time finding another nursing job.

Although you can't undo what's already been done, you should resign from this case. Once you become emotionally entangled, as you have, you shouldn't be caring for the patient. You're no longer an objective nurse. If you can't get a transfer, find a job at another hospital. Give no reason. No one has to know why you've transferred or resigned. And you'll be free to be more objective—and less guilty—about your whole situation.

Not having to care for the man's wife and not having to worry about losing your job should take some of the burden off your shoulders.

What can be done about a nurse who's having an affair with a patient's husband?

Q For the last 8 months, one of the nurses in our nursing home has been openly having an affair with a patient's husband. The patient had a cerebrovascular accident, but now she's becoming more alert, and we think she's starting to realize what's going on.

How could she *not?* This nurse is in the room whenever the husband visits, and I've actually seen the two of them holding hands in front of the patient.

Frankly, we'd *prefer* to mind our own business, but we're concerned about the patient's emotional health.

We asked our supervisor to talk to the nurse, but so far she hasn't. We think she's afraid the nurse might quit. (We're chronically understaffed because of the nursing shortage in this area.)

We don't mean to sound self-righteous, but things like this *shouldn't* happen among professionals, should they?

A Unfortunately, things like this *do* happen among professionals—although the behavior is totally unprofessional.

Morality may play a part here, but a more important consideration is the effect of this romantic liaison on your co-worker's overall job performance and her treatment of the patient. Holding hands with a patient's husband in front of the patient certainly is *not* helping the patient. If your co-worker's spending so much time with the husband, chances are she's neglecting her other patients.

At any rate, someone should speak to this nurse. Since your supervisor won't, go through the proper channels until you find someone interested in the patients' well-being as well as staff shortages.

If administration decides to fire this nurse for poor professional conduct and judgment, she could have a hard time getting another nursing job. The cause for her dismissal would remain on her permanent record. (In some states her actions would be grounds for having her license revoked.)

No one knows what action, if any, your administration will take. They might warn the nurse and then transfer her to another floor—away from the patient and the patient's husband during working hours. What she does on her own time is *her* business.

What's the risk of attending a wine-and-cheese party while on duty?

Q I work on the long-term unit of a community hospital. Twice a month, the patients are invited to an afternoon wine-and-cheese party in the activities room, and the morning-shift nursing staff members are invited to spend their last half hour on duty at the party (they leave the department as soon as the 3-to-11 nurses arrive). The administrator says it's okay for the nurses to join in the festivities and drink wine and eat with the patients, yet according to hospital policy, a staff member can be dismissed for "possessing or being under the influence of alcohol."

> *"I just don't feel right about on-duty nurses drinking with patients, and I've said so."*

As charge nurse, I'm concerned about who's liable if any of the nurses are needed for an emergency during the half hour, or if one of them has a car accident on her way home after the party. True, this party is one of the few extras the staff enjoys. But I just don't feel right about on-duty nurses drinking with patients, and I've said so. Now they think of me as a spoilsport. What do you say?

A A wine-and-cheese party for the patients is a terrific idea. They need a little diversion, and they're not heading anywhere in a car afterward.

But nurses drinking wine on duty and in uniform? No way, José. Nobody needs an alcoholic drink to have a good time and to socialize with the patients. And with all the attention being directed toward drunk driving and shared liability for those serving the alcohol, hospital administration could be asking for trouble.

More than liability is at stake here. How about professional image? Nurses in white uniforms are very "public" people, and patients' families or the patients themselves many times can't tell who's on duty and who's not. One untoward incident and the whole institution, if not the whole nursing profession itself, suffers.

So bravo. It's not easy to put a damper on a popular activity. That's why, as the saying goes, it's lonely at the top.

Social workers

Are they qualified to take over medical and psychiatric functions?

Q We're facing some disturbing problems at the children's psychiatric hospital where I've been nurse-manager for several years.

About a year ago, the administration began adding to the number of social workers (MSWs), while cutting back on our medical staff's time with the children.

What's happening now is that the social workers seem to be arbitrarily taking over medical and psychiatric functions. They try to dictate what medications a child should receive, but they're blocked by the nursing staff, which refuses to take medical orders from nonmedical personnel.

As a way of resisting the medications prescribed by doctors, the social workers absent the children at medication times. We tried to arrange for the social workers to take the medications with them when they plan to be off the grounds with the children. But this remedy hasn't worked—and we continue to have serious difficulties administering the children's prescribed medications.

The social workers seem to be taking over in the therapeutic area by deciding which children should have psychotherapy—and by deciding whether the therapy should be given by a psychiatrist or by a social worker. They're also making psychiatric diagnoses, and placing these in the children's files.

We nurses have met with the social work staff to iron out the problem, and we've talked to the hospital administrator. Nothing has changed.

S

Now, we'd like to know:
• Are social workers qualified to decide what medications a child needs?
• What can we do about the constant absenting of children at medication times?

> *"The social workers seem to be arbitrarily taking over medical and psychiatric functions."*

• Are MSWs qualified to decide who needs psychotherapy—and to give therapy themselves?
• Are they qualified to make psychiatric diagnoses that become part of a child's permanent record?

A The situation you describe is a blatant power struggle between the nursing and the social work departments, with the children caught in the middle.
• No one can prescribe except a doctor—unless he wants to be sued later. Prescribing medications is strictly a doctor's prerogative.
• Since a nurse is responsible for administering medications as ordered, she must inform the doctor if his treatment plans and prescribed medications are not being followed.
• Unfortunately, the issue of who makes a psychiatric diagnosis is a fuzzy one; the definition of psychiatric diagnosis varies from agency to agency. But putting a diagnosis into a permanent file may be risky—unless you are an MD. Patients have been checking their files in recent years—and if they can prove the diagnosis is wrong, the social workers could find themselves in court.

The issue of *who* gives psychotherapy is also fuzzy and confused. In many agencies, psychiatric social workers, psychologists, and psychiatric nurses are *all* qualified to give psychotherapy.

As a last word, you're dealing with highly sensitive issues. So whatever you do to resolve the problem, try to avoid taking any action that will harm the real victims of the power struggle: the children.

Spelling

What can be done about a care coordinator's poor spelling?

Q The care coordinator at our home health agency is a terrible speller. She misspells the doctors' names and the medications they order. The latter can be serious because so many have similar spellings to begin with. When we tried pointing this out to the coordinator, she got angry.

What would you do?

A Here's a suggestion: Type out a list of the most frequently ordered medications in your practice. Post a memo on the bulletin board saying something like: "Lately we've had some close calls for medication errors because of misspellings. Here's a handy reference list of medications to help you check your spelling when you're writing orders and charting."

Don't make too big a deal of this or criticize the coordinator behind her back. She'll probably start double-checking once the list is up (bad spellers know who they are). And a friendly and professional approach may spell the difference between success and failure of your efforts.

Sphygmomanometer

What's the best way to test its accuracy?

Q Now that I've retired from hospital duty, I've volunteered my nursing services at a local blood pressure clinic. To save the clinic the expense, I bought my own sphygmomanometer at a major department store. The sphygmomanometer's electronic, uses a 9-volt battery, lights up at the systolic reading, blinks until the diastolic reading, and is designed for self-operation.

My volunteer work begins next month, and I'm wondering what's the best way to test the accuracy of my new sphygmomanometer.

A Find a willing subject and take his blood pressure reading with standard testing equipment. Then take a second reading immediately, using your electronic sphygmomanometer. Repeat the process a couple of times. If the results of both readings are the same, you can be fairly certain your new equipment works properly. (Assuming, of course, that the standard equipment you used was accurate.)

As an extra precaution, call a medical supply house in your area and describe the equipment to them. Tell them the name of the manufacturer, and read the specifications that came with the appliance. Ask if they'd recommend this sphygmomanometer for use in a community blood pressure clinic.

You sound like you're going to have an active retirement. And it's commendable to find you going into your volunteer activities with the professional's concern for accuracy. By the way, hang onto your receipt just in case.

Sponge count

Would a nurse be liable if a doctor blames her for his mistake?

Q A few weeks ago, one of our surgeons—who allegedly left a sponge in a patient's abdomen—was sued for negligence. He's blaming the nurse who counted the sponges after he removed them, because she'd told him that the count was correct. Is she liable?

A No. Some state supreme courts have affirmed that removing and accounting for sponges is the surgeon's duty. Failing to remove a sponge—or any surgical instrument—constitutes negligence. So even if he delegates counting to a nurse, the surgeon is still liable if the patient is harmed by a sponge that he overlooked. What's more, he's liable even if delegating the sponge count is standard practice in his area.

> *"A surgeon being sued for leaving a sponge in a patient's abdomen is now blaming the nurse who counted them."*

The bottom line? A surgeon can't shift blame to a nurse by saying that she'd told him he'd removed all the sponges. Legally, he's responsible; she serves only as a double check.

Sports medicine

Would it be risky to examine participants at karate matches?

Q I've been asked to give nursing care and advice at a series of local karate tournaments. I'd be providing first aid and giving my opinion about whether injured participants are fit to continue their matches. I'd be paid for my services.

I haven't found any information about my liability in a situation like this. Should I agree to help out?

A Absolutely not. You're being asked to make medical, not nursing, diagnoses—and that's clearly outside the scope of your practice. For that reason, your malpractice insurance probably wouldn't cover you if you were sued. And because you're accepting a fee, the Good Samaritan act wouldn't protect you either.

Staff development

Any suggestions for an independent instructor?

Q I'm an RN working as an independent staff development instructor. Because hospitals are becoming increasingly cost-conscious, I thought my services could be an inexpensive answer to their staff education needs. So I prepared several programs and have more in the works. But so far, only two hospitals have requested my services.

What am I doing wrong? I always thought if you invented a better mousetrap, clients would beat a path to your door.

A The trick is for *you* to beat a path to a potential *client's* door. Hospitals won't know about your services unless you tell them.

Here's how to promote yourself more effectively: Meet with area hospital administrators to discuss their staff education needs and the ways your programs (or customized programs you'll develop) can serve them. Then convince them that you'll be an effective (and economical) instructor. Be sure to get feedback from everyone you meet with—whether they're currently in the market for your services or not—so you can evaluate your strategy.

By the way, health care providers are becoming more competitive, so don't be concerned that promoting your services is unprofessional or too commercial. And good luck.

Staff relations

How can a nurse get her subordinates to stop acting like patients?

Q As unit manager on a large surgical unit, I'm spending too much time shuffling work assignments to suit individual employees.

I have one nurse, for example, who can't give meds because it requires too much walking and she has "bad feet." Another, currently pregnant, makes constant demands for light assignments, all her patients in one room, help with lifting, and so on. Last month, I was coping with a nurse with a sprained back. Truthfully, I'm fed up with treating my staff like patients. Any suggestions?

A There are two extremes of thought on this problem. The first is exemplified by the unit manager whose attitude is: The patients are the ones in the beds. No changes. Period. This hardnosed approach spares her a lot of decision making and paperwork. The time she saves, however, is spent trying to locate floaters to fill in for her regular staff who absent themselves for minor ailments.

The other extreme is the supervisor so undiscriminating in weighing requests that she winds up with some of her staff goldbricking, others complaining about favoritism, and a schedule in chaos.

But it doesn't have to be either of these extremes. The fairest thing— to your staff and to you—is to judge each request on its individual merits.

Take the nurse with "bad feet." This sounds like a chronic problem, meaning that she will never be able to take her turn. She is, therefore, unable to perform the duties specified in her job description. Is this fair to the other nurses, being paid the same salary, who have to cover for her? Employees with chronic problems limiting their working capacity could be transferred to different positions where their problems wouldn't present difficulties.

The nurse in question, for example, might go to a smaller unit or a desk job where the walking would be minimal and she could function fully. Not only would this simplify your scheduling, but the nurse would probably be happier too. A genuine professional does not want people doing her "favors."

S

She's proud of her ability and wants to know that she's holding up her end.

The other cases you mention, the pregnant nurse and the one with the sprained back, are somewhat different. Every employee has occasional problems for which we must make temporary adjustments— especially if the employee is a good worker.

And every good supervisor will go out of her way to make those temporary adjustments. Who can appreciate this better than you—a supervisor *and* an employee?

Standards of care

Is a nationwide nursing standard another pie-in-the-sky ideal?

Q Recent news stories report that court decisions in nursing malpractice lawsuits are now being based on national, not local, standards of nursing care.

Naturally, I want to be sure my care plans (and practice in general) meet *national* standards of care. But I don't understand how the American Nurses' Association's (ANA) specialty standards can apply to specific medical/surgical nursing situations in various hospitals across the country.

Is standardized nursing care nationwide another pie-in-the-sky ideal? Or is it something that will actually have an impact on how we perform our daily nursing care?

A You'd better believe it will have an impact. In fact, any nurse whose practice doesn't measure up to national standards may have much to be concerned about. Two trends—toward uniform nursing educational requirements and standardized medical treatment regimens—support the courts' increasing bias toward national standards.

The ANA specialty standards don't address specific patient diag-

noses. But by using them as a model, individual nursing service departments can develop specific patient care and goal-outcome standards that do meet national standards for optimal care. These outcome standards can then also be used for nursing audit purposes.

Remember, though, that standards, even the best of them, are guidelines—not laws. Here's where your professional nursing judgment comes into play. If you have to bypass a standard (say, an asepsis principle during an emergency situation), tell your immediate supervisor as soon as possible and make sure she approves of your decision. And be sure that you can justify your actions with sound reasoning.

Considering the number and diversity of hospitals, and state and regional differences, standardizing nursing care *is* a complex problem. Specialty nursing organizations have been grappling with that problem for some time. Only now is the focus on professionalism and individual liability provoking the interest of *all* nurses. Any nurse with enthusiasm for excellence should volunteer for the policy committee at the hospital where she works.

Staph infection

Is someone who gets it a carrier for life?

Q I'm a student nurse and I'm worried about my future in nursing. Here's why: For the second time this year I've had a boil caused by a staphylococcal infection.

Two doctors gave me different opinions. One said that I'm a *Staphylococcus aureus* carrier for life; that my career is in jeopardy; and that, if I'm smart, I won't let anyone at the hospital where I work know. The other doctor said not to worry—I won't be the only carrier.

Will you please tell me what's going on and what preventive measures I can take?

A Your future in nursing's not about to go down the tubes because of a boil. Or even two. There's no way, not even with extensive testing, to determine that you'll be an *S. aureus* carrier for life.

The fact is, at any given time, approximately 30% to 50% of hospital personnel will produce positive results in a nasal culture for *S. aureus.* Some of these are noncarriers. Others can be intermittent carriers when they have an infection. Some are persistent, asymptomatic carriers. Nasal culture surveys can detect asymptomatic carriers, but determining whether and when these carriers will actually transmit *S. aureus* is very difficult. So a reasonable approach would be to emphasize vigilance in recognizing and treating *S. aureus* infections in personnel and patients.

The persons most likely to disseminate *S. aureus* through direct contact, however, are those with skin lesions. Obviously, then, someone with a boil caused by *S. aureus* should avoid patient care until the infection is resolved.

Here are some general suggestions: See an infectious disease specialist who can determine the etiology of your specific problem and suggest appropriate treatment; pay particular attention at all times to good handwashing practices between patient contacts; use an antimicrobial soap for bathing during the time of infection.

Have patience. Your future in nursing is bright.

Stat doses

When should the next dose be given?

Q We're arguing over stat doses on our pediatric unit. Medication times are:
- t.i.d.: 10 a.m., 2 p.m., 6 p.m.
- q.i.d.: 10 a.m., 2 p.m., 6 p.m., 10 p.m.
- q6h: 6 a.m., 12 noon, 6 p.m., 12 midnight.

Now, here's the problem: If a doctor calls in at 10 p.m. and orders a medication stat, repeated every 6 hours, when do we give the next dose? At midnight so there's no danger of missed doses? Or at 4 a.m., 10 a.m., and so on, with the nurse taking responsibility for the unusual schedule?

A The answer depends on the drug, the dose, the doctor, and the patient. You can't solve this problem with a rigid policy.

Don't give a dose at midnight, 2 hours after the stat dose, without the doctor's approval. However, there are several other possibilities: One is to ask the doctor if you can delay the stat dose till 11 p.m. and the next dose till 6 a.m. That way, you'll only have one 7-hour interval before you resume your usual schedule. Because most drugs are given during a certain time period (for example, between 11:30 a.m. and 12:30 p.m.) rather than at the exact time they're scheduled (such as 12 noon), this usually won't make much difference.

If the doctor wants the stat dose exactly at 10 p.m., you might give the next dose at 5 a.m., and the third at 12 noon. This would put you back on schedule after two 7-hour intervals.

Of course, the most obvious solution is to give the drug every 6 hours after the stat dose, as the doctor ordered. There's usually nothing sacred about the 6-12-6-12 schedule. But if it *is* on your unit, use one of the above alternatives.

Status epilepticus

How long can a seizure go on before irreversible effects occur?

Q Most nights, I'm the only RN working on our medical/surgical unit. If a patient develops status epilepticus, how long can the seizure go on before irreversible effects occur? Do I have time to transfer the patient to the critical care unit? Or should I try to handle the situation myself, including administering I.V. diazepam (Valium)?

A You can't decide to withhold nursing treatment because you're short-staffed. Status epilepticus is a major medical emergency. If you have a doctor's order for I.V. diazepam, administer it.

Permanent neuronal damage probably won't occur if the status epilepticus ends within an hour or within a half hour for a child. But you can't wait the limit before taking any action; you should stop the seizures as quickly as possible. Transferring the patient would take too long.

When a patient has repeated episodes of status epilepticus, some respiratory arrest at the height of each seizure produces venous congestion and hypoxia of the brain. Move the patient to a semiprone position, administer antiseizure medication and oxygen, and use a manual resuscitation bag during periods of respiratory arrest.

If you know that your unit hasn't enough staff to care for a patient who has uncontrolled seizures, try to have him transferred before you have a crisis. It's safer for this patient and the others as well.

Sterilization

Can dressings or an irrigation set be sterilized in a microwave oven?

Q Can I sterilize dressings or an irrigation set in a microwave oven? I'm a public health nurse, and occasionally come across a microwave oven in a home I'm visiting. If I *could* use the microwave for sterilizing purposes, I'd certainly find it convenient.

A The answer is no. You cannot sterilize in the microwave oven. The gauze dressing, which is "transparent" to microwaves, would not disintegrate; it wouldn't even heat. The plastic or rubber elements in the irrigation set might melt.

Is it acceptable to soak a copper stylet and a laryngoscope blade in an emesis basin?

Q I recently started working weekends in a busy emergency department. Halfway through the shift last night, I noticed a copper stylet and a used laryngoscope blade soaking in a green, soapy solution in an emesis basin. Is this acceptable for sterilization? No one here seemed to know. What do you say?

A Obviously, someone in a hurry put the equipment in the soaking solution and forgot about it. You should have dumped the solution and started over.

The Association of Operating Room Nurses' standards recommends that one of the following methods be used: sterilizing by gas or steam or soaking for 20 minutes in an aldehyde solution. If used properly, this method will kill all organisms except spores forming in the soak itself.

The green solution was probably an aldehyde solution, but guessing isn't good enough when it comes to taking care of equipment. Make sure your department has written guidelines for cleaning and sterilizing equipment.

Is there any way to wrap autoclaved instruments so they'll stay sterile?

Q I work in a small labor and delivery unit where nurses are responsible for wrapping all supplies to be autoclaved. We double-

S

wrap trays in surgical wraps and put small instruments into plastic pouches. We're told that these supplies are sterile for a month; so whether we use an instrument or not, after a month we wrap and autoclave it again.

The trouble is, we stock a lot of instruments we rarely use. Is there any way we can wrap them so they'll stay sterile longer than a month?

A Definitely. You can keep supplies sterile up to 6 months in two different ways. One way is to put items in special sterilizing pouches before sterilization and then heat-seal the pouches after sterilization. Or you can wrap items in muslin or water-repellent paper and seal them in a plastic bag (you can even use a fresh trash bag) immediately after removal from the autoclave. This should save wear and tear on you and on your rubber and plastic instruments. (Too much sterilization can deteriorate rubber and plastic.)

However, items that aren't sealed in plastic pouches or bags *don't* stay sterile longer than a month.

Be sure to mark all sterile supplies with the expiration date and rotate supplies by putting newly sterilized items at the back of the shelf. Once a week make a habit of checking for outdated supplies and removing these from the shelves for resterilization. To save money *and* space, avoid "stock piling" supplies you seldom use.

Stethoscopes

Where can someone get free or low-cost ones?

Q We teach each patient in our cardiac care unit how to take his own apical pulse. Then he can keep a check on his heart rate himself after he's discharged. But some of our patients are on fixed incomes and an expensive stethoscope just doesn't fit into their budgets. Do you know where we can get some free or low-cost stethoscopes for our patients?

A To start, all stethoscopes are *not* equal—in price, that is. Take a look in any nursing catalog or a uniform and supply store. You'll find plenty of good, low-cost (under $15) stethoscopes there.

If even these stethoscopes are out of your patients' financial reach, you might get free stethoscopes one of these ways:
• Call your local chapter of the American Heart Association (AHA). Tell them your plan to get stethoscopes for your patients. The AHA often supports projects such as yours with grants. Ask them to consider your project as a possible recipient of this grant money.
• Your local church, community, or women's group may be looking for a pet project. Get in touch with one of these groups to see if *your* project fits their bill. (And, while you're at it, don't forget the resources of your own hospital's women's auxiliary.)
• You might also call a local support group for stroke or heart surgery patients (such as the Zipper Club). Perhaps they've already sponsored a similar project and can tell you how to get yours started.

Stomatitis

Are there benefits to using lemon and glycerin swabs?

Q At our hospital, we've begun to question the benefits of using lemon and glycerin swabs to treat stomatitis associated with cancer chemotherapy.

What's your advice?

A Don't use them. First of all, the glycerin may absorb moisture from mucous membranes, drying out the patient's mouth. And second, the citric acid or flavoring used in the lemon ingredient may further irritate inflamed mucous membranes.

To clean a patient's mouth before and after chemotherapy, try using a simple rinse, such as water, saline, saline and sodium bicarbonate solution, or a 1:6 solution of hydrogen peroxide and water.

Stress

Is it unrealistic to stay in nursing and still expect that feeling of "a good job well done" at the end of each day?

Q After 26 years of being a housewife (no children) I decided I wanted a career, and entered an AD program from which I graduated with honors. Four months after I started my first job as the 3-to-11 shift charge nurse in a small hospital, my husband sued for divorce. It was a great shock, and my personal problems at that time plus the stress of the new job were too much. On a doctor's advice, I changed to a staff-nurse job in a nursing home. The pay wasn't good but I was reasonably happy there for 11 months. My mother's terminal illness forced me to move back to my hometown and for the past 7 months, I've been charge nurse on the 11-to-7 shift in an acute care hospital.

Although I give maximum effort during working hours, I spend between ½ and 1½ hours overtime every day (no extra pay) just to make sure my most elementary obligations are fulfilled. Even then, that's not always possible and I have worries about something hastily done. When I get home, I'm exhausted and dread facing the next day. It's been suggested that I'm too conscientious, but how else can you be when you're responsible for other people's well-being—even their lives.

Maybe I should be in some other kind of work. But I'm 51 years old and completely dependent on a weekly paycheck. There's no way I could start training for some new career.

Is it unrealistic of me to stay in nursing and still expect that feeling of "a good job well done" at the end of each day—that I could go off duty with my mind at peace?

A If there's anybody who deserves—absolutely needs—a sense of job satisfaction and peace of mind, it's you. Emotionally, you know better then anyone else what stress you've recently been through. But, academically, did you know there's a way to measure that stress?

Researchers in a psychiatric study devised a point system that rates stress-triggering changes in a person's life. If the points total 300 or more, the person is considered under severe stress. When you see how your recent experiences total up, perhaps you'll get a clearer perspective on your present and future goals:

Leaving housewife career 36
Beginning school 26
Ending school 26
Taking first job 36
Divorce 73
Change in financial status 38
Change in social status 18
Change to second job 29
Mother's illness 44
Change in residence 20
Change to present job 29

That's a walloping 377 points! And that's just from changes dictated by your personal life. Daily *professional* stress is something you hardly need more of, so changing your career is the last thing we'd advise. We do think, however, that you should consider changing *jobs.*

We'd like to suggest you start right away checking out possibilities in office nursing, occupational health nursing, school nursing, private clinics, or day-care centers. Make no mistake. These jobs are not featherbeds; they're hard work. But there's a difference between hard work and pressure.

You sound like a very conscientious person. And employers are always looking for workers who are dependable, conscientious, and mature (not just in age, but in outlook). Once you start looking, you'll probably be able to find something more suitable to your talents and present emotional needs.

Student health problems

Should a diabetic or epileptic student be assigned to a patient who's totally dependent on a nurse for care?

Q As a nursing instructor, I'm concerned about student nurses who have severe health problems of their own. Don't these health problems interfere with their ability to provide safe nursing care?

One of my students, who's a brittle diabetic, was recently found almost unconscious in the hospital elevator. She had no warning that a reaction was setting in, she said. Another of my students is epileptic, and had a generalized tonic-clonic seizure while observing in the endoscopy room. This student didn't know she was epileptic. Because of the severity of her seizure and her failure to breathe, a Code Blue was called.

How can I assign either the diabetic or epileptic student to a patient who's totally dependent on a nurse for care? Couldn't the onset of the student nurse's physical crisis compromise a patient's safety? Yet, if I don't assign the student with physical problems the same tasks as other students, I'd be depriving her of basic background training—perhaps even preparing her for future failure on the job.

It's up to me to ensure patient safety, protect students' rights, and maintain the standards of the nursing profession. The dilemma is more than I can resolve by myself. What advice can you offer?

A You *do* have a difficult problem. Begin by seeing that the diabetic and epileptic students are brought under better medical control. Many hospitals employ RNs who are known epileptics, but only after they have evidence that they are well-controlled by medication. The student you cite is obviously *not* under medical control. Any student with a major physical problem should provide the instructor with written confirmation from her doctor that the problem *is* under control.

But you yourself should assess the student's insight into her problem. Because she's a nursing student, don't assume she understands her illness thoroughly. Ask your supervisor to arrange for counseling for the diabetic student who needs some guidance on the management of her diabetes.

Rarely does a diabetic have *no* warning signs of hypoglycemic attack. If she does ignore the warning signs, you or the counselor must intervene to forestall repeated incidents.

Working with the epileptic student is more complex because seizures may occur without warning. Since you're responsible for this student in the nursing situation, talk with the student's personal doctor about your concern. Knowing that emotionally stressful situations can precipitate the student's seizures, assign her to such tasks only after receiving the approval and moral backing of the student's doctor.

If this approach is not successful, and you still think the student might, at some point, jeopardize the patient's safety (and perhaps her own), seek legal counsel to clarify your responsibility and liability.

In the meantime, protect the patients, the student nurse, and yourself. Assign the student *cautiously*.

Students

Is it an infringement of students' rights to insist they give each other injections?

Q I'm an instructor in an associate degree nursing program. We've always had the students practice giving injections to each other, but last semester one of the students refused to participate, saying I was infringing on her rights.

Am I infringing on the students' rights? Do I have a right to insist that a student participate?

A Most nursing schools have the students practice on each other once, by injecting 0.5 ml of sterile saline subcutaneously. Some nursing schools also have a second practice session on I.V. techniques: The students don't inject anything, just stick and aspirate blood to ensure they're in the vein.

Student refusals are rare. One instructor reported only two refusals among 700 students: One refused to stick another student, and the other refused to be stuck. The instructor didn't insist, and the two students managed to learn the technique without the practice.

What about student rights? You can try telling students they shouldn't expect to practice on a sick patient unless they're willing to let others practice on them.

Practicing on a person is most important. A student can practice on oranges and animals and synthetic materials, but sticking a needle through another person's skin for the first time is a major psychological hurdle. If the students don't cross that hurdle by practicing on each other, their first injection

with a real patient is likely to be traumatic for everyone. That's not fair to the patient.

What about liability? There surely wouldn't be any ill effects—the equipment is sterile, and the practice is supervised.

Continue having the students practice on each other. If a student resists despite encouragement and support, excuse her from the exercise. You could let the extra student practice on you.

Substance abuse

How should a nurse handle a paraplegic who drinks and smokes marijuana while she's caring for him?

Q As a private-duty nurse, I work 8-hour shifts in patients' homes. Last week when I began caring for a paraplegic patient, he refused his medication and most treatments. The only treatment he accepted was for a painful pressure sore. During my second day on duty, he started smoking marijuana right in front of me, and twice he asked me to get him rum and colas.

I fixed the drinks because I felt sorry for him, and he was in his own home. But I have mixed emotions about my own rights and my professional responsibility. When I opted for private duty over hospital work, I never expected to run into this. What do you suggest I do?

A Start by counseling your patient on what's important to keep him healthy—why he needs his medication and how your care will prevent further problems. That nasty pressure sore, which he can see and feel, could be your best argument against his smoking marijuana. Explain that marijuana depresses the white blood cell count and could increase his susceptibility to infection. And infection—of pressure sores, the urinary

tract, and lungs—is one of the leading causes of death for spinal cord-injured persons.

Moderate drinking may be okay, but alcohol abuse can be especially dangerous for him. Blackouts or sitting for hours in a stupor can only cause more complications; loss of movement in joints can't ever be cured.

Have a heart-to-heart talk with him; offer to arrange a care conference with his doctor so he can ask about drinking or getting a prescription for marijuana. If rum and colas are okay, he should mix his own. Call in a psychiatric nurse consultant. Your patient may be turning to drugs and alcohol to ease his frustrations and loneliness. There's an excellent book for spinal cord-injured patients entitled *Spinal Network: The Total Resource for the Wheelchair Community* by Sam Maddox (Boulder, Colo.: Spinal Network, 1988).

Now about your own protection. Marijuana use is illegal, and you can't be an innocent bystander without jeopardizing your license. Explain this to your patient. If his doctor won't prescribe marijuana, and he wants you to continue caring for him, he'll have to stop using it while you're there.

Substitutions

What if they involve changes in the medication administration schedule?

Q At the hospital where I work, the pharmacy stocks only cefazolin (Ancef) to fill all orders for first-generation cephalosporins. A recent memo instructs us to transcribe all orders for cephalothin (Keflin), cephapirin (Cefadyl), or cephradine (Velocef) every 6 hours as Ancef every 8 hours.

I'm concerned that substitutions involving changes in the administration schedule leave too much room for error. What do you think about this practice?

A Consolidating inventories is in itself a perfectly appropriate measure to fight escalating costs. But you're not the one who should be rewriting the orders.

Here's how the system should work during the transitional phase.

The pharmacy and therapeutics committee specifies in the formulary which single product will fill all orders for drugs in a given family (e.g., cefazolin for first-generation cephalosporins).

You transcribe every order exactly as the doctor writes it.

The *pharmacy* revises orders for drugs that aren't stocked and processes them.

After receiving the substituted drug, you write the new drug name, dose, and administration times on the medication administration record. You also double-check the pharmacy's instructions before giving the drug.

Everyone needs some time to adjust and become familiar with the mechanics of the change. But set a deadline. By that time, the doctor should be prescribing only the drugs that are on hand.

Suctioning

Is it safe for nurses to suction postoperative tonsillectomy and adenoidectomy patients?

Q We pediatric nurses suspect we could be in for potential trouble. Here's why.

The laryngologists at our hospital requested that we be permitted to suction postoperative tonsillectomy and adenoidectomy patients by inserting a suction catheter 2 to 6 inches (5 to 15 cm) into the nose to remove old blood clots. First of all, we're concerned about damag-

ing the surgical site and causing hemorrhage. Besides that, the pediatric unit is quite a distance from both the operating suite and the emergency department, and a doctor may not be readily available.

We want to refuse, but first we'd like an expert's opinion on the safety of RNs performing this function.

A Refuse. For all of the reasons you cite. A suction catheter can cause trauma to the nasal mucosa or surgical site and induce bleeding that could require nasopharyngeal packing or surgical ligation.

Hemorrhage is not an uncommon postoperative complication of tonsillectomy and adenoidectomy. Furthermore, insertion of a catheter into the nasopharynx may also lead to cardiac dysrhythmias or laryngospasm under certain circumstances.

If this reasoning isn't convincing enough, the remoteness of the pediatric unit and unavailability of a doctor are additional hazards. Your hospital's legal department should back up your refusal to take responsibility for this risky procedure.

Suicidal nurse

Must a history of suicidal depression be reported on an application for licensure endorsement?

Q After 5 happy years in nursing, I left to raise a family. I haven't worked these 10 years since. Two years ago, I became suicidal and was hospitalized for 5 months.

Now, we're moving to the opposite end of the country where no one knows us. My application for licensure endorsement in this new state asks if I've had a major physical or mental illness within the past 5 years. And if so, explain fully.

My three questions are these: What is meant by "explain fully"? (I can't believe the source of my depression is anybody else's business.)

What legal processes can I follow if my application is denied?

Since no one in my nursing background (school and work references) knows of my illness, why should I admit it at all? Who would be the wiser?

A Professional licensing boards are charged with protecting the health, welfare, and safety of the people. To fulfill this function, they are empowered to demand *all* information reflecting on an applicant's ability to practice her profession.

> *"Two years ago, I became suicidal and was hospitalized for 5 months...now, I'm trying to get licensed in another state."*

Some states ask only about past convictions for a felony. If your state asks about a history of mental illness, then "explain fully," means exactly that: a full disclosure of your emotional illness. The board then has the right to make its own investigation and can demand access to all records.

A board usually revokes, suspends, or refuses to grant a license only in cases involving conviction of a crime. It can do so, however, if it believes an applicant's illness could pose a danger to patients. A nurse's emotional problems, for example, could impair her ability to exercise proper judgment.

You can see, then, that your depression is justifiably the business of the board but what its decision is will depend on the exact nature of your illness and recovery.

If you happen to be denied licensure, you can ask the board to give its reasons. You would then be entitled to a hearing before the board with the right to present evidence and cross-examine witnesses. Depending on the jurisdiction, you might or might not be allowed to have a lawyer present as a consultant or actual advocate. You should know, however, that courts very rarely reverse a board's judgment, even though they may not agree with its decision.

Who would be the wiser if you lied on your application? The answer is, first of all, *you*. So, please, don't even consider it.

By lying, you, as an honest citizen and responsible professional, would place yourself in a position entirely alien to you.

Emotional illness is no crime. Nor does it necessarily disqualify a person from nursing. But failure to disclose information on an official application *could* subject you to a criminal charge of perjury. It *could* be grounds for revoking your license.

Telling the truth may present complications and cause some delay, but you should apply for your license honestly.

That way, you can return to your profession—now or in a few years—with your mind at peace, fully confident of adding many more happy years to those early ones in nursing you mention so fondly.

Good luck.

Suicidal patients

Can a nurse refuse to care for them?

Q At our general hospital, we have no psychiatric unit, so doctors often admit patients who have attempted suicide to our open medical unit. If such a patient injures or kills himself while in our care, who will be liable?

Have I a right to refuse to care for these patients and still retain my job?

A The presence of suicidal patients on an open unit of a general hospital poses many problems—practical, medical, and legal. Legally, both the hospital and attending physician could be liable if such a patient injures or kills himself while hospitalized. The determination of liability would depend on many things: whether the history of previous suicide attempts was known, whether maximum preventive measures were taken, whether the patient could have been transferred to a more appropriate facility, and so on.

When you work with a suicidal patient, you will, of course, make sure to institute all protective measures for the patient that fall within the realm of your professional duties. By recording chronologically on the patient's chart all your observations of and concerns for the particular patient, you further protect yourself from civil liability for malpractice. You should also advise your nursing supervisors, the administrator, and attending physician of your concerns. Put these communications in writing and keep a copy for yourself.

As to your last question, if you're asking if you can refuse to care for suicidal patients and still retain your job *on the same unit,* the practical administrative problem would preclude that.

But if you find the care of suicidal patients too nerve-racking, surely your administration would honor your request for transfer to another unit.

Suicide

How should it be handled?

Q A patient recently confided in one of my co-workers that he was contemplating suicide, then asked her not to tell anyone. She immediately alerted his family, his doctor, and the rest of the unit's staff. I'm not sure how I would have handled this situation. What's the right thing to do?

A Sometimes you have to betray a patient's confidence to protect his safety. In this case, your co-worker did the right thing. Legally and ethically, she couldn't promise to keep quiet because her patient's welfare was too important. And she shouldn't have had to shoulder the burden alone. Protecting a patient from suicide is a team effort.

Where does one draw the line between an attempt and a gesture?

Q Our hospital recently resurrected a dormant emergency department (ED) policy requiring us to report all suicide attempts to the police. I know that in my state we have to report an attempt involving the use of a firearm. But what about a suicide attempt involving drug overdose or other means? Notifying the police has serious drawbacks and raises some tough questions.

For example, I would draw the line between a genuine suicide attempt and a suicidal *gesture* that's actually an unconscious cry for help. If a highly disturbed adolescent swallows 15 aspirin tablets, this probably won't kill him. But must I tell the police that this young boy tried to take his life?

Another puzzling element is informed consent. Doesn't a patient have the right to know *before* I interview him that I intend to report to the police? Once he hears the word "police," he'll clam up and become cautious. But if I'm to help him, he has to confide in me.

What do you make of all this?

A The policy of reporting all suicide attempts would discourage the suicidal person from going to the ED for the help he so desperately needs. There are also some auxiliary issues: What do you do about the unconscious patient, or about *hearsay* reports from the person who brings the drug-overdose patient into the hospital?

You should obtain informed consent before notifying police of a patient's attempted suicide by drug overdose. However, when a firearm has been used in the suicide attempt, you *don't* need an informed consent. (Because your particular state law requires reporting all gunshot wounds to the police, you're protected under this law from any possible breach of confidentiality. In a suicide attempt by drug overdose, you'd have no comparable protection under the law.)

The implications of this resurrected policy must be thoroughly examined by representatives of the hospital's administration, the medical and nursing staffs, the legal department, and the local police. (By the way, do the police really *want* all these calls?)

Nobody has anything to *gain* by renewing this old policy. But the patient stands to *lose* the most: He's losing the opportunity for professional help at a time of deep personal crisis.

Sump tubes

How can solution be kept from draining out of the blue air-port lumen?

Q On our intensive care unit (ICU), we use sump tubes for nasogastric feedings and often have problems with solution draining out of the blue air-port lumen. We've tried to correct this by keeping the pigtail of this lumen above the patient's midline. When this fails, we clamp the lumen, but we're wondering if this could harm the patient.

A Sump tubes are designed for applying suction, so they're not the best choice for feedings. When necessary, however, you can use a sump tube for a short-term feeding. And it's okay to clamp the blue lumen during the feeding because the tube isn't attached to suction.

However, when you're using a sump tube for gastric suction, never clamp the smaller blue lumen while the tube is attached to suction. This blue air-port lumen vents the larger suction-drainage lumen to the atmosphere, and this constant flow of atmospheric air moderates the suction in the tube, preventing mucosal damage and traumatic suction levels.

Supervision

How can a nurse acquire some new growth without leaving a job?

Q I'm a diploma graduate of the late 1960s, and I've worked for 7 years at a large teaching hospital. During the first 3 years, I was steadily promoted from one position to another, including unit manager of the medical/surgical unit. Then I reluctantly accepted a promotion to supervisor of the oncology department.

It didn't take too long to realize that I was in over my head in my new position. I requested transfer back to the medical/surgical unit, as a staff nurse, until my self-confidence and esteem returned.

Months passed, and I applied for a patient-teaching position. The same administrator who encouraged me before now said, "There are no upper-level positions for you in this hospital because you failed as a supervisor."

Not one to make waves, I continued working as a staff nurse for the next few years, always receiving excellent evaluations and praise for exceeding job requirements and being a good role model and resource person. Still no promotion.

I need some new growth and challenge, yet I hate to leave a job I've held for so long. Any suggestions?

A Sounds as if you expect a lot *of* but not enough *for* yourself. Any marketer would agree that, as an employee, you're a saleable package: experienced, motivated, loyal.

Here are some suggestions: Forget the past and focus on where you are at *this* point in your career. Sit down and write a career profile like this: "I've worked here (x number of) years; nursing and the people I work with are important to me, just as I know my contribution to this hospital is valuable. I've successfully completed (name an accomplishment you're proud of). I want to continue working here, but I need a change and a challenge. The positions I'd like to be considered for are (job titles)."

Prepare copies for the personnel department, your immediate supervisor, and the director of nursing. Before sending documentation, however, tell them what you're doing and ask to meet with them after they've had a chance to review your statements.

Remember that administrators, like all of us, can become comfortable. Having an excellent, nonassertive worker slotted in a certain job is like money in the bank. Being noticed, speaking up, getting ahead (or recognizing when it's best to move on to another job) is partly *your* responsibility as an employee—and your reward for a job well done.

Supervisor

Should a nurse be concerned when her hospital no longer has night supervisors?

Q I spent 10 years at home raising my family, and now I'm returning to nursing. I've been offered a night-shift staff position at a nearby hospital, but I have serious doubts about the job. The hospital no longer has night supervisors on the premises; although a supervisor is on call, I'm leery of working under these conditions. Am I unduly concerned? Is this now common practice?

A The no-night-shift-supervisor policy hasn't been common practice up to now—but many hospitals are looking into this and other management changes because of the nursing shortage.

Some hospitals that *say* they no longer have night supervisors actually do have "supervisors" with different job titles and slightly different functions. For example, some unit managers have been given more responsibility and preparation for the increased responsibility. They cover the weekend day shift—and occasionally the evening shift—with backup from an on-call supervisor. So unit managers are now dealing with problems once handled by the on-site supervisor.

The new approach has been a successful—and safe—alternative to on-site weekend and evening supervisors. But if you sense that there's no one with strong management skills in the unit where you'll be working, you'd better ask these questions before accepting the job:
• Is there one person on every shift (somebody who's *on* the premises) responsible for making decisions?
• How available is the supervisor on call? Does she live several minutes—or hours—away? Who calls her in?
• Does the hospital have clear, written policies and procedures for managing crisis situations?

And there's one question only *you* have the answer to: After your long absence from nursing, how comfortable will you be in a less structured, less "supervised" environment? Would closer supervision be the security blanket you need in your first months back?

Use the answers to these questions to help you make your decision. This is just the first of many nursing judgments you'll be making now that you've returned to nursing. Good luck—and welcome back.

Surgical lifts

If a patient gets hurt, where does a nurse stand legally?

Q In the recovery room where I work, the unit manager has decided that we *must* use a certain surgical lift, rather than the conventional carrier, to return patients to their beds. She believes the lift is lighter to push and easier on patients.

> *"The unit manager has told us to use the surgical lift or get out of her department."*

I can agree with these points. But I don't think the lift is safe, because it's so lightweight and has no side rails. The unit manager has said we can do it her way or get out of her department. So I'll be using the lift—for now.

But if something happens to a patient while I'm using this piece of equipment, where do I stand legally?

A Technically, if your hospital has a written policy or procedure for returning patients to their beds, your immediate responsibility is to follow that procedure, as written.

But if you do this, you still won't be sure how safe the lift is. If one of your patients *does* fall off the lift, it's surely your responsibility—not that of the unit manager.

So if you and other nurses feel that using the lift is truly unsafe, why not get together and draft policies for the patients' care and safety? But until the matter is resolved we suggest that, for safety's sake, you'd better use a patient strap with the lift.

Suturing

Could it be opening a nurse up to a lawsuit?

Q For 5 years, I've been office nurse to a very fine physician. Professionally, he's taught me many new things—including suturing.

He now has me cover for him when he's called out, and on these occasions I've often done minor suturing.

At a recent nursing seminar, the lecturer was a lawyer. In his discussion, he described my job situation to a "T". Then he said that any nurse doing such suturing was leaving herself wide open for a lawsuit.

I reported this to the doctor. He said that, as long as he's taught me to suture correctly and I do it in his office, I have nothing to worry about because he'll be responsible for me.

I'd appreciate another opinion, though.

A Suturing is not ordinarily an accepted nursing procedure and, therefore, ordinarily may not be performed by nurses.

There are, however, certain circumstances under which a nurse *may* suture. For example: if the nurse is a nurse practitioner or nurse clinician practicing where state statutes permit her to suture; or if the nurse is a particular part of a health care delivery team (say, an operating room nurse) who works under the immediate direction, control, and supervision of a physician.

Since you aren't performing under either of these circumstances, you are in legal jeopardy and subject to disciplinary action by your licensing board.

S

Undoubtedly your employer means well for you. Once he understands the legalities involved, he'll surely make proper arrangements for medical services when he's out of the office.

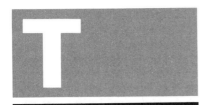

Talwin

Isn't the patient left with unexplained headaches and a dependence on Talwin?

Q I love my new job in the emergency department (ED), but one doctor's standing orders worry me. For 15 years, this doctor has prescribed pentazocine lactate (Talwin), 30 mg I.M., for a particular patient who complains of chronic headaches. I'm concerned because the prescription's never changed, and the patient reports to the ED almost daily for his injections. I wonder: Isn't this dependency?

My supervisor says, "don't rock the boat by refusing to give the injections. You'll just upset the doctor." But where does that leave the patient—except with unexplained headaches and a dependence on Talwin?

When I did discuss this with the doctor, he said it "bothered" him, too, but he wouldn't change the orders. I don't want to make an issue by refusing the doctor's orders, but do I have an alternative?

A Seems like your patient's prolonged "headache" has turned into a headache for you, too. Don't refuse to give the injections. Instead, put the issue in writing and send it through the proper hospital channels. You may have to go as far

as the doctor in charge of the ED. Be sure to point out that the situation is upsetting the ED staff—who do not consider these injections a true "emergency."

Going through channels may help *you*, but meanwhile, what about your patient? *Why* has he had a "headache" for 15 years? Ask his doctor for permission to schedule a psychiatric or mental health consultation for the patient.

Although the current prescription for Talwin is a schedule IV controlled substance and has a relatively *low* potential for abuse, that doesn't mean there's *no* potential for abuse.

"Making an issue" of the patient's injections may be uncomfortable for you, but remember: finding the cause of your patient's headache may be the best way to get rid of yours.

Tape recording

Could a patient's tape recording be held against nurses in a lawsuit?

Q We've just found out that the husband of one of our patients has been secretly tape-recording our bedside conversations. Now we're afraid he's planning to use the tapes in a lawsuit against us. Do we have any recourse?

A Tell him you don't want your conversations recorded. Then document that you've objected in your nurse's notes.

Unless sanctioned by court order, tape-recorded conversations generally aren't admissible as evidence (except when all parties know they're being recorded and consent to it). Because you didn't give permission to be recorded, the patient's lawyer couldn't use these tapes as evidence in any subsequent lawsuit.

You should wonder, though, why this patient's husband feels he has to record your conversations. Per-

haps he and his wife have a concern that isn't being addressed. Schedule a bedside conference and invite him, your manager, and the patient's doctor to attend. If he and his wife feel their concerns are being taken seriously, they'll be less likely to consider a lawsuit—and the electronic eavesdropping should stop.

Does it prevent freedom of speech?

Q A recently hired co-worker is a good nurse, but she's causing a lot of problems for the other staff members (and for me, in particular) at the nursing home where I work.

Last week, she began bringing a tape recorder on those nights when I relieve her after her shift is finished. Sometimes she conceals the recorder, other times she doesn't.

> *"My co-worker has been tape-recording conversations on the unit. I thought there was freedom of speech in America."*

But more than once, I've noticed the "recording" button depressed, and I can't be sure how many times she's taped my conversation. When I complained to my supervisor about this, she advised, "Just don't say anything you don't want recorded."

Is this America or what? I think I've lost my freedom of speech, and I don't like being recorded.

A Then don't let this co-worker bug you (in more ways than one). First of all, did you ask her *why* she's taping your conversations? You mention that she's new on the job. Could it be that she wants a record of what she has said to you for her own protection? Instead of wearing yourself out wondering, why not just ask her over a

T

friendly cup of coffee? After all, this is America.

Chances are nothing sinister's afoot. But if your co-worker's answers don't satisfy you, let her know—in a written, dated note, with copies for you and administration—that you do *not* want her, or anyone, to tape what you say without your permission. When you have job-related information worth sharing, you will. And if she wants to tape it, you'll expect her to keep the recorder in full view.

What if an LPN forgets to use the tape recorder or the machine doesn't work?

Q Policy in the hospital where I work allows LPNs and unit secretaries to tape telephone orders from doctors. This is supposed to save time for the RN. But occasionally an LPN or unit secretary will accept an order without remembering to use the tape recorder. Or if the machine's on the blink, the LPN or secretary will nevertheless go ahead and accept the doctor's order. But in both instances, failure to tape-record the doctor's order is contrary to policy.

If you were the RN on duty, what would you do about such an order?

A An order that hasn't been taped is unacceptable. Period. To adhere to your hospital's policy, you must use the tape to verify the conversation and be sure the order's correct.

You have two options when you're faced with an untaped order: You can call the doctor yourself (in which case no time's been saved after all), or you can have the person who should have turned on the recorder in the first place call the doctor back—and this time, be sure to *use* the recorder.

If failure to tape orders becomes a chronic problem, everyone involved should review hospital policy—emphasizing the risks of *not* adhering to a policy designed to protect both the hospital and the staff.

Telemetry system

Is it a good idea if patients are a long distance away?

Q I'm unit manager of a small intensive care/coronary care unit (ICU/CCU), and I foresee a problem.

Here it is: Our hospital's planning to purchase a four-bed telemetry system to use for a selected group of patients who require monitoring but who don't need the "intensive" care of the ICU/CCU. According to the plan, the telemetry monitors would be placed on the regular ICU/CCU, but the patients themselves would be on a medical/surgical unit some distance away.

"We'll have to rely on telephone communication if one of the ICU/CCU patients should run into problems."

We're frequently short staffed and unable to leave the ICU/CCU—so we'll have to rely on telephone communication with the medical/surgical unit if one of these patients should run into problems.

I'm *not* enthusiastic about this proposed plan. How about you?

A You have a right to be concerned with this arrangement. But the fact is, many hospitals now use the system you describe. It *can* work if there's good communication between the nurses in ICU/CCU and those on the medical/surgical unit.

Also there's a need for special preparation, *before* the telemetry monitors are installed, for those nurses responsible for handling emergencies once the system's in use.

You're wise to get the problem straightened away beforehand—not to wait for some critical minute when a patient's life could be at risk.

Telephone advice

Is there a risk of liability?

Q At the health maintenance organization (HMO) where I work, part of my responsibility is giving telephone advice. I'm supposed to triage calls and encourage patients who aren't seriously ill to try home treatment. I was told that, without this screening, the doctors would be deluged with patients because office visits are free to HMO members.

I understand the doctors' problem, but I'm worried about my own liability. Any advice?

A In a nutshell, you can avoid liability problems by understanding your role, following approved protocols, documenting, and advising each caller to seek medical treatment immediately if his symptoms persist or worsen.

Your role in telephone triage is limited to assessing the patient's problem, making a nursing diagnosis, and recommending intervention. All three depend on your nursing knowledge, protocols, and the severity of the patient's complaint. When an unusual question comes up or a problem needs medical advice, contact the doctor and document your action.

In fact, document all calls in a telephone log. Include the patient's name (and his parent's name, if appropriate), date, time, chief complaint, a very brief summary of advice you gave, plus your name. This log could prove invaluable if any legal problems develop. (Patients are likely to recall the phone conversations, but you might not. And without documentation, you can't prove or disprove what you said.)

For help in developing protocols, try *Nurses' Guide to Telephone Triage and Health Care* by the Group Health Cooperative of Puget Sound (Baltimore: Williams & Wikins, 1985). This book was designed to help ensure quality triaging by nurse practitioners and by RNs in clinics, HMOs, or doctors' offices.

What are the legal risks of giving advice over the phone?

Q I work in the emergency department (ED) of a major pediatric hospital that treats as many as 150 to 200 children a day. Lately we've been having a problem with an inordinate number of telephone calls. Most of the callers are parents who want detailed medical advice on some problem a child's having.

Because our hospital administration believes that answering these calls is excellent public relations for the hospital, we're expected to take every call that comes in.

The time the calls take is the least of my worries. I'm worried about the legal implications of our giving medical advice over the telephone. We have no protocol to follow— and that leaves most of us feeling we might be putting ourselves in legal jeopardy by giving out advice about a child we haven't seen.

The nurses in our ED would value your opinion.

A The usual broad definition of nursing practice offers no guidance on giving advice to a patient or a parent by telephone. But yes, telephone consultations can frequently be a source of both medical and legal entanglements for the hospital and the hospital professionals.

Try the following safeguards to lessen the risk of any legal problems:
• Start by establishing a set of guidelines for the more routine inquiries about a child's sore throat or diarrhea. This should ensure your giving uniform and consistent advice. The established guidelines should also provide protection if your advice is ever questioned. Be sure that the guidelines have been approved by the hospital policy committee.
• When faced with an unusual telephone request—one that is totally outside the established guidelines—enlist the aid of the doctor on duty in the ED, and be careful to document the facts of his involvement.
• Be sure to record *every* call received in the ED in a log kept solely for this purpose. Note the parent or patient's name, the date and time of the call, the chief complaint you were asked about, and a brief summary of the advice you gave. Initial each entry in the log. This kind of evidence could prove invaluable if litigation ever developed.
• *All* conversations should be concluded by urging the caller to seek medical treatment promptly if the child does not improve or if any untoward symptoms should occur.

Telephone orders

How can anyone prove the doctor gave them?

Q The doctors in our small community hospital recently found out that a second nurse listens in when we take their phone orders. We started this practice for our own protection because we've occasionally had doctors deny giving certain orders.

You can imagine our amazement when the director of nursing issued a memo banning this practice. The doctors complained to administra-

tion that the nurses are "stacking the deck against them." As usual, the director of nursing didn't stick up for us.

Now, if a doctor denies an order he gave, we're out in left field. Any thoughts on this?

A It's hard to believe the director of nursing didn't go to bat for you. Double-checking phone orders—standard practice throughout the country—isn't intended as an affront to any doctor. It just ensures that the nurse got the order right (which, incidentally, protects the *doctor,* too).

Go back to the director of nursing and ask for a staff meeting to discuss the phone order policy from your side of it.

Until then, here's an alternative: Take the phone orders and ask another nurse to read your notes back to the doctor. Or just read them back yourself. Document your action, and note specifically that the doctor confirmed the orders as read.

You've got enough day-to-day stresses on the unit. You don't need more discord over the phone.

Should narcotic injections be given in the ED solely on a doctor's telephone order?

Q In the emergency department (ED) of our small community hospital, our nurses routinely take doctors' telephone orders for narcotic injections.

What usually happens is that when a patient comes in complaining of a headache, a staff doctor is consulted by phone, and he orders a narcotic. The patient receives his injection, then leaves without ever seeing a doctor. Supposedly, the doctor will come by the next day to sign the verbal order he gave. But many doctors here "forget" this step.

Several months ago, one of the ED doctors reported this practice to the hospital administration and said he felt it was ill-advised and illegal. The administration responded with a letter to *all* staff doctors indicating that the ED would continue to honor telephone orders for narcotic injections. After that, our nurses were told to continue taking and carrying out telephone orders as a service to staff doctors. (We were also told doctors would sign their telephone orders the next day.)

Can you give me the facts? I'd like to refuse to give narcotic injections under these circumstances, but I need some backup.

A The practice you describe is a controversial one whose legality has not yet been determined. But you asked for support. Here it is: Accepting and following a doctor's telephone order for a patient he never sees is unsafe.

Document these telephone orders as they occur (with fact only; leave your opinions aside) and then send a memo with the facts and reasons for your concern through proper channels. If you're attempting to change your hospital's policy, why not join forces with the ED doctor who's already protested against the unsafe practice? Since this matter's controversial, you'll need all the troops you can muster.

Telephoning

Could a nurse get fired for insisting that the relief nurse phone the doctor?

Q For the past several months, I've been the night charge nurse of a surgical/oncology unit. Although I need my supervisor's permission to telephone doctors after midnight, this hasn't been any problem until recently. That's because the relief supervisor—an old-school nurse who came back from retirement to work part-time—always disagrees when I think a doctor should be called. I typically end up insisting on phoning.

You can imagine my consternation when the director of nursing told me the relief supervisor had complained, and she warned me that I'm risking termination if those complaints continue. The next day, I talked with my regular supervisor, who urged me to ignore the incident. I'd like to, but my confidence is shaken, knowing the word of a relief nurse could get me fired. What do you say?

A A director of nursing might not fully understand the unique pressures and disagreements occurring on the night shift— especially if she never worked that shift. Send her a follow-up letter, stat. You might say, "I have several concerns about our conversation, and I want to explain how I see my position as charge nurse on the 11-to-7 shift." Explain, then give two examples of patients who were in trouble and why you felt it imperative to call the doctor. Don't make this a power play; state your own observations and conclusions, and avoid mentioning the relief supervisor's actions in this letter.

Ask your regular supervisor to meet with you and the relief supervisor to explore your different perceptions of the telephone policy so you can find a middle ground. If the relief supervisor continues to veto your calls, explain why you think the doctor needs and wants to be called. Then document your conversation.

Terminal illness

Was it wrong to not relay a conversation to the doctor?

Q Last week, we admitted a terminally ill cancer patient to our medical/surgical unit from the emergency department. During morning rounds, his doctor ordered me to discontinue the I.V. line being used to administer fluids because, he said, the patient had told him several months before that he didn't want any artificial measures used to prolong his life.

As I removed the catheter, the patient asked me why. Wouldn't this mean he might die sooner? Is an I.V. what the doctor considers a life-prolonging measure in cases like his? When I said yes, his wife became upset; she said they didn't consider the I.V. an artificial means of prolonging life. I urged them to talk with their doctor.

Before I could leave the room, the patient asked several questions about survival rates for cancer patients, the pain they experience, and the effectiveness of different types of analgesics. I answered as objectively and gently as possible. At the end of our discussion, the patient said not to call his doctor, to just follow the original order. He had enjoyed a good life; he didn't want a long and painful death. The next day, the patient died.

Later, when his doctor heard about my conversation, he was furious and reported it to the director of nursing. They both accused me of overstepping my nursing role.

I did what I thought was right for the patient. What's your opinion?

A You're not the culprit here. You answered questions for a patient; you supplied no new or different diagnostic information; you were hardly overstepping nursing bounds. If the doctor had kept the patient updated as he should have, you wouldn't have been put on the spot.

In the future, if time allows, tell the patient that you would like his doctor to address these concerns. Add that you will call his doctor in and will stand by to help clarify the answers.

By insisting that the doctor talk directly to the patient, you'll make sure he's aware of the patient's anxiety. And you won't be *shielding* him from his responsibility to his patient.

In some states without right-to-die legislation yet on the books, many hospitals set up grand rounds to discuss what each team member can do to assure maximum consideration and comfort for the terminally ill. Why not suggest one where you work?

Termination

Can the staff save a director who's forced to quit?

Q Recently—and without warning—our director of nursing was asked to resign. Despite a series of budget cuts and the hostility of some staff physicians, this woman has been an effective, progressive leader. Nursing service can't afford to lose her. From unit managers to unit secretaries, we want to fight this move. What's the best way?

A Your chances of changing this administrative decision are slim. Circumstances surrounding a forced resignation are usually kept highly confidential. That means you probably don't know all the reasoning behind the decision. Lots of hearsay and speculation, no doubt, but for an effective protest, you need *facts*.

This is not to suggest you do nothing. There are other facts you *can* cite with authority: the director's effective leadership, and the continuing support she commands among nursing service, for example.

Type up a statement to this effect by way of introducing a petition that the director be retained. Circulate this statement for the staff's signatures, then send copies to the administration and to the director of nursing herself.

What happens then, remains to be seen. Even if you don't get the administration to change its decision, you still have the comfort of knowing you did everything you could. And, believe us, the director of nursing will remember forever that her staff, at least, understood—and valued—her worth.

Test anxiety

Any suggestions?

Q After passing the state boards on my second attempt, I swore never to put myself through so much torture again. Now, bowing to pressure from my manager, and after working 6 years as a pediatric nurse, I plan on taking the certification exam.

During the summer, I studied a specialty text and did practice tests, but I'm still a nervous wreck. Any suggestions?

A Start by reminding yourself that you've already passed the major tests determining your career direction. Certification exams, although hardly a piece of cake, are practice-based. And if you have the work experience and continuing education to qualify as an exam candidate, you already have the necessary skills to pass the examination.

Some pretest jitters are normal—and helpful (they get the adrenaline pumping). But you can control damaging anxiety by using some general study and test-taking techniques. Take a review course; if none are available and several of you will be taking the exam, your administrators might consider offering one free. Form a study group—the interaction can help you identify "blind spots" and bolster your morale. And consider paying a co-worker who's already certified to give your group some tutoring sessions.

When taking the test, read the instructions thoroughly. Pace yourself; answer 60% of the questions by midpoint of your allotted time so you'll have extra time for difficult questions. If you'll be scored for right answers only, answer every question. When you're stumped, cross out wrong or unlikely choices, then try to make a logical guess. If you want to come back to a question, put a reminder check in the margin.

Don't look for patterns on the answer sheet or try to read between the lines. Watch for the words "always" or "never" in questions or answers. Hint: Correct answers tend to contain qualifiers such as "sometimes" or "most." When a case study's involved, the correct answer usually matches the point of view expressed in the question; if there are several questions about the case, read a few ahead; you may get clues to the correct answers.

Of course, check your sheet one final time to erase stray marks and make sure you haven't skipped any questions. Don't overscrutinize and begin to doubt your answers. Nurses have a great deal of intuitive knowledge—let it work for you.

Tetanus injections

Should nurses give them routinely and without a doctor's order?

Q I've just started a job as an occupational health nurse in a company with 2,000 employees, and I've already hit the first snag.

My predecessor used to routinely administer tetanus booster injections for certain minor injuries that didn't require a doctor's treatment. The employees now expect me to follow the same practice; they come to see me for a tetanus injection after a dog bite, a skin puncture, and so on.

The problem is that the previous nurses didn't—and I don't—have a medical order to give these injections, not even a standing order.

T

I certainly want to help keep employee sick time to a minimum, but I'm concerned about giving injections without a doctor's order. Am I legally jeopardizing myself and the company by continuing this practice?

A You certainly are putting yourself in jeopardy. Giving injections without a written medical order is not only illegal, but also unethical. Administering tetanus injections may seem like a routine procedure—until you consider all the possible complications that *could* arise.

Why not check your state's nurse practice act to see what your legal limitations are? Then have a straight talk with your company's management; tell them you can administer medication *only* in accordance with a doctor's written order. Explain that as an occupational health nurse, your responsibility in treating employee injuries is to administer first aid, to refer the employee to his family doctor, and to give whatever palliative treatment is necessary.

This would be a good moment to point out that the company should be paying for your malpractice insurance coverage—if it's not already doing so.

A company's not legally obligated to provide treatment or pay for employee's *nonoccupational* injuries. These injuries—even the minor ones—should be treated by the employee's family doctor.

Theft

What can be done if a woman refuses to let the staff put her jewelry in safekeeping?

Q We recently admitted a frail elderly woman to our medical/surgical unit, largely because she couldn't remain at home alone. (Her husband had been admitted to the hospital with pneumonia 2 days earlier.) When this woman arrived, I noticed she was wearing a ring and offered to put it in safekeeping for her. "Don't you touch it," she snapped.

We'd been warned about how obstinate and difficult this woman could be, but she didn't appear either confused or disoriented. So I left the ring on her finger. I felt that since she was clearheaded, she had a right to make that decision.

I reported the incident to my unit manager and to the RN who was replacing me, and noted in the nursing Kardex that the patient was anxious to keep her ring. Then I went off duty for a week's holiday.

When I returned, I was confronted by the woman's husband—now recovered. He was irate: He said the ring was missing and accused the staff of stealing it. He'd already called the police and reported the value of the ring at $20,000.

The nurse who had replaced me when I left on my holiday was the only other person who remembered seeing the ring. We've both given our statements to the police, and we'll probably have to go to court. What could I have done to avoid this unpleasant scenario?

A You did all that could be expected. You acted as any reasonably prudent nurse would act to protect her patient's property:
• You determined that the patient was conscious and competent.
• You informed her that safekeeping was available for her valuables.
• You reported the incident to your supervisor and documented it.

In the future, you might want to state in writing why you believe the patient is competent, and note that when you offered to safeguard the valuables, the patient refused. Enter such a report in the nurses' notes rather than in the Kardex.

The hospital's (and your) responsibility is to provide an opportunity for reasonable security, not to guarantee that the patient's property won't be stolen.

Time

How long should preparing and dispensing medications take?

Q I graduated from nursing school in 1947. Right now I work in a nursing home, and one of my jobs is giving medications. I arrive for work at 7 a.m. Report lasts until about 7:25, and then I prepare medications for all 49 patients. I give the insulin injections first—before the breakfast trays arrive at 8:15. Then, while the patients eat, I start preparing for the next medication rounds.

I've just learned that breakfast is being moved up to 7:30 a.m., but I can hardly keep up with the pace as it is. My supervisor says I'm already "too slow," but I don't know how I can work any faster and still be accurate.

Can you tell me how long preparing and dispensing my medications should take? I have 112 different drugs to dispense to 49 patients. Some drugs are stored in the refrigerator and others are in a locked cabinet. Some pills have to be crushed; others, broken in half.

Things sure have changed since I graduated. I think my supervisors are asking too much of me. Do you agree?

A Setting up the medication cart, getting the system ready (cards in order and so on), and then crushing and pouring the medications can take anywhere from 30 minutes to an hour. And that's not counting dispensing time, which, with 49 elderly patients, will take at least another hour—depending on how alert and cooperative your patients are.

Clearly, you're under a lot of pressure, but before you throw up your hands, try this: Prepare just the insulins and medications that need to be given before or with breakfast *first.* Then, after breakfast, set up the other medications.

If this system doesn't work for you (it might not, since so much depends on your style of work and your other responsibilities), talk to other nurses; see what tips they have to offer. Ask your supervisor if she can make some practical suggestions.

You might also want to take a fresh look at your system of giving medications: Dispensing according to a unit-dose system should be safer and easier in this situation.

A nurse in a hurry is more apt to make a mistake than a nurse working at a comfortable pace. So let your supervisors hear about your problem *before* you make a mistake. And when you get discouraged, remember that the fundamental part of nursing—*caring* for your patients—hasn't changed since you graduated in 1947.

Time clocks

Why should other employees be penalized because a few employees forget to punch in and out?

Q This morning, the hospital where I work posted this notice on all time clocks: "Effective next Monday—Forget to punch? Forget your pay. Signed time slips will no longer be accepted."

Before, on the rare occasion that I forgot to punch in, I just filled out a time slip and had my charge nurse sign it to verify the time I started work that day. Now, with this new policy, I can lose an entire day's pay for being in a hurry and forgetting to punch in on the time clock.

Why should I or anyone else be penalized for the few employees

who make a practice of this? Can management really do this?

A Yes. Management is within its right to enforce its personnel policies, and if it says that you get paid only for the time listed on your time card, that's how you get paid.

Finding that rather flip notice couldn't have been pleasant, but somehow, nothing grabs our attention like the prospect of losing money. And although you may not like the method or the message, you're at least in no doubt about how to avoid the problem. One other thing you should do, however, is mention your feelings at your next staff meeting.

Management should know how the employees view the style as well as the content of its latest communiqué.

Time off

How can a team leader handle a nursing assistant who wants to leave early when it's busy on the unit?

Q I'm team leader on a medical/surgical unit. One day last week a nursing assistant told me she had to leave work earlier than usual because her grandson was having surgery. She said the nursing supervisor had just given her permission.

My first impulse was to say, "Well, *I* won't give you permission because you waited until the last minute." But of course I understood why she wanted to be with her family, and the unit *was* quiet that day. So I said we could get along without her.

As the assistant was leaving, another nurse reported that one of the assistant's patients had been incontinent and that both he and his bed were a mess. I told the assistant that we'd take care of her patient, that she could go. But then several other patients developed problems, and the "quiet" unit didn't stay that way.

As a result, everyone on my team got angry at everyone else. The nursing assistants were angry at me for allowing their co-worker to leave early, leaving them to do her work. *I* was angry at the supervisor for not consulting me, and I was angry at everyone on my team for making a fuss.

> *"The nursing assistants were angry at me for allowing their co-worker to leave early, leaving them to do her work."*

Maybe I shouldn't have allowed the nursing assistant to leave. Maybe I should've insisted that she take care of her patient first. If you'd been in my shoes, what would you have done?

A Unfortunately, you got caught in the middle of a difficult situation. If the nursing assistant had asked for the time off a week in advance, you could have probably arranged for extra coverage. At the very least, the other nursing assistants would have been prepared for some additional work.

The assistant should have come to you first with her request, and the nursing supervisor should have consulted you before giving the assistant permission to leave. To make sure this won't happen again, discuss it with the supervisor.

If the patient's incontinence occurred while the nursing assistant was still on duty, she should have taken care of the patient herself. If it happened just as she was leaving, the other staff members should have been willing to take over.

Patient care has to be a *team* effort. When the assistant left the floor (whether she gave advance notice or not), the rest of the staff should've pitched in to cover for her. Who knows when *they'll* want their turn at being concerned grandmothers?

How can nurses ensure that they get it?

Q I'm one of four RNs working the 7-to-3:30 shift in a busy operating room (OR). Lately, we've had so many emergency cases at night that we've each been working on call one or two nights a week, plus every fourth weekend. We get paid for on-call time and overtime.

What we *don't* get is any guaranteed time off after being on call. Oddly, a weekend on call is considered time off, no matter how many hours we work.

Morale in our department has been very low. We sent a grievance letter to the administration requesting time off after being on call. This was denied, for financial reasons. The director of nursing rubs salt in the wound by telling us, "It was your choice to work in the OR."

We're tired of getting the runaround, and we're just plain tired. What can we do to get the time off we need?

A Realistically, an OR nurse can't expect a day off after *every* on-call worked. But you *do* deserve a break.

Here are some suggestions: Ask to come in at 9 a.m., instead of 7 a.m., after a night on call. Also, suggest that a room with a cot be set up in the hospital so you can sleep right there after you've finished a night-call case. When you have to be in the OR again the next morning, at least you'll save the travel time.

If you take this advice and you're still losing sleep, sit down with the OR unit manager and work out a better rotation schedule. You might try to get Monday off automatically if, and only if, you've worked during your on-call weekend. (Make sure the other three RNs know you won't be in that Monday. If you do show up, it'll be a bonus.)

As a last resort, bring the problem to the attention of your director of nursing and of your hospital administrator. You have some strong "financial" arguments on your side: turnover, "burnout," and OR mistakes can be *very* costly indeed.

You're working in a most demanding area. Good luck resolving your problem.

Tipping

Is it ethical to accept gifts from patients?

Q In 6 years of nursing, I've been offered anywhere from $1 to $50 in tips. Some of the patients, I hardly know—others, I knocked myself out for; some were rich, some poor; some I loved, others I dreaded. But in no case have I ever accepted the tip. This has caused such bad feelings: I'm embarrassed, the patients and their families are embarrassed—some deeply hurt. I've honestly come to wonder if it might not be the generous gesture on my part just to accept the money with thanks. How do you handle this?

A Common practice is for a customer to offer a gratuity for fulfilling his *requests* or *demands*. A nurse, however, through her uniquely professional training, assesses and meets a patient's *needs*. Keeping this difference in mind, then, she can ethically accept only her pay.

This is the proper professional stance. Unfortunately, you can't count on patients' knowing—or observing—*your* professional standards. What you must do is consider each patient's tip with the same specificity you provide in his nursing care. Judge his manner. Is he offering you a tip because he thinks one is expected of him? Tell him he just gave you the best tip, the only tip you can take, by getting well again. But what of the elderly pensioner who gratefully slips a quarter in your hand as she's leaving? Clearly, this gesture means a great deal to that patient, and it leaves you with no choice but to accept. In a question of ethical priorities, the patient's dignity and well-being must always supersede your personal feelings on professional conduct.

The simplest thing for everyone is to decide what to do with any tips that can't be gracefully refused. Ask your unit manager to make a ruling on this. Some hospitals have unit funds in which all tips are pooled to buy textbooks or equipment or coffee-break treats for that department. Others have a "sunshine" fund to supply toys for pediatrics or shaving kits for the needy.

Your question made no mention of personal gifts, which can also be considered a form of tipping. This suggests that you've already recognized an important difference. Money is a universal form of exchange that can be as correctly offered to a maitre d' as to a paper boy. But a personal gift, to which someone has given special thought and effort, is an intimate interaction between two people. To decline such a gift can only appear as a rejection of the giver, and you should accept it in kindness and good grace. The fact that the gift is usually not your size, your style, or your scent is of no importance. This is one time when it is, indeed, the *thought* that counts.

Naturally, a personal gift calls for a written "thank you." But, remember, a tip, even when pooled, is still a gift and should also be acknowledged in writing.

Tongue blades

Should they be used when a patient has a seizure?

Q At the hospital where I work, seizure precaution protocol includes taping a padded tongue blade above the patient's bed. Recently, however, I read that tongue blades are no longer used when a patient has a seizure. If that's so, should we modify our current policy? What's the latest information?

A Opinions differ on this one: Some experts believe nothing should be placed in the patient's mouth during a seizure, but others prefer using soft objects such as a rolled washcloth, a padded tongue blade, or an oropharyngeal airway, which can also be used for suctioning.

The important point is to act quickly. If you put anything into the patient's mouth, do it before his jaws clamp down— never pry clenched teeth apart. Keep the object forward in the mouth so he doesn't gag or vomit. (An oropharyngeal airway can trigger gagging and vomiting, so never tape the airway in place; this prevents the patient from rejecting it.) Keep the patient on his side to prevent aspiration of mucus and vomitus.

A periodic review of all procedures is always a good idea, so why not ask your policy committee to take a new look at its recommendations?

They're lucky to have someone as concerned as you on staff.

TPN

Doesn't changing the tubing three times a day increase the risk for infection and the cost?

Q The policy on total parenteral nutrition (TPN) in the unit where I'm working requires us to change the tubing with each new bottle of TPN solution. Yesterday, when one of our patients received a TPN infusion at 125 ml/hour, we ended up making three tubing changes in one day. I can't help wondering if this doesn't increase the risk of infection. And how about the

mounting expense, in this current cost-conscious period?

At other hospitals where I've worked, we made tubing changes every 24 hours.

Is there an overall rule for this situation?

A The frequency of tubing changes for TPN will depend upon the fluids you're infusing.

If you're infusing fluids of different consistencies—such as amino acid solution (serous) followed by a fat emulsion (milky), it would be better to change the tubing with *each* bottle, even though this would mean opening the system. Here's the reasoning.

If you infuse fluids of different consistencies through the same tubing, you increase the chance of contaminating the system.

When you're infusing fluids of the same consistency—such as glucose solutions—you can safely change the tubing every 24 to 48 hours.

This is a good rule of thumb to know. Good luck.

How much of the contents should be infused?

Q Total parenteral nutrition (TPN) bags often exceed 1,000 ml by the time all the constituents are mixed in. So what do we do when the order reads, "1 liter over 12 hours"?

Infuse 1,000 ml and dump what remains, or infuse the entire contents?

A Infuse the entire contents to ensure that the patient receives the prescribed amount of additives. Don't be concerned about infusing 1 liter in 12 hours; concentrate instead on infusing approximately 85 ml per hour. Set the pump and time-tape the bag. And when the bag is finished, record the time and amount infused.

Is it safe to run TPN, lipids, and packed red blood cells at the same time?

Q On our unit, we have many patients receiving continuous infusions of total parenteral nutrition (TPN), and 10% to 20% lipid solutions. Many of them have central venous access devices, including triple-lumen catheters and double-lumen catheters.

We know that blood products such as packed red cells should never be directly "piggybacked" into an already infusing line of TPN, but we're not sure whether running TPN and lipids through one lumen of a catheter and packed red blood cells through the other lumen at the same time is safe.

Our pharmacy and blood bank people say the high dextrose solution in the TPN could cause clumping, clotting, and hemolysis of the red blood cells. But others we've checked with say concurrent administration is the purpose of multilumen catheters.

We'd sure like to clear up this debate.

A Infusing red blood cells and TPN products simultaneously in a double- or triple-lumen catheter is safe, if these catheters contain separate side-by-side lumens.

You could, however, run into a problem when TPN and blood cells are administered in a double- or triple-lumen catheter that is a single catheter with two or three exit openings. Slight mixing of infusate can occur within the catheter. Minimal cell clumping could occur from direct contact of blood cells and hypertonic TPN solutions—especially if the blood is infused at slow rates. (The normal rate for a unit of whole blood or packed cells is 2 hours.)

The safest procedure with these catheters would be to stop the TPN while the blood infuses. Flush the entire line before and after the blood

T

administration with 20 ml of sterile normal saline. If you can't stop the TPN, administer the blood through a peripheral vein; if venous access isn't possible, get a doctor's order to administer the blood and TPN solutions concurrently through the catheter.

Should Intralipid be mixed with TPN solutions?

Q A doctor on our unit orders fat emulsions (Intralipid) to be run I.V. piggyback simultaneously with total parenteral nutrition (TPN). I remember reading in the past that fat emulsions shouldn't be mixed with TPN solutions. Is that still valid? If so, are these orders safe?

A Yes, that's still valid. A usual ratio is a 3:1 admixture (3 parts TPN to 1 part Intralipid).

As you know, TPN fluids are a likely medium for bacterial growth, so sepsis is always a risk. For this reason, the National Intravenous Therapy Association recommends a closed system as much as possible. Now that mixing fat emulsions with TPN has approval, piggybacking these solutions shouldn't be necessary.

Tracheostomy

Is it safe to take out both cannulas for an hour?

Q As a nurse in a home health agency, I sometimes care for patients who've been sent home from the hospital with a tracheostomy.

I'm responsible for evaluating how well the patient and family can suction and care for the tube. But last week I came across something unexpected: A doctor ordered me to do tracheostomy care on one of his at-home patients by cleaning both the inner and outer cannulas. To do this, he wanted me to remove both cannulas, leave them out for an hour, then reinsert them.

I questioned this unusual order, but the doctor informed me that this was the current trend and part of the process of weaning a patient from the airway.

> *"The doctor wanted me to remove both cannulas, leave them out for an hour, then reinsert them."*

Are you familiar with this new trend? Do you consider this the proper way to clean a double-cannula tracheostomy? Would I be subject to any legal risk by following this doctor's order?

A The doctor's way was *not* the way to handle this situation.

Here's the accepted procedure: The inner cannula is removed routinely for cleaning, but the outer cannula should be removed only when it's necessary to insert a fresh one. In this case, the outer cannula should be removed for only a few minutes—just long enough to insert the new one. Whenever this procedure is done, replacement equipment should be readily available along with the proper equipment for an emergency, and the person doing the procedure should be skilled both in removing and replacing the tracheostomy tube.

Weaning implies a step-by-step process—not an abrupt removal of the cannulas. Weaning can be properly achieved through the use of special fenestrated tubes or one-way valve attachments—or by plugging the tube with a tracheostomy button for gradually increasing periods of time—until the final removal of the tracheostomy tube seems called for. At the time of removal, the equipment and personnel we've described above *must* be kept immediately at hand.

This is accepted procedure and can be verified in a manual on respiratory nursing. Any other practice *could* have troublesome legal implications.

Tranquilizers

Should a nurse take them to reduce nervousness at work?

Q I'm an AD graduate with 4 years' experience. More than anything I want to be a good nurse, but I cannot seem to work efficiently. I seem to get nervous just when I'm needed most. I get flustered and forget to do things. I've gone from one hospital job to another, lasting the probation period...and that's that.

Finally, I got my present job as a float nurse. I've been here 7 months and, at one point, thought I was gaining confidence. But then I noticed my efficiency decreasing again. Last night, the unit manager was upset over the care I was giving a postop patient. I really tried to make up for my forgetfulness but the supervisor called me to her office before I went off duty and asked me about my "negligence." Then she made a reference to my nervousness. I am not taking any medications and am in excellent health otherwise. I was once advised to take tranquilizers but I don't believe in them. Not in my job.

I have a lot of continuing education units. I just don't know what's wrong.

A If "Physician, heal thyself" is fair enough advice, then so is "Nurse, assess thyself." Look at what you're saying. You "cannot seem to work efficiently...get nervous when you're needed most...get flustered and forget to do things...

notice your efficiency decreasing again...try to make up for your forgetfulness...are questioned about your negligence and nervousness." When you put that all together, haven't you answered your own question about what's wrong?

Doesn't it seem to you that you have some problem that causes you to become abnormally anxious when you're working under tense conditions? You don't say *who* advised you to take tranquilizers, but consider your reaction. Surely a blanket dismissal of such a proven valuable medication is out of keeping with your nursing education. If tranquilizers can help you through periods of stress—they have helped millions of others—then perhaps you should consider them. But first go to a doctor whose judgment you respect. Explain your problem just as you explained it here—and follow his advice, even if it means tranquilizers.

From your question, you seem to be an honest and conscientious nurse. Now you must try to be as open-minded and dedicated in your care of yourself as you would be in your care of a patient.

Treatment delay

Are time-saving steps in the ED safe?

Q In the intensive care unit (ICU) where I work, a new policy has our nursing staff worried. Administration wants to cut the time that emergency department (ED) nurses must spend on a new admission. So for any patient who's scheduled for transfer to the ICU, we're supposed to accept admitting orders over the phone from the attending doctor while the patient is still in the ED.

But sometimes the patient won't arrive in our unit until hours later, depending on bed availability. We're concerned that medications and other important treatments aren't

being given to this patient because we're holding the orders until he arrives in the unit.

What do you think about this?

A The answer is simple: Admitting orders should be called in to the unit where the patient *is* so they can be carried out. Obviously, staff members working with the patient know his condition and how to set priorities.

Ask administration for a review of this new policy. What seems on paper like a timesaving move for the ED nurses could result in damaging delays for the patient.

Treatment error

Should a nurse always tell her patient the truth?

Q While I was on a coffee break, a chronic obstructive pulmonary disease patient of mine was mistakenly taken to the gastroenterology laboratory for an endoscopic procedure. Before I discovered the error, he was premedicated with I.V. midazolam (Versed). Luckily, the procedure hadn't been started when I called the lab, and he was returned to the unit.

Because he hadn't been receiving oxygen while in the lab, he was having trouble breathing. So after resuming oxygen therapy, I started a theophylline (Theo-Dur) drip, as ordered.

The patient, who routinely took oral theophylline, later asked why he was getting the drug I.V. I told him that his doctor had ordered the change and that he should talk to him for more details.

I wanted to tell him the whole truth, but I wasn't sure where I stood legally. What should I have done?

A Generally, honesty is the best policy. In fact, some courts have held that health care providers are obligated to tell patients when

errors occur. So you should have followed up on the question.

Your first step should have been to ask his doctor how he wanted to proceed. Then you or he would have talked with the patient. If he disagreed about telling the patient and you felt the error was serious enough, you could have taken the matter to the unit's medical director. Either way, you should have carefully documented the conversation in your own records.

Treatment refusal

Could a nurse be held liable if she forgot to get the patient to sign a waiver?

Q I just started working in a busy emergency department. One night, a group of young men brought in a 20-year-old friend—obviously against his will. Although he had a large, bleeding cut across his eyebrow, he loudly refused even routine first aid. Finally, the attending doctor told me to let him leave. I did, but I forgot to ask him to sign our waiver first. Now I'm scared. Could I be held liable if the patient developed complications after he left?

A Relax. You aren't liable for a competent adult patient who refuses medical care. That's his right, even if you and the doctor recommend treatment.

Although this patient didn't sign the hospital's waiver, you're protected if you carefully documented relevant facts and observations. The doctor's progress notes should back you up.

In the future, quickly determine your patient's competence as you take his history and get his consent for treatment. If he refuses, make sure the doctor explains the benefits and risks of the proposed treatment. Document the conversation

T

in your notes. Finally, following hospital policy, ask him to sign the waiver form before he leaves and add it to his chart.

How can a nurse help the family and keep her job?

Q Sometimes I'm caught between a doctor's orders and the patient's wishes. For example: A few days ago, the daughter of a cancer patient told me that her elderly father doesn't want any more chemotherapy and that she agrees with his decision. She also told the doctor. But he told me he wouldn't write an order to discontinue treatment.

I don't know what to do next. The daughter still doesn't know the doctor hasn't written the order. Should I tell her what's happened and suggest she see a lawyer or get another doctor? Or should I keep quiet? I want to help my patient and his family, but I want to keep my job, too.

A You have a duty to safeguard your patient's right to refuse treatment. But don't close down the lines of communication.

To help your patient without creating unnecessary conflict between him and his doctor, chart each specific statement he makes about his treatment wishes. Be sure to keep your notes factual and nonjudgmental. For instance, you could chart: "The patient told me, 'I've had enough. I want to stop this chemotherapy.'"

Next, enlist your unit manager's help. Share your charting with her, and explain why you think the matter should be pursued. Then talk with the doctor about his obligation to honor his patient's request. If necessary, also ask for support from the unit's medical director, the chaplain, or the hospital's ethicist.

Finally, you might suggest that the patient sign a living will, which allows him to express his preference about the treatment he wants.

It also allows him to designate a proxy to carry out these wishes if he should become unconscious or incompetent. If the patient signs a living will, make sure it becomes part of his medical record.

How can a nurse protect her patient's rights and address parents' concerns?

Q The doctor has recommended chemotherapy and an amputation to stop the spread of cancer in my 18-year-old patient's leg. The patient agrees to the chemotherapy but refuses to accept amputation. His parents want me to talk him into it. I agree that the doctor's advice is sound, but I don't want to pressure my patient. What can I do to protect his rights *and* address his parents' concerns?

A At 18, your patient is an adult who's both legally and ethically justified in making his own treatment decisions—including the decision to refuse all or part of the therapy his doctor recommends.

Your patient needs your support. Make sure he understands the facts about his condition, and talk with him about why he's agreed to one treatment but not the other. Are his reasons based on fact, fantasy, or fear? (Remember, to an 18-year-old, the prospect of losing a leg may be more frightening than dying.) You can give the doctor valuable insights by carefully and nonjudgmentally charting your conversations, using direct quotes whenever possible.

Most important, don't let your patient view the situation as a battleground where everyone he loves is against him. Try to be as fair, honest, and respectful as you can when you discuss his decision. And let him know that you'll be there to support him at all times, no matter what he decides.

Should a nurse have a patient sign a release form if he refuses sutures and wants adhesive skin closures instead?

Q The following episode took place in the emergency department (ED).

The resident on duty was about to suture a patient's minor skin laceration, but the patient wanted the wound closed with adhesive skin closures. The nurse stepped in and told the patient that he could have the adhesive skin closures, if he insisted, but that he'd have to sign an against medical advice (AMA) release. In these circumstances, she added, his insurance company would not cover this emergency department visit. The resident did not speak up, either to agree or disagree with the nurse. The patient, intimidated by the nurse's stand, agreed to the suturing.

I'd say having a patient sign an AMA release every time he refuses a medication or a test is improper nursing or improper use of the AMA form. But I could find nothing definitive about this in our written hospital policy.

And then, about the business of a patient's bill not being covered if he signs the AMA form: Neither the health insurance manager nor the insurance billing department in our hospital could give me a clear-cut answer.

Can you give me a more satisfactory answer?

A You're right to ask—and right to look askance. The nurse's behavior in the ED was *not* acceptable nursing practice. Every patient has the right to be informed of the proposed treatment *and* the right to refuse the treatment, even if the nurse or other health care professional is convinced the recommended treatment is in the patient's best interest.

If, after an explanation, the patient in the ED still wanted adhesive skin closures, not sutures, he should have *had* adhesive skin closures. The nurse's job was not to be insistent and arbitrary, but to enter the facts of the case in the patient's record.

This is the wrong use of the AMA form; the patient did not object to being *treated,* he objected only to the *form* of treatment.

The ED nurse was altogether wrong on the matter of insurance coverage. First, she was wrong to use "no medical coverage" as a means of persuading the patient to accept the sutures. And second, she didn't have her facts right: The insurance sources in most states (including Blue Cross and Blue Shield) say that if treatment were given, the insurance carrier *would* provide coverage—even if the patient chose a treatment other than that recommended by the staff. Of course, whatever the treatment, it has to be covered in the patient's insurance agreement in order to warrant payment.

The nurse was attempting to act in what she thought was the patient's best interest. But she overlooked a fundamental patient right: the right to make the final decision about his own treatment.

What if the doctor and a relative ignore a patient's wishes?

Q A couple of months ago, I cared for an 82-year-old woman with sick sinus syndrome. On admission, her heart rate was 50 beats/minute and her doctor wanted to insert a permanent pacemaker. She refused. She told me she'd made peace with her family and God and she was ready to die. Her doctor was furious, but he had to go along with her decision.

When her heart rate dropped to 38 beats/minute and she became confused, he convinced her son to consent to the procedure. I protested, but the doctor went ahead anyway.

I can still remember my patient's anger when she recovered from the anesthesia. I was upset, too. What could I have done to prevent the doctor and her son from ignoring her wishes?

A You and your manager should have gone to the medical director with documentation of your conversations with the patient. She'd made her wishes very clear. The doctor, in an overly zealous attempt to save her life, violated her right to refuse treatment.

Why did the patient's son sign the consent form? He may not have understood his mother's wishes or her right to refuse treatment. Perhaps he felt confused or pressured by the doctor. Or he may have believed that by refusing treatment for his mother, he'd be abandoning her. Whatever his reasons, the situation underscores the importance of family communication *before* a patient loses the ability to speak for herself.

In the future, observe family dynamics and identify the person who could take the lead in discussing the patient's desire to refuse heroic measures. If the patient can't communicate, you could say to the family: "Did you know that your mother felt very strongly about refusing this procedure? She and I discussed it several times. Our hospital supports the patient's right to make this choice." You might also ask the hospital's chaplain, patient advocate, or medical ethicist to get involved. This objective input could help the patient and family resolve conflicts.

One more thing: When a patient wants to refuse treatment, suggest that he sign a living will or give durable power of attorney to someone who understands his wishes. Either step will help protect his rights. You can support him by documenting your conversations about refusing treatment. This will show that he discussed his wishes with you.

Troubled husband

How can a nurse help her husband?

Q Although I've had considerable success in my nursing career (my present salary is $21,000), my life was incomplete until 4 years ago when at the age of 32, I met and married the most handsome, brilliant, charming, gentle, and good man.

He's still all of these things, but he's also an alcoholic, a transvestite with strong homosexual fantasies, and a pathological liar. My entire life's savings are gone ($15,000 alone to save him from jail after a business deal involving forged legal papers). I no longer turn over my pay to him and that causes more trouble between us.

I've begged him to go to Alcoholics Anonymous or to a therapist but he won't hear of it. I've considered divorce but the thought of this man's good, even wonderful, traits stops me from proceeding. I'm at my wit's end. I don't know what to do. Please answer me.

A Dear friend, your three obvious options are: to continue living as you are—albeit, unhappily; leave your husband; or stay with him only on the condition that you both obtain professional help.

Apparently without your realizing it, you've already discarded the first option by taking two positive steps to change your situation. You've retaken control of your salary, and you've sought advice.

The second option, to sever a marital relationship of 4 years standing, is one that should be exercised only after you've had professional counseling. So your best bet is your third option: insist that you, as a couple, get professional help.

If you cannot get your husband to go, *please* see a therapist yourself—a marriage counselor or psychiatrist. You need—and will surely profit from—the direct support and advice of a professional counselor.

Truthfulness

Should a nurse give her opinion about a doctor if a patient asks?

Q Every so often, a patient asks me, "Is my doctor any good?" When a doctor's reputation isn't that great, I don't know what to say. I'm not talking about an incompetent doctor, just one who's not particularly gifted. I usually evade the question, but I'm afraid that puts more doubts in the patient's mind. I don't feel right about lying, but telling the truth is out, too. What do you suggest?

A Find out what's behind the patient's question. What qualities does he want to know about when he asks if a doctor is "good"? Some patients would rate technical skills highest; others, compassion and the ability to communicate.

Perhaps the best response to the question is another question: "What's on your mind?" or "What makes you wonder?" This invites him to ask health-related questions that may be relevant to his care and your patient teaching.

But if he believes he isn't getting good care from his doctor, discuss his concerns with him. If he has reason to worry, you may have to pursue the matter through channels.

Tube feeding

Should only gravity be used when tube feeding a newborn?

Q I'm the newest staff member on the pediatric unit of a well-thought-of hospital. But I need a bit of help. Some of the nurses on the

unit say I should use only gravity when tube feeding a newborn. Others say I can gently push the feeding formula.

What do you think?

A You really shouldn't have to push the feeding formula if the tube is in the correct position. If you're having problems with the flow rate, try holding the tube higher. This should increase the flow rate of the feeding formula.

Pushing the feeding formula can cause diarrhea in a newborn. You're better off appreciating the gravity of the situation.

Tuberculosis

Can students refuse to be tested more often than the state law requires?

Q The school of nursing where I'm enrolled requires all nursing majors to receive a yearly tuberculin (Mantoux) test. Our state law requires tuberculin testing only every 2 years for nursing home personnel and only every 3 years for public health nurses working in the town's tuberculosis clinic, so I wonder about the necessity for this *annual* testing.

Here are my questions: Can we, as students, refuse to be tested more often than state law requires? Can we possibly suffer ill effects from repeated testing?

A To answer your last question first: literature from the American Thoracic Society shows no indication that annual tuberculin testing can cause ill effects. True, there are warnings and precautions, but not against annual testing.

Testing at your school is in line with what other nursing schools are doing. Other schools *are* testing students annually. If annual tuberculin testing is part of your school's

written policy, you must comply with that policy or risk disciplinary action.

You probably have little cause for worry, but certainly question the policy. Ask your administration for the reasoning behind annual testing. Perhaps the answer will put your mind at ease.

Should annual chest X-rays be required when other tests prove negative?

Q At the hospital where I work, nurses are required to have an annual chest X-ray to screen for tuberculosis (TB)— even when the results of other tests for TB prove negative. I'm so leery of *any* possible risk of radiation exposure that I question this routine X-ray.

Do you think the annual X-ray is necessary if other test results are negative?

A You've got some big guns on your side when you object to routine X-ray screening for tuberculosis.

The Centers for Disease Control (CDC) does *not* recommend annual routine X-rays. However, it *does* recommend a tuberculosis surveillance program for employees in hospitals. This includes giving all employees the tuberculin (Mantoux) test.

Retesting at regular intervals should be determined by the degree of epidemiologic risk. This means that in a hospital with a high quotient of tuberculosis, repeated Mantoux tests would be in order; but in hospitals with less risk, such repeat testing would be unnecessary.

What does CDC recommend if a new or prospective employee shows a positive or significant reaction (an induration of 10 mm in diameter or more) to the initial tuberculin test? That person, according to CDC, should be X-rayed and considered for a year of preventive treatment, consisting of the drug isoniazid (INH), 300 mg daily, in either tablet or liquid form. Repeated X-rays are *not* recommended, and repeated skin tests would be pointless: Once someone reacts to the test with an induration of 10 mm or more, future testing will always show significant results.

Tuberculosis is an atypical disease: Evidence of infection (as shown, for example, by the skin test) does not always equal presence of *active* disease. That's why preventive therapy is so important; it's designed to protect both the health professional and the patient.

But if active disease is present, the employee should be treated with multiple antitubercular drugs.

The CDC policy is in line with the latest recommendations of the American College of Radiology (ACR), which say chest X-rays should be discontinued as part of a routine preemployment examination. In the ACR's judgment, the radiation exposure, cost, and inconvenience outweigh the limited benefits.

One state's department of health services agrees with the CDC and the ACR. The manager of the TB control program said X-ray should not be used as a screening tool because "someone can have TB a long time before it shows up on an X-ray. So routine X-rays become a waste of money and a hardship for the patient." The program recommends the Mantoux test, which they feel has a good track record of accurately indicating the presence or absence of infection.

Before you write a memo to your administration citing these powerful resources, check your facts. Does your hospital's policy *require* an annual chest X-ray, no matter what? Or does it accept the Mantoux test as an alternative?

If your hospital's still determined to demand the annual X-ray, it's obviously out of step. So you can take your stand with confidence.

Should there be more instruction on this?

Q Our small teaching hospital has a new protocol for combating tuberculosis (TB) among staff members: Any employee with a positive purified protein derivative (PPD) skin test receives a 12-month prescription for isoniazid (INH). And that's it. They're not examined, tested, or followed up on any further. We don't have an employee health nurse to instruct the staff on isoniazid's purpose and adverse reactions, so the task falls to me, the nursing staff development instructor. What's your opinion on this new protocol?

A A positive reaction to a PPD test doesn't always indicate *active* TB. It may indicate only *exposure* to the bacilli.

When a hospital employee has a positive PPD, a complete medical workup is necessary. Definitive diagnosis of TB necessitates both a chest X-ray and sputum test, and before treatment the doctor sometimes performs other studies, such as a biopsy. The treatment of choice could be isoniazid, but a positive PPD test by itself does not warrant yearlong medication without follow-up.

Tuition assistance

Can anyone get tuition aid after dropping out of college before?

Q The hospital where I work has a tuition aid fund for employees who continue their education. When I applied for this, I was told that I wasn't eligible because I'd once started college and dropped out. This is true, but the reason I dropped out was financial, not academic, difficulty. Is there anything I can do about it?

A Each institution sets its own rules for educational grants. If your employer's rules preclude help to anyone who had once started and then left college, it seems to us you have three steps to follow. The first is to go to the institution's governing board and try to get them to change the rule—or make an exception in your case. The second is to investigate other institutions' educational funding rules to see if you can find one whose policies are more favorable to your situation. The third is to send $8.95 and a stamp for the National League for Nursing pamphlet, *Scholarships, Fellowships, Educational Grants, and Loans for Registered Nurses,* to National League for Nursing, Ten Columbus Circle, New York, NY 10019.

Twins

Should they be placed in the same incubator for their phototherapy?

Q A set of twins in our nursery became jaundiced and were put under bilirubin lights. But much to my surprise, the resident ordered that they be placed in the *same* incubator for their phototherapy. I think crowding the two babies together like that will cut down on the amount of skin surface exposed to the bili lights and will expose them to more infections. How, for instance, can we stick to the infection control policy of washing our hands between each patient?

Everyone thinks the babies look cute together and can't understand my concern. Am I being ridiculous?

A "Cute" is definitely not the word for the situation you describe. The American College of Obstetricians and Gynecologists recommends at least 20 square feet (1.8 square meters) of space for *each* baby, with at least 2' (60 cm) of space surrounding each incubator.

T

That certainly doesn't support the resident's two-in-one order.

The twins' exposure to the light would probably not be significantly reduced. However, from a safety standpoint, two active babies sharing the same space could knock off each other's mask. In addition, you're right to be concerned about infection control when handling babies in such close quarters: Poor handwashing technique is the single most common vehicle for transmitting organisms and increasing the incidents of colonizations and infections in nurseries.

Until there's valid evidence that putting twins in the same incubator won't harm them, they should be separated.

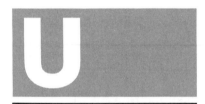

Understaffing

Can you recommend how a nurse can cope?

Q Understaffing at our community hospital is so severe that night after night, I'm the only RN on our medical/surgical unit. Last night, after 4 unbelievably hectic hours, I broke down and screamed at a nursing assistant. When my nurse coordinator heard about it, her only comment was: "I know how bad it is, but do the best you can."

I love nursing, and I'm determined to stay with it and give my patients the best care possible. However, if I'm going to survive in this job during the nursing shortage, I'll have to find some coping strategies. Any suggestions?

A You've already taken the first survival step: You've decided that you want to stick it out. Waffling between staying and leaving a job

is exhausting. But don't be too passive in accepting the bleak staffing situation. At least continue to put in written requests for more help so that administration doesn't take a laissez-faire attitude.

> *"Last night, after 4 unbelievably hectic hours, I broke down and screamed at a nursing assistant."*

Here are some suggestions to help you cope in the meantime:
• Identify and eliminate time-wasting habits, and avoid those around you who constantly complain.
• Plan your most difficult tasks for your most energetic hours so you can get those tasks out of the way with minimum stress. (If you have any doubt as to when you're at your best, track your energy levels several times a day for 2 or 3 weeks, using a scale of 1 to 10, with 10 representing your peak.)
• Ask administration for more non-nursing staff to free you from non-nursing tasks.
• Listen to your body; it will tell you when you're physically tensing up. Here's a trick to help you tune in to it: Pick out a familiar sound that you hear on your unit (an elevator door opening, an intercom message), and use it as your signal to pause for a moment and consciously relax. If your neck and shoulders are tense, do simple head and shoulder rolls; if you have a headache, massage your temples.
• Listen to your thoughts, too; weed out irrational worries, and try to keep your concerns in perspective. And while you're at it, credit yourself for the important work you're doing.
• After hours, get some fun exercise—and try not to take your work worries home with you.

Finally, if things don't improve on the job, consider working a different shift or transferring to another

unit—or even another hospital. Administration will have to get the message eventually.

How can a nurse complain without losing her job?

Q I'm going into my seventh year as the *only* nurse on the night shift of a state university health service, which provides both infirmary and outpatient services for students and employees. I've always enjoyed my job, but now I'm running into a problem.

Here it is: On my shift, I care for the patients in the infirmary as well as outpatients. I also complete the charts of the 65 to 100 patients seen throughout the day. In addition, I do routine preparations for the next day, such as sterilizing equipment and taking inventory.

All this keeps me hopping. But now there's more, and the "more" may be more than I can handle. The administrator has set up a statistical project that entails coding patient diagnoses with computer numbers. He did the coding himself until he got bored with it, then delegated the job to me.

When I objected to adding computer work to the duties I already had, he implied if I continued to object, either I'd be fired or the clinic would be closed nights—thereby eliminating my job.

I need your advice: What can I do *without* losing my job?

A If you're going to make a stand for yourself and your job, you'll need to do some good groundwork. Start by checking your job description. Exactly what did you agree to do? Are routine administrative chores such as computing the diagnosis statistics included or excluded? (Night nurses have the reputation for being not fully occupied, and so traditionally get stuck with a lot of detail work spilling over from the day shifts.) And you know the big trap in health care: If a job needs to be done—and there's no one else to do it—give it to a nurse.

If you don't have a job description, ask for one. It may be your best defense against tedious administrative extras.

Take notes for a week on how you're allocating your time. Clock the hours spent caring for patients, completing the charts, sterilizing equipment, and taking inventory. When you get this information together, does it prove your point: that you were doing 9 or 10 hours' work in 8 *before* the computer responsibility was added?

If you're going to argue for relief, be ready to prove the computer work takes time from *nursing* duties.

Also, remember that the most persuasive arguments won't wash when presented argumentatively. No one—especially a boss—enjoys being backed into a corner. Give him room to maneuver and figure out for himself that you can't do it all.

If, after your best reasoned efforts, you find yourself in a no-win situation with your administrator, you may have to decide whether to stay and adjust to what you consider is unjust, or leave and look for another job.

Without sounding like somebody's grandmother, if the circumstances force you to make a move, who's to say it won't be a move for the better?

How can nurses be more supportive of one another?

Q The surgical department where I work is hectic, with long hours, short staffing, no support from the doctors, and quick turnover in nursing personnel. The nurses who survive this pressure cooker give great patient care, but we have very little camaraderie or support for one another. Nurses put down nurses and often snap out in front of other people—even patients. And if you need a day off and

want someone to switch schedules, forget it.

There's got to be more to life—and work—than this. What can I do to help save this unit?

A You've probably heard that it doesn't take Wonder Woman to bring about change on a unit. But sometimes it sure looks that way. If you're willing to take on the job, it's worth a try.

Call a full staff meeting with the specific goal of exploring the whys and wherefores of your present situation. And request that a managerial or psychiatric nurse consultant sit in to make suggestions. Brainstorm possible solutions. For instance, resolve to document staffing needs and to ask for additional nurses to lighten the burden. Discuss specific ways the doctors could be more supportive, and send your conclusions to the medical chief of the department. And last, but perhaps easiest, sponsor some social activities outside the hospital. Your staff members may just be too busy to get to know each other at work. But given the opportunity, they might even come to *like* one another.

For a while after the meeting (or several meetings, if that's what it takes), expect some exaggerated politeness and artificial behavior. That's okay. It takes time to change what's ingrained. But resolving to make gradual, small changes is the first step in the right direction.

Should a nurse be expected to work a third shift?

Q After coming off a double shift on a medical/surgical unit, my manager asked me to work *another* shift because someone had called in sick. I could barely function at that point, so I refused. I went home and tried to sleep, but I kept thinking about the patients who needed care. Was I ethically responsible for staying to give that care?

A No one should have to bite the bullet repeatedly in a staffing crunch. You were right to refuse a third shift. Did your manager know you'd already put in 16 hours? You could have said something like, "I can't work another shift because I've already worked two in a row. I'm physically exhausted, and I can't think straight." Worn-out nurses shouldn't be caring for patients who may be more alert than they are.

Ensuring adequate staffing is everyone's responsibility. That includes you and your co-workers as well as hospital and nursing administrators. So if the problem continues, take action. With input from your co-workers and manager, make a list of standards for safe patient care. Topping that list should be a statement that nurses won't be asked (or allowed) to work longer than two consecutive shifts.

Identify the reasons for the problem, and suggest possible solutions. Then, you and your manager should request a meeting with administrators to work toward your goal: ensuring safe patient care.

You might also take a closer look at the psychological stressors you're feeling, such as guilt. Where does your guilt about refusing a third shift come from—an outside source (nursing administrators who are pressuring you to work, for example) or your own attitudes (perhaps a feeling that you aren't living up to what a "good nurse" should be)? Once you acknowledge your feelings, you'll be free to say, "I'm right to refuse a third shift. I'm proud of myself for willingly working a second shift and coping well in a crisis."

Should the ED help an arriving patient into the wheelchair or let the family member do it?

Q Can you solve a small problem for me? I'm the only RN in the emergency department (ED) of our semirural hospital. When a patient

U

who's too ill to walk arrives at the emergency entrance, the member of the family or the friend who's with the patient usually asks me for a wheelchair.

When this happens, I'm never sure what to do: Should I take the wheelchair out myself and help the patient into it? Or should I let the family member or friend put the patient into the wheelchair and bring him in?

> *"I'm never sure whether I should help the patient into the wheelchair or let the family member or friend bring him in."*

I don't feel comfortable leaving my ED patients unattended—even for a few minutes. But I would like to attend to the patient on his way in.

Since I can't be in two places at once, what do you suggest?

A The answer depends upon your hospital's policy. Some hospitals won't assume responsibility for the patient until he comes through the door. Some hospitals prohibit a nurse from leaving the ED to assist an incoming patient. Ambulance staff must be called, if necessary, *just* to bring a patient through the door into the hospital.

This does seem a bit extreme, but the underlying goal makes sense: If the nurse is the only one on duty, she doesn't belong on the street—away from her patients. (She should send the unit secretary as a last resort, rather than go herself and leave the department unattended.)

But your problem's bigger than you think. If you can't help an incoming patient because you're the only nurse on duty, you probably have other critical times in your ED that call for you to be in two places at once. It can't be done.

A one-nurse ED is unsafe—no matter how small your hospital may

be. Why not put the problem on your supervisor's doorstep—before you encounter a situation where a patient (or *two* patients) are at risk?

What should be done in emergency situations?

Q Our small community hospital is having great financial problems. Staffing at night is so low that we're worried. We have an RN and one other staff member (either an LPN or nursing assistant) in each department—intensive care, medical/surgical, and the emergency department (ED), plus one supervisor who covers all three.

What happens if we have a code? Although we have an ED doctor on duty, the RN from one department can't leave for a code in another. (The enormity of the problem hit home the other night when a code occurred right before the evening-shift nurses left.)

Our director of nursing knows the situation; she just can't add more staff for emergency situations. Do you agree with our concerns? And what do you suggest?

A Your situation's tough, but it's not surprising in these days of rising costs and nursing shortages. Fortunately, that one close call alerted you to plan for such emergencies, as rare as they may be.

Here's what you can do: Make sure that all nurses are proficient in code procedures. If everyone's prepared properly, three people can conduct a code smoothly. For instance, if a code happens on your unit, get your supervisor and the doctor (who will have to work during the code, not just call orders). Have an RN from another unit assume an "on-call" role; she'll respond if the LPN or nursing assistant on your unit needs help with a nursing procedure while you're on the code.

Very important: Post a "map" outlining what role each person will assume during a code. Staging code drills and evaluating your performance will help reduce anxiety and confusion during the real thing.

If you find yourself in this bind repeatedly, ask your supervisor if your hospital could set up a system of nurses who'd be paid to come in on call and float where needed during the disrupted shift.

"Be prepared" is more than a Boy Scout motto. In an emergency code situation, planning ahead could save a life.

Who's responsible if patients are injured because of understaffing?

Q I work on the seven-bed intensive care unit (ICU) of a small community hospital. Because the postanesthesia room isn't staffed between 3 p.m. and 7 a.m., we're asked to monitor postanesthesia patients during that time. But when we're understaffed, we can't watch any of our patients as closely as we should.

We're uncomfortable about taking on these extra patients because we can't guarantee a safe nurse-patient ratio. If any of our patients suffer because we're understaffed, who's responsible?

A A court could find both the hospital and the nurse involved liable for a patient injury. Here's why: When you accept a patient, the courts expect you to give the level of care that any reasonably prudent nurse would provide. If you can't do that, you shouldn't accept the patient. But the court could also find the hospital responsible for failing to maintain safe staffing levels.

Your best defense is to speak up, loud and clear. If you can't care for postanesthesia patients adequately, tell your manager immediately. Keep your tone nonconfrontational

U

and say that you want to help out if you can. But emphasize your concerns about how this situation jeopardizes patient safety. Then document the conversation in a memo and send a copy to the hospital's risk manager.

Also ask your manager to meet with you and your co-workers to consider solutions to the staffing problem, such as hiring an extra nurse for the evening. When she doesn't have postanesthesia patients, that nurse could float to other units.

Incidentally, if a nurse anesthetist has administered the anesthesia, *she* should remain with the patient, according to the standards of the American Association of Nurse Anesthetists. Until she can entrust him to a qualified nurse—that is, someone who's specifically trained to care for postanesthesia patients—she's responsible for the patient's care. On an understaffed ICU like yours, where nurses can't provide appropriate monitoring, that means the nurse anesthetist should stay with the patient until his vital signs are stable.

Would a step down be a blot on a career record?

Q Eight years ago, I was lucky enough to get a job as staff nurse in a small rural hospital—the only one within commuting distance for me. I was soon raised to team leader, then appointed unit manager.

In the beginning, I loved it. Over the past 3 years, however, the paperwork has increased so much that I'm nothing more than a desk jockey.

We're chronically understaffed and, with no unit secretaries, I can't even delegate any of the paperwork.

My work day now seems like drudgery and I long to be a team leader again.

Such a change would cause work for the administration (getting a re-

placement, shuffling schedules), and I've seen what happens to such cases. The "offender" is punished by getting all the scut jobs—constantly floated, and so on.

My greater worry, though, is that if we ever move and I need references for a new job, won't this "stepdown"—albeit voluntary—look bad on my record? I'd appreciate your thoughts.

A There's nothing wrong with your desire to leave administration and return to direct patient care. If this is where you find the greatest job satisfaction, you're entitled to—indeed, should be encouraged in—your preference.

Would a potential employer see a voluntary step-down as a blot on your career record? No. Dismiss that worry from your deliberations.

Before you apply for the actual change, though, discuss your feelings with someone in administration. Explain about the burden of paperwork and (administrators perk up at this kind of reasoning) point out the wastefulness of paying a unit manager's salary for work that should be done by a unit secretary.

If you get no help, though, make the change. As for getting stuck with the scut work, any hospital that's chronically understaffed is going to need a good team leader—to team lead.

Unemployment compensation

Can it be collected when there's such a nursing shortage?

Q For the past several years, I've worked as a utilization review coordinator. The other day, a discharge planner and I were discussing the problem we'd have returning to hands-on nursing if we ever lost our jobs. Most nursing departments

wouldn't hire someone who hasn't been involved in patient care for over 2 years. But my friend tells me we can't collect unemployment compensation when there's such a nursing shortage. Because we're licensed nurses, we can't even file for it.

Is that true? What can you tell me about the system?

A Nurses who meet the usual eligibility requirements of other workers won't be denied unemployment compensation because they're nurses. Generally speaking, you're eligible if you're unemployed through no fault of your own—whether you've been laid off or fired for not having the required skills. And your eligibility isn't affected if you have any other money (other than wages) coming in.

You're ineligible if you are self-employed, if you quit your previous job without sufficient reason, or if you were fired for committing a willful act.

> *"My friend tells me we can't collect unemployment compensation when there's such a nursing shortage."*

Because of the great demand for nurses, the Job Service Office would probably get you a job sooner than the 6 months usually allowed for unemployment compensation. But you wouldn't have to take just any job you're referred to. For instance, if you can prove you don't have current skills, you might turn down a job in a highly skilled unit. However, you'd probably take one calling for limited nursing skills if the employer provided orientation. You can turn down jobs that are unreasonably hard to get to or that offer significantly less pay than your previous jobs.

If you actually find yourself in this situation, try discussing the specifics of your case with your local un-

U

employment office. Knowing that you're eligible can be a benefit in itself.

Uniforms

Are nurses' caps still in favor?

Q My best friend went back to nursing school to become an RN after working 17 years as an LPN. For all those years, she dreamed about wearing an RN's cap, so even though I've heard that most nurses don't wear them anymore, I'd like to give her one as a graduation gift—even if she just hangs it in her closet. I'm not concerned about the cost—I just don't know how to go about getting the right cap.

A If your friend wants the cap as a symbol of her achievement, then it's a great gift. Although nursing caps have fallen out of favor these days, some nurses still wear them. In fact, there's a wonderful story about some surgical nurses who had their manager's cap bronzed as a retirement gift because they knew how much that cap meant to her.

"I'd like to give my friend an RN's cap for graduation but I don't know how to go about getting the right cap."

Phone the dean of studies where your friend is completing her nursing program; she'll tell you whether there's an official cap representing the school and how you can get one. Otherwise, you can buy a "generic" nursing cap at a uniform store for a modest cost.

Whatever you choose, you've already given your friend the best gift—you've encouraged her over the years to follow her dream.

Can a nurse yell at another nurse if she's not in uniform?

Q I really enjoy my work as a nursing assistant in a large metropolitan hospital—except for one thing. One of the nurses takes out her stress on us—me in particular. Yesterday, before she got her coat off and her cap on, she started yelling at me in front of everyone to hurry up with the breakfast trays.

I didn't answer her back or show in any way how I felt. Now I'm wondering: Can she yell at me when she's not in full uniform? Is this legal?

A Legal, yes; courteous, not very. A nurse gets her authority and responsibility from her license and job description—not from her uniform. That skill doesn't excuse bad manners and even worse "people skills."

Next time, wait for a lull in the verbal barrage and say something like this: "I'm sure you have something important to say to me. But yelling makes me too nervous to hear the message. I'd welcome the chance to discuss this with you in private." Be sure to keep your self-control. Talk slowly and carefully, and use appropriate body language.

If you can keep your cool (while the nurse is losing hers), chances are your message will come through soft and clear.

Is it sanitary for nurses to wear their uniforms on the street?

Q I'm a British nurse who visited my Yankee cousins in the United States this past summer. I was surprised to see so many American nurses wearing their uniforms in the streets, on buses, in stores, and so on. Surely this practice is unsanitary. I even saw one nurse wearing her uniform—with a stethoscope around her neck—in the supermarket!

A As you noticed, uniform practices aren't, well, uniform on both sides of the Atlantic. Most British hospitals have locker areas where nurses can change from street clothes to freshly laundered uniforms furnished and maintained by the hospital. And British nurses generally put on aprons when performing tasks that might soil their uniforms.

In the United States, most nurses do travel to work in their uniforms. If working in a general nursing area, they'll work in the uniform worn from home. After work, they return to the community in the same uniform.

No studies have linked this practice with increased infection rates; neither is there evidence of lowered infection rates in the British hospitals as a result of their uniform precautions.

The differences in dress, though, aren't as wide as the ocean that separates the United States and your country. Some U.S. hospitals do provide lockers and changing rooms for their staff nurses. And in the hospital areas with a high risk of infection (renal units, operating rooms, recovery rooms, and the like), nurses *do* change from their street clothes or the uniform worn from home into a scrub gown supplied by the hospital.

Remember that it's not the uniforms but the handwashing that counts: Many studies have stressed handwashing as one of the chief keys to infection control.

The number of nurses wearing uniforms on the street may not be as large as you think. Some of the "nurses" you saw may have been waitresses or beauticians—many of whom also wear white uniforms in the United States.

U

Unit manager

Are they a "thing of the past?"

Q After many years at home, I've just returned to nursing part-time at a community hospital where, I was surprised to learn, they employ no unit managers. When I asked about this, I was told, "Unit managers are a thing of the past."

That's a new one on me. How do you explain the demise of the unit manager?

A As Mark Twain once said, "The reports of my death have been greatly exaggerated." In hospitals using task-oriented or team-nursing systems, unit managers are very much in evidence. In hospitals using the primary nursing system, however, the title "unit manager" probably won't appear on name tags. That's because primary nursing assigns one nurse to each patient. That nurse is responsible for *all* of that patient's care— including certain duties (such as making sure doctors' orders are followed) that unit managers in other systems usually handle. But *someone,* no matter the title—nurse-manager, supervisor, clinical co-ordinator, or even unit man-ager—must still oversee the department and manage its admin-istrative needs.

So if your hospital uses the pri-mary nursing system, the title "unit manager" may indeed be a thing of the past—at your hospital. But unit managers are still very much alive, well, and busy in many other hos-pitals.

How can a nurse keep a job she's happy with?

Q I'm a diploma school graduate, 45 years old. For 10 years I've been an assistant unit manager, and I'm more than content. I love my job: I work at a desk 3 days a week doing staffing schedules and help-ing the unit manager with paper-work, discipline problems, and evaluations. On the other 2 days, I work directly with patients. My work record has been excellent, and I *know* I get along well with both the nursing and medical staffs.

Here's the problem in my quasi-paradise: When the present unit manager retires next year, I'm afraid I'll be told to earn my BSN degree and prepare myself to be-come the next unit manager.

I don't *want* to go back to school, and I have absolutely no desire to be the unit manager. But I'm afraid if I don't go that route, I'll be trans-ferred to another unit or returned to general duty.

How can I be sure of staying on my unit and continuing to do what I do best?

A There's no cut-and-dried an-swer to your problem. So be-fore you make your plans, you should see the whole picture.

Many nurses are not interested in climbing the career ladder and prefer staying where they are. Like you, these nurses feel comfortable and competent at their present level, and take satisfaction in working di-rectly with patients.

However, if you choose to sit tight, expect pressure from above and below. You could find yourself under pressure from administration to improve your qualifications—or move out of the managerial posi-tion.

About the pressure from below: You'll find younger nurses coming along who can give good care (just as you do), but who are also ex-cellent managers *and* have one or more degrees.

The competition out there is get-ting stronger all the time. On the other hand, it's understandable you wish to do what you do best and feel most comfortable with.

In making your choice, try taking a personal inventory. Collect all your past evaluations; list the qual-ities that rated commendations— your steadiness, enthusiasm, judg-ment, concern for the patients, and so on. Also list the continuing-education courses you've taken over the past 10 years.

If you have a sympathetic super-visor, take your inventory to her and discuss your dilemma. Remind her (in case she needs reminding) of your value to the unit.

The final decision's up to you. You are in charge of your own life, and making decisions is both your great responsibility and your great priv-ilege.

How can nurses persuade administration to keep a unit manager?

Q A few months ago, Dottie, our unit manager, discovered she had multiple sclerosis (MS). She's only 27 years old, and this is her first supervisory job.

Although she doesn't have any symptoms that interfere with her work, her doctor advised her not to work 5 days a week. Too much phys-ical exertion might exacerbate her symptoms.

So for the past month, Dottie's been working 4 days a week—but 10 hours a day. And our unit's still running smoothly.

But this week, Dottie was offered a position in staff development. Well, she wasn't actually *offered* the job, she was informed by the director of patient care services that a unit manager *must* work 5 days a week, with no exceptions. Although the new salary would be equal to her present salary, Dottie doesn't want the new job. She wants to continue caring for patients.

Dottie's a great unit manager, and we don't want to lose her. Our di-rector of nursing feels the same way, but unfortunately, she takes her or-ders from the director of patient care services.

What can we do to keep Dottie as a unit manager? We're willing to fight for her if we have to.

U

A Of course you're willing to fight for a good nurse and good friend. But even though she doesn't want the staff development job, and you don't want her to take it, an administrative job might be better for Dottie.

Besides having flexible hours, the job would certainly be less stressful, and less physically demanding. And as you know, emotional and physical stress exacerbate the symptoms of MS.

When the doctor told Dottie to stop working 5 days a week, what he probably really meant was, start working part-time. Compressing 40 hours' work into 4 days *doesn't sound like part-time.*

But if Dottie's intent on continuing as unit manager, she'll need her doctor's support. If he agrees to Dottie's work schedule, then you and the rest of the staff can go ahead. Document the excellent work Dottie's done as unit manager. Stress that so far her performance and the unit's level of patient care haven't been hurt by her illness. Then take your documentation up through the usual channels of communication.

But if you really care about Dottie, look ahead. Although her illness might not affect her nursing performance, if she continues to work as hard as she's done in the past, her performance might affect her illness—adversely.

Unlicensed nurse

Should another nurse tell on her?

Q Three months ago, I started working as an LPN in a nursing home. When the unit manager introduced me to my co-workers, one of the LPNs pretended not to know me—even though we were in training together. The reason? She flunked out. I guess she's afraid I'll tell someone she's not licensed.

She's very bright, and I don't want to ruin her life. But I feel guilty keeping this secret. What should I do?

A This is a dangerous secret to keep. Hiring an unlicensed nurse—knowingly or unknowingly—is illegal. In most states, practicing nursing without a license, illegally selling or obtaining a diploma or license, and aiding and abetting these practices are gross misdemeanors.

The American Nurses' Association Code for Nurses directs you to safeguard patients who are threatened by incompetent, illegal practitioners. Act quickly: Not only is the nursing home risking its licensure, it also may be compromising patient care by allowing an unqualified person to practice nursing.

To make sure you have the facts straight, talk with your former classmate. Avoid an accusatory tone—after all, she may have nothing to hide. Maybe she earned her diploma elsewhere. Or she might be working as a nursing assistant, not an LPN.

Of course, she may not tell you the truth. She could refuse to talk to you at all. If you still have doubts, go to the unit manager. Ask her to report your suspicions to the home's administrators so they can investigate her background.

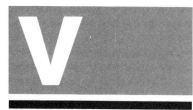

Vacation

Can the administration force an employee to take vacation time?

Q I work for a profit-making hospital where the nurses don't have an employment contract—and aren't represented by a union. My unit is being moved to another area of the building. My supervisor tells us the move will take 2 weeks, and she's given us the choice of either taking our vacation during that time or going without a paycheck until the move is completed.

Some choice. I don't *want* to take my vacation now nor do I want to go without pay. Can the administration force me to choose?

A No. Under the conditions you describe, the hospital is acting illegally. Try to get administration to put the choices they're offering in writing. If you can't get a written statement, write down the choice of options as you understand them, then ask administration to clarify, verify, or deny what you've written. Make a copy for your file.

When your supervisor asks for your decision, explain that neither option appeals to you and ask for an official statement confirming that you're being laid off for the 2-week period. The hospital pays taxes for unemployment compensation, and you should file for unemployment compensation. You could qualify for a week's payment. That's better than nothing—and might make your hospital take notice.

Is it fair to base holiday pay on 8 hours instead of the 10 hours worked?

Q Our hospital recently shifted to 10-hour days and 4-day work weeks. Now, we've been told that holiday pay will be based on an 8-hour day. I think this is very unfair because nurses who work on the holiday will work (and be paid for) 10 hours. The plan also means that a week with a holiday in it will cost RNs nearly $15. Do we have any recourse?

A This sounds like a clash between a *new* schedule and an *old* budget.

The shift to a 10-hour schedule didn't increase the payroll for total

U

work time because each nurse still works a 40-hour week. But the new schedule could cost the hospital a lot of money for holiday pay. Here's why:

Under the old system, you worked 32 hours in a week containing a holiday (4 days × 8 hours per day) and received 8 hours of holiday pay. So a holiday week cost the hospital only 8 hours of "unearned" pay per nurse.

Under the new system, you work only 30 hours in a holiday week (3 days × 10 hours). From your point of view, the hospital should pay for 10 hours on the fourth day so that you'll receive as much as you do in a regular week. From the hospital's point of view, paying 10 "unearned" hours per nurse may be prohibitively costly.

If your hospital employs 100 nurses at $17.50 per hour, paying for 10-hour holidays is going to cost the hospital $3,500 more under the new system ($17.50 × 2 hours × 100 nurses). If your hospital gives each nurse the usual 7 paid holidays per year, the new schedule will cost $24,500 per year more than the traditional 8-hour day schedule.

Both you and the hospital have legitimate arguments, although they should have been settled before the new system was adopted. Perhaps the hospital adopted the new schedule in the middle of the fiscal year and can't pay for 10-hour holidays this year because they aren't budgeted. Or perhaps it never intends to pay.

You should certainly follow through with your side of the argument to find a fair way to handle those problematical 2 hours.

Vaccination

What is b-Capsa I?

Q As a nurse in a pediatrician's office, I've recently had to give infant patients a vaccine called b-Capsa I. Because we've never used this product before, I'm wondering if you can tell me something about it.

A The pediatrician in your office has done his homework on this one. The Food and Drug Administration has approved the first vaccine to prevent *Haemophilus influenzae* type b, the most common cause of bacterial meningitis in children under age 5. Called by the trade name b-Capsa I for *Hemophilus* b polysaccharide, the vaccine gets its name from the organism that causes the disease. The vaccine is recommended for all children 24 months and older, and for those age 18 to 23 months at high risk (children attending day-care facilities, for example). Because the adverse effects are minimal, the vaccine is considered quite safe.

Every year roughly 12,000 cases of meningitis are reported, and approximately one third of the victims suffer neurologic damage or die. So you see, this vaccine is a real breakthrough.

Vaginitis

What is the treatment of choice?

Q Our emergency department doctors don't agree about the treatment of *Gardnerella vaginalis,* so we're having trouble answering our patients' questions. What is the treatment of choice? Do asymptomatic partners need treatment? And is *G. vaginalis* a sexually transmitted disease?

A Researchers haven't established that this type of infection is always sexually transmitted. According to current thinking, gardnerellae act synergistically with anaerobic bacteria to produce bacterial vaginitis, which is characterized by a nonirritating, odorous, thin, grayish-white vaginal discharge.

The Centers for Disease Control (CDC) considers oral metronidazole (Flagyl) the drug of choice, but opinions vary about the regimen. Several studies of women evaluated 7 to 10 days after therapy suggest that a single 2-gram oral dose of metronidazole is as effective as a 7-day regimen of a 400- or 500-mg oral dose twice daily; however, other studies show that patients taking the single dose have an increased likelihood of recurrence several weeks after therapy's completed.

The CDC doesn't recommend treating asymptomatic male partners. Treating the sexual partners of a woman with symptomatic *G. vaginitis* won't reduce her chances for recurrence.

Caution: Pregnant patients shouldn't take metronidazole at all. And any patient taking metronidazole shouldn't drink alcohol during treatment or for at least 24 hours after taking the last dose.

Ventilator patients

Is it safe to use manual ventilation during the time patients are in X-ray?

Q Patients in our neurosurgical intensive care unit who are on ventilators must sometimes go to the X-ray department for computed tomography scans or arteriograms.

Our policy is to supply the patient with oxygen via a manual ventilation bag while he's on his way down to X-ray. Regulations require that an RN accompany and monitor the patient. The ventilator is usually transported with the patient, and once he's in the X-ray department, his ventilator is reconnected and remains connected until the patient's ready to return to the unit.

But we're running into a problem: Occasionally a respiratory therapist will leave the ventilator in the unit and use manual ventilation (bagging) during the entire time in

V

X-ray. Our therapists defend this practice. They say it's safe and saves time. Besides, they contend, they have the *right* to make this decision.

I'm not so sure. I feel responsible for our patients, and I'd feel more secure if they were maintained on their ventilators.

Who's right?

A *You're* right. Following your established policy is better for everyone involved. Manual ventilation could inhibit accurate assessment of the patient's respiratory response and result in unnecessary respiratory distress.

There's another concern: During the X-ray procedure, whoever is manually ventilating the patient would be unnecessarily exposed to radiation. With repeated exposure, the effect could become cumulative.

To solve the problem and return to your safer practice, send a documented memo through nursing and hospital administration channels. Then request a meeting with your immediate supervisor, the director of nursing, and the director of respiratory therapy to evaluate the problem. The best possible outcome for all concerned would be a standardized procedure, in writing, designed for the protection of the patient *and* the staff. Care, not convenience, is the object here.

Where should weaning be done?

Q A new hospital policy calls for transferring stable ventilator patients from the intensive care unit (ICU) to our medical/surgical unit. Last week, we got orders to wean one of these patients; he had no order for cardiac monitoring, nor was a monitor available. Because of our setup, we couldn't observe this patient from outside his room (either through a window or closed-circuit TV). So the other nurse and I had a hectic time taking care of him and

giving barely minimal care to our other patients.

Although we dislike making waves when a policy's so new, we're concerned for *all* of our patients. What do you suggest?

A Any ventilator patient with orders for weaning is usually sent back to the ICU for the day or so it takes to wean him. On a medical/surgical unit with limited staffing, you haven't the time or the setup to continually observe the patient being weaned and still take appropriate care of your other patients.

To ensure safe patient care, all stable ventilator patients admitted to your unit should be put on cardiac monitors and assigned to rooms near the nurses' station so you can observe them more easily.

Make waves.

Verbal abuse

How can a nurse handle a doctor's temper?

Q One of the doctors who admits patients to the hospital where I work has a terrible temper. Just last week, he exploded when a volunteer dropped a glass of orange juice in a patient's room. Then he chewed *me* out in front of the patient and his family. To add insult to injury, my manager told me to let it pass—the hospital needs his business. How can I handle this problem?

A You certainly don't have to grin and bear it. Nobody should have to put up with the abusive behavior you've described.

This doctor is expressing his anger and frustration by making those around him feel inadequate and powerless. If he's charming one moment and in a rage the next, you may feel as if you're constantly "walking on eggs" to avoid another confrontation.

So let the doctor know that his behavior isn't acceptable. Next time

something triggers an explosion, ask him if you can speak with him privately. Then say something like this: "Doctor, I know you're upset about (whatever). But when someone yells, I lose what the person is saying."

Explain to him that patient care is suffering because the staff is on edge. Speak slowly and carefully, and make sure you're specific and objective when you discuss the problem.

Then suggest a solution: "I'd like to work with you to improve our communication. The next time a problem develops, let's step away from other people and discuss it in a reasonable manner."

Also document the conversation in your personal records. If you have to go through channels to resolve future conflicts with the doctor, your notes will back you up.

You may even need a team approach to the problem. Meet with other nurses on the unit and decide how you'll handle this doctor. To present a united front, each staff member should use the same response to his outbursts. Pretty soon, he'll get the message that you won't tolerate his abusive behavior any longer.

Verbal orders

Could a nurse be liable for a doctor's mistake?

Q An emergency department (ED) doctor gave a verbal order for lidocaine. After I administered it, the patient's blood pressure dropped rapidly and he became cold and clammy. The ED doctor said the patient didn't really need the drug, so I shouldn't have given it to him.

Fortunately, the patient recovered quickly. But if he'd been seriously injured, would I have been liable for the doctor's mistake?

A That depends. First and foremost, would the doctor admit to giving the order? If he denied it, your word would be pitted against his. Then you'd have to prove that ED policy allows you to accept verbal orders.

Second, after the doctor gave the order, how much time elapsed before you administered the drug? If you gave it immediately, you'd be in a better position than if you delayed. In the intervening time, the patient's condition could have changed dramatically. That underscores the importance of carefully charting what you do in response to a verbal order.

Finally, in your nursing judgment, was lidocaine indicated for this patient? If so, you acted properly. Remember, you're legally required to follow a doctor's order unless you feel it's inappropriate and potentially harmful.

How can doctors be persuaded to put their orders in writing?

Q One doctor in our emergency department (ED) insists on giving verbal orders—not just in emergencies, but all the time. When we couldn't find a written policy on verbal orders, my manager and I talked with the ED's medical director. At first he was very noncommittal—then he and two other ED doctors started giving verbal orders, too. What's more, none of these doctors ever go back and document anything. So orders for medications, treatments, and so on appear with only nurses' signatures. How can we resolve this situation?

A Verbal orders should be reserved for true emergencies only. Using them in *non*emergencies is asking for trouble.

Like you, a doctor has a legal duty to follow a reasonable standard of care. That includes maintaining adequate written documentation in the patient's record. Neglecting to cosign a verbal order is irresponsible. And it's risky for you, because you have no way of proving that the doctor ordered the medication or treatment.

What about the chance that you could misinterpret an order? Malpractice lawsuits involving this issue usually center on illegibly written orders. But verbal orders are even trickier. You must correctly hear what the doctor ordered, record it on the chart, then administer the medication or treatment. That's too many steps and too many opportunities for an error.

Finally, there's an economic angle: Many third-party payers won't reimburse the hospital unless the medication or treatment was clearly ordered by a doctor.

To correct this dangerous situation in your hospital, first talk with other staff nurses to find out who'd be willing to protest this practice openly. Then, request a meeting with nursing and hospital administration, the ED's medical director, and the hospital lawyer. At this meeting, you should discuss the issues we've just raised. Ask for a hospital policy requiring doctors to write their orders in all situations except extreme emergencies and to cosign any verbal orders within a specified time.

Without a hospitalwide policy, you'll have a tough time convincing the ED doctors to break their bad habit.

Should a unit manager present an instruction as a verbal order from a doctor and then refuse to record it on the chart?

Q I'm a very confused and frustrated nurse on the midnight shift at a chronic care hospital. Here's why.

When I came on duty one night last week, I found a note from our unit manager clipped to a patient's 24-hour report sheet. The note said that the patient's doctor had given a verbal order for a new medication.

> *"I'm a very confused and frustrated nurse on the midnight shift at a chronic care hospital."*

On checking the doctor's orders sheet for the day, though, I saw that the new order hadn't been added. I did give the patient the new medication, but I also wrote on the unit manager's note, "Please record order on doctor's orders sheet," initialed the request, and left the note attached to the 24-hour report.

When the unit manager came on duty that morning, I was finishing my charting at the nurses' station. She read my request on her note, crumpled it up, and threw it in the trash bin without saying a word to me. As she walked away, I retrieved the note.

Incidentally, this particular unit manager frequently makes disparaging remarks about the night shift, and her manner toward us has fostered serious hostilities.

Two days later, the new order still wasn't written on the doctor's orders sheet. I reported the facts to our supervisor, who brought the problem to our senior nursing supervisor and director of nursing. They said the unit manager had done nothing out of the ordinary.

Okay, that's what they say—but I say a unit manager doesn't have the right to present an instruction as a verbal order from a doctor and then refuse to record it on the chart. What do you say?

A Your "write-in" campaign was right on target. The unit manager who took the doctor's verbal order was responsible for recording it on the appropriate hospital forms. And she should have gotten the order countersigned as soon as possible. You're wise to be careful about following any order that's not recorded.

Your "incidental" comment about the unit manager's attitude toward the midnight staff could be the real problem.

Perhaps you and like-minded coworkers could suggest ways to cool the growing hostility. For instance, you could hold a monthly staff development meeting for representatives of all shifts—so each shift could understand the other's problems better. Perhaps a "pep talk" on good communication would help.

In short, your next campaign should focus on having the staff on all shifts talk to each other more—and write less.

Vibrators

Couldn't they cause a venous thrombosis?

Q I'm currently doing private-duty nursing for a 74-year-old man with emphysema.

My patient has a doctor's p.r.n. order for using a vibrator on his chest and back to loosen mucus in his lungs. He also uses the vibrator on his legs and feet to relieve "shooting pains and a burning sensation" that are, he says, an aftereffect of back surgery several years ago. He wants me to do this for him while I'm on duty.

His doctor says I can use the vibrator on the patient's legs as a comfort measure.

I'm concerned that vibration will cause a venous thrombosis leading to a pulmonary embolism, but I can't find anyone who'll comment one way or the other. Can you give me an expert opinion?

A The vibrator won't *cause* a venous thrombosis, but it could aggravate an existing thrombus. So before you use the vibrator, look for

these signs of thrombus: localized pain, redness, heat, swelling, fever. If none of these signs exist, you can feel comfortable going along with the patient's request.

Visitation rights

What do you do when relatives disagree about who may visit a comatose patient?

Q At our skilled nursing facility, we have a 30-year-old auto crash victim who's been in a semicomatose state for 2 years. Recently, his ex-wife and three young children started visiting, and his face lights up when the children appear—a reaction he's never shown before.

When the patient's parents found out about these visitors, though, they were furious. In front of everyone, they told the director of nursing they don't want the ex-wife and children visiting their son—period. Fortunately for the patient, they continue to come anyway but telephone first to find out if he's alone. If the patient's parents do arrive unexpectedly, the director of nursing asks the ex-wife and children to leave right away. The last time this happened, the youngest child cried all the way to the parking lot.

Can't we nurses do more than just document the patient's reactions in our notes? Administration refuses to become involved, claiming there are legal implications. We think a care conference is needed with the parents and ex-wife attending. What do you think?

A You should proceed with discretion. Your motives are undoubtedly of the highest, but getting involved in family dynamics without knowing all the facts can be risky business. As you well know,

the "referee" in a family quarrel is often the one who ends up with the bloody nose.

Not that you have to play a spectator role. Yes, do call a care conference, but limit attendance to the nursing staff, administration, and the patient's doctor (who hasn't been mentioned). Pool your information. What motivated the ex-wife to bring the children to visit? Why do the parents object? Would they relent if they knew how beneficial these visits are to their son? Ask administration to explain any legal implications. Are the parents court-appointed guardians? Is there a court order against visits by the ex-wife? If so, how can this be modified and by whom?

Appoint a spokesperson from the nursing team who will handle *all* future confrontations. Consistency's important here, as is the caring example you're setting. It should help shift the focus away from past history and onto your patient's future.

Visiting hours

How can nurses ensure compliance?

Q Our intensive care unit (ICU) has strict visiting hours, and most families willingly comply. But last week, one patient's wife and daughter refused to leave. They insisted that he wanted them to stay. In the end, we had to call security to evict them, which upset everyone. How could we have handled this better?

A Negotiation and compromise are the keys to resolving a problem of this sort. First, assess family members' anxiety. Are they unnecessarily concerned about their loved one? Certainly if his prognosis were grim, you'd let them stay as long as they wished. But if he weren't in such critical condition, you'd want to find out why his relatives were so worried.

With that information, you could give them the facts they need to resolve their fears. Finally, you should agree on a compromise. You could allow them extra time with their loved one, with the understanding that you'd need uninterrupted time for nursing care after that.

Visitors

How do other nurses keep their cool with pesty visitors?

Q For family reasons, I've switched from the night shift on a medical/surgical unit to its evening shift. I like it and find that things go well until visiting hours—then it's worth your life to get your work done. The visitors are always asking for additional care for the patients or information about the patients' conditions, or are requesting to see the doctor. They're much more trouble than the patients. I mean the people are pests!

How do other nurses keep their cool when working under these circumstances?

A First, consider emotional adjustment—yours and the visitors. You've just come from a shift on which you have rare contact with visitors to one with even more visitors than the day shift, and usually fewer nurses to handle them. That's going to take a little adjustment.

The visitors—family, friends—have just come from their familiar environment to the strangeness of the hospital; then they find their loved one displaced out of his normal role of a well person into the ranks of the sick. These threatening changes call for a lot of adjustments on the part of the visitors. Adjustments that *you* can help them with. And yes, you *can*—once you stop thinking of visitors as pests.

You know, for many years, psychiatric nurses have had a well-deserved reputation for successfully dealing with patients' families. This is, in part, because psychiatric nurses long ago recognized that the patient is most successfully treated when we view him in the context of his total environment. And his family and friends (those visitors) will usually be the primary factor in his environment.

Why can't you adopt this attitude in your work setting? Try thinking of the patient *and* his family as part of your total responsibility. After all, when a patient asks for additional care or information about his condition, or requests to see his doctor, you don't consider him to be a pest. You accept these requests as part of your work. These very same attitudes and skills you use in dealing with anxious patients are just as applicable with visitors.

Once you view the visitors' requests as part of the patient's total picture, you won't find them so annoying. This easing of your resentment is bound to communicate itself to the visitors who can very well respond with a lessening of anxiety (and requests) on their part.

Another positive advantage of better rapport with visitors is that you'll find discharge planning and patient and family teaching *so* much easier.

And that's a plus you won't find hard to adjust to.

Is it legal to give the family member of a deceased patient an oral or intramuscular dose of some tranquilizer?

Q As a nurse in the critical care unit, I must deal with families experiencing shock and grief after the death of a family member. Often, the patient's doctor will write an order on the deceased patient's chart for the nurse to give the family member an oral or intramus-

cular dose of some tranquilizer. Whenever I carry out one of these orders, I worry. Is it legal? After all, the family member is *not* my patient.

A Most nurses run into this situation sooner or later. But very few hospitals have a written policy to protect the nurse who gives medication to a family member.

As you pointed out, the family member's not a patient and hasn't signed consent forms. Suppose he or she were to have an adverse reaction to a tranquilizer? Or have an accident driving home under stress *and* under the influence of the sedative you'd administered? Both you and the doctor could wind up in the courtroom.

Check your hospital's policy and procedure manual as well as your job description. If your hospital doesn't have a written policy permitting the nurse to give medications to family members, tell your supervisor about the problem. She can take it up with hospital administration. The higher-ups may not even be *aware* that doctors *do* order medication for family members after a patient's death.

In general, sedation will only delay the grieving process. In the hospital setting, there are usually people around to be supportive, so a sedative may not be really indicated. If, however, the doctor orders a tranquilizer, you have three alternatives:

1. Urge your hospital to write a policy stating a doctor *can* order medication for a family member, but that the doctor himself must dispense the medication.

2. Urge your hospital to write a policy that allows the doctor to order medication and the nurse to administer it to a family member; but the hospital takes responsibility if the patient suffers an adverse effect.

3. In extreme cases, refer a highly distraught family member to the

V

emergency department. He'll have to sign a consent form in the emergency department, and then he'll be a *real* patient.

Is it reasonable to check a visitor's blood pressure and weight if they ask?

Q Recently I transferred from a medical center to a 35-bed community hospital. I've had some surprises, but the one last week took the prize. A visitor to the hospital wrote an angry letter to the hospital administrator, complaining that I'd refused to check her blood pressure and weight.

Her complaint is true: She was visiting a cardiac patient, and when I went into the room to weigh the patient and take her blood pressure, the visitor said, "Take mine, too, will you?" I said I was sorry but that we weren't allowed to do that, and left the room. I didn't know whether we were allowed or not. Frankly, I was so surprised when she asked that I didn't know what to say. When I repeated the conversation to my supervisor, she thought it was funny.

Unfortunately for me, the visitor happens to be a big contributor to the hospital. As a result, I've been reprimanded, and we've been told to check blood pressures and weigh anyone who asks.

Do you think this is reasonable?

A The policy may be reasonable but the reprimand certainly wasn't. From your supervisor's reaction, your hospital probably *didn't* have a policy of providing such a service, so you were right to refuse it. The administrator should have supported your response when the visitor complained. When the administration unfairly reprimanded you, the director of nursing should certainly have defended you.

If you meant by the "reprimand" that you were just criticized verbally, you may want to forget the whole thing. But if you were officially reprimanded—an action that may affect your chances for promotion and merit raises—you should certainly follow your hospital's grievance procedure and get the reprimand withdrawn.

Is the new policy reasonable? The hospital certainly needs to give the policy careful thought: Is there need for this service, or is some other organization (such as a public health agency) already meeting the need? How many requests for this service are likely? Does the present nursing staff have time to handle these requests?

If the community needs the service and the staff is able to provide it, the medical and nursing directors should define the policy carefully, including specific guidelines concerning:
• how the hospital should inform the community that the service is available
• what the nurses should tell a visitor who has a high blood-pressure reading
• where they should refer someone with a high reading.

What can be done about visitors' rude behavior?

Q I've been an intensive care unit (ICU) nurse for 8 years. We've always issued printed sheets outlining the standard ICU visiting privileges (one person, 5 to 10 minutes every hour, at the discretion of the nurse) and the purpose of these rules.

Over the past 2 years, we've noticed a growing disrespect for the rules. Families feel free to walk into the unit almost anytime and they become hostile when asked to wait outside. Rudeness has become the norm, and visitors think nothing of snapping orders at a nurse who is already busy with another patient. They use the visitors' lounge as a forum to criticize the care we give and stir up other families.

I can't tell you the number of times our poor administrator has been plagued with absurd complaints ("My daughter had to wait 10 minutes for a nurse—I timed her. And you call this an intensive care unit?" As later unfolded, two of the staff were on dinner break, the rest of us had an emergency procedure, and the daughter's need was for facial tissue! That's a fact.)

Has anybody else experienced this change in attitude?

A Judging from the number of hospitals that have changed from the old standard ICU hours, a lot of other nurses must have experienced your problem.

Today, many ICUs follow this schedule: two visitors for 15 minutes at 10-2-7 or at 10-1-4-7. All visits, of course, are still at the discretion of the nurse.

Why should this new schedule work better than the old? Look at it from the viewpoint of the families.

Unlike us, most people would never willingly choose a hospital as a place to spend 8 hours a day. Yet that's what the old schedule forces them to do. The 50 minutes between patient visits is seldom enough time to let families leave the hospital premises to pursue their normal business. So, in a sense, they're chained to the waiting room. The reward for this enforced "imprisonment" is a mere 5 or 10 minutes with their loved one, which, in their anxiety, often seems more like 5 or 10 seconds. Further, they're not only distraught about their loved one's condition, but many of them are downright horrified at some of the necessary procedures being carried out.

In the hothouse atmosphere of an ICU waiting room, commonly shared fears and anxieties not only can be magnified, but also completely distorted. Under these conditions, even sensible people become unreasonable and hostile.

V

The new hours, by directing longer intermissions between visits, allow the visitors to pick up the threads of their normal lives. They can leave the hospital between visits and channel their emotions in the more usual, constructive manner.

> *"Rudeness has become the norm, and visitors think nothing of snapping orders at a nurse who is already busy with another patient."*

The 15-minute visits themselves seem more satisfactory. When the family see that 15 minutes is just about the limit an intensely ill patient can handle, they leave agreeably rather than with feelings of having been deprived. Give the new schedule a try.

Even under the best of circumstances, of course, you'll run into some troublesome people. When you do, remind them, "Look, every minute I have to spend with you is one less minute I get to give to your loved one."

And of course, for the absolutely impossible visitors, call the security guards. After all, you're the nurse. *They're* the police.

What should be done if a visitor aggravates the patient's problem?

Q Every so often, a visitor upsets one of our patients. When this happens, we're never sure how to handle the problem—especially if the visitor is a family member.

Just last week, a patient who was recovering from a myocardial infarction was visited by his sister. When I walked past my patient's room, he and his sister were obviously having an argument. He was so upset I politely asked his sister to leave. She left in a huff. But she returned the next day—and the whole episode was repeated.

Luckily, the patient's sister was in town for only 2 days, so the problem resolved itself. But I'm not sure what I would've done otherwise. What's the best way to handle a sticky situation like this?

A Tactfully, but assertively. When you noticed your patient and his sister arguing, you should've asked the sister to step outside the room. Then you might've said something like "The conversation between you and your brother seemed to be upsetting him, and right now, he needs to stay calm and quiet. If you have a family problem, perhaps you could wait until he feels better."

Then remind your patient that he needs to avoid stress, and ask him if he'd prefer *not* to see his sister. If he still wants to see her, you'll have to go along with his decision. But if he *doesn't*, reassure him that you and the staff will take responsibility—he won't have to worry about hurting anyone's feelings.

Inform the sister and the rest of the family of your decision. Then put a note on the patient's door: "All visitors please report to the nurses' station before entering."

When your patient's feeling better, ask him if he wants the restriction lifted. He may be ready and able to run his own interference.

Vital signs

What can be done when a nurse suspects that vital sign readings are being faked?

Q Most of my 8 years as an RN have been spent in acute care. But with two young children, all I can manage now is working weekends in a 75-bed nursing facility near my home.

I've run into a disturbing problem: I've noticed a discrepancy between the vital signs I take on weekends and those recorded during the week. One patient's pulse measures 42 to 52 beats/minute. During the week, his pulse is recorded as 70 to 72 beats/minute. Then there's a second patient whose pulse measures from 120 to 140 beats/minute. But when I check the records, I find his pulse recorded as 80 to 82 beats/minute during the week. (This patient told me he's *always* had a rapid heartbeat.)

I began to suspect that vital signs weren't being taken during the week—but being recorded nonetheless as "normal." Since both of these patients are taking digoxin (Lanoxin) and antihypertensive drugs, vital signs are truly vital for monitoring drug effects.

When our director of nursing went on vacation and I filled in for her, I confronted the two nurses who seemed responsible for the contradictory measurements. They assured me they *were* taking vital signs, but had nothing to say when I asked for an explanation of the discrepancies in our measurements.

I didn't press the matter any further, but when the director of nursing returned, I discussed the problem with her and with the nursing home administrator. We agreed on a nurses' meeting to discuss the issue.

Two weeks have passed, and no meeting has been scheduled. What can I do now?

A If nurses are recording vital signs that were never taken, obviously this is a serious matter. Is it possible, however, that these patients are going to physical therapy on weekday mornings (and not on weekends)? If so, no wonder the pulse rates change Monday through Friday.

On the other hand, if the two nurses *were* responsible for the in-

V

accurate measurement (remember, you don't *know* this for sure), your direct confrontation has to be counter productive: What would you expect from the nurses but denial?

Your objective is to remedy a situation that's potentially dangerous to patients. So go back to square one and do the following:

• On Monday morning, talk to the unit manager about the problem: Deal solely with the discrepancies you've observed.

• File an incident report if you find discrepancies continuing.

• Suggest that the director of nursing reinforce the importance of taking accurate vital signs.

What is the accepted range for newborns during the first 24 hours?

Q What is the accepted range for vital signs of newborns during the first 24 hours, and how frequently should we check them?

A A minimal schedule for monitoring vital signs in normal neonates is every 15 minutes for at least 1 hour, every 2 hours for the next 8 hours, and every 4 hours up to 24 hours.

Ranges for vital signs will vary according to the number of hours since birth and the infant's behaviors (sleeping, crying, and so forth). Core body temperature is usually 96° to 99.5° F (35.5° to 37.5° C). Pulse and respirations range from 120 to 140 beats/minute and 30 to 60 breaths/minute, respectively. Count for a full 60 seconds to detect irregularities in rate or rhythm; check the heart rate apically with a stethoscope.

Finally, although it may not be routine procedure where you work, you should take a newborn's blood pressure to establish a baseline. The average systolic blood pressure is from 50 to 70 mm Hg, and diastolic pressure is from 25 to 45 mm Hg.

Vocal cord paralysis

Has a change in endotracheal intubation increased the incidence?

Q Recently, I had abdominal surgery that went fine, but I experienced paralysis of my left vocal cord from the endotracheal tube and cuff. After 3 months, my voice is almost back to normal, but it was one scary experience. In 12 years of nursing, I can't remember this happening to anyone with scheduled nonneck surgery. Yet when I checked with a lawyer, he said that vocal cord paralysis of up to 3 months is considered an assumed risk of intubation and not at all unusual.

> *"I was very surprised that I experienced paralysis of my left vocal cord from the endotracheal tube and cuff when I had surgery."*

Has a change in technique caused an increase in the incidence of vocal cord paralysis? Or am I just more aware of the problem?

A Intubating technique remains unchanged. It's just that the larynx is subject to injury throughout intubation. Some injuries are sequelae of pressure on the recurrent laryngeal nerve by the tube or cuff of the tube. (Low-pressure cuffs usually help prevent this problem.)

The most common postintubation complaint is sore throat (16%), followed by severe sore throat (3%), hoarseness (2.5%), sore throat with severe hoarseness (0.8%), and lost voice (0.4%). More women (because of the thinness of their mucosa) experience these symptoms than men.

Volunteering

Could a nurse-volunteer be held liable?

Q I'm one of two licensed professionals on the board of directors for our community's volunteer suicide-prevention organization. Although my master's degree in psychiatric and mental health nursing makes me a "mental health professional," I don't answer the crisis telephone or train volunteers. But I do give lectures on suicide for the organization.

Our lawyer says the board doesn't need liability insurance. He's basing his recommendation on cost concerns and the existence of a Good Samaritan law in our state. I'm wondering, though: As a professional, could I be sued by family members who blame me for not stopping a suicide, or who claim I put ideas into a teenager's head during a talk at his school?

A It's a sad commentary on our litigious society when someone who's volunteering for a worthwhile cause has to worry about being sued. Unfortunately, your fears are well-founded.

You *can* be sued as a professional—even though you're working as a volunteer without pay. Should you be sued, the plaintiff's lawyer would attempt to show that you were acting as a professional, and so should be held to the same standards of care as any other professional nurse.

Your state's Good Samaritan law wouldn't cover you. Usually, these laws protect health care professionals only when they're giving care at the scene of an emergency. Lectures in the community don't fall into that category.

You need personal liability insurance, which should cover you any time you're sued in a professional capacity. To protect yourself further, consider keeping a list of those who attend your lectures (if possible) and general notes to prove what you said. That way, you'd have backup if a plaintiff misrepresents something that you said.

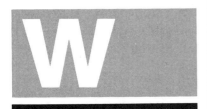

Waiting

How long is too long to keep a nonemergency patient waiting?

Q Patients who come into our office usually have to wait a half hour or more before the doctor sees them. And although they don't complain to him, I overhear their angry comments to one another. How long is too long to keep a nonemergency patient waiting?

A There's no law, but a 15-minute wait—no longer—seems reasonable. Anything longer warrants an apology (from you) and a brief explanation. Occasionally, of course, an emergency can't be deferred, but if a half-hour wait is the norm, your appointment schedule should be revamped—without delay.

Walking report

Isn't it cruel to disturb the sick for report?

Q Just recently, our medical/ surgical unit initiated walking report. Both the night and the oncoming staff go into the patient's room, switch on the overhead light, and give report, usually before 7 a.m. I think it's cruel to disturb the sick for *our* report. One patient made his opinion clear when he said, "I'm not coming here again."

My sister works for a competing hospital; she says that walking report went out with bell-bottoms. What do you say?

A Now, with diagnosis-related groups, a patient spends less time in the hospital, and the nurses face more demanding care for sicker patients. Within that tighter time frame, walking reports become counterproductive.

Other reasons for not holding walking report are the disturbance to the patient (as you pointed out) and the inhibiting effect on the nurses who can't speak as freely as they do in a sit-down conference.

Remember, though, you'll always have a few instances when the whole staff could improve care and benefit themselves by observing the dressings, tubes, and so on of an especially sick patient. Or you might have an occasional patient who needs to feel he's participating in his own care. Be flexible, and schedule walking report for these patients.

Wandering patient

Could threatening a patient be considered assault?

Q Recently, one of the residents at the nursing home where I work wandered downstairs in the middle of the night. After trying unsuccessfully to get him back to his room, my co-worker said to him, "If you don't go upstairs right now, I'll take you back in the elevator." This man is afraid of elevators, so he complied immediately. I know my co-worker thought she was doing what was best for him, but I'm concerned about her making threats. Could that be considered assault?

A That depends. In most jurisdictions, assault is defined as an action or behavior used to threaten physical or psychological injury or fear. As you noted, your co-worker had good intentions, so she probably wasn't guilty of assault.

Still, you're right to question her methods—a nursing intervention shouldn't exploit a patient's fears.

What is a nurse's responsibility if a patient sustains an injury?

Q One of my patients, a 74-year-old woman, has started getting out of bed in the middle of the night and wandering the halls. She fell once (without injuring herself), so we got an order for restraints. When her son found out, he convinced the doctor to write an order for no restraints. He wants his mother to maintain a sense of independence, so he doesn't want her restrained.

I appreciate his feelings, but I'm concerned about his mother. I'm also worried about my liability if she were injured. What should I do?

A As long as the doctor's order is clearly documented, you wouldn't be responsible for any injuries the patient might sustain during her late-night wandering.

But you must question an order that doesn't seem appropriate. First, talk to your patient's son. He may not realize that his good intentions could harm his mother.

If he still stands firm against restraints, go to her doctor and discuss the situation. In her chart, document the problem and any conversations you've had with the doctor or the son. That may get the doctor moving because he won't want her chart to show that he didn't address a problem he knew about.

You can try to curb your patient's travels by checking on her more frequently. Make sure her bedrails are up, her bed is in the lowest position, the wheels are locked, and her call light is within easy reach.

W

Who's responsible if a patient harms himself or somebody else?

Q I've just taken a job at a 25-bed acute care hospital in the Rocky Mountains. I'm enjoying the scenery, but I've already run into a problem.

Let me explain: Since there are no other nursing facilities for geriatric patients within a 100-mile (160-km) radius, we must handle the care of these patients.

Currently, we have six long-term geriatric patients; almost all have organic brain syndrome. Incidentally, I mean *long-term.* Several of these patients have been here almost 10 years.

What concerns me is a 76-year-old male patient who has adult-onset diabetes mellitus, an amputation of his left foot, and severe confusion. More than once he's left our facility without permission. We never know whether we'll find him entangled in barbed wire, hitchhiking out on the highway, or ordering a steak dinner (without money) in a downtown restaurant.

Just yesterday he stole an employee's car (the keys shouldn't have been in the car, I know), and drove more than 25 miles (40 km) over an unpaved mountain road—in first gear. A sheriff's deputy found the patient and returned him to us.

We don't have either the facilities or the staff to keep this patient out of harm's way, but nevertheless, this man with wanderlust *is* my patient. Who's responsible if he harms himself or somebody else? I'm wondering: Could I end up in court or lose my license?

Our administrator insists that the patient's responsible for himself. What do you say?

A There's no easy solution to your problem. But both the nursing staff and the hospital *do* have a legal duty to maintain a safe and adequate standard of care for each patient. Certainly this standard becomes difficult to maintain when the patient's confused and being cared for in an inappropriate setting.

But once the hospital accepts such a patient, it's obligated to provide an *appropriate* setting.

> *"We never know if we'll find the patient entangled in barbed wire, hitchhiking out on the highway, or ordering a steak dinner somewhere."*

The harsh fact is the hospital *and* the nursing staff run the risk of being held liable if the patient injures himself or someone else when he wanders off.

Since you're faced with a legal and moral obligation to protect your patient, check frequently on his whereabouts when you're on duty, and document this information. For example, note "4:40 p.m.: patient watching TV in his room." Also fill out incident reports whenever his whereabouts are unknown.

If the patient has no relatives, have his doctor or the hospital administration bring the county welfare department in on the problem. If a welfare investigation determines that the patient's not legally competent, he could become a ward of the court or the state. Once that happens, you can take steps (if you have to) to find a more protective environment for this patient.

Do not overlook protecting yourself. Do the prudent thing: Write a documented memo stating your concerns (and ask other nurses to sign it, too). Send the memo through channels; at the same time, request a meeting to review safety measures that might forestall further incidents.

You've certainly walked into a challenging situation, but you sound like you intend to handle it.

Water pitchers

Should they be left at the bedside of patients on fluid restriction?

Q We have a conflict about whether or not to leave water pitchers at the bedside of oriented patients on fluid restriction.

What do you say?

A The only person who can tell you the answer to this one is the patient himself. One patient may need a policeman: If you pour his water allowance into his pitcher and leave it at his bedside, he'll drink the whole amount in the first hour. Then he'll beg for more. Another patient may welcome the independence of monitoring for himself how much he's allowed hour-by-hour during the shift.

It helps to remember that you're not going to change a patient's long-standing personality in the short time you have him as a patient. He knows for himself what he's like—ask him, and act accordingly.

Pitcher at the bedside or not, make sure any patient on fluid restriction realizes that every milliliter he drinks counts. At home, he'll have to take over monitoring fluid intake for himself whether he wants to or not.

Weapons

Should a nurse turn over a weapon she finds in a patient's coat pocket?

Q A colleague in the emergency department was recently assigned to an unconscious patient who'd been injured as he was fleeing the scene of a robbery. She was going through his coat pockets to look for ID when she found a gun. She immediately turned it over to a police officer. Was that the right thing to do?

A Yes and no. Because she wasn't actually looking for evidence, she could legally remove the gun without violating the patient's constitutional right to protection against unreasonable search and seizure.

> *"The nurse was going through the patient's coat pockets to look for ID when she found a gun."*

But she shouldn't have given the gun to the officer. She should have turned it over to her manager, who would have decided how to handle it. If her manager had given it to the officer, she would have asked for a receipt.

What if your colleague *had* been asked to search for evidence? She could have legally done so if the officer had presented a search warrant or if the patient had been under arrest.

Of course, hospital policy will guide your actions. At some hospitals, a nurse in this situation would call security immediately and a security officer would take over. She wouldn't be allowed to touch the weapon. You might ask your manager to review hospital policy with the staff so you'll be prepared for the next time something like this happens.

If you can obtain or take charge of evidence, remember these points:
• Identify and label the evidence.
• Give the patient a receipt for all personal belongings you take. Also keep a copy of this receipt for hospital records.
• Preserve the evidence in its original state; that is, protect it and handle it as little as possible.
• Obtain the signature of anyone who handles evidence that's in your custody.
• Ask for a receipt when you give it to the police.

Weight loss

Can a nurse legally monitor it without a doctor's supervision?

Q I'm a nurse in a public health agency where I see patients who may or may not have their own doctors. I'll often encounter obese patients who aren't receiving any medical attention at all or whose doctors have given them only vague orders to "lose weight."

I'd like to help these patients lose weight, but I'm concerned about my legal standing: Can a nurse legally monitor weight loss without infringing on medical territory— whether or not the patient is under medical care?

A Since many states have expanded their nurse practice acts in the last decade, patient education on weight loss is probably accepted nursing practice. You'd probably risk legal problems *only* if you were to deal with medications.

But be on the safe side. Check with your employer, state department of public health, and state nursing board to learn what regulations each has on monitoring weight loss. For example, must your patient be under a doctor's orders?

Be sure of your ground: If you were to inadvertently violate existing regulations, *you'd* have a lot to lose.

Withholding information

Were we justified in keeping the truth?

Q A woman who was in a car accident with her teenage son was admitted to our medical/surgical unit with fractured ribs, con-

tusions, and abrasions. Nearly hysterical with worry, she kept asking us about her son's condition. Unfortunately, he died in the emergency department (ED) shortly after she was transferred to our unit. We decided not to tell her until her husband arrived to give her emotional support. When she finally learned the truth, she cried out, "Why did you lie to me?"

Were we justified in keeping the truth from her? What else could we have done?

A In this case, you probably made the right decision. Physically and emotionally, your patient's husband was in better shape to receive the news first, then decide how and when to share it with his wife.

When you withhold information temporarily, though, you should avoid misleading the patient or giving false hope. For instance, don't say, "I'm sure he's okay" or "He has one of the very best doctors." Instead, you could say, "I've called the ED, and I'm expecting the doctor to call when he's free." You might add, "Your son is in critical condition. I've called your husband, and I hope to have more information for you as soon as he arrives."

But those answers won't satisfy every patient. For some, hearing the truth is better than hearing nothing and sensing the worst—especially if the patient's anxiety compromises his own recovery. If you feel that's the case, consult with the patient's doctor, tell the patient, then call in the hospital chaplain to provide extra support.

What should be done if a nurse feels uncomfortable about it?

Q One of my patients recently had a biopsy for prostate cancer. Although the test was positive, the man's wife asked the doctor not to disclose the results. So, the doctor told the patient that the results were "inconclusive." I'm very uncomfortable about this. What should I do?

A Your observations and assessment can be valuable in helping to resolve this problem. Because the doctor was so vague, the patient is bound to start asking for more details—"Will they have to do the test again?" "When can I get out of the hospital?" or "Why did my doctor say I might have to have surgery?" Carefully document his questions, along with any anxiety the patient expresses over the lack of information about his biopsy and prognosis.

Armed with this documentation, discuss the situation with the doctor. He may have a good reason for withholding the test results at this time. For example, the patient may have a history of severe depression associated with bad news.

In most circumstances, though, a patient has the right to expect full disclosure of information about his medical condition. He needs a complete, accurate explanation before he can give informed consent for any treatment the doctor contemplates. He may also need to make plans for the future, such as writing a will, signing a living will or durable power of attorney for health care, or delegating financial responsibility.

If you feel the patient isn't getting the information he needs to make informed decisions, you may have to get your manager involved.

What should be done if a patient's accusing the staff?

Q A week ago, we got the results of a patient's liver biopsy: widespread metastases from her cervical cancer. Her doctor wants to wait until she's stronger before he tells her. When she asks us, we're supposed to tell her the results aren't back yet. But now she's accusing us of keeping something from her. What should we do?

A Most nurses are uncomfortable about lying to a patient. But many recognize what's called "therapeutic privilege," that is, withholding some or all of the truth in the patient's best interest.

In this case, you may want to call a patient care conference to discuss your concerns. The doctor might explain some evidence in her medical or psychological history indicating that she can't handle the results right now.

Weigh all the information against these ethical considerations:
• You have a moral duty to tell your patient the truth, except when doing so would endanger her life or mental health.
• She should know the truth so she can take steps to plan her future.
• Her growing suspicion is causing anxiety and distrust that may hinder her recovery.
• Recent studies show that most patients who have life-threatening illnesses want to know their prognoses.

Withholding treatment

How can a nurse be sure she's acting in her patient's best interest?

Q I work in a small midwestern hospital. One of my patients is 93, terminally ill, and unaware of her surroundings. She's fed by a nasogastric tube and receives antibiotics for infections.

Because I believe these treatments just prolong the dying process, I'm uncomfortable administering them. How can I be sure I'm acting in my patient's best interests?

A In the kind of situation you describe, nurses can rarely be "sure" they're acting in a patient's best interests. That's what makes it so difficult.

As the patient's advocate, you have to rely on the answers to these questions: What's her prognosis? Is she likely to regain consciousness? Does she seem to be suffering? What does her family want? And most important, what would *she* want?

If you know that she previously expressed a desire *not* to be kept alive under these circumstances, talk to her doctor and suggest that he discuss discontinuing treatment with the patient's family members. With their support, he may agree to end those treatments that only postpone death. Because of the rising number of malpractice suits these days, the doctor really has to make sure patients (if possible) and their families fully understand and agree to the life-support measures he has in mind.

Of course, your patient may have no family to speak for her. That's why you should help establish an ethics committee at your hospital. You need clear policies about heroic measures, patient rights, and informed consent.

Besides setting policies, an ethics committee will give you a forum for expressing similar concerns in the future. You shouldn't have to shoulder these ethical burdens alone.

Should a nurse be a witness to her patient's request?

Q One of my patients—a woman with end-stage renal disease—wants to stop her dialysis treatments. She says they seem more like torture than treatment. Now she wants me to witness her request to withhold the treatment. I'm not sure I want to help her die this way. Can you give me some guidelines for making my decision?

A Perhaps the best guide is to ask yourself this: *What would I want a nurse to do for me in this situation?* Then consider these questions: Can the patient's disease be cured? Is she a candidate for renal transplantation? If not, does she say she's ready to die? Does she believe the pain, risks, and cost of her treatments outweigh the benefits?

In this case, honoring your patient's right to refuse dialysis treatment wouldn't mean abandoning her altogether. She'd need plenty of palliative care (including pain and symptom management) and emotional support. So your nursing skills—particularly your ability to comfort—would still be important.

Witnessing

What is a nurse's responsibility in witnessing wills?

Q Occasionally, patients in the nursing home where I work ask me to witness their wills. I've always agreed. But now, another nurse says I shouldn't sign a will unless I've read and understood it. I've never read the wills I've witnessed because I think they're private. Just what is my responsibility?

A Your co-worker is wrong. You *don't* have to know, understand, or approve of the contents of a will before witnessing it. In general, your signature on a will means three things: that the will writer acknowledges the will as his, that he appears competent, and that he's not under duress.

If you ever have doubts about witnessing a signature, contact the nursing home's lawyer for advice.

Work load

Any suggestions for adjusting to a slower pace?

Q In my first job after graduation, I was team leader on a 43-bed medical/surgical unit of a large teaching hospital. I was personally responsible for twenty of the patients, and I had two nursing assistants and one LPN to help me, if I was lucky.

I put in a tough first year: overtime three and four times a week; 10-minute lunch breaks, and chronic staff turnover and shortages.

I've just escaped from that "pit," and now I'm working in a smaller private hospital with half the responsibilities I had in the first job. Sound good?

The truth is I'm having trouble adjusting to the slower pace. I miss the hustle-bustle of the past year. I had plenty of problems, and the job was hard, but I learned a great deal— and became an independent, self-motivated nurse.

I'd welcome a word of wisdom from you.

A Don't be hard on yourself for your seemingly contrary reaction. Many bright, young, energetic nurses have to choose between a hectic, challenging, overdemanding job and a more routine, slower paced job.

You can probably sense which job suits you better—at a particular time. But of course the "right" answer for you should be a good mix.

Maybe you can try to do some mixing on your own: Add a professional challenge to your present job by putting your overflow energy into completing a degree or by taking some continuing education courses. When you hear about new procedures that are being introduced or an interesting staff development presentation at the hospital you just left, why not request permission to "sit in"?

Or if these suggestions seem too much like patchwork, look for a job that could combine the best of the two extremes. How about a job at a smaller university-affiliated hospital? (This just might provide the stimulation of your former job, yet at the same time provide better staffing and a more reasonable pace.) Or look into a job in a hospital clinic, which should mean Monday through Friday hours—with weekends to yourself.

You do have choices. But whichever way you go, keep your ambition and enthusiasm in good working order. They'll serve you well, whatever job you take.

How can anyone cope with added charting responsibilities when already overworked?

Q Our director of surgical nursing told us that we RNs must make notes on all our patients—every day and every shift. This is in addition to the charting customarily done by LPNs and nursing assistants.

Does this new administrative ruling makes sense to you? We currently practice "crisis nursing"— running from one problem to the next. The 50-bed general surgical unit I work in cares for acutely ill preoperative and postoperative patients. Typical staffing for the day shift is two RNs, two medication-qualified LPNs, one nonmedication-qualified LPN, and three nursing assistants. The night shift has only one RN.

The additional charting our director insists upon will cause serious neglect of other (and I think more important) patient care duties. But our noncompliance with the new ruling would probably result in disciplinary action.

How can we get the director to listen to us?

A Your first step should be to ask the administration *why* they introduced the new charting requirement.

Even when you find out, you'll still have a problem. No matter what the administration's reasoning is, two RNs in your spot aren't going to have time to do the charting *and* take care of their patients.

W

You may not like the next step—because it means *more* documentation for you—temporarily.

For the next 2 or 3 weeks a group of your nursing staff should document activities, patient load, hours of nursing care required, and amount of time spent documenting. Try to discover how the situation at your hospital compares to nurse-patient ratios at nearby hospitals. (The accepted standard for "reasonable work load" is that followed by hospitals with similar patient populations in similar localities.)

Send your documented report up through nursing channels. Be sure to stick to facts and observations only. Don't add any opinions or conclusions—no matter how accurate you think they are.

Once administration has had a chance to review the written report, ask for a meeting to discuss the problems facing your unit, particularly the problems of staffing and charting.

True, this approach demands a lot of work and courage. But we think it's the way to improve the situation.

Grumbling to your co-workers may make you *feel* better, but documentation should be a better route to your document-minded nursing administration.

How should it be handled if it's unfair?

Q I've read several nursing articles lately on how to delegate work to your staff. The problem is that I'm the delegatee—not the delegator. And our unit manager delegates so much that I end up running my legs off while she sits behind her desk. This doesn't seem fair, and I find myself grumbling about it as I work. Any suggestions?

A Stop grumbling, and let your fingers do the walking. Look in the hospital policy manual for the job descriptions of both a unit manager and staff nurse. You may find

that the unit manager is delegating exactly what she's supposed to. And just by reading her job description, you'll get a better perspective on her work load, which may be heavier than it looks.

However, if you find you're routinely being assigned responsibilities that aren't in your job description, ask to meet informally with your unit manager. Focus your discussion on your job description and how it relates to your heavy work load. Stay away from accusatory "you" messages ("*You* assigned extra duties."). It certainly won't help your cause any to engage in a personality duel with your unit manager.

Here's an approach you might try: "My work load is very heavy. (Give some examples.) I'm finding it difficult to accomplish all that I'm supposed to, let alone taking on tasks that aren't in my job description. (Give examples of assignments that aren't in your job description or that complicate your work schedule.) I'm hoping that a review of my assignments will show that I need some relief, and soon."

Wait for a few days. If your message hasn't gotten through and the problem continues, tell your department supervisor. It's her job from there.

If an incident occurs, would the LVN or RN be responsible?

Q Because no registered nurses are available for weekend duty in the hospital where I work, the nursing office now designates a licensed vocational nurse (LVN) as the weekend charge nurse on several units. I'm an RN filling in as a substitute on a unit where an LVN is in charge.

I don't mind this somewhat odd arrangement because I don't feel qualified to be in charge of a unit I don't know well. But if an incident

should occur that later develops into a court case, would I be considered responsible—since I'm the RN with more education than the LVN in charge?

A Relax. The simple answer is: The LVN would be responsible. Why? Because you haven't agreed to any supervisory duties, and the LVN has. She was *officially* in charge. You were not.

However, simple answers often have modifying ifs, ands, and buts: This case is no exception. In most states, licensed vocational or practical nurses are defined by the law as practicing under the "direction of a registered nurse." This restriction usually means that there's an RN on the unit to supervise the LVN. (This is sometimes broadly interpreted to mean that the RN doing the supervising isn't *on* the unit but is somewhere in the hospital.)

Your hospital seems to be taking this view of supervision. The bottom line is that the person who designates the LVN as charge nurse is considered the "supervisor." This "supervisor" could conceivably be found liable for negligent supervision if the LVN should be found not qualified or competent to handle the assignment.

But you should have concerns other than legal. Where do you go if you have problems? Who'll give you information, support, and guidance if a patient needs sudden critical attention? If you have no one and nowhere to turn, you could be in trouble. Resolving *this* problem has to be your big priority.

What's so important about a patient classification system?

Q As a part-time float nurse working in a hospital that's chronically understaffed (so what else is new?), I've got plenty to keep me busy. Now, on top of everything else, I'm required to rate our patients' nursing needs—using preassigned numerical scores for each need—as part of the hospital's patient classification system (PCS). Because I work only part-time and float from unit to unit, I'm usually not as familiar with the patients' needs as other nurses are. Is it any wonder that it takes me 45 minutes to 1 hour to rate the patients' needs correctly?

I don't understand what's so important about a PCS. I'd say the last thing we need is more paperwork. Maybe if we spent less time *rating* patients' needs and more time *attending to* their needs, we could scrap the whole system. For my own peace of mind, could you shed some light on the thinking behind this system?

A You're certainly not alone in your feelings about paperwork. Many nurses believe it takes valuable time away from their patients.

But a PCS, when used properly, can provide solid evidence to back up departmental requests for increased staffing come budget time. By presenting the information documented in a PCS, nursing administrators can support their contention that they just don't have enough nurses to go around to meet patients' needs. And if that leads to the hiring of a few more nurses, then the patients may benefit directly.

You shouldn't be hearing all this for the first time, however. Someone should've explained the purpose of a PCS to you during your orientation. And as a part-time float nurse, you shouldn't be classifying the needs of all the patients in your unit—just those of the patients you've cared for yourself.

Ask for a staff development program on the value of a PCS. A nurse who understands patients' needs and the political issues involved in making budgetary decisions should give the program. Once nurses realize how a PCS can help solve the problem of constantly working shorthanded—and how much their patients stand to gain as a result—they'll take a more favorable view of this particular form of paperwork.

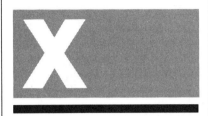

X-rays

Shouldn't nurses be monitored for radiation exposure?

Q I work in a small hospital's intensive care unit (ICU). Recently I sent this memo to administration: "ICU personnel are being exposed to radiation when they assist with patients having portable X-rays done, especially at night when only one technician is on. The National Radiation Council says that persons exposed to radiation should be monitored. Employers should inform personnel about their exposure risks. The hospital may be at risk of lawsuit by former employees who develop cancer. I feel that $2.00 to $2.50 per month per person is cheap insurance for the hospital and peace of mind for the staff."

Administration's answer: "Step outside the room or away from patient; wear a lead apron; and if pregnant, step outside the room completely."

What kind of answer is this? All I was asking for is a monitoring badge.

A If the point of your memo was that you wanted a monitoring badge, you should have enclosed a decoder in the envelope. As James Thurber said, "A word to the wise is not sufficient if it doesn't make any sense."

Remember, when you want to be understood and answered, say what you mean. Double-Check (that's capital C) every memo: Is it Clear, Concise, Complete, Correct, and Calm? If not, rewrite it—or don't expect a satisfying answer.

By the way, ask your *radiologist* for a monitoring badge.

What safeguards should be taken?

Q We're concerned about the danger of radiation exposure when we accompany our patients to the X-ray department or the fluoroscopy lab. What safeguards do you suggest we take?

A When you're working anywhere near radiation, the one fixed rule is: Always be careful. The basic safety principles are *time, distance,* and *shielding.* Spelled out, this simply means that the less time you spend in the vicinity of the radiation, the farther away you stay, and the more thoroughly you shield yourself from it, the less you'll be risking exposure.

When you *do* accompany a patient who's having X-rays, set up the equipment, see that he's comfortable—and then *leave the room.* If you *can't* leave the room during the course of your patient's X-rays or during the insertion of his pacemaker (which is done under fluroscopy), stand as far back as possible, and make sure you wear a lead apron, which completely covers the front of your body. Don't think you're being a sissy when you insist upon an apron. You have the right to be protected.

If you feel you're exposed to a dangerous amount of X-rays over a period of time, request the badge worn by an X-ray technician. This will enable you to check periodically on the amount of radiation you've been exposed to.

The National Council on Radiation Protection and Measurements

(NCRPM) publishes several radiation safety guides for hospitals, clinics, and laboratories. Request their list of publications by writing to NCRPM at 7910 Woodmont Ave., Suite 800, Bethesda, MD 20814.

Perhaps you'll be reassured to learn that, according to an NCRPM spokesman, radiation equipment is checked more often than any other type of hospital equipment, and that most states require a periodic inspection.

What's the best protection for pediatric nurses?

Q As a pediatric nurse, I'm occasionally asked to hold a child while X-rays are taken.

Although I don't have to do this more than three or four times a year, I still worry about the possible danger of radiation exposure.

When I raised the question, the unit manager arranged for us to wear lead aprons while holding the children. But I still feel this isn't a complete solution to the problem.

Do you think I'm being overly cautious?

A No, you're not. Any radiation exposure can be hazardous, even the occasional exposure you describe.

Minimize your exposure by rotating this duty with other nurses (except with a nurse who might be pregnant, of course). Also, ask the hospital to provide you with exposure-meter badges for additional protection.

And speaking of protection, you don't mention wearing rubber gloves. Make sure you wear these as well as the lead rubber apron.

If taking these precautions still doesn't give you a thorough sense of security, make your concerns known to the administration, and ask for a review of hospital policy on this matter.

Sure, getting a good X-ray is important for making a diagnosis. But *not* exposing you and other nurses to radiation is equally important.

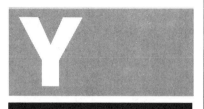

Youthful appearance

How can a nurse with a young-looking face be convincing?

Q Although this may sound funny, I think my face is hampering my career growth. At 30 years old, I have one of those young-looking faces that doesn't instill confidence in my colleagues. They never stop treating me like a kid even though I've worked here longer than many of them. At staff meetings, no one pays attention to my suggestions or gives me credit for good ideas. Short of going to a plastic surgeon, how can I let the people I work with know I have a lot to offer?

A Your youthful appearance is a problem that time will surely solve (just ask Estée Lauder or Elizabeth Arden). Of course, we can understand why some people meeting you for the first time may be put off. But if your colleagues keep treating you like a kid, there's probably more to your credibility gap than meets the eye. Better look for some ways you can add maturity to your professional *image,* not your visage.

For starters, add to your credentials—seek certification, attend seminars, or take courses toward an advanced degree. Work on learning some special skill that's needed on the unit—become the resident "expert" your colleagues will turn to for help. At staff meetings, sit opposite the chairperson so you'll be heard and noticed. Volunteer for specific tasks. And offer ideas, such as self-scheduling, that will get your co-worker's attention and support.

Of course, your body language sends its own message. Practice speaking in a firm, low voice, and when you introduce yourself to new colleagues, make direct eye contact and give your full name—save your nickname for after hours.

Finally, smile. It'll bring some wrinkles to your face everyone will welcome.

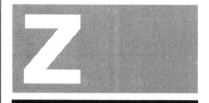

Z-track injections

Can they be used for a number of different I.M. injections?

Q In nursing school, I was taught to use the Z-track method for administering iron dextran preparations. My co-worker says this method is now considered appropriate for other I.M. injections. Do you agree?

A If you use the Z-track method only to administer iron dextran preparations, you may be overlooking a good thing. A nurse-researcher found that Z-track injections cause fewer and less severe skin lesions and, in many cases, less pain than standard I.M. injections. The Z-track method is good to use especially when patients receive frequent injections over extended periods of time.

Index

A

Abortion, 1
Academic degrees of health care providers, 65
Acquired immunodeficiency syndrome
blood transfusion and risk for, 5-6
patient confidentiality and, 6
protection against contracting, 6, 8.
See also HIV antibody test, reliability of.
ribavirin therapy and, 8
self-healing and, 6
volunteer caregivers and, 7
will to live and, 6-7
Admission of patient to emergency department, 3
Advanced Cardiac Life Support test, failure of, 2. *See also* Baccalaureate clinical examination, failure of *and* State board examination, retaking of.
Affectionate behavior
between nurse and patient, 3-4
between visitor and patient, 3
Agency contract, acceptance of permanent job as breach of, 4-5
AIDS. *See* Acquired immunodeficiency syndrome.
Alcoholic. *See also* Drug abuser.
doctor as, 8-10
nurse as, 10-11
patient as, 11-12
recovering nurse as counselor for, 10
visitor as, 12-13
Allergy bracelets, preparation of, 13
Allergy injections, 13-14
Allergy tests, administration of, 14
Aloe products, ethics of recommending, 14-15
Alternative therapy, nurse's recommendation of, 15
Alzheimer's disease, caring for patient with, 15
American Nurses' Association's code, violation of, 17
Amputee as nurse, 16
Anesthetic administration as nursing procedure, 17
Anger, seeking help to resolve, 18
Angioplasty, assisting with, 18
Antibiotics, overuse of, 18-19
Antiembolism stockings, use of, 19
Apgar scores, repeat testing for, 19
Apnea monitoring for neighbor's baby, 19-20. *See also* Friendly advice.
Arterial puncture, responsibility for, 20
Aseptic technique, doctor's compliance with, 20
Assault and battery, forcing of medications as, 207-208
Assignment, refusal to comply with, 118

Associate degree program, clinical experience and, 40-41
Autologous blood transfusion, precautions for, 21-22. *See also* Blood transfusion.

B

Baccalaureate clinical examination, failure of, 22. *See also* Advanced Cardiac Life Support test, failure of *and* State board examination, retaking of.
Bad news, telephone notification of, 43-44
Barium preparations, responsibility for administering, 22-23
Bedside charting, legal risks of, 104
Bladder, drainage of, 23-24
Blind nurse, talking textbooks for, 24
Blind patient, labeling of, 24
Blood pressure measurement during ambulance ride, 15-16
Blood return, checking central line for, 34
Blood specimen collection without consent, 148-149. *See also* Informed consent.
Blood transfusion. *See also* Jehovah's Witness.
AIDS risk and, 5-6
autologous, 21-22
conscientious objection to, 26
febrile patient and, 25
needle size for, 26
recording of, as intake, 100
starter I.V. solution and, 25
from unlabeled bag, 25-26
Body donation, registry for, 27. *See also* Organ donation.
Body odor, sensitivity to, 27-28
Bomb threats, procedure for handling, 28
Burnout
changing jobs as result of, 30
coping with, 29-30
hospice nursing and, 30

C

Call lights, watching for, 30-31
Cancer treatment, 31-32
Cardiac patient
hospital vs. medical center care for, 32
replaying CCU experience, 33-34
Cardiopulmonary resuscitation
adequacy of instruction in, 58
expression of opinion on, 57-58
refusal to perform, 58
Career choices, middle-age nurse and, 32-33

Care plans, computerized, 45
Cast removal, legal implications of, 33
Catheterization
long-term, catheter choice for, 33
sterile vs. clean technique for, 33
Central line, 34
Certification
compensation for, 136
recommendations for, 17
Challenge, need for, 289
Changing jobs, burnout and, 30
Chart access, 34. *See also* Patient privacy *and* Patients' rights.
Charting, backdated, 95, 96, 97
Chemical dependency, job outlook for nurse with, 178-179
Chemotherapeutic drugs
administering, 36-37
guidelines for handling, 35-36, 37-38
Chemotherapy
administration of, 36-37
bone marrow status and, 37
reasons for continuing, 31-32
safe practices for, 35-36, 37-38
Chicken pox, relieving itching from, 38
Child abuse
photographs of, 247
reporting reasonable evidence of, 38-39
Childbirth
fundal pressure in, 39
patient's rights and, 39, 40
Child's death, notifying parents of, 63.
See also Pediatric cancer, preparing parents to cope with.
Clinical experience, associate degree program and, 40-41
Code
documentation of, 98-99, 103-104
training needed to respond to, 41
College degree programs, appraisal of, 114
College infirmary. *See also* School's medication policy.
administration policies for, 42-43
understaffing in, 43
Committee, defining role as member of, 7-8
Complaints, expression of, 119
Compliance, cultural biases and, 44-45
Confidentiality
AIDS patient and, 6
among peers, 45, 48. *See also* Nurse as substance abuser.
breach of, 45, 46-49
doctor-patient, violation of, 45-46
protection of, 46
Conscientious objection, hospital policy on, 26
Consultation, reviewing hospital policy on, 56

Contact lenses, pain from prolonged wearing of, 56
Continuing education
home study program and, 56-57
license renewal requirements and, 57
Conviction, reporting of, 272
Copyright requirements, 57
Coronary care unit, understaffing of, 150-151
Co-worker
difficult, dealing with, 70-71
poor performance of, 71-72
Crash cart
accessibility of, 59-60
maintenance of, 60
Credentials, sequence for listing, 65
Cremation, respecting patient's wishes for, 60
Cross-contamination, infection control and, 159-160
Crowding, hospital policy on, 60-61
Cultural biases and compliance, 44-45
Cytomegalovirus, risk of contracting, 61

D

Deaf nurse, 62
Death education, sourcebook for, 63
Death. *See also* Dying children, working with.
dealing with, 63-64
doctors' acceptance of, 64
impending, 169
notification of, 62-63
pronouncement of, 254
Defibrillation, adequacy of training for, 64-65
Departmental hierarchy, liability and, 65-66
Deposition, guidelines for giving, 66
Depressed nurse, 66-67
Dermatitis, avoiding aggravation of, 68
Diabetes educator, certification requirements for, 68
Diabetic regimen, noncompliance with, 69
Dilatation and curettage, performance of, 61-62
Diphenhydramine as transfusion reaction preventive, 23
Director of nursing, qualifications for, 119. *See also* Termination of director, opposition to.
Discharge assessment, timing of, 79
Discharge orders, liability for, 78
Discharge planning, patient acceptance of, 78-79
Discharge teaching, 78
Discouraged nurse, 79-82
Discretion, need for, 82
Discrimination
against male nurses, 82-83
against patient on medical assistance, 83-84
in employment, 82
Dismissal, justification for, 84-85
Dispensing medication, liability for, 85-86

Doctor
as alcoholic, 8-10
difficult, dealing with, 72-74
disagreement among, 152
libelous remarks by, 73-74
negligence of, 214-216
personal habits of, 28
responsibility of, 263-264
unprofessional behavior of, 86-87
verbal abuse by, 314
Doctor-patient confidentiality, violation of, 45-46
Doctor-patient relations, 86
Doctor's orders, 211
careful reading of, 89-90
vs. hospital's written policy, 87, 93
improper use of, 91-92
legal responsibility to carry out, 89
vs. patient's wishes, 87-88
questioning of, 90-91, 92-94
renewal of, 88-89, 92
verbal, 88, 90, 91, 314-316. *See also* Telephone orders.
Documentation. *See also* Nurse's notes.
alteration of, 96-97
backdated, 95, 96, 97
at bedside, 104
for billing purposes, 94-95
of code notes, 98-99, 103-104
correcting errors on, 102-103
cosigning of, 104
doctor's progress notes and, 99-100
importance of full signatures on, 94
inclusion of vulgar language in, 101
incomplete, 95, 96, 97
reconstruction of, 98
reference to patients in, 96
registering disagreement on, 99
signing of, 98, 102
staff information on, 100, 101-102
standardization of symbols in, 104-105
summary of, 100
use of abbreviations in, 98
Do-not-resuscitate order. *See* "No code" order.
Double effect, principle of, 7
Drafting of nurses, 105
Drainage tubes, preventing infection from, 105
Draping policies, foreign-educated nurses and, 23
Dress code, 105-106
Dressings
frequency of changing, 106
initialing and dating of, 106
Driver, hazardous, 147
Drug abuser. *See also* Alcoholic.
health care worker as, 107-108
patient as, 107, 108-109
Drug-addicted nurse, licensure and, 108
Drug addiction, 108-109. *See also* Alcoholics; Drug-addicted nurse, licensure and; Patient as drug abuser; *and* Nurse as drug abuser.

Drug administration, unclear orders and, 109-110
Drug dosage, questioning of, 90-91
Drug incompatibilities, legal responsibility and, 110
Drugs, generic vs. trade name, 204
Drug samples, legal implications of dispensing, 110
Drug screening test
false-positive results of, 111
witnessed specimens for, 111
DTP vaccines, recommended regimen for, 111-112
Dying children, working with, 31. *See also* Death.
Dying patient, 112-113. *See also* Body donation, Death, *and* Organ donation.
relieving suffering of, 7

E

Educational grants, rules for, 305
Elder abuse, reporting suspected cases of, 114
Electrocardiograms, learning to interpret, 114-115
Emergency department
agency nurses in, 117. *See also* Nursing agency.
detaining patients in, 115
dispensing drugs in, 115. *See also* Patient as drug abuser.
malingering patients in, 117
parents in, 115
private patients in, 116-117
responsibility for patient in, 117
understaffing of, 115-116
working overseas in, 116
Emotional illness, licensure and, 287-288
Emotional involvement with patient, 117-118. *See also* Affectionate behavior between nurse and patient.
Emotional support of patient, 118
Employment recommendation, 259-260
Endoscopy, use of Versed for, 120
Endotracheal intubation
of dead patient, 121-122
drug administration and, 121
by emergency medical technicians, 120-121
of newborns, 120
by nurse, 121-122
Enemas, time interval between, 122
English-Spanish guide for medical personnel, 43
Enteral feedings, coloring of, 122-123
Enteral pump, turning off of, 129
Epidural catheters, administering medication through, 123
Epileptic nurse, 123-124
Equipment bag technique, 124
Euthanasia, patient request for, 124
Exhibitionism by patient, 124-125
Expiration date on medication, 125
External degree program, 22

Externs, responsibility assigned to, 125-126
Eye, removal of foreign body from, 126
Eye patch, patient driving with, 126

F

False accusation, removal from record, 126-127
Falsifying records, 127
Family members, involvement in patient care, 127-128
Family questions about patient, 128
Febrile patient, blood transfusion and, 25
Feeding tubes
  clogging of, 128-129
  confirming placement of, 129
Felony charge, nursing licensure and, 129-130
Fetal monitoring of twins, 130
Fibrotic area as injection site, 130
Fingernails, artificial, 130
Fire drills, evacuation of bedridden patients during, 131
First names, use of, 211-212. See also Informality.
Flexion deformity, prevention of, 131
Flirting, professional image and, 131
Floating
  intensive care unit and, 153
  liability for making mistakes and, 132
  preparation for, 131-132
  reducing stress of, 132
Florence Nightingale, cause of death of, 132-133
Fluid challenge, urinary output as basis for, 205
Food and Drug Administration testing, enlisting patients for, 128
Foot care in nursing home, 134
Footprinting of newborn, 154
Forced absence, 134. See also Vacation time, forced.
Forcing treatment on patient, 135
Foreign object, removal from eye, 126
Formula feedings for breast-fed infants, 135
Friendly advice, 21
Fundal pressure, safe use of, 39

G

Gastrostomy tubes, catheter used to replace, 135-136
Generic substitute, avoiding confusion with, 136
Gifts, acceptance of, 136-137. See also Tipping by patient.
Gloves
  for CPR, 137
  for instrument transfer, 137
  vinyl vs. latex, 137
Glucose levels, emergency treatment of, 137

Good Samaritan acts, implications of, 137-138
Gossip, 138-139. See also Confidentiality.
Graduate nurse
  administration of medication by, 139
  liability for mistakes, 139
Grief, family coping with, 139-140
Group dynamics, 7-8
Growth, need for, 289
Guardianship, 140
Guest-patient, charting care of, 140

H

Harsh treatment of patients, reasons for, 141. See also Burnout.
Heart rate measurement during ambulance ride, 15-16
Heel sticks for newborns, 141-142
Hematoma, treatment of, 142
Hemorrhage, postoperative, 249-250
Heparin injection, 142-143
Heparin locks, preventing clots in, 143
Hepatitis B carrier
  CDC guidelines for, 143
  as CPR performer, 143-144
  working with, 144
Hepatitis B vaccine, pregnancy and, 144
Hexachlorophene preparations for infant bathing, 23
HIV antibody test
  disclosure of results of, 145-146
  mandatory, 145
  reliability of, 5-6
Holiday pay, basis for, 312-313
Home health care. See also Nursing agency.
  laypersons' guide to, 147
  liability for, 146-148
  master's degree programs for, 4
  payment for, 146
  responsibilities of RN in, 147, 148
Homosexuality, documentation of, 149
Hospice nursing, burnout and, 30
Hospital manual, guidelines for, 149
Hypochondria in nurses, 150
Hypothermia blanket, setting for, 150

I

I.D. badges, 153-154
I.M. injection
  deltoid muscle as site for, 154
  drawing air into syringe for, 154
Incidental professional service, 192
Incident report
  reasons for filing, 154-155
  removal from files, 155
Incompetent colleague, 155-156
Incompetent patient, 156. See also Driver, hazardous.
Incontinence pad, need for, 156

Indwelling urinary catheter
  frequency of changing, 158
  precautions for insertion of, 157
    before pelvic ultrasonography, 156-157
  sterile technique for, 157-158
  taking bath with, 156
Infant bathing, hexachlorophene products for, 23
Infection control, 158-161
Infiltration, treatment of, 142
Informality, 161-162
Information, patient's need for, 244
Informed consent
  alteration of, 53
  disagreement between parent and child and, 55
  durable power of attorney and, 50
  failure to obtain, 54-55
  implied, 50
  incompetent patient and, 50-51, 53, 54
  legality of nurse obtaining, 49, 50-51, 52
  legality of premedicated patient signing, 51
  patient's right to explanation and, 52-53
  rescheduled surgery and, 51-52
  signing blank form for, 53
  specificity of, 54
  for tape recordings, 54
  updating of, 55
Initials after name, 267. See also RN after signature.
Injections, administration to child, 162. See also I.M. injection.
Injured nurse, 162-163
Inquisitiveness of patient, 163-164
Insecurity of new nurse, 164
Instructor's liability, 164-165
Insulin
  administration by nonlicensed assistants, 166
  dispersal of particles in, 166
  giving to fellow workers, 166
  I.M. vs. S.C. administration of, 166
  mixing of, 165, 166-167
  prompt administration of, 165
Insulin syringes, reuse of, 68
Insurance
  adequate coverage by, 167
  physical examinations for, 167-168
Intensive care unit
  floating and, 153
  inexperienced nurses in, 152
  monitoring patients in, 151-152
  prolonged patient stay in, 152-153
Interviews
  inappropriate questions in, 168-169
  personal questions in, 168
Invasion of privacy, chart access and, 34. See also Confidentiality.
Isolation, 169
I.V. bags. See also I.V. therapy.
  changing of, 172
  marking on, 169-170

I.V. infusion pumps, blood cell damage and, 170. *See also* I.V. therapy.
I.V. lidocaine therapy, discontinuing, 170. *See also* I.V. therapy.
I.V. therapy, 170-173
  air in tubing in, 171-172
  base solution used in, 172
  disconnected line in, 172-173
  disconnecting tubing in, 170-171
  drug abuser and, 172
  long-term, 171
  reading fluid levels in, 170-173
  responsibility for premixed admixtures in, 173
  strengthening veins for, 172

J

Jehovah's Witness, blood transfusion and, 173. *See also* Blood transfusion.
Job application, reporting of hearing deficit on, 173-174
Job benefits, loss of, 174
Job change, exploring possibilities for, 174
Job description, updating, 174-175
Job dissatisfaction, 175. *See also* Burnout.
Job evaluation
  disagreement with, 176-177
  of friend, 176
  overdue, 177
  suggestions for writing, 175-176
Job hunting, 177-179
Job loss, economic situation as cause of, 178
Job offer, checking out, 119-120
Job rejection, dealing with, 179
Job responsibility, 179-185. *See also* Floating.
  carrying out therapy as, 184
  delegation and, 180
  determining area of, 180-182, 183
  double shifts and, 180
  private-duty nurse and, 182
  standing orders and, 181
  supervising as, 182-183
  transfer of patients as, 183-184
Job selection for new graduate, 185
Job title, authority and, 185-186. *See also* Nurses' titles, changing terminology for.
Joint Commission on Accreditation of Healthcare Organizations
  announced visits by, 2
  lying to, 1-2
Jurisdiction, accepting out-of-state doctor's orders and, 186

K

Kerosene heaters, respiratory problems and, 186
Kidnapping, prevention of, 186-187

L

Labor, questionable inducement of, 134-135
Laboratory values as nursing responsibility, 187
Language barrier, informed consent doctrine and, 187
Lateness as psychological problem, 188
Laughter, benefits of, 267
Lawsuits, 188-189
Laxative, inappropriate, 189
Leadership, building confidence in, 190
Legal guardian, 140
Legal responsibility
  alcoholic patient and, 11-12
  allergy injections and, 13-14
  during apnea monitoring for neighbor's baby, 19-20
  for carrying out doctor's orders, 89
  deterioration of patient's condition before admission and, 3
  drug incompatibility and, 110
  live-born aborted fetus and, 1
  lying and, 2
  narcotics law violator and, 8-9
  psychiatric assessment and, 20-21
Liability, 190-192
Libelous remark by doctor, 73-74
License reinstatement, 193. *See also* Licensing by endorsement.
License revocation, circumstances for, 193-195
Licensing by endorsement, 192. *See also* License reinstatement.
Lie-detector test, restrictions for using, 195
Life support, termination of, 195-196
Light handles as cause of contamination, 56
Lights-out policy, enforcement of, 254
Live-born fetus, abortion and, 1
Lonely patient, 196-197
LPN, improving image of, 197
Lying, legal risks of, 2

M

Male nurse
  discrimination against, 82-83
  as responder to security problems, 41-42
Male student, role model for, 197. *See also* Male nurse.
Malpractice insurance, off-duty nursing and, 236
Management position
  improving chances for, 197
  nonnurse in, 197-198
Manipulative patient, dealing with, 198
Marijuana smoking by patient, 198-199
Marital relationship, troubled, 303-304
Married couples working together, 199
Mastectomy patient, blood pressure measurement and, 24-25
Master's degree programs for home health care, 4

Meal-break policies, 28-29
Medical assistance patient, discrimination against, 83-84
Medical assistants, nurse practice act and, 199-200
Medical records
  as legal document, 35
  patient's right to, 35
Medical student's orders, 200
Medicare reimbursement for doctor's visit, 200
Medication changes, doctor's countersignature on, 201
Medication confusion, separating tablets to avoid, 201
Medication error, 201-203
  correction of, 95
  documentation of, 100-101
Medication orders, 203-207
  countersigning of, 206-207. *See also* Medication changes.
  delay in filling, 205, 206
  writing of
    by medical students, 204-205
    by nurses, 203-204
Medication practices, questionable, 18-19
Medication risks, informing patient of, 205-206
Medication
  administration as assault and battery, 207-208
  adverse effects on, 200-201
  borrowing of, 28
  dispensing time for, 296-297
  expiration dates for, 209
  for home hospice patients, 208
  liability for preparation of, 208-209
  sending patient home with, 208
  transporting of, to patients' homes, 209
Meningitis, vaccine to prevent, 313
Mercury, accidental ingestion of, 209-210
Military service, drafting nurses into, 105
Mood swings, nurses and, 210
Morale, improvement of, 210-211
Mortar and pestle, cleaning of, 40
Mouth-to-mouth resuscitation, AIDS protection and, 41
Moving, motivation for, 177-178
Multidose vial, contamination of, 211
Multiple-choice tests, improving scores on, 113-114

N

Nail polish as source of infection, 130
Narcotic injections, administration of, 192
Narcotics counts, 212
Narcotics for home hospice patients, 208
Narcotics record, 212
Nasogastric feeding, airway suctioning and, 212-213

Nasogastric tubes
  charcoal administration through, 213
  insertion of, 213
  replacement of, 213
Nasopharyngeal airway use in incontinent patients, 213-214
Needle size for transfusion, 26
Negligence, 214-216. *See also* Patient abuse.
Neonatal intensive care unit, staffing standards for, 216
New admission, assessment of, 21. *See also* Patient's condition, deterioration of.
Newborn
  endotracheal intubation of, 120
  footprinting of, 154
  screening of, 141-142
  transportation of, 225
  tube feeding of, 304
New techniques, resistance to, 163
Night shift nurses, duties of, 141
Night supervisor, need for, 289-290
Nipple pinching, reaction to pain and, 216-217
"No code" order, policy for, 217-223
Noises, mysterious, 223
Nourishment, patient refusal of, 260
Nuclear accident, potassium iodide and, 223-224
Nurse
  affectionate behavior of, 3-4
  as alcoholic, 10-11
  amputee as, 16
  blind, 24
  deaf, 62
  depressed, 66-67
  discouraged, 79-82
  as drug abuser, 107-108. *See also* Drug addicted nurse.
  epileptic, 123-124
  feelings of adequacy in, 80
  hearing deficit in, 62
  middle-aged, career choices for, 32-33
  insecurity of, 164
  vs. nursing assistant, 80
  overbearing, 234
  penicillin allergy and, 13
  personal hygiene habits of, 27, 58-59
  pregnant, 250-251
  refusal of, to give transfusion, 26
  retirement of, 118-119
  as working mother, 238-239
Nurse anesthetist, anesthetic administration by, 17
Nurse-attorneys, job availability for, 188
Nurse-doctor conflict, 224
Nurse-manager, difficult, 74
Nurse practitioner, standards for, 224-225
Nurse's notes. *See also* Documentation.
  charting of, 99-100
  editing of, 103

Nurses' pledge, 225
Nurses' titles, changing terminology for, 225. *See also* Job title, authority and.
Nurse-volunteer, liability of, 320-321. *See also* Good Samaritan acts.
Nursing, late entrance into, 225-226
Nursing agency
  acceptance of permanent job and, 4-5
  how to start, 5
  quality care and, 5
Nursing assistant vs. nurse, 80
Nursing home
  community dining in, 226
  independent judgments in, 226-227

O

Observation of nurses as research project, 227-228
Observation of procedures, patient privacy and, 242
Obstetric nursing, 228-230
Occupational health nursing, 230-231
Off-duty nursing, 231
Office management in medical practice, 69-70
On-call policy, legality of, 231
Operating room
  abandonment in, 232
  narcotics box in, 231-232
Operating room nurse, training for, 233
Opinions, acceptance of, 7-8
Orderly, difficult, 75
Organ donation, 232-233. *See also* Body donation.
Orientation to new job, 79-80
Ostomy care, 233
Otoscope, infection control precautions for, 233-234
Overbearing nurse, 234
Overdose
  charting time of, 234-235
  naloxone for, 235
Over-the-counter products, orders for, 235-236
Overtime, 236-237. *See also* Off-duty nursing.
Oxytocin drips, dosage for, 237

P

Pacemaker, nurse with, 237-238
Pain medication, patient's request for, 238
Paramedic, medical command for, 238
Parenting, nursing and, 238-239
Parking problems at hospital, 239
Particulate matter, I.V. injection of, 16
Patient
  as alcoholic, 11-12
  difficult, 75
  as drug abuser, 107, 108-109
Patient abuse, 239-240. *See also* Negligence.

Patient advocacy, 74, 240-241. *See also* Patients' rights.
Patient-centered nursing, 241-242
Patient classification system, importance of, 326-327
Patient departure against medical advice, 271
Patient injury, liability for, 242
Patient privacy, 242-244
Patient safety, recovery room stretchers and, 267
Patient's condition, deterioration of, 3. *See also* New admission, assessment of.
Patient's property, protection of, 296
Patients' rights, 244. *See also* Patient advocacy.
  childbirth and, 39, 40
Patient transfer, 245
Pay
  increase in, 245-246
  for on-call time, 246
Payroll deduction for donation, 246
Pediatric cancer, preparing parents to cope with, 246
Pediatric cancer patients, working with, 31
Pediatric intensive care, qualifications for, 158
Peer evaluation, 246-247
Penicillin allergy, nurse and, 13
Permanent job acceptance as breach of agency contract, 4-5
Personal disability, nurse with, 247
Personal hygiene habits, nurse and, 27, 58-59
Personal journal in malpractice suit, 247
Physical ailments, scheduling nurses with, 281-282
Picketing, hospital reaction to, 248
Piggybacking, 248
Pilfering
  prevention of, 248-249
  reporting, 249
Placebos, 249
Police request for blood specimen, 148-149. *See also* Informed consent.
Postpartum depression, helping patient with, 67-68
Postpolio syndrome, 250
Potassium chloride, ulceration of vein walls and, 170
Power of attorney, 140
Preemployment examination, preparation for, 250
Pregnant nurse, safety for, 250-251
Pressure sore, controlling, 251
Prison nursing, capital punishment and, 251
Private-duty nursing
  doctor's attitude toward, 252
  for family members, 253
  staff nurses and, 251-253
Private home care, implications of, 257

Prolixin injections, frequency of administering, 253
Promotion, effect on relationships, 253-254
Pronouncing death, 254
Psychiatric assessment, legality of nurse performing, 20-21
Psychiatric nursing, 254
Psychiatric patient
in community college program, 42
preparation for handling, 255
suicide threat of, 254-255
Pulmonary artery catheter
monitoring of patient with, 255-256
moving patient with, 256
Pulse dosing, 256
Pupil response check as nursing responsibility, 227
Pupil size, measurement of, 256

Q

Quadriplegia, body surface area calculation and, 257
Quality of care, nursing agency staffing and, 5
Quota system pay, 257-258

R

Radiation monitoring, 258
Radium implants, responsibility for, 258
Recreation program, volunteers for, 258-259
References
reliability of, 259
unfavorable, 179
Refusal, nurse's right of, 266
Relatives, conflicts involving, 260-261
Religious beliefs, treatment decisions and, 261. See also Patients' rights.
Reporting
of nursing error to patient, 262
unworkable system for, 262
Restraints, doctor's order for, 264
Retired nurse, 118-119
Retirement village, health care in, 265
Return to nursing, preparation for, 265-266
Ribavirin therapy, AIDS and, 8
RN after signature, 99. See also Initials after name.

S

Scare tactics and children, 133
School nurse, covering for, 267-268
School's medication policy, 268. See also College infirmary.
School transcripts, review of, 268
Scrub gowns, benefits of wearing, 268-269
Search of belongings, 243, 269
Secrets, 270. See also Confidentiality.

Security problems, male nurse as responder to, 41-42
Sedated child, supervision of, 270
Sedated patient, discharge of, 76
Self-confidence, lack of, 271
Self-discharge, 271
Self-esteem, improving, 271-272
Self-healing, AIDS and, 6
Self-hypnosis, teaching of, 149-150
Self-medication, legal risk of, 272
Self-treatment, 8. See also Acquired immunodeficiency syndrome, patient confidentiality and.
Sexual intimacy, deprivation of, 243
Sexual preference, documentation of, 149
Sick leave, 272-274
Signing doctor's name, legality of, 274
Silver nitrate application in newborn's eyes, 274
Sleep
awakening stable patients from, 275
documentation of, 275-276
for nursing home patients, 274-275
Smoking, 276
Socializing
with doctor, 277-278
with patients, 276-277, 278-279
while on duty, 279
Social workers, medication decisions and, 279-280
Specimens for drug screening test, witnessed, 111
Spelling, importance of, 280
Sphygmomanometer, testing accuracy of, 280
Sponge count, liability for, 280-281
Sports, examination of participants in, 281
Staff development instructor, promoting services of, 281
Staff relationships, improvement of, 75-76
Standards of care, 282
Standing orders, malpractice action and, 89
Staph infection carriers, 282
Stat doses, schedule for, 282-283
State board examination
failure of, 133-134
retaking of, 27. See also Advanced Cardiac Life Support test, failure of and Baccalaureate clinical examination, failure of.
Status epilepticus, preventing damage from, 283
Sterilization
recommendations for, 283
using microwave for, 283
wrapping to prolong, 283-284
Stethoscopes for patients, 284
Stomatitis, treatment of, 284
Stress, changing jobs to reduce, 284-285
Student health problems, 284-285
Student rights, 286
Student status, notation of, 99

Subclavian vein as insertion site for central line, 34
Substance abuse by patient, 286. See also Alcoholic.
Substitutions, medication administration schedule and, 286-287
Suctioning
of tonsillectomy and adenoidectomy patients, 287
use of saline solution with, 204
Suffering, relief of, 7
Suicidal patient
refusal to care for, 288
restraint of, 264
Suicide, reporting attempts of, 288-289
Suite sharing, cross-infection risk and, 159-160
Sump tubes used for feedings, 289
Surgical lift, safety of, 290
Suturing as nursing procedure, 290-291

T

Talwin, dependence on, 291
Tape recording conversations, 291-292. See also Telephone orders and Verbal orders.
Technique, discrepancies in, 5
Telemetry system, effectiveness of, 292
Telephone advice, legal risks of giving, 292-293
Telephone orders, 18-19, 293-294. See also Verbal orders.
Telephoning doctors, policy for, 294
Temper, seeking help to control, 18
Terminally ill patient, concerns of, 294-295
Termination of director, opposition to, 295
Test anxiety, 295
Testimony of nurse against nurse, 86
Tetanus injections, doctor's order for, 295-296
Time clocks, 297
Time off, 297-298
Tipping by patient, 298. See also Gifts, acceptance of.
Tongue blades, seizure precautions and, 298-299
Total parenteral nutrition, administration guidelines for, 299-300
Tracheostomy care, 300
Tranquilizers for nurse, 300-301
Transfer of patient, 245
Transfusion reaction, diphenhydramine as preventive against, 23
Transporting patient, liability for, 76-77
Traveler's diarrhea, prevention of, 69
Treatment delay, 301
Treatment error, telling patient about, 301
Treatment refusal. See also Religious beliefs, treatment decisions and.
patient's rights and, 302-303
waiver for, 301-302
Truthfulness, 304
Tube feeding of newborn, 304

Tuberculosis, testing for, 304-305
Tuition assistance, rules for, 305
Twins sharing incubator, 305-306

U

Understaffing, coping with, 306-309
Unemployment compensation, nursing
  shortage and, 309-310
Unfair labor practices, filing claim of,
  262-263
Uniforms, 310
  washing of, 158
Unit manager, 311-312
  incompetent, 261-262
Unlicensed nurse, reporting of, 312

V

Vacationers in emergency department,
  resentment of, 263
Vacation time, forced, 312. *See also*
  Forced absence, paid.
Vaginitis, treatment of, 313
Ventilator patients
  weaning of, 314
  in X-ray department, 313-314
Verbal abuse from doctor, 72-73, 314
Verbal orders, 314-316

Versed and endoscopy, 120
Vibrator, venous thrombosis and, 316
Visitation rights of relatives, 316
Visiting hours, compliance with,
  316-317
Visitor
  affectionate behavior of, 3
  as alcoholic, 12-13
  giving medications to, 317-318
  providing services for, 318
  resentment of, 317
  rude behavior of, 318-319
Vital signs
  faking reading of, 319-320
  newborns, 320
Vocal cord paralysis, endotracheal intubation and, 320
Volunteer caregivers, AIDS patients
  and, 7

W

Waiting time for nonemergency patient,
  321. *See also* Treatment delay.
Walking report, value of, 321
Wandering patient, responsibility for,
  321-322
Water pitcher for patient on fluid restriction, 322
Weapon on patient, removal of,
  322-323. *See also* Search of belongings.

Weight loss, monitoring of, 323
Will to live, AIDS and, 6-7
Withholding information, 323-324
Withholding treatment, 324-325. *See
  also* Refusal, nurse's right of.
Witnessing wills, 325
Working mother, nurse as, 238-239
Work load, 325-327
Written orders for patient on pass, need
  for, 77-78

X

X-rays, safeguards against exposure to,
  327-328. *See also* Radiation monitoring.

Y

Youthful appearance, overcoming disadvantages of, 328

Z

Z-track injections, 328